Feline Reproduction

Feline Reproduction

Edited by

Aime K. Johnson DVM, DACT

Auburn University College of Veterinary Medicine
Department of Clinical Sciences
Auburn, Alabama, USA

and

Michelle Anne Kutzler MBA, DVM, PhD, DACT

Oregon State University
Department of Animal and Rangeland Sciences
Corvallis, Oregon, USA

CABI

CABI is a trading name of CAB International

CABI
Nosworthy Way
Wallingford
Oxfordshire OX10 8DE
UK

Tel: +44 (0)1491 832111
Fax: +44 (0)1491 833508
E-mail: info@cabi.org
Website: www.cabi.org

CABI
WeWork
One Lincoln Street
24th Floor
Boston, MA 02111
USA

Tel: +1 (617)682-9015
E-mail: cabi-nao@cabi.org

A catalogue record for this book is available from the British Library, London, UK.

ISBN-13: 9781789247084 (paperback)
9781789247091 (ePDF)
9781789247107 (ePub)

DOI: 10.1079/9781789247107.0000

Commissioning Editor: Alexandra Lainsbury
Editorial Assistant: Kate Hill
Production Editor: Marta Patiño

Typeset by SPI, Pondicherry, India

Contents

Acknowledgement

The editors would like to thank the future Dr Tanya Robinson for her tireless efforts and assistance in editing during her summer break. Without her, this work would not have been possible. The editors would also like to thank the technical staff at Scott Ritchey Research Center, Jessica Cannon, Melissa Korbley, and Jordan Doss, for their assistance in obtaining many images used in this book. Lastly, the editors would like to thank the cat breeders who contributed cases and images for this book.

Contributors

Editors

Aime K. Johnson DVM, DACT
Auburn University College of Veterinary Medicine, Department of Clinical Sciences, Auburn, Alabama, USA.
Email: akj0001@auburn.edu

Michelle Anne Kutzler MBA, DVM, PhD, DACT
Oregon State University, Department of Animal and Rangeland Sciences, Corvallis, Oregon, USA.
Email: michelle.kutzler@oregon.edu

Contributors

Carla Barstow DVM, MS, DACT
Highland Pet Hospital, Lakeland, Florida, USA.
Email: dr.barstow@tampavet.com

Marco Cunto DVM, PhD, Assoc. Prof
Animal Reproduction Unit, Department of Veterinary Medical Sciences, Alma Mater Studiorum, University of Bologna, Bologna, Italy.
Email: marco.cunto@unibo.it

Diane Delmain DVM, DABVP Feline
Auburn University College of Veterinary Medicine, Department of Clinical Sciences, Auburn, Alabama, USA.
Email: dmd0038@auburn.edu

Jamie M. Douglas DVM, MS
Auburn University College of Veterinary, Department of Clinical Sciences, Auburn, Alabama USA.
Email: jmd0125@auburn.edu

Alain Fontbonne DVM, PhD, MSc, HDR, Prof., DECAR
Centre d'Etudes en Reproduction des Carnivores, Ecole Nationale Vétérinaire d'Alfort, Maisons-Alfort Cedex, France.
Email: alain.fontbonne@vet-alfort.fr

Natalie S. Maticka DVM, MS, MANZCVS, DACT
Guide Dogs Queensland, Bald Hills, Australia.
Email: matickan@vt.edu

Cristina Gobello DVM, PhD, Prof, DECAR
Director Center of Reproductive Physiology, Veterinary Sciences, National University of La Plata and National Research Council, La Plata, Argentina.
Email: cgobello@fcv.unlp.edu.ar

Sandra Goericke-Pesch DVM, Dr. med. vet., Prof., DECAR
Reproductive Unit – Clinic for Small Animals, University of Veterinary Medicine Hannover, Foundation, Hannover, Germany.
Email: Sandra.Goericke-Pesch@tiho-hannover.de

Fiona K. Hollinshead BVSc, PhD, DACT
College of Veterinary Medicine and Biomedical Sciences, Colorado State University, Fort Collins, Colorado, USA.
Email: Fiona.Hollinshead@colostate.edu

Jacob A. Johnson DVM, DACVAA
Auburn University College of Veterinary Medicine, Department of Clinical Sciences, Auburn, Alabama, USA.
Email: jaj0005@auburn.edu

Cindy Maenhoudt DVM, DACT, DECAR
Centre d'Etudes en Reproduction des Carnivores, Ecole Nationale Vétérinaire d'Alfort, Maisons-Alfort Cedex, France.
Email: cindy.maenhoudt@vet-alfort.fr

Jennifer B. Nagashima PhD
Center for Species Survival, Smithsonian Conservation Biology Institute, Front Royal, Virginia, USA
Email: NagashimaJ@si.edu

Zuzanna Niewiadomska DVM
Centre d'Etudes en Reproduction des Carnivores, Ecole Nationale Vétérinaire d'Alfort, Maisons-Alfort Cedex, France.
Email: zpniewiadomska@gmail.com

Budhan Pukazhenthi BVSc, MS, PhD
Center for Species Survival, Smithsonian Conservation Biology Institute, Front Royal, Virginia, USA.
Email: PukazhenthiB@si.edu

Juliette Roos DVM, DECAR
Ecole Nationale Vétérinaire d'Alfort, Centre d'Etudes en Reproduction des Carinvores, Maisons-Alfort Cedex, France.
Email: roos.juliette@gmail.com

William F. Swanson DVM, PhD
Center for Conservation and Research of Endangered Wildlife (CREW), Cincinnati Zoo and Botanical Garden, Cincinnati, Ohio, USA.
Email: bill.swanson@cincinnatizoo.org

Riley E. Thompson DVM, PhD
Department of Clinical Sciences, Colorado State University, Fort Collins, Colorado, USA.
Email: Riley.Thompson2@colostate.edu

Lindsey M. Vansandt DVM, PhD
Center for Conservation and Research of Endangered Wildlife (CREW), Cincinnati Zoo and Botanical Garden Cincinnati, Ohio, USA.
Email: Lindsey.Vansandt@cincinnatizoo.org

Daniele Zambelli DVM, PhD, Prof, DECAR
Animal Reproduction Unit, Department of Veterinary Medical Sciences, Alma Mater Studiorum, University of Bologna. Bologna, Italy.
Email: daniele.zambelli@unibo.it

1 Reproductive Anatomy and Puberty in the Queen

MICHELLE ANNE KUTZLER

Department of Animal and Rangeland Sciences, Oregon State University, Corvallis, Oregon, USA

1.1 Anatomy in the Queen

The reproductive anatomy in the queen consists of the vulva, vestibule, vagina, cervix, uterus, uterine tubes, ovaries, and mammary glands (Fig. 1.1).

The vulva consists of two vertical lips connected by a dorsal commissure, located just below the anus (Fig. 1.2). The vulvar lips come together evenly without gaping (Roberts, 1986). In newborn kittens, the distance between the anus and vulva is <5 mm in females (Fig. 1.3a), compared to >10 mm between the anus and prepuce in males (Fig. 1.3b). During estrus, the feline vulva may enlarge slightly and become edematous but otherwise undergoes little physical change (Fig. 1.4) (da Silva *et al.*, 2006). In addition, the vulva may be slightly smaller in spayed females when compared to unaltered queens. The queen has major vestibular glands (about 5 mm in size) located in the lateral walls of the vestibule, with small openings on the vestibular floor (Schummer *et al.*, 1979). During estrus, a clear vulvar discharge may occur, but this may not be observed given the hygienic behavior of the cat (da Silva *et al.*, 2006). The vulva and the vestibule are the only reproductive organs in the queen that are well innervated by sensory new fibers (Roberts, 1986).

The length of the feline vestibule and vagina are of approximately equal length (Roberts, 1986), and each is up to 4 cm long (McEntee, 1990a). Unlike other species, the queen does not have a true hymen that separates the vestibule and vagina (Roberts, 1986). The urethral orifice opens onto a urethral tubercle, which is elevated off the floor of the vestibule. The feline vagina tapers to a width of 1 mm in diameter near the cervix (Watson and Glover, 1993), and this is the site of semen deposition during mating. The feline cervix is poorly defined compared to other species and is characterized by thickened walls with transverse folds (Roberts, 1986), that protrudes as a prominent papilla into the vagina directed ventrocaudally (McEntee, 1990a). The feline cervix also contains glands (Schummer *et al.*, 1979). The patency of the cervical canal changes during the estrous cycle, such that it is only open during estrus and at parturition (Chatdarong *et al.*, 2001, 2002; da Silva *et al.*, 2006) (Fig. 1.5).

The cranial vagina, cervix, uterus, and uterine tubes (oviducts) begin to develop from the paramesonephric (Müllerian) ducts when the feline embryo is at a crown–rump length of 1.2 cm and is completed when the embryo is at a crown–rump length of 3.2 cm (Inomata *et al.*, 2009). Queens have a bipartite uterus that is characterized by a short uterine body (up to 2 cm long) and long uterine horns (up to 10 cm) and weighs about 1.5 grams in the nonpregnant state (Latimer, 1939; Chatdarong *et al.*, 2005; Aspinall, 2011) (Figs 1.6 and 1.7). However, the size of the feline uterus depends on the queen's size, age, and parity, as well as the stage of the estrous cycle or pregnancy (Gatel *et al.*, 2020). Research in our laboratory has demonstrated a positive correlation between age (2–6 months old) and uterine weight (Fig. 1.8), which has been shown in rodents to be associated with increasing estradiol secretion (Medlock *et al.*, 1994). The increase in uterine weight is likely associated with an increase in the number and depth of endometrial glands that begin at 8 weeks of age (Lopez Merlo *et al.*, 2017). In addition, the feline myometrium thickens after puberty and both the endometrium and myometrium thicken during the follicular phase (Chatdarong *et al.*, 2005; Mehl *et al.*, 2017).

The shape of the feline uterine horns also changes depending on the ovarian cycle, such that

DOI: 10.1079/9781789247107.0001

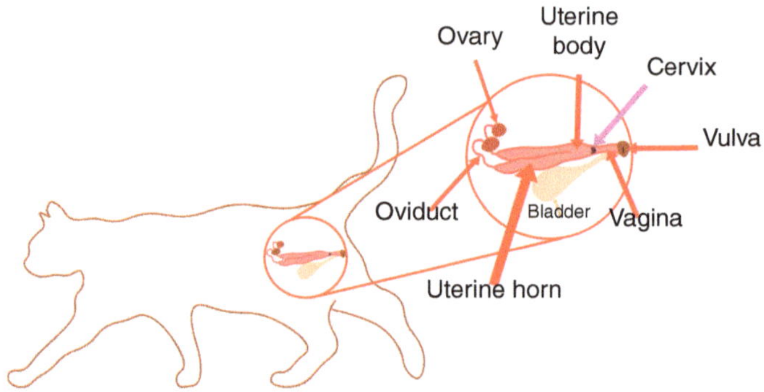

Fig. 1.1. Diagram of the feline female reproductive tract. (Diagram courtesy of Dr Jamie Douglas.)

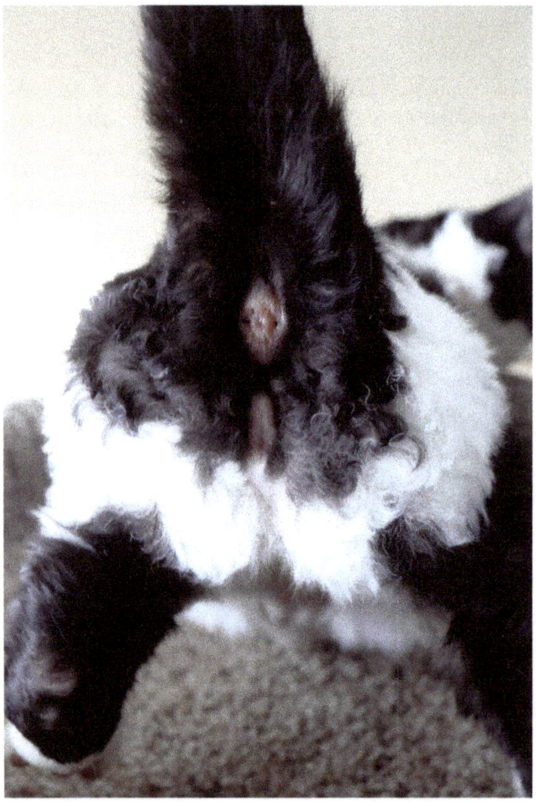

Fig. 1.2. The vulva consists of two vertical lips connected by a dorsal commissure, situated just below the anus. (Photo courtesy of Tina Chittick.)

they appear straight during the follicular phase and are moderately curved during the luteal phase (Fig. 1.9) (Chatdarong *et al.*, 2005). Changes within the endometrial glands during the follicular and luteal phases are also evident (Dawson, 1950). During anestrus, the feline endometrial glands are straight, short, and narrow. During proestrus and estrus, the endometrial glands dilate, and the surface and glandular epithelium increases in height and presence of mitotic figures. During the luteal phase, the endometrial glands enlarge and become tortuous. Ultrasonographically, the uterine body can be identified between the urinary bladder and colon as a homogeneous, hypoechoic tubular structure surrounded by a thin hyperechoic line (Fig. 1.10). In most examinations, a thin hypoechoic line is apparent between the endometrium and myometrium (Gatel *et al.*, 2020). The lumen of the nonpregnant uterus is observed as a thin hyperechoic line in the center of the uterus.

The feline uterine tube opens into the uterus through a low papilla that protrudes into the uterine lumen (McEntee, 1990b). The feline uterine tube is tortuous, 4–9 cm long, and includes the fimbria, infundibulum, ampulla, and isthmus (Roberts, 1986). At ovulation, oocytes are picked up by the fimbria, transported into the conical-shaped infundibulum, and to the ampulla. The junction of the ampulla and isthmus is the site of fertilization when sperm are present. Secretions within the uterine tubes provide an environment for gamete survival, fertilization, and the first few days of embryonic life (Momont, 2018). Unlike the dog, the feline mesosalpinx does not contain adipose tissue. The ovarian bursa only partially encloses the ovary on the lateral side (McEntee, 1990b). The entrance of the ovarian bursa is bounded dorsally by the proper and suspensory ligaments of the ovary and ventrally by the fimbriae of the uterine tube (Schummer *et al.*, 1979).

The feline ovary is oval shaped and 8–9 mm long (Schummer *et al.*, 1979; McEntee, 1990c) (Fig. 1.11).

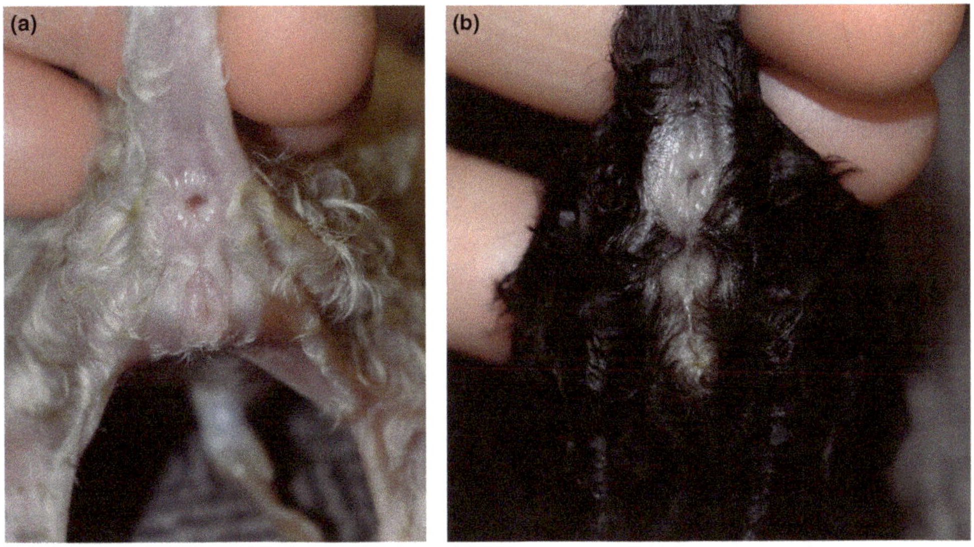

Fig. 1.3. The perineum of newborn kittens. **(a)** In females, the distance between the anus and vulva is <5 mm in females. **(b)** In males, the distance between the anus and prepuce is >10 mm. (Photo courtesy of Tina Chittick.)

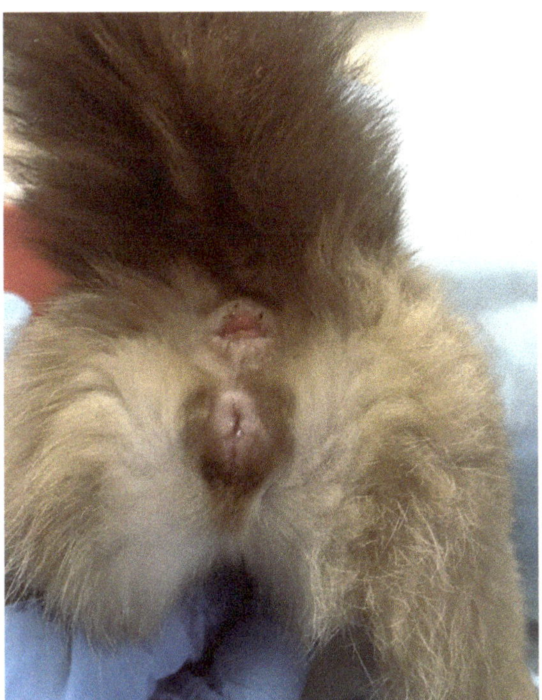

Fig. 1.4. During estrus, the feline vulva may enlarge slightly and become edematous but otherwise undergoes little physical change. (Photo courtesy of Dr Aime Johnson.)

The ovarian bursa contains no fat (Roberts, 1986). Supernumerary ovaries have been reported and can be identified as two ipsilateral ovaries located approximately 1 cm apart within the broad ligament (Anonymous, 1977). The ipsilateral supernumerary ovaries are each smaller than the contralateral ovary, but their total mass exceeds that of the contralateral ovary. The gross appearance of the ovary varies with the stage of the estrous cycle (Wildt, 1980). During seasonal or lactational anestrus, the ovarian surface is smooth and pre-antral follicles are only visible histologically. As the follicular phase (estrus) approaches, three to seven follicles enlarge, and the rest undergo atresia. Most follicular development occurs in the two-day interval just prior to the onset of estrous behavior (Wildt and Seager, 1978). The feline ovaries can be located caudal to the caudal pole of both kidneys, firmly fastened just beneath the third and fourth lumbar vertebrae (Roberts, 1986). The left ovary is commonly located lateral to the descending colon whereas the right ovary tends to be adjacent to small intestinal loops (Gatel *et al.*, 2020). Feline follicles are 2–3 mm in diameter at the time of ovulation (Foster and Hisaw, 1935) and can be visualized using transabdominal ultrasonography (Fig. 1.12).

Histologically, cat ovaries can be distinguished from other domestic animal species by the abundance

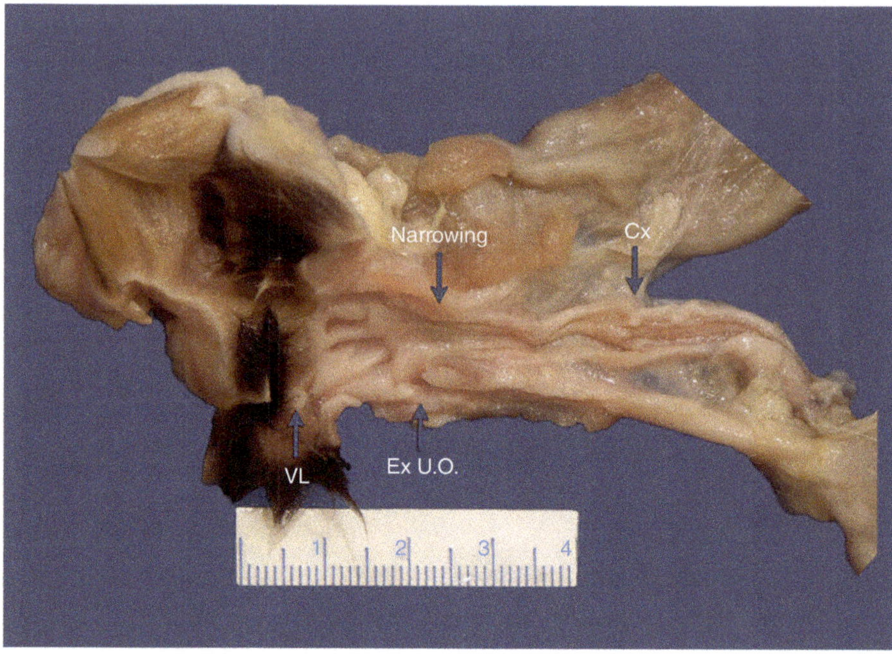

Fig. 1.5. Dissected view of the caudal reproductive tract of the queen. VL, vulva; Ex U.O., external urinary orifice; Cx, cervix. (Image courtesy of Dr Rob Lofstedt and the Library of Reproductive Images (LORI).)

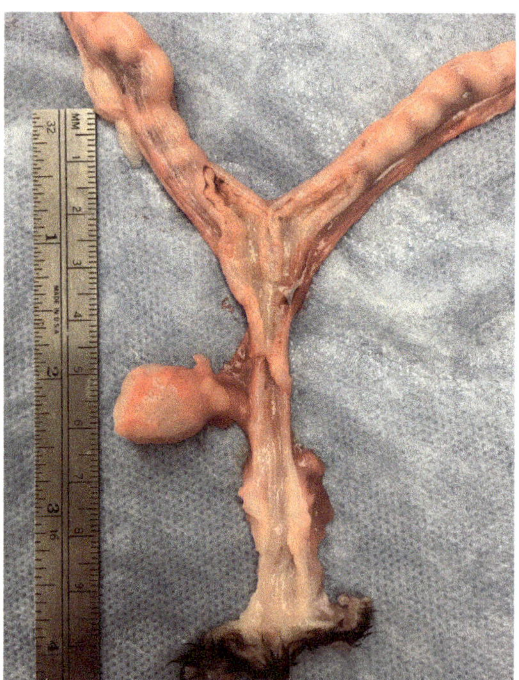

Fig. 1.6. The dissected feline reproductive tract. (Photo courtesy of Dr Aime Johnson.)

of primordial follicles beneath the tunica albuginea (Bristol and Woodruff, 2004). Primordial follicles are characterized by having a single layer of flattened pre-granulosa cells directly surround an oocyte that is 20–30 µm in diameter (Bristol-Gould and Woodruff, 2006) (Fig. 1.13A). Primary follicles are larger than primordial follicles, have a zona pellucida with single layer cuboidal of granulosa cells, and a basement membrane separating the granulosa cells from the ovarian stroma (Bristol-Gould and Woodruff, 2006) (Fig. 1.13B). Secondary follicles have more than one granulosa cell layer and a theca cell layer on the opposite side of the basement membrane (Fig. 1.13C). In prepubertal queens, there are over 300 primordial follicles, 25 primary follicles, and 9 secondary follicles per mm^2 of ovarian cortex, which does not change significantly after puberty (Mehl *et al.*, 2017). Tertiary follicles are large and range in size from 400–1000 µm in diameter. In addition to increased layers of theca cells, the main feature of a tertiary (antral) follicle is the appearance of a fluid-filled antrum (Fig. 1.13D).

Queens generally have four pairs of bilaterally symmetric mammary glands (cranial thoracic, caudal thoracic, cranial abdominal, and caudal

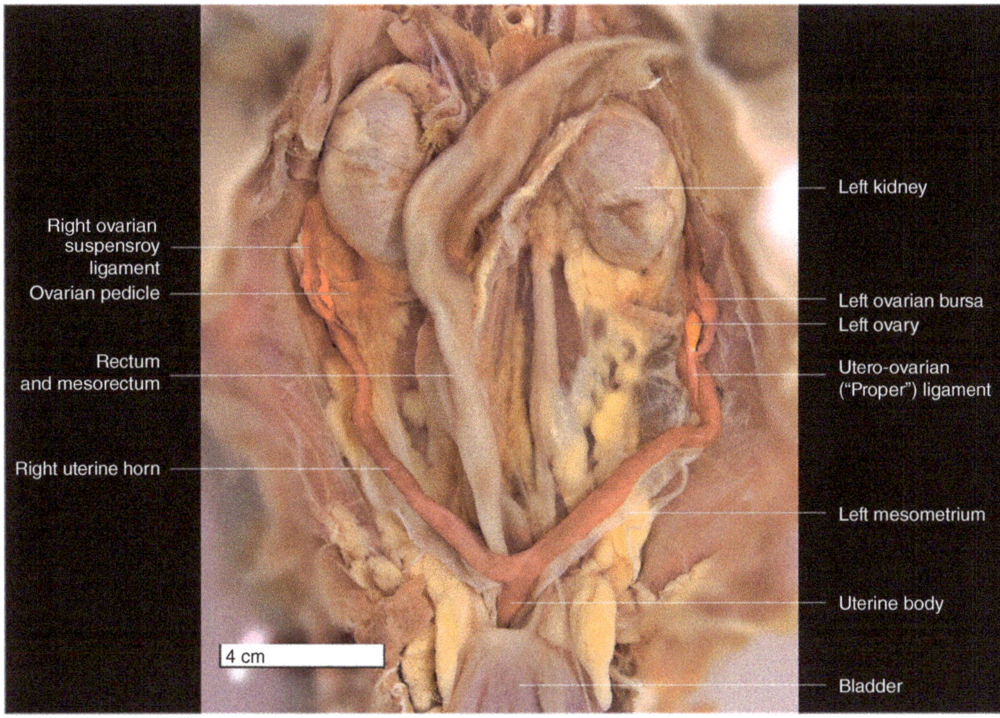

Fig. 1.7. Dissected female reproductive tract in situ. (Image courtesy of Dr Rob Lofstedt and the Library of Reproductive Images (LORI).)

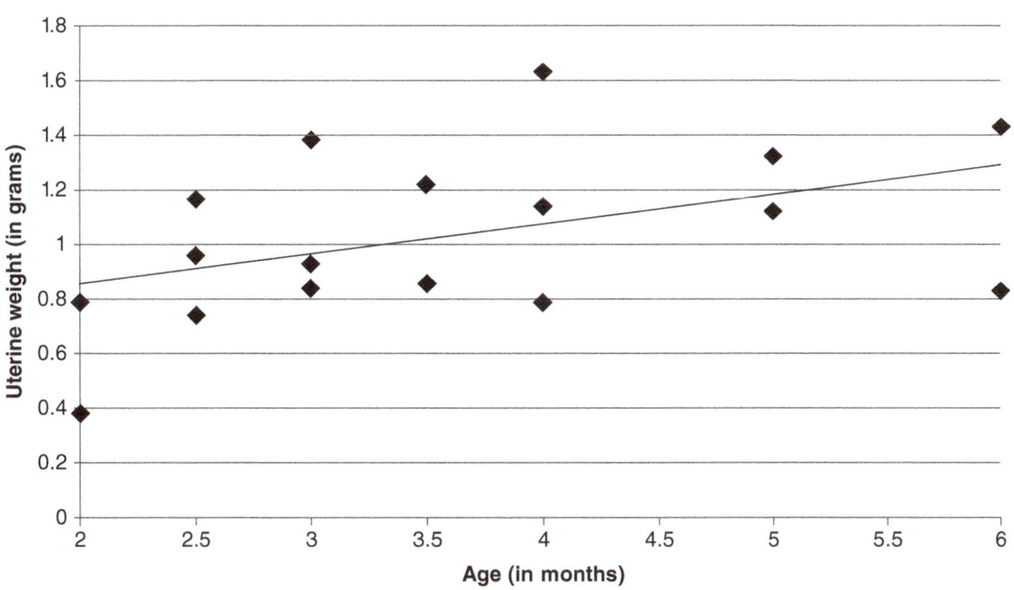

Fig. 1.8. Graph showing the age in months and the uterine weight in grams. The uterine weight increases as the cats age and approach puberty. (Image: author's own.)

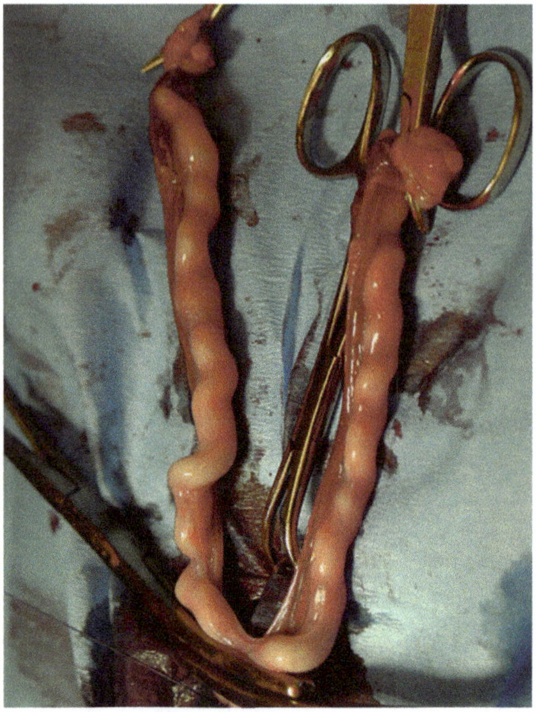

Fig. 1.9. The feline uterine horns have a moderately curved shape during the luteal phase. (Photo: author's own.)

abdominal) (Fig. 1.14) (Silver, 1966). Each mammary gland is made up of multiple lobes that are drained by four to eight ducts into individual openings on each teat (Schummer *et al.*, 1981; Hughes, 2021). Non-function accessory teats can be found occasionally in the inguinal region and are not connected to any mammary tissue but should not be confused with supernumerary teats that are functional (Schummer *et al.*, 1981; da Silva *et al.*, 2006). Feline mammary tissue expresses both estrogen and progesterone receptors and stimulation of these receptors at puberty and during pregnancy result in mammary epithelial proliferation and mammogenesis, respectively (Mol *et al.*, 1996; de las Mulas *et al.*, 2002; Millanta *et al.*, 2005). During lactation, the concentrations of milk components (e.g. total solids, crude protein, fat, lactose) vary significantly by mammary gland (teat) location as well as stage of lactation, diet, and litter size (Jacobsen *et al.*, 2004).

1.2 Puberty in the Queen

The word *puberty* is derived from the Latin word *pubescere*, which means 'becoming covered with hair'. This literal translation is anthropocentric because the change in hair covering observed in humans does

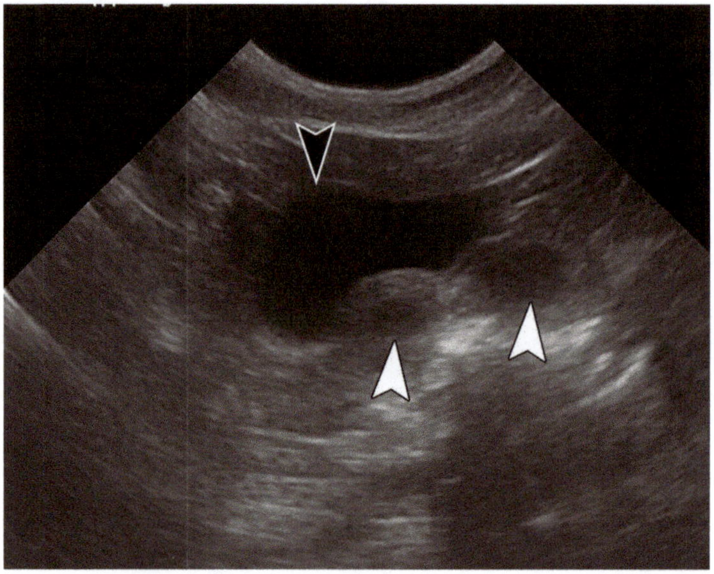

Fig. 1.10. Ultrasound image of a cross section of both horns of the uterus (white arrows) just dorsal to the bladder (black arrow). (Photo courtesy of Dr Aime Johnson.)

not occur in other mammals. The onset of puberty in female domestic animals is typically attributed to either the onset of the first estrus or the first ovulation. Because queens are induced ovulators, the former is more appropriate for this species. If spayed before puberty, final skeletal maturation associated with puberty still occurs but will be delayed (Stubbs *et al.*, 1996).

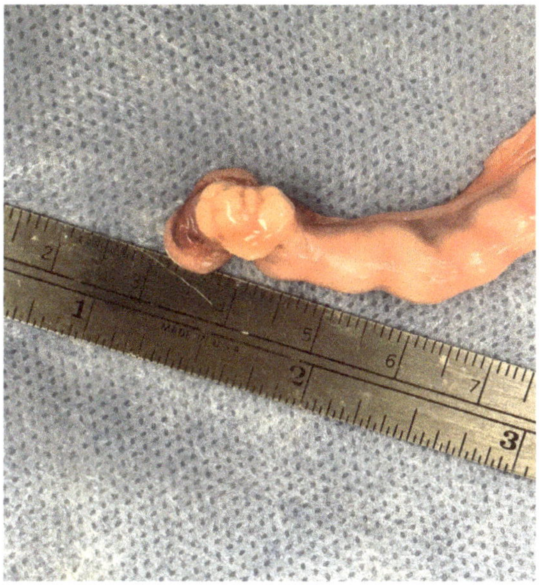

Fig. 1.11. The dissected feline ovary showing multiple corpora lutea. (Photo courtesy of Dr Aime Johnson.)

There is significant variation in the rate at which a mammal matures reproductively. In domestic queens, puberty occurs at 181–560 days (mean ± SD: 345.0 ± 0.9 days) and significantly earlier in kittens born between March and June in the Northern Hemisphere compared to all other times of the year (Tsutsui *et al.*, 2004). However, more recently puberty was reported to occur at 13.3 ± 0.4 weeks of age (Faya *et al.*, 2013) and our laboratory reported ovulatory-sized follicles in cats as young as 2 months old (Bohrer *et al.*, 2016). Feline ovarian weight increases rapidly as their body weight approaches 1 kg, around 100 days of age (Uchikura *et al.*, 2010). Like ruminants, the increase in ovarian weight is accompanied by an increase in the number and size of secondary and tertiary follicles (Desjardins and Hafs, 1969; Mahdi and Kahlilli, 2008). The average body weight at puberty is 2.5–3.0 kg (about 80% of the adult body weight) (England, 2010). In addition to body weight, the onset of feline puberty is affected by other intrinsic factors (e.g. breed) as well as extrinsic factors (e.g. environment, season) (Jemmett and Evans, 1977; Romagnoli *et al.*, 2019). Many short-haired breeds

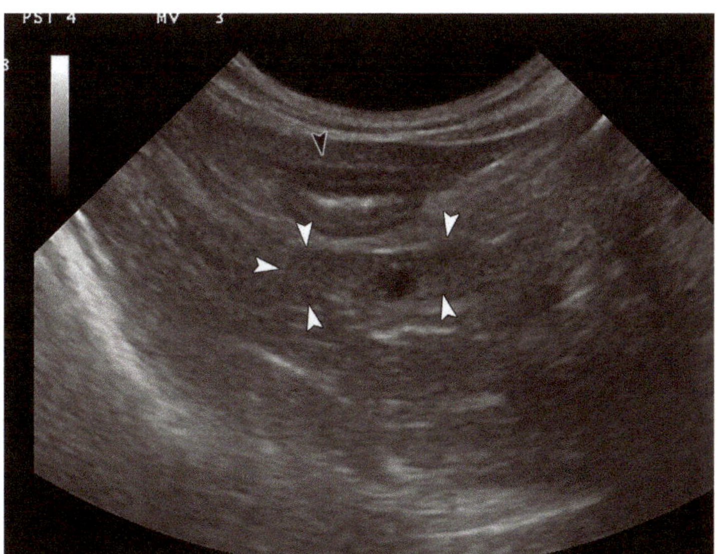

Fig. 1.12. Ultrasound image of the right ovary (white arrowheads) with a mature follicle (2 mm anechoic structure within the ovary). A loop of small intestine is visualized ventral to the ovary (black arrowhead). (Photo courtesy of Dr Aime Johnson.)

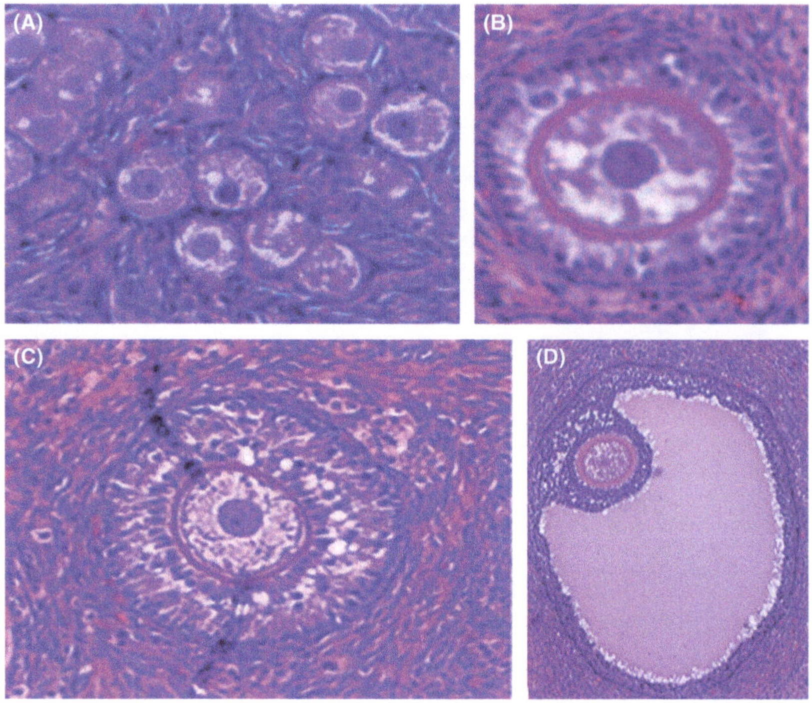

Fig. 1.13. Histologic images from the feline ovary. **(A)** Primordial follicles are characterized by having a single layer of flattened pre-granulosa cells directly surround an oocyte that is 20–30 μm in diameter. **(B)** Primary follicles are larger than primordial follicles, have a zona pellucida with single layer cuboidal of granulosa cells, and a basement membrane separating the granulosa cells from the ovarian stroma. **(C)** Secondary follicles have more than one granulosa cell layer and a theca cell layer on the opposite side of the basement membrane. **(D)** Tertiary follicles have several layers of theca cells and a fluid-filled antrum. (Images: author's own.)

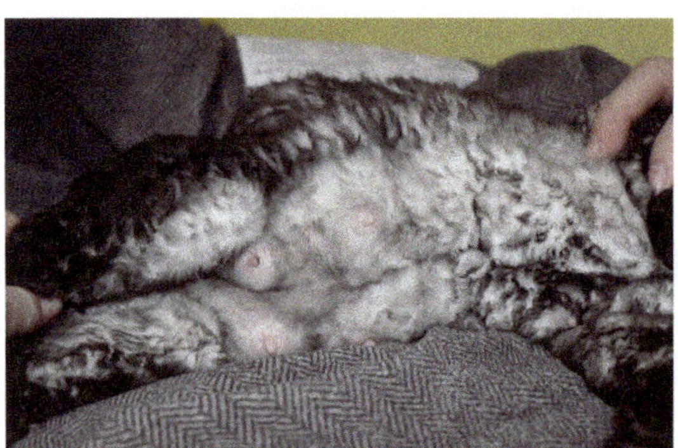

Fig. 1.14. Queens have four pairs of mammary glands. (Photo courtesy of Tina Chittick.)

(e.g. Burmese, Orientals, domestic short hairs) reach puberty earlier than long-haired breeds (e.g. Persian and related breeds) (Malandain *et al.*, 2006; England, 2010) (Table 1.1). Free-roaming cats tend to reach puberty earlier than pet cats (England, 2010); whereas indoor pet cats without contact with other cats reach puberty later (Malandain *et al.*, 2006). Photoperiod plays an important role determining the onset of puberty in queens. A period of extended daylight (at least 12 hours per day) is required for follicular activity in

Table 1.1. Onset of puberty in the normal queen of reported breeds. Modified from Johnston (1989)

Breed	Age at pubertal estrus
Abyssinian	7–14 months
Birman	10–18 months
Burmese	4–19 months
Himalayan	4–16 months
Manx	9–18 months
Siamese	4–20 months
Domestic short haired	4.5–15 months
Domestic long haired	6–18 months

the cat (Hurni, 1981). When the photoperiod is shortened, melatonin and PRL secretion are increased, resulting in a cessation of follicular activity (Levya *et al.*, 1989). For this reason, queens born in late fall will in general go through puberty at a younger age than those born during other times of the year (Malandain *et al.*, 2006). Failure to show estrus by 2 years of age warrants investigation (Malandain *et al.*, 2006).

1.3 References

Anonymous (1977) Third ovary in a cat. *Modern Veterinary Practice* 58, 199.

Aspinall, V. (2011) Reproductive system of the dog and cat. Part 1 – the female system. *Veterinary Nursing Journal* 26, 43–45. doi: 10.1111/j.2045-0648.2010.00013.x

Bohrer, E., Patton, K., and Kutzler, M. (2016) Early onset of reproductive capacity in free-roaming, unowned cats. *Proceedings from the 8th International Symposium on Canine and Feline Reproduction*. Paris, France. [abstract].

Bristol, K. and Woodruff, K. (2004) Follicle-restricted compartmentalization of transforming growth factor beta superfamily ligands in the feline ovary. *Biology of Reproduction* 70, 846–859.

Bristol-Gould, S. and Woodruff, T. K. (2006) Folliculogenesis in the domestic cat (*Felis catus*). *Theriogenology* 66, 5–13.

Chatdarong, K., Lohachit, C., Ponglowhapan, S., and Linde-Forsberg, C. (2001) Transcervical catheterization and cervical patency during the oestrous cycle in domestic cats. *Journal of Reproduction and Fertility* Supplement 57, 353–356.

Chatdarong, K., Kampa, N., Axnér, E., and Linde-Forsberg, C. (2002) Investigation of cervical patency and uterine appearance in domestic cats by fluoroscopy and scintigraphy. *Reproduction in Domestic Animals* 37, 275–281. doi: 10.1046/j.1439-0531.2002.00348.x

Chatdarong, K., Rungsipipat, A., Axnér, E., and Linde-Forsberg, C. (2005) Hysterographic appearance and uterine histology at different stages of the reproductive cycle and after progestagen treatment in the domestic cat. *Theriogenology* 64, 12–29. doi: 10.1016/j.theriogenology.2004.10.018

da Silva, L. D. M, da Silva, T. F. P., Rodrigues Silva, A., and Mattos, M. R. F. (2006) Fisiologia Reproductiva Felina. In: Wanke, M. M. and Gobello, C. (eds) *Reproduccion en Caninos y Felinos Domesticos*. Inter-Medica S.A.I.C.I., Buenos Aires, Brazil, pp 247–266.

Dawson, A. B. (1950) The domestic cat. In: Farris, E. J. (ed.) *The Care and Breeding of Laboratory Animals*. Wiley, New York, pp 220–225.

de las Mulas, J. M., van Niel, M., Millân, Y., Ordâs, J., Blankenstein, M. A., *et al.* (2002) Progesterone receptors in normal, dysplastic and tumourous feline mammary glands. Comparison with oestrogen receptors status. *Research in Veterinary Science* 72, 153–161. doi: 10.1053/rvsc.2001.0542

Desjardins, C. and Hafs, H.D. (1969) Maturation of bovine female genitalia from birth through puberty. *Journal of Animal Science* 28, 502–507.

England, G. C. W. (2010) Physiology and endocrinology of the female. In: England, G. and von Heimendahl, A. (eds) *BSAVA Manual of Canine and Feline Reproduction and Neonatology*, 2nd edn. BSAVA, Glouchester, England, pp. 1–12.

Faya, M., Carranza, A., Miotti, R., Ponchón, T., Furlan, P., *et al.* (2013) Fecal estradiol-17β and testosterone in prepubertal domestic cats. *Theriogenology* 80, 584–586. doi: 10.1016/j.theriogenology.2013.05.026

Foster, M. A. and Hisaw, F. L. (1935) Experimental ovulation and the resulting pseudopregnancy in anoestrous cats. *Anatomical Record* 62, 75–93.

Gatel, L., Rault, D. N., Chalvet-Monfray, K., de Rooster, H., Levy, X., *et al.* (2020) Ultrasonography of the normal reproductive tract of the female domestic cat. *Theriogenology* 142, 328–337. doi: 10.1016/j.theriogenology.2019.10.015

Hughes, K. (2021) Comparative mammary gland postnatal development and tumourigenesis in the sheep, cow, cat and rabbit: Exploring the menagerie. *Seminars in Cell and Developmental Biology* 14(20), 186–195. doi: 10.1016/j.semcdb.2020.09.010

Hurni, H. (1981) Daylength and breeding in the domestic cat. *Laboratory Animals* 15, 229–233.

Inomata, T., Ninomiya, H., Sakita, K., Kashiwazaki, N., Ito, J., *et al.* (2009) Developmental changes of Müllerian and Wolffian ducts in domestic cat fetuses. *Experimental Animals* 58, 41–45. doi: 10.1538/expanim.58.41

Jacobsen, K. L., De Peters, E. J., Rogers, Q. R., and Taylor, S. J. (2004) Influences of stage of lactation, teat position and sequential milk sampling on the composition of domestic cat milk (*Felis catus*). *Journal of Animal Physiology and Animal Nutrition* (Berlin) 88, 46–58. doi: 10.1046/j.1439-0396.2003.00459.x

Jemmett, J. E. and Evans, J. M. (1977) A survey of sexual behavior and reproduction of female cats. *Journal of Small Animal Practice* 18, 31–37.

Johnston, S.D. (1989) Premature gonadal failure in female dogs and cats. *Journal of Reproduction and Fertility* Supplement 39, 65–72.

Latimer, H.B. (1939) The prenatal growth of the cat. VIII. The weights of the kidneys, bladder, gonads, and uterus, with the weights of the adult organs. *Growth* 3, 89–108.

Levya, H., Madley, T., Stabenfeldt, G. H. (1989). Effect of light manipulation on ovarian activity and melatonin and prolactin secretion in the domestic cat.

Journal of Reproduction Fertility Supplement 39, 125–133.

Lopez Merlo, M., Faya, M., Priotto, M., Barbeito, C., and Gobello, C. (2017) Development and proliferation of feline endometrial glands from fetal life to ovarian cyclicity. *Theriogenology* 99, 119–123. doi: 10.1016/j.theriogenology.2017.05.030

Mahdi, D. and Kahlilli, K. (2008) Relationship between follicle growth and circulating gonadotropin levels during postnatal development of sheep. *Animal Reproduction Science* 106, 100–112.

Malandain, E., Little, S., Casseleux, G., Shelton, L., Pibot, P., and Paragon, B. M. (2006) *Practical Guide to Cat Breeding*. Aniwa SAS, Lyon, France, pp. 63–132.

McEntee, K. (1990a) Cervix, Vagina, and Vulva. In: McEntee, K. *Reproductive Pathology of Domestic Mammals*. Academic Press, Inc., San Diego, California, pp. 191–223.

McEntee, K. (1990b) The Uterine Tube. In: McEntee, K. *Reproductive Pathology of Domestic Mammals.* Academic Press, Inc., San Diego, California, pp. 94–117.

McEntee, K. (1990c) The Ovary. In: McEntee, K. *Reproductive Pathology of Domestic Mammals.* Academic Press, Inc., San Diego, California, pp. 31–51.

Medlock, K., Forrester, T., and Sheehan, D. (1994) Progesterone and estradiol interaction in the regulation of rat uterine weight and estrogen receptor concentration. *Proceedings of the Society for Experimental Biology and Medicine* (New York) 2, 146–153.

Mehl, N. S., Khalid, M., Srisuwatanasagul, S., Swangchan-Uthai, T., and Sirivaidyapong, S. (2017) Comparison of the ovarian and uterine reproductive parameters, and the ovarian mRNA and protein expression of LHR and FSHR between the prepubertal and adult female cats. *Reproduction in Domestic Animals* 52(2), 41–44. doi: 10.1111/rda.12926

Millanta, F., Calandrella, M., Bari, G., Niccolini, M., Vannozzi, I., *et al.* (2005) Comparison of steroid receptor expression in normal, dysplastic, and neoplastic canine and feline mammary tissues. *Research in Veterinary Science* 79, 225–232. doi: 10.1016/j.rvsc.2005.02.002

Mol, J. A., van Garderen, E., Rutteman, G. R., and Rijnberk, A. (1996) New insights in the molecular mechanism of progestin-induced proliferation of mammary epithelium: Induction of the local biosynthesis of growth hormone (GH) in the mammary gland of dogs, cats and humans. *Journal of Steroid Biochemistry and Molecular Biology* 57, 67–71. doi: 10.1016/0960-0760(95)00251-0

Momont, H. W. (2018) The gonads and genital tract of cats. Available at: https://www.merckvetmanual.com/cat-owners/reproductive-disorders-of-cats/the-gonads-and-genital-tract-of-cats (accessed 10 December 2020).

Roberts, S. J. (1986) *Veterinary Obstetrics and Genital Diseases (Theriogenology)* 3rd edn. Roberts, S. J. (published by the author), Woodstock, Vermont, pp. 3–13.

Romagnoli, S., Bensaia, C., Ferré-Dolcet, L., Sontas, H. B., and Stelletta, C. (2019) Fertility parameters and reproductive management of Norwegian Forest Cats, Maine Coon, Persian and Bengal cats raised in Italy: a questionnaire-based study. *Journal of Feline Medical Surgery* 21, 1188–1197. doi: 10.1177/1098612X18824181

Schummer, A., Nickel, R., and Sack, W. A. (1979) In: Nickel, A., Schummer, A., and Seiferle, E. (eds) *The Viscera of the Domestic Mammals*, 2nd edn. Springer Verlag, Berlin, pp 304–389.

Schummer, A., Wilkens, H., Vollmerhaus, B., and Habemehl, K. H. (1981) In: Nickel, A., Schummer, A., and Seiferle, E. (eds) *The Anatomy of the Domestic Animals* (Volume 3: The Circulatory System, the Skin, and the Cutaneous Organs of the Domestic Mammals). Springer Verlag, Berlin, pp 469–475.

Silver, I. A. (1966) The anatomy of the mammary gland of the dog and cat. *Journal of Small Animal Practice* 7, 689–696. doi: 10.1111/j.1748-5827.1966.tb04394.x

Stubbs, W. P., Bloomberg, M. S., Scruggs, S. L., Shille, V. M. and Lane, T. .J. (1996) Effects of prepubertal gonadectomy on physical and behavioral development in cats. *Journal of the American Veterinary Medical Association* 209, 1864–1871.

Tsutsui, T., Nakagawa, K., Hirano, T., Nagakubo, K., Shinomiya, M., *et al.* (2004) Breeding season in female cats acclimated under a natural photoperiod and interval until puberty. *Journal of Veterinary Medical Science* 66, 1129–1132. doi: 10.1292/jvms.66.1129

Uchikura, K., Nagano, M., and Hishinuma, M. (2010) Evaluation of follicular development and oocyte quality in pre-pubertal cats. *Reproduction in Domestic Animals* 45, 405–411.

Watson, P. F. and Glover, T. E. (1993) Vaginal anatomy of the domestic cat (*Felis catus*) in relation to copulation and artificial insemination. *Journal of Reproduction and Fertility* Supplement 47, 355–359.

Wildt, D. (1980) Laparoscopic determination of ovarian and uterine morphology during the reproductive cycle. In: Morrow, D.E. (ed.) *Current Therapy in Theriogenology*. W.B. Saunders Company, Philadelphia, Pennsylvania, pp. 828–832.

Wildt, D. and Seager, S. (1978) Ovarian response in the estrual cat receiving varying doses of hCG. *Hormone Research* 9, 114–150.

2 Feline Estrous Cycle

LINDSEY M. VANSANDT

Center for Conservation and Research of Endangered Wildlife (CREW), Cincinnati Zoo and Botanical Garden, Cincinnati, Ohio, USA

2.1 Seasonality

The queen is seasonally polyestrous and will repeatedly cycle during a breeding season, unless interrupted by ovulation, pregnancy, or disease. Cyclicity is initiated when the length of daylight increases, and anestrus occurs following a reduction in daylight hours. Because seasonality is affected by photoperiod length, geographic location (i.e. latitude) has a strong influence on the degree of seasonality. Cats in equatorial zones may breed throughout the year. As latitude increases from the equator, the breeding season is shortened such that cats at the polar circles will cycle for approximately 6 months (Hurni, 1981). In northern temperate zones, the cat breeding season usually begins around February (range: January–March) and ends by September (range: June–November) (Schmidt, 1986). Breed, or more precisely the specific adaptions of a breed, can also influence photoperiod sensitivity. Long-haired breeds tend to show a shorter, more-defined breeding season than short-haired breeds (Jemmett and Evans, 1977). Periods of high heat and/or humidity can affect cyclicity by increasing the interestrous interval (Concannon and Lein, 1983).

For cats housed exclusively indoors without natural light (such as in a laboratory setting), exposure to a minimum of 10 hours of artificial light equivalent to a 100-watt bulb in a 4 × 4-meter room can maintain cyclicity year-round (Shille and Sojka, 1995). However, a light:dark cycle of 12:12 hours, which is similar to equatorial conditions, has been demonstrated to yield the most productive year-round cyclicity (as defined by percent of successful breedings per week) (Hurni, 1981). If a shortened and more-defined breeding season is desired, 2 months at 9:15 hours light:dark followed by 14:10 hours light:dark will significantly increase the number of litters born 5 to 6 months following the change to 14 hours of light. Cats maintained in a home setting are often exposed to both natural and artificial light. Because the artificial lighting in a home setting is not constant, it may not result in predictable ovarian cycles and anecdotally, most intact pet cats do not cycle October–December.

2.2 Ovulation Physiology

Although the domestic cat is classified as an induced ovulator, spontaneous ovulation has been documented (Lawler *et al.*, 1993; Gudermuth *et al.*, 1997; Graham *et al.*, 2000; Pelican *et al.*, 2005; Binder *et al.*, 2019). The percentage of females that demonstrate spontaneous ovulation vary greatly from study to study (35–87%), as does the rate of spontaneous ovulation, with some females rarely spontaneously ovulating, and other females consistently ovulating without copulatory stimuli. Anecdotally, it has been reported that factors such as advanced age, group-housing, and the non-copulatory presence of a male (e.g. visual, olfactory, and vomeronasal contact) may increase the rate of spontaneous ovulation. However, spontaneous ovulation has been documented in young queens, queens that are singly housed, and queens without any male exposure. It has also been suggested that high rates of spontaneous ovulation contribute to the cystic endometrial hyperplasia-pyometra complex in cats, mediated through extended periods of progesterone influence on the endometrium. In one case study, 45% of cats evaluated for inflammatory uterine disease or infertility had active corpora lutea due to spontaneous ovulation at the time of investigation (Lawler *et al.*, 1991).

In the canonical induced ovulation reflex, vaginal stimulation from the tomcat's spined penis during the act of copulation is transmitted via a spinal afferent nervous pathway to the queen's hypothalamus, causing a release of gonadotropin-releasing

DOI: 10.1079/9781789247107.0002

hormone (GnRH) and a subsequent pulsatile release of luteinizing hormone (LH) from the anterior pituitary gland. The LH surge can occur within 10 minutes of copulation and the amplitude is correlated with number of copulations. Peak LH levels occur 4 hours after 8–12 copulations. The peak level of LH is significantly lower if the queen only breeds four times during the 4-hour period, and further reduced with only one breeding (Concannon *et al.*, 1980). In the aforementioned study, 50% of estrual females ovulated after a single breeding whereas every queen ovulated following four or more copulations.

The occurrence or absence of ovulation appears to be the result of differences in the amount of LH released following mating, and not due to differences in the response of the follicles to comparable LH levels, as serum LH is only elevated in queens that ovulate (Wildt *et al.*, 1980). There is a large degree of within-animal and among-animal variation in the amount of LH released following a single mating (Concannon *et al.*, 1980) or multiple matings (Wildt *et al.*, 1981). Furthermore, ovulation appears to be an all-or-none phenomenon, as the number of mature follicles (defined as ≥2 mm in diameter) observed during the pre-ovulatory period correspond to the number of corpora lutea post-mating (Wildt *et al.*, 1980).

The copulation-induced LH-release neuroendocrine pathway is subject to fatigue. If the queen is limited to three copulations per day, there is a major LH surge on the first day, a smaller surge on the second day, and a negligible surge on day three (Wildt *et al.*, 1980). For unrestricted copulations, there is a rapid suppression of LH release within 2–4 hours of the first mating that will persist for 48–72 hours (Concannon *et al.*, 1989). During this refractory period, matings are able to elicit a postcoital response from the queen and treatment with physiologic doses of GnRH may induce a pronounced spike in LH levels. These data suggest that the decreased responsiveness during the refractory period is caused by a depletion of hypothalamic GnRH and/or local negative feedback of GnRH on further GnRH release.

Queens bred on the first day of behavioral estrus typically require at least 48 hours to ovulate (Wildt *et al.*, 1981). Queens bred on day two typically ovulate 30–36 hours later (Swanson *et al.*, 1994), and queens breed on days three or four complete ovulation by 32 hours post-coitus (Shille *et al.*, 1983). Differences in ovulation timing could be due to a reduced follicular maturity and level of LH-responsiveness in the earlier day of estrus (Wildt *et al.*, 1981).

2.3 Phases of the Estrous Cycle

The estrous cycle of the queen has five defined phases: proestrus, estrus, interestrus, diestrus, and anestrus. Each phase is associated with distinct changes in hormones and behavior. Changes in vaginal cytology do occur but are not as clearly demarcated as they are in the bitch (Mills *et al.*, 1979). Additionally, the queen enters estrus more abruptly than the bitch. For these reasons, vaginal cytology is not as commonly used in queens. Transabdominal ovarian ultrasonography has been described to monitor follicular growth but is also not commonly employed in the cat (Malandain *et al.*, 2011).

2.3.1 Proestrus

This phase is associated with an increase in follicle size and rising estradiol levels. Follicles appear as indistinct dark areas, approximately 1 mm in diameter, on the surface of the ovary. Proestrus is defined behaviorally as the period preceding estrus in which the queen is sexually attractive to a tom but will not permit coitus. The queen will often rub her head and neck against objects, vocalize frequently, and roll over on her back (Michael, 1961). In stark contrast to the bitch, overt signs such as vaginal bleeding, vulvar swelling, and consistent changes in vaginal cytology are not observed. Clearing (a slide that shows an absence of noncellular debris, mucus, and decrease of coalescence of cells) of the vaginal smear is the most sensitive and earliest indicator of follicular activity and occurs in approximately one-third of cats during proestrus (Shille *et al.*, 1979). Recognition of this phase can be difficult because behavioral signs may be subtle and the duration is short, typically lasting less than 24 hours. In one study, proestrus was seen in only 27 of 168 cycles and averaged 1.2 ± 0.8 days in length.

2.3.2 Estrus

Following a short proestrus, queens enter the estrous phase, characterized by the female permitting mounting and coitus. Estradiol rises rapidly from a basal plasma level of approximately 15 pg/ml to ≥20 pg/ml as the ovarian follicles grow into distinct, vesicular structures measuring ≥2 mm in diameter and protruding from the surface of the ovary. In a typical cycle, the queen will have two to seven mature follicles, and follicular number does not differ between queens that have been mated and queens that have not (Wildt *et al.*, 1981). There is considerable individual variation in peak estradiol levels, with plasma concentrations ranging from 25–80 pg/ml (Shille *et al.*, 1979; Wildt *et al.*, 1981).

Estrus behavior lags behind the rise in estradiol, with only 8% of cats showing behavioral estrus on day 1 (as defined by >20 pg/ml plasma estradiol), but 80% of cats will show such behavior by day 4 (Shille *et al.*, 1979). Mounting activity by the tom or stroking of the flanks and perineal region by a handler may elicit lordosis posturing (bent forelegs with elevation of the hind quarters and lateral tail deviation) and treading of hind feet. Other behaviors may include intense vocalization, frequent urination, and increased restlessness. While an estrual queen typically displays obvious personality changes, there is a great deal of individual variation in what behaviors are expressed. Queens that are particularly affectionate can exhibit many estrus behaviors during times of non-estrus, including lordosis.

Both the absence of and extended expression of estrus behavior have been observed in queens. Absence of apparent estrus behavior has been suggested to occur in cats that are timid and/or on the lower end of the social hierarchy (Shille *et al.*, 1979); however, a lack of behavior has been observed in cats not exhibiting this personality type and cats that fail to exert signs in one season may exhibit signs in another one. Extended estrus behavior can occur from overlapping waves of maturing follicles, which subject the female to a persistently high level of plasma estrogen. However, prolonged behavior can be observed in cats with distinct, repeated follicular waves as well. It remains unclear why some queens experience a lack of coordination between plasma estrogen levels and estrus behavior (Feldman *et al.*, 2014).

As estradiol rises, superficial vaginal cells (partially cornified with signs of nuclear degeneration) remain constant (40–60%) while anuclear cells (fully cornified) increase from 5% to 40% and intermediate cells (partially cornified with intact nuclei) decrease from ~45% to <10% by day 4 of estrus (Fig. 2.1). Parabasal cells (non-cornified) are

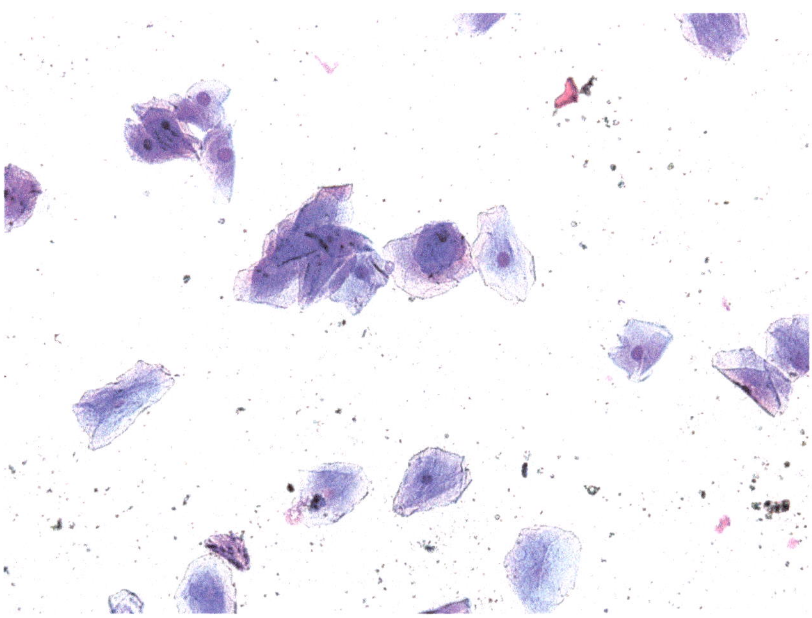

Fig. 2.1. Vaginal cytology of a queen in estrus. Greater than 50% of the cells are cornified (95% in this image). Many retain their nucleus, but the nucleus is small and pyknotic. In the queen, red blood cells and white blood cells are not typically seen on vaginal cytology. (Image courtesy of Dr Aime Johnson also included in VISGAR.)

generally low throughout the feline estrous cycle (1–6%) but are completely absent on days 4–7 of estrus. Clearing occurs in the majority of cats (~90%) during estrus (Fig. 2.2), and smears will remain cleared for five days following the end of estrus (Shille *et al.*, 1979). Feline vaginal cytology also differs from the bitch in that red and white blood cells are rare in the queen. Red blood cells are more typical early in estrus while white blood cells are more typical later in estrus, rising with the non-cornified cells. In one report, only cats with a vaginal bacterial overgrowth presented with red blood cells on their vaginal smears (Mills *et al.*, 1979).

The duration of estrus, as defined by the interval of time when plasma estradiol remains above 20 pg/ml, has been reported to be 7.4 ± 2.3 days in length (range 3–16 days) (Shille *et al.*, 1979). The amount of time that estradiol remains elevated is unaffected by coitus or ovulation. However, it is a point of contention whether coitus and subsequent ovulation may affect the duration of estrus behavior. Ovulation has been reported to shorten estrus behaviors (Scott and Lloyd-Jacob, 1955). Coitus (irrespective of ovulation) has been reported to lengthen estrus behaviors (Shille *et al.*, 1979). Finally, coitus with or without ovulation has been reported to have no effect on the duration of behavioral estrus (Wildt and Seager, 1980; Wildt *et al.*, 1981). The seemingly contradictory results of these studies may be attributed to differences in mating protocols, particularly with regards to when during the estrus phase breeding was allowed. If copulation can potentiate behavioral estrus, such an effect may only occur if mating is delayed until late in the estrus phase (Wildt *et al.*, 1981).

2.3.3 Interestrus

In the absence of ovulation, the queen enters the interestrus phase. The mature follicles undergo atresia and plasma estradiol levels drop to <20 pg/ml. This phase is characterized behaviorally by a return of the queen to her normal behavior. The queen will not typically attract a tom during this phase but will display passive or active resistance if a male does attempt to mount her. Vaginal smears are dominated by intermediate cells (48%), a decreased percentage of superficial cells (~46%), and non-cellular debris during this phase (Shille *et al.*, 1979) (Fig. 2.3).

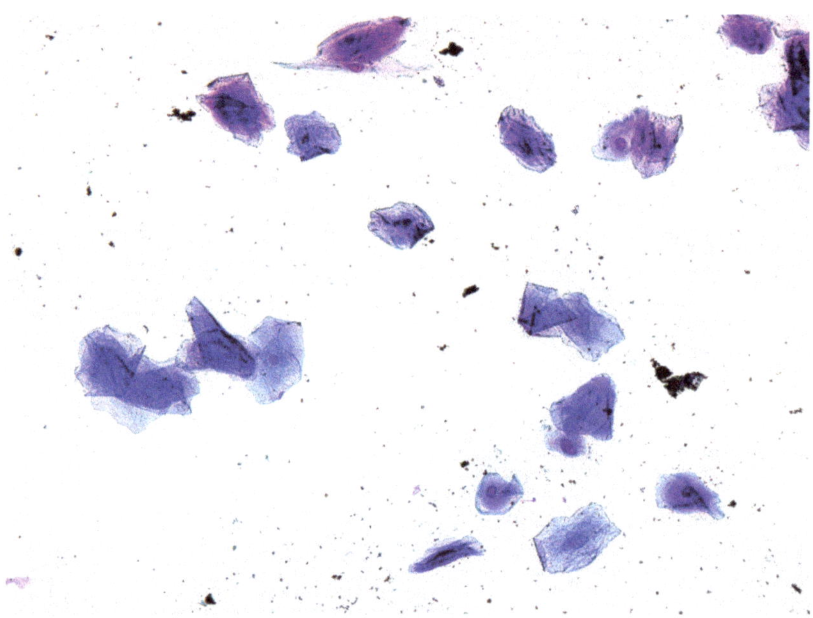

Fig. 2.2. Vaginal cytology of a queen in mid estrus. This queen has mostly cornified epithelial cells and most lack their nucleus. (Image courtesy of Dr Aime Johnson also included in VISGAR.)

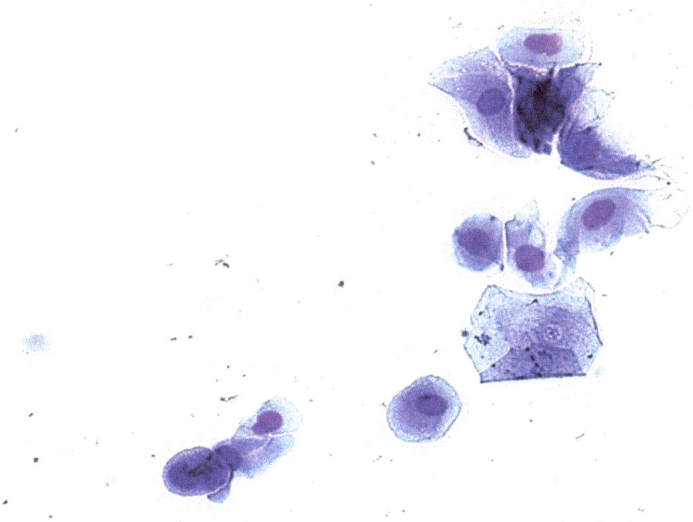

Fig. 2.3. Vaginal cytology of a queen in interestrus. Note the cornified cell intermixed with intermediate and parabasal cells. The percentage of cornified cells would be less than 50%. (Image courtesy of Dr Aime Johnson also included in VISGAR.)

The average length of the interestrus interval is 8.1 ± 3.1 days (Shille *et al.*, 1979), but there is considerable variation among individual queens, with ranges of 3–21 days reported (Jemmett and Evans, 1977; Shille *et al.*, 1979). Breeding without ovulation will not affect the duration of this phase (Shille *et al.*, 1979).

2.3.4 Diestrus

If ovulation occurs (due to coitus, vaginal stimulation, or occurring spontaneously), the queen will enter the diestrus phase, commonly referred to as the luteal phase. The queen will not perform estrual postures and is unresponsive to the male, similar to the interestrus phase. Vesicular ovarian follicles (2.5–3.4 mm in diameter) become more vascularized, develop a central hyperemic stigma, and release follicular contents onto the ovarian surface (Dawson and Friedgood, 1940; Wildt and Seager, 1980; Shille *et al.*, 1983). Within 24–48 hours after ovulation, corpora lutea develop as raised, reddish-orange structures, reaching their maximum diameter (3.6-4.5 mm) by 10-16 days post-ovulation (Dawson and Friedgood, 1940; Wildt and Seager, 1980; Wildt *et al.*, 1981). Vaginal cytology during the luteal phase is characterized by small intermediate and parabasal cells (Fig. 2.4).

The cat produces no pre-ovulatory surge in progesterone (Wildt *et al.*, 1981), which is in contrast with many other similar species such as the rabbit (an induced ovulator; Shaikh and Harper, 1972) and the dog (a carnivore, Concannon *et al.*, 1977; Wildt *et al.*, 1979). Plasma progesterone begins to rise 1–2 days following ovulation from <1 ng/ml to peak levels of 25–90 ng/ml by 14–22 days post-ovulation (Paape *et al.*, 1975; Verhage *et al.*, 1976; Wildt *et al.*, 1981). If the female is not pregnant, progesterone will remain elevated for 36–38 days (Paape *et al.*, 1975; Shille *et al.*, 1979; Wildt *et al.*, 1981), with the corpus luteum gradually regressing to form a persistent, yellow luteal scar. Queens usually begin a new estrous cycle within 7–14 days of corpus luteum regression, making the entire non-pregnant luteal phase approximately 40–50 days (Paape *et al.*, 1975; Wildt *et al.*, 1981). Progesterone concentrations may peak slightly later in pregnant females (>20 days post-ovulation) and at a slightly higher level (Verhage *et al.*, 1976), but progesterone has a high degree of individual variation and cannot

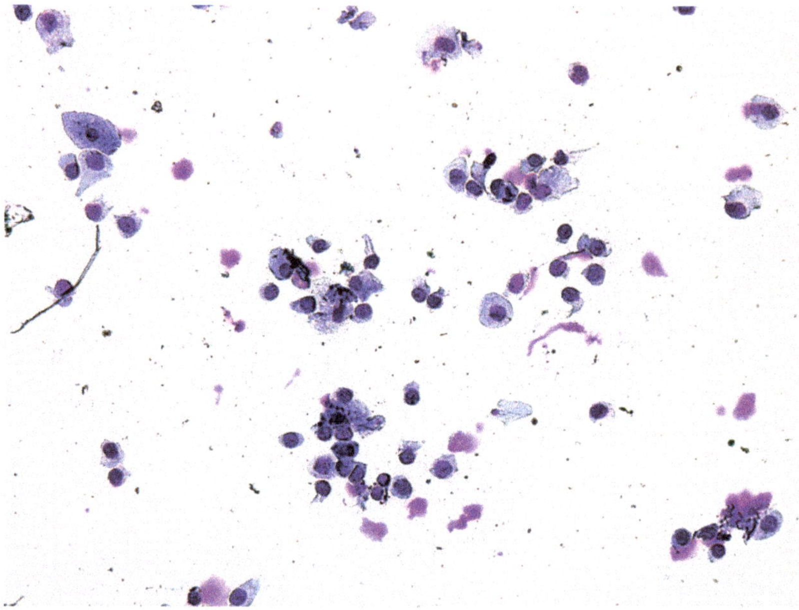

Fig. 2.4. Vaginal cytology of a queen in diestrus. This cytology is characterized by small intermediate and parabasal cells. (Image courtesy of Dr Aime Johnson also included in VISGAR.)

be used as a reliable indicator of pregnancy status until approximately 40 days post-ovulation, when progesterone levels fall in the non-pregnant females.

During a non-pregnant luteal phase, queens do not show any of the physical or behavioral changes (e.g. weight gain, mammary development, nesting) typically seen in pseudopregnant dogs. As opposed to many other carnivores such as the dog (Smith and McDonald, 1974) and the ferret (Heap and Hammond, 1974), which have similar durations in luteal phases irrespective of pregnancy status, the duration of a non-pregnant luteal phase in the cat is considerably shorter than that of pregnancy (36–38 days versus 63–67 days) (Verhage *et al.*, 1976; Jemmett and Evans, 1977; Schmidt *et al.*, 1983). Collectively, these differences make the term pseudopregnancy inappropriate for the cat.

Estradiol drops quickly to 8–12 pg/ml during the first five days following mating and typically remains low (Verhage *et al.*, 1976). However, ovarian follicular activity can occur during diestrus. In one study, the mean number of mature follicles observed was 2.1 ± 0.4, which was significantly less than the number seen at day 1 of estrus (Wildt *et al.*, 1981). None of the follicles observed during diestrus ovulated, but the presence of mature follicles often corresponded with a modest to significant increase in plasma estradiol. Thus, it appears that periods of follicular growth and regression occur continuously in the domestic cat, irrespective of stage in the estrous cycle.

2.3.5 Anestrus

Anestrus is the period of reproductive quiescence. As described in seasonality (Section 2.1), the breeding season is affected by photoperiod length and hence geographic region. Anestrus typically begins in October and ends in January or February in the Northern hemisphere. Behaviorally and hormonally, anestrus is similar to interestrus. Plasma estradiol and progesterone remain basal and the queen does not attract males or display any estrual behaviors. Also, similar to interestrus, vaginal smears are dominated by superficial cells (~46%), intermediate cells (48%), and non-cellular debris (Shille *et al.*, 1979).

2.3.6 Summary

In summary, the non-mated queen will cycle between estrus and interestrus phases. The mated queen that ovulates will either become pregnant where the luteal phase is approximately 2 months, or not become pregnant where the queen will enter a luteal phase that lasts between 40–50 days (see Figures 2.5–2.8).

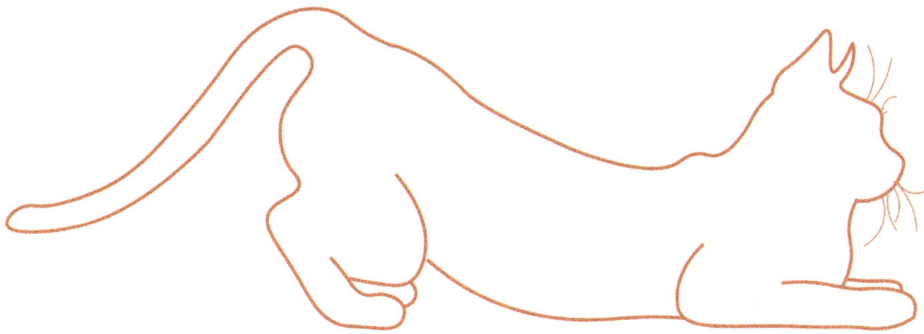

Scenario 1: Female in heat, no mating

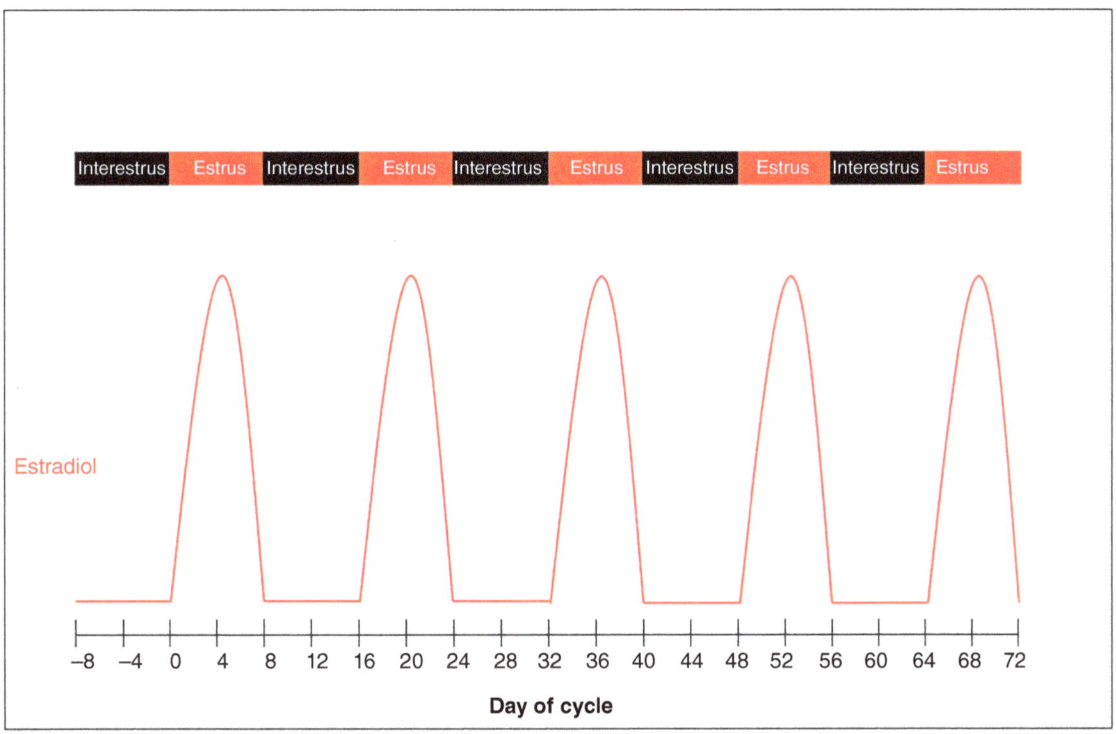

Fig. 2.5. In heat, no mating: the polyestrus queen will remain in proestrus/estrus for 8 days. In the absence of ovulation, the queen will enter an 8-day interestrus interval before returning to estrus. (Image courtesy of Dr Jamie Douglas and Dr Lindsey Vansandt.)

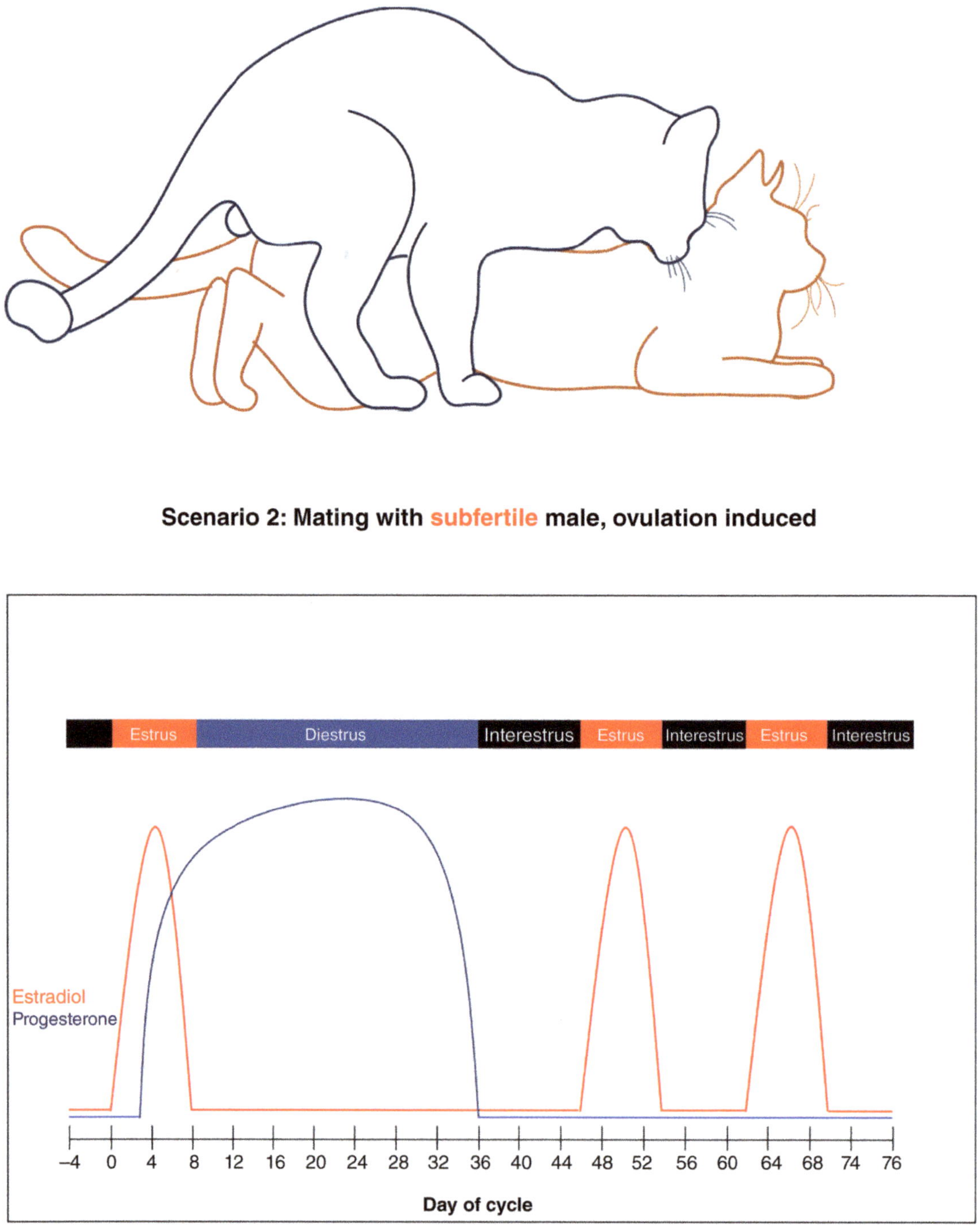

Fig. 2.6. Mating with a subfertile male: an ovulation without subsequent fertilization results in a progesterone elevation of 36-38 days. The queen will return to estrus in 7-14 days following corpora lutea regression. (Image courtesy of Dr Jamie Douglas and Dr Lindsey Vansandt.)

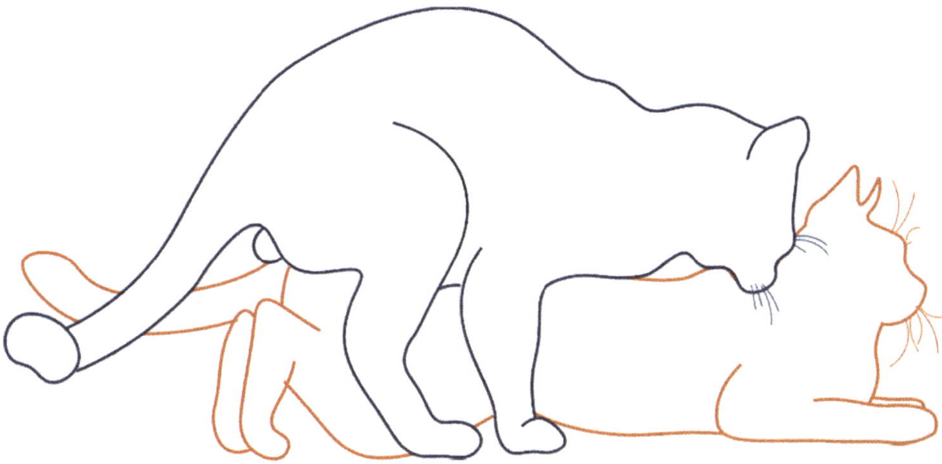

Scenario 3: Mating with fertile male, ovulation induced

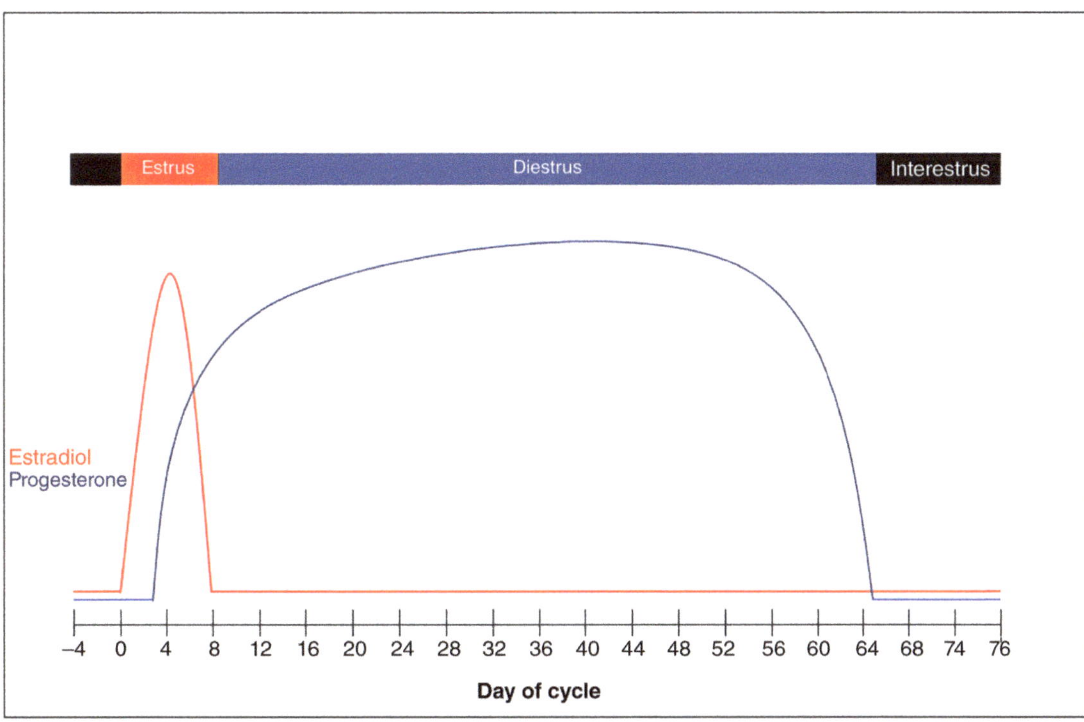

Fig. 2.7. Mating with a fertile male: an ovulation with fertilization and full-term pregnancy results in a progesterone elevation of 63-67 days. Progesterone decreases shortly before queening. (Image courtesy of Dr Jamie Douglas and Dr Lindsey Vansandt.)

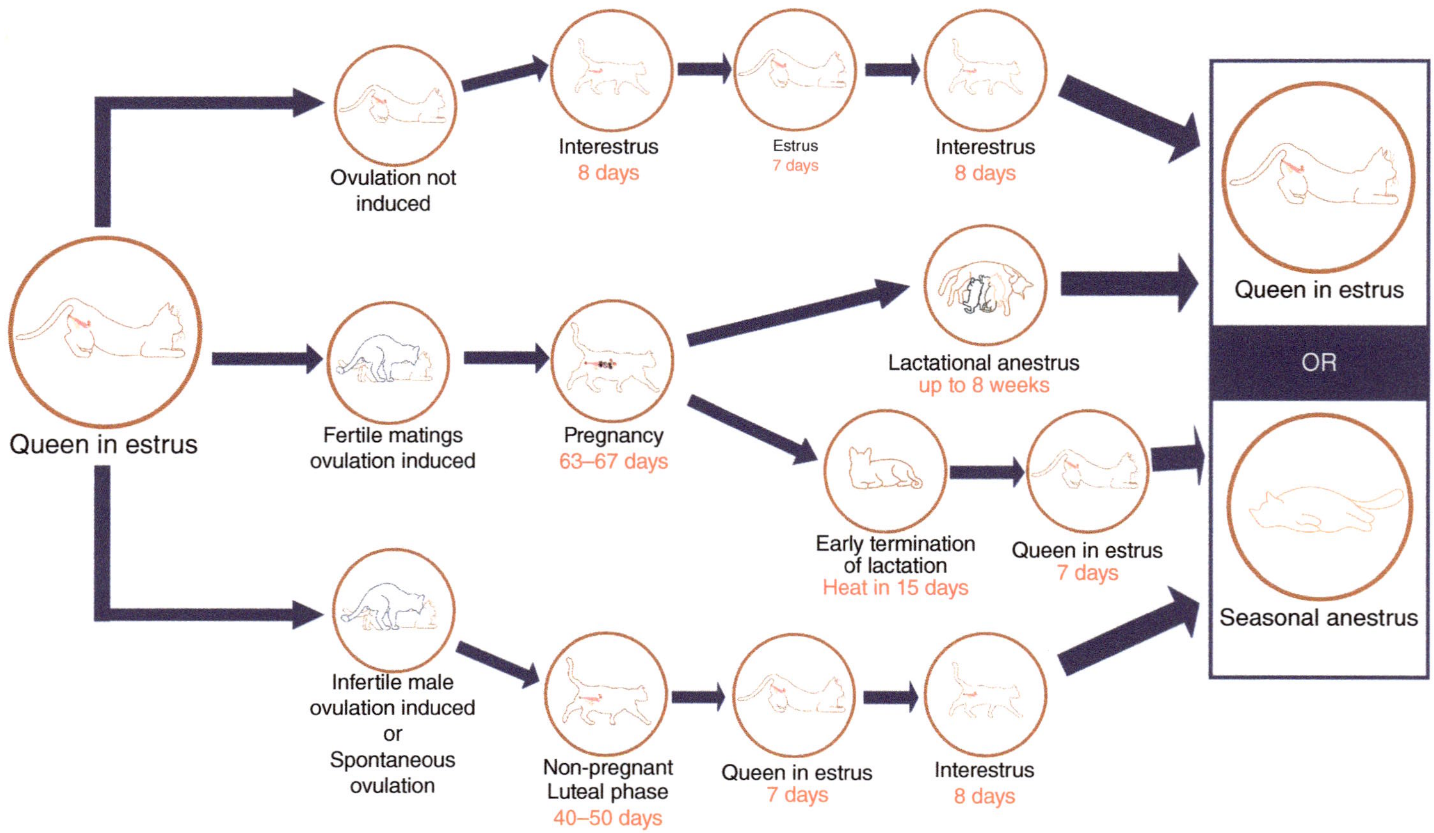

Fig. 2.8. Flow chart showing the feline cycle. (Image courtesy of Dr Jamie Douglas.)

2.4 References

Binder, C., Aurich, C., Reifinger, M., and Aurich, J. (2019) Spontaneous ovulation in cats—Uterine findings and correlations with animal weight and age. *Animal Reproduction Science* 209. doi: 10.1016/j.anireprosci.2019.106167

Concannon, P. and Lein, D. (1983) Feline reproduction. *Current Veterinary Therapy, Small Animal Practice* 8, 932–936.

Concannon, P., Hansel, W., and Mcentee, K. (1977) Changes in LH, progesterone and sexual behavior associated with preovulatory luteinization in the bitch. *Biology of Reproduction* 17, 604–613. doi: 10.1095/biolreprod17.4.604

Concannon, P., Hodgson, B., and Lein, D. (1980) Reflex LH release in estrous cats following single and multiple copulations. *Biology of Reproduction* 23, 111–117. doi: 10.1095/biolreprod23.1.111

Concannon, P., Lein, D., and Hodgson, B. (1989) Self-limiting reflex luteinizing hormone release and sexual behavior during extended periods of unrestricted copulatory activity in estrous domestic cats. *Biology of Reproduction* 40, 1179–1187.

Dawson, A. B. and Friedgood, H. B. (1940) The time and sequence of preovulatory changes in the cat ovary after mating or mechanical stimulation of the cervix uteri. *Anatomical Record* 76, 411–430. doi: 10.1002/ar.1090760405

Feldman, E. C., Nelson, R. W., Reusch, C., and Scott-Moncrieff, J. C. (2014) *Canine and Feline Endocrinology*. Elsevier Health Sciences, Oxford.

Graham, L. H., Swanson, W. F., and Brown, J. L. (2000) Chorionic gonadotropin administration in domestic cats causes an abnormal endocrine environment that disrupts oviductal embryo transport. *Theriogenology* 54, 1117–31. doi: 10.1016/s0093-691x(00)00420-9

Gudermuth, D., Newton, L., Daels, P., and Concannon, P. (1997) Incidence of spontaneous ovulation in young, group-housed cats based on serum and faecal concentrations of progesterone. *Journal of Reproduction and Fertility* Supplement 51, 177–184.

Heap, R. and Hammond, J. (1974) Plasma progesterone levels in pregnant and pseudopregnant ferrets. *Reproduction* 39, 149–152. doi: 10.1530/jrf.0.0390149

Hurni, H. (1981) Daylength and breeding in the domestic cat. *Laboratory Animals* 15, 229–233. doi: 10.1258/002367781780893803

Jemmett, J. and Evans, J. (1977) A survey of sexual behaviour and reproduction of female cats. *Journal of Small Animal Practice* 18, 31–37. doi: 10.1111/j.1748-5827.1977.tb05821.x

Lawler, D., Evans, R., Reimers, T., Colby, E., and Monti, K. (1991) Histopathologic features, environmental factors, and serum estrogen, progesterone, and prolactin values associated with ovarian phase and inflammatory uterine disease in cats. *American Journal of Veterinary Research* 52, 1747–1753.

Lawler, D., Johnston, S., Hegstad, R., Keltner, D., and Owens, S. (1993) Ovulation without cervical stimulation in domestic cats. *Journal of Reproduction and Fertility* Supplement 47, 57–61.

Malandain, E., Rault, D., Froment, E., Baudon, S., Desquilbet, L., *et al.* (2011) Follicular growth monitoring in the female cat during estrus. *Theriogenology* 76, 1337–1346. doi: 10.1016/j.theriogenology.2011.06.002

Michael, R. P. (1961) Observations upon the sexual behaviour of the domestic cat (*Felis catus* L.) under laboratory conditions. *Behaviour* 18, 1–24.

Mills, J. N., Valli, V., and Lumsden, J. (1979) Cyclical changes of vaginal cytology in the cat. *The Canadian Veterinary Journal* 20, 95.

Paape, S., Shille, V., Seto, H., and Stabenfeldt, G. (1975) Luteal activity in the pseudopregnant cat. *Biology of Reproduction* 13, 470–474. doi: 10.1095/biolreprod13.4.470

Pelican, K., Brown, J., Wildt, D., Ottinger, M., and Howard, J. (2005) Short term suppression of follicular recruitment and spontaneous ovulation in the cat using levonorgestrel versus a GnRH antagonist. *General and Comparative Endocrinology* 144, 110–121.

Schmidt, P. M. (1986) Feline breeding management. *Veterinary Clinics of North America: Small Animal Practice* 16, 435–451. doi: 10.1016/S0195-5616(86)50052-8

Schmidt, P. M., Chakraborty, P. K., and Wildt, D. E. (1983) Ovarian activity, circulating hormones and sexual behavior in the cat. II. Relationships during pregnancy, parturition, lactation and the postpartum estrus. *Biology of Reproduction* 28, 657–671, doi: 10.1095/biolreprod28.3.657

Scott, P. P. and Lloyd-Jacob, M. (1955) Some interesting features in the reproductive cycle of the cat. *Proceedings of Society for the Study of Fertility*, pp. 123–129.

Shaikh, A. A. and Harper, M. J. (1972) Ovarian steroid secretion in estrous, mated and HCG-treated rabbits, determined by concurrent cannulation of both ovarian veins. *Biology of Reproduction* 7, 387–397. doi: 10.1093/biolreprod/7.3.387

Shille, V. and Sojka, N. (1995) *Feline Reproduction. Textbook of Veterinary Internal Medicine.* 4th edn. W.B. Saunders Co., Philadelphia, Pennsylvania, pp.1690–1698.

Shille, V., Lundström, K. E., and Stabenfeldt, G. (1979) Follicular function in the domestic cat as determined by estradiol-17 β concentrations in plasma: relation to estrous behavior and cornification of exfoliated vaginal epithelium. *Biology of Reproduction* 21, 953–963. doi: 10.1095/biolreprod21.4.953

Shille, V., Munrot, C., Farmer, S. W., Papkoff, H., and Stabenfeld, G. (1983) Ovarian and endocrine responses in the cat after coitus. *Reproduction* 69, 29–39.

Smith, M. S. and McDonald, L. (1974) Serum levels of luteinizing hormone and progesterone during the estrous cycle, pseudopregnancy and pregnancy in the dog. *Endocrinology* 94, 404–412. doi: 10.1210/endo-94-2-404

Swanson, W. F., Roth, T. L., and Wildt, D. E. (1994) In vivo embryogenesis, embryo migration, and embryonic mortality in the domestic cat. *Biology of Reproduction* 51, 452–464. doi: 10.1095/biolreprod51.3.452

Verhage, H., Beamer, N., and Brenner, R. (1976) Plasma levels of estradiol and progesterone in the cat during polyestrus, pregnancy and pseudopregnancy. *Biology of Reproduction* 14, 579–585. doi: 10.1095/biolreprod14.5.579

Wildt, D. and Seager, S. (1980) Ovarian and uterine morphology during the reproductive cycle. In: Morrow, D. (ed.) *Current Therapy in Theriogenology*. 2nd edn. W.B. Saunders Co. St Loius, Missouri.

Wildt, D., Panko, W., and Seager, S. (1979) Effect of prostaglandin F2α on endocrine-ovarian function in the domestic cat. *Prostaglandins* 18, 883–892, doi: 10.1016/0090-6980(79)90125-4

Wildt, D., Seager, S., and Chakraborty, P. (1980) Effect of copulatory stimuli on incidence of ovulation and on serum luteinizing hormone in the cat. *Endocrinology* 107, 1212–1217. doi: 10.1210/endo-107-4-1212

Wildt, D., Chan, S., Seager, S., and Chakraborty, P. (1981) Ovarian activity, circulating hormones, and sexual behavior in the cat. I. Relationships during the coitus-induced luteal phase and the estrous period without mating. *Biology of Reproduction* 25, 15–28. doi: 10.1095/biolreprod25.1.15

3 Manipulation of the Estrous Cycle

Cindy Maenhoudt[1] and Sandra Goericke-Pesch[2]

[1]Centre d'Etudes en Reproduction des Carnivores, Ecole nationale Vétérinaire d'Alfort, Maisons-Alfort, France; [2]Reproductive Unit – Clinic for Small Animals, University of Veterinary Medicine Hannover, Foundation, Hannover, Germany

3.1 Introduction

The female cat (the queen) is indeed a species with some particularities. While the control of the luteal phase allows in most species the manipulation of the estrous cycle, in this species the approach is different. As described in Chapter 2, the season plays an important role in the estrous cycle of domestic cats. The queen is considered a seasonally polyestrous and facultative induced ovulator. Therefore, the control of reproduction will be based on two main approaches: (i) the manipulation of the daily photoperiods and/or the hormone related to the photoperiodic regulation: melatonin; and (ii) the control of gonadotropin hormones. Hence, treatments mimicking the physiology of the normal cycle can cause the inhibition or stimulation of follicular activity and ovulation in domestic cats.

3.2 Estrus Induction

3.2.1 Photoperiod and social stimulation

Controlling of the photoperiod is one of the most efficient and oldest techniques (Dawson, 1941; Scott and Lloyd-Jacob, 1959) to induce cyclicity in the queen since cats are stimulated by longer photoperiod exposition. The benefits of the use of photoperiod stimulation are the low cost and the absence of side effects. In fact, queens exposed to equatorial or near-equatorial photoperiods (Johnston *et al.*, 1996; da Silva *et al.*, 2006) and queens kept under artificial light for longer than 14 hours/day (Leyva *et al.*, 1989a) show estrus all year-round with no influence of season on the estrous cycle. However, under continuous light (24 hours), the frequency of cycles can decrease.

Reproduction in the queen can, therefore, be controlled by the length of hours of light, directly related to the geographic localization in relation to sun exposure (Hurni, 1981; Feldman and Nelson, 1996) or to the artificial source of light. The increase in hours of daylight leads to increased sexual activity (Cline *et al.*, 1980; Pope, 2000). The influence of light exposure can also be observed in the temperate areas (Northern hemisphere), with a more pronounced seasonal effect. In these regions, queens will show anestrus from October to December (Romagnoli *et al.*, 2019) when the daylight is declining. However, seasonality has less influence on queens living in a house environment than free roaming ones (Jemmet and Evans, 1977). Several authors (Jemmet and Evans, 1977; Schmidt, 1986; Tsutsui and Stabenfeldt, 1993; Pope, 2000) observed the influence of artificial light on seasonality and the effect of the breed.

The length of light exposure is somewhat controversial, but 14 hours of light seems to be ideal to stimulate the hypothalamic–pituitary axis (Romagnoli, 2003). However, reproductive cyclicity has been obtained in female domestic cats exposed to artificial lighting for 12 hours (Hurni, 1981; Corrada and Gobello, 2000). Considering natural conditions in the equatorial regions and cyclicity of queens during the whole year, perhaps 12 hours of lights might be enough to induce estrus in the queen (da Silva *et al.*, 2006). Indeed, the duration of light/day influenced the number of follicles and the concentration of 17β-estradiol. Different protocols of light have been studied as summarized in Table 3.1.

Another aspect that seems to influence the success of the induction of estrous activity is a previous anestrous period before the stimulation of the estrous cycle. Exposing the queens to a long daily dark phase or a reduced number of hours of light/day (<8 hours; Leyva *et al.*, 1989a), seems to optimize the response to a new estrous cycle once the exposure is increased to 12 hours of light/day. The time

DOI: 10.1079/9781789247107.0003

Table 3.1. Overview of various light protocols to induce estrus in the queen. (Author's own table.)

Light exposure	Percentage of queens in estrus	Particularities	References
12 h of light/day	Enough to restart sexual activity	After a period of 30 days in the predominant dark phase (9 h light: 15 h dark)	Hurni (1981)
Exposed to 12 h of lighting in 24 h for one month, then 14 h of lighting in 24 h until estrus was detected (n = 6)	5/6 (85%) In the presence of estrous female 3/4 (75%) In the presence of a tomcat 3/4 (75%)	Two neon tubes giving 150 lux furnished the programmed lighting system	Michel (1993)
13 h of light/day, distributed in 12h of light, and 1h of light during the dark phase	5/6 (85%)		
13 h of light/day, distributed in 12 h of light, and 4h of dark and 1 h light and 7 h dark	5/6 (85%)		
Minimum of 14 h of bright artificial light per day	May take several weeks for estrous cycles to resume	Increase in number of females in estrus	Little (2012)

to respond to the light system decreased significantly if a 1-hour flash of light is provided during the dark period (Michel, 1993).

Social interactions appear also to have an impact on estrous induction. The cohabitation of cycling queens with prepuberal or non-cycling female cats seems to have a positive effect on estrous manifestations (Michel, 1993; Corrada and Gobello, 2000; Romagnoli, 2003) most likely due to the action of pheromones. Queens are also sensitive to the male effect (Michel, 1993). The presence of a tomcat will have a positive effect in non-cycling queens by decreasing the frequency of estrus without clinical signs and in accentuating the expression of estrus (Romagnoli, 2003). Even the response to the light system can be directly affected by social interactions. The number of days of 14 hours of light exposure to the first signs of estrus was significantly less when an estrous queen or an active male were introduced (22.3 ± 0.6 days) as compared to the light system alone (44.6 ± 0.6 days) (Michel, 1993).

In practice, the best option is to add light before sunset to extend the day to 12–14 hours of exposure with 300 lux and introduce an estrus female or a tomcat. Cyclicity should begin within 30–45 days.

3.2.2 Hormonal treatment

An alternative method to induce estrus is hormonal treatments. Different protocols are available with variable success rates. The aim of the hormonal treatment is to mimic the cascade that controls the reproductive cycle of female cats. Therefore, the base of the treatments is the use of follicle-stimulating hormone (FSH) responsible for folliculogenesis and luteinizing hormone (LH) necessary to induce ovulation (Feldman and Nelson, 1996; Johnston *et al.*, 2001). In general, the domestic cat responds well to gonadotrophic treatment, but there is an important variation and irregularity in the response. The ideal protocols for domestic cats have not yet been established (Pope, 2000) due to individuality and variation in the hormonal concentration, purification and time of stimulation in relation to the estrous cycle. To avoid interference of progesterone resulting from spontaneous ovulations or altered response to gonadotropins due to the stage of follicular activity, anestrous induction with progestin seems to be the first step before the use of hormonal therapies since inactive ovaries respond better to stimulation protocols (Michel, 1993; Mattos *et al.*, 2001; Pelican *et al.*, 2008). Using 0.088 mg/kg of oral altrenogest (Regumate®, Merck Animal Health) once daily for 38–45 days will ensure most cats will respond to induction protocols. An interesting finding was the distinction of two cat populations, induced or spontaneous ovulators, since they showed a difference in ovarian physiology and in the response to gonadotropin stimulation. In a study conducted by Pelican *et al.* (2008), once stimulated by eCG (150 IU) followed by 100 IU of human chorionic gonadotropin (hCG) 84 hours later, queens which are more prone to have spontaneous ovulations showed longer follicular phases (~11 days) than the ones characterized by induced ovulation (~5 days). The physiologic differences seem to be related to the number and/or availability of gonadotropin receptors. Progestin (Levonorgestrel) pre-treatment induced similar responses on the follicular activity after stimulation with eCG/hCG (~9 days) regardless of the type of ovulation of the queens. Progestin (levonorgestel) had no luteolytic action but was capable of suppressing a new follicular growth and led to baseline ovarian activity and prevented ovulation. Therefore, progestin imprint (by endogenous or exogenous exposition) changes the ovarian follicular environment and increases the sensitivity to gonadotropin stimulation. The mechanism is unclear but most likely is associated to the population of receptors or at least the sensitivity to gonadotropin.

The main products used are equine chorionic gonadotropin (eCG) with both FSH and LH function, porcine FSH (pFSH), human FSH (huFSH), human menopausal gonadotropin (hMG), and human chorionic gonadotropin (hCG) often used to induce ovulation. Different protocols from specific clinical trials are summarized in Table 3.2. All the injections should be done intramuscularly (IM) or subcutaneously (SQ) to reduce the risk of an anaphylactic reaction.

Signs of estrus are normally observed 3 to 5 days from the first injection. Although different protocols give good results, the association of FSH with hCG has limitations since the multiple injections are not ideal, requiring frequent restraint and increasing stress. Therefore, the use of eCG is more practical since only one single injection is necessary. Two protocols seem to be optimal: (i) the use of 2 mg of FSH daily until the onset of estrus signs (normally from 3 to 7 days), followed by natural mating or 250 IU of hCG (Johnston *et al.*, 2001); and (ii) eCG at the dose of 100–150 IU one single time followed by 50–100 IU of hCG 5 to 7 days later to induce ovulation (Romagnoli, 2006).

The biggest limitation toward the use of hormones is the side effects most likely due to an overstimulation of the ovaries. Exogenous gonadotropins affect the endocrine environment by developing a new follicular wave leading to increased estradiol levels (hyperstimulation) and an extra ovulation with increase in progesterone levels. These disruptions of the endocrine environment can interfere with early embryonic development and transport, and consequently the pregnancy rate. The use of eCG is currently associated with the presence of follicular cysts and anovulatory follicles. Signs of estrus can also be weak or imperceptible (Dresser *et al.*, 1987). The presence of follicular cysts seems to be responsible for the low fertility observed in the hormonally-induced estrus (Pope, 2000) because of a hormonal imbalance modifying the oviductal motility and/or uterine environment.

Another limitation of the hormonal therapy is the possibility of the production of neutralizing antibodies against eCG and hCG directly impacting the response to the treatment (Pelican *et al.*, 2006). However, if long intervals are allowed between stimulations (at least 4 months), follicular production seems not to be affected (Swanson *et al.*, 1996).

3.2.3 GnRH Agonists

Gonadotropin-releasing hormone (GnRH) is a hypothalamus-derived decapeptide. Physiologically, the efficacy of GnRH to stimulate pituitary activity for gonadotropin secretion is based on pulsatility. GnRH injections every 70–90 minutes for more than 8 days are required in the bitch to induce a fertile estrus (Kutzler, 2007). These frequent injections are a major limitation making protocols using GnRH and its agonists not suitable for clinical use for estrus induction in cats (and dogs). To overcome this problem, subcutaneous infusion pumps with pulsatile release are administered in human medicine with good success rates. The costs and the need for surgical removal make this option unsuitable for cats too. GnRH agonist implants provide the possibility of continuous release and are currently registered as deslorelin implants (2.1/4.7/9.4 mg) for the use in veterinary medicine in different areas of the world. Zambelli *et al.* (2015) used a 4.7 mg deslorelin implant and successfully induced estrus in 13/13 cats (100%) with 7/13 queens exhibiting behavioral estrus. The peak of estrus, based on the presence of 100% cornified superficial cells, was 5.0 ± 2.2 days (range: 4–11 days) after implant administration. No side effects were observed. Three of these cats were inseminated twice, resulting in 100% pregnancy rate indicating that estrus induction with a deslorelin implant is a practicable option in queens. In the bitch, premature luteal failure resulting in pregnancy loss had been described following the use of deslorelin implants (Kutzler *et al.*, 2009; Maenhoudt

Table 3.2. Overview of protocols used in specific clinical trials with different hormones to induce estrus in the queen. (Author's own table.)

Drug	Protocol	Female selection	Results	References
FSH-p	2 mg/day 5 days	Inactive ovaries (no CL, no follicles or follicles <2 mm) 2 mg/day for 5 days	Estrus within 5/6 days in 93% (28/30 queens)	Goodrowe *et al.* (1986)
FSH-p + hCG	FSH-P every 24 h for 6 days (equal doses/5 days and half or one-third of the FSH-P on the 6th day) + hCG (two doses at d6 and d7) Dose FSH-P varies from d1–d5 = 0.5 to 1.5 mg/day d6 = 0.25 to 0.5 mg Dose hCG varies from none to 500 IU at d6 and 750 IU at d7	Healthy female queens not observed in heat for 7 to 10 days	All treatments were able to stimulate the ovaries and induce ovulation. The most desirable results were from the treatment of 0.75 mg of FSH-P for 5 days and 0.25 mg at d6 followed by two injections of 375 IU of hCG at d6 and d7	Dresser *et al.* (1987)
FSH-p + hCG	Induction of estrus using FSH-p (IM injection) of 2 mg on day 1 followed by 1.0 mg until signs of estrus (up to 4 days) Ovulation was induced by 500 IU of hCG (IV)	22 mixed breed cats in seasonal anestrous 10 females used as donor animals 12 females used as recipient – received the ovulation protocol	Estrus was induced in 86.4% of the queens (19/22). Duration of estrus 3 to 9 days Ovulation in all females (9/9) showing estrous signs	Tsutsui *et al.* (1989)
FSH-p + hCG	pFSH injected SQ in decreasing doses from 1–6 mg/day for 4 days On the 5th day, hCG at the dose of 100 IU was injected IM	Interestrous domestic female cats housed in a controlled light system of 14:10 h light:dark ratio. Estrous behavior monitored 3 to 4 days/week and vaginal cytology once/week Ovariectomy at 26 ± 1 h of hCG and collection of oocytes	Presence of mature follicles in all treated animals	Pope *et al.* (1993)
FSH-p (ultra pure) without any luteinizing hormone activity + hCG	Three different doses SQ of 2.5 IU (G1), 10 IU (G2) and 30 IU (G3) divided into five daily doses 1 IU = 10 µg of pure FSH-p At d6 half of FSH-p dose together with 250 IU of hCG and 24 later 250 IU of hCG (SQ)	18 domestic female cats housed in a controlled light system of 14:10h light:dark Pre-pubertal queens (n = 9) Adult queens (n = 9) without signs of behavioral estrus Embryo recovery by uterine lavage (d11 to d13)	Estrus was induced in all females except one pre-pubertal queen in G1 Ovulation rate % and embryo recovery (x ± sd) were respectively: 0% pre-pubertal queens For adult queens: G1 = 72.9%, 2.6 ± 2 G2 = 43.6, 15.3 ± 12.4 G3 = 35.3%, 8.6 ± 6.1	Verstegen *et al.* (1993)
huFSH + hCG hMG (15 IU of FSH and LH) + hCG	G1-GA(n = 5) four injections of 7.5 IU of huFSH/day (IM) or G2 GA (n = 4) four injections of 15 IU of huFSH/day (IM) and 12 h + 1 later an injection of 100 IU hCG (IM) G3 GB (n =6) four injections of 15 IU huFSH/day (IM), and 12 h + 1 later an injection of 0.1 ml saline (IM)	Adult domestic shorthair cats housed under 8-h light/l6-h dark cycle Selected female by video endoscopy (follicles ≤1 mm in diameter, no CL, and/or uterine tone)	Follicles increased in size up to 2.0 to 2.9 mm) in G1, G2, G3, and G5 (with one follicle larger than 3 mm) In G4, the follicular growth was less important with no follicles bigger than 1.9 mm	Orosz *et al.* (1992)

	G4 GC(n = 6) control group, saline injection replaced the huFSH and 12h + 1 later an injection of 100 IU hCG (IM) G5 GD(n = 8) five daily doses of hMG (15 IU of FSH and LH) and 34 h later an injection of 100 IU hCG (IM)	Laparoscopy for collection of oocytes was done 27 to 34 h after the administration of hCG or saline	Aspirated oocytes/ovary: G3 and G4 = none G1 and G2 = 6.4 ± 1.7 G5 = 10.64 ± 2.9 Fertilization rate was close to 20% in all groups with aspirated oocytes	
eCG + hCG	150 IU (IM) on day 1 followed by 100 IU 80 h later 84 h later 88 h later 92 h later 96 h later	45 queens with no follicular development or luteal tissue (n = 9/group)	No effect on the mean number of ovarian follicles, but less mature oocyte in hCG at 92 h and 96 h Observation of more oocytes that are degenerated at 96-h treatment.	Donoghue *et al.* (1992)
eCG + hCG	100 IU eCG IV (G1), 100 IU eCG IM (G2), 75 IU hCG IV (G3) 75 IU hCG IM (G4), or 100 IU eCG IM and 80 h later injection of 75 IU hCG (IM). (G5)	20-catheterized anestrous queens (n = 4 per treatment based on lighting controlled 12L/12D) with no CL and absence of mature follicles (≥2 mm)	Behavioral estrus in 95% of females following IV or IM administration of eCG or hCG, within 2–3 days, with queens receiving IV injections entering estrus –1 day earlier ($p < 0.05$) than queens injected IM Ovulation was observed in 25% (1/4) in G1, G2 and G3, 50% (2/4) in G4, and 100% (4/4) in G5 All anovulatory females had at least ten mature follicles	Swanson *et al.* (1997)
eCG + hCG FSH + hCG	Donor animals 100 UI eCG – d1 50 UI eCG – d2 50 UI eCG – d3 500 IU hCG – d7 to induce ovulation Recipient animals 2 mg of FSH (IM) – d1 followed by 1 mg/day (IM) until onset of estrus or the first day of estrus 500 IU hCG – d7 to induce ovulation	24 mixed breed queens in seasonal anestrus	Estrus in 5/5 donor queens. Estrus in 18/19 queens – 3 to 6 days after the first dose of FSH-P (4.4 ± 0.3 days), estrous duration 5–14 days (9.4 ± 0.7 days)	Tsutsui *et al.* (2000)
eCG + hCG	Single-dose 150 IU eCG and 80–84 h later a single injection of 100 IU hCG	16 females in estrus detected by vaginal cytology to stimulate follicular activity and ovulation	Ovulation observed in all females with average of 13.5 and 20 luteal bodies	Santana *et al.* (2012)
FSH-p	Females with inactive ovaries (no CL, no follicles or follicles < 2 mm) 2 mg/day for 5 days	Estrus within 5/6 days 93% (28/30 queens)		Cline *et al.* (1980)

Indication, selection of the queens and the success rates by authors.

et al., 2012, 2018) resulting in the recommendation to remove the implant around/following ovulation and to follow progesterone in pregnancy. Likely to avoid similar problems, the implant had been surgically removed in all three cats (Zambelli *et al.*, 2015).

3.2.4 General consideration

Although queens are still being defined as induced ovulators, the observation of spontaneous ovulation seems to be more frequent than previously described. Therefore, one important piece of information before any attempt to induce estrus is to know the level of progesterone since the presence of progesterone will prevent estrus induction.

3.2.5 Conclusion

Different methods of estrous stimulation are available for use in domestic cats. Although many protocols are still experimental, they can be potentially used in pet-owned animals and cattery breeders. Breeders commonly use light protocols as a method to induce and maintain cyclicity. Even though inducing estrus by hormonal therapy is not so demanded by owners, it is a possibility to consider this in the clinical setting. The administration of protocols with FSH or eCG and hCG to induce estrus and ovulation in queens is an important tool to develop better methods to apply to endangered or exotic feline species. The GnRH agonist implants inducing estrus and ovulation in a single application might be the approach of the future.

3.3 Estrus Suppression

Besides the control of free-roaming cat populations, a concern for the veterinary profession all over the world, estrus suppression is a common request from cat owners. Contraception is defined as a reversible method of blocking fertility, whereas estrus suppression is defined as a lack of estrus behavior by blocking or suppressing the follicular phase. Estrus suppression methods need to combine safety, be trustworthy, reversible, and be adapted to the owner's expectation, but also be well adjusted to the physiology of the species. Medical estrus suppression could be indicated in cases where anesthesia would be a risk, such as queens suffering from cardiac and kidney pathologies. The temporary suppression of cyclicity in a queen is a request of many cat breeders. For example, Maine Coon queens might show dysorexia or even anorexia during heat, which can lead to a remarkable loss of body condition that is not ideal when breeding is finally desired (personal observation). Some countries and registries only authorize three litters in a 2-year period, so estrus suppression can help control breeding. Although in high demand, the choices for reversible estrus suppression in domestic cats are limited. The oldest methods available for this purpose and the only one currently approved are progestins (oral or injectable) with important side effects depending on the dose and the frequency of administration. The other option for longer inhibition of cyclicity is GnRH agonist implants. Melatonin (oral or implant) seems like a good alternative for short-term estrus suppression as well as the manipulation of duration of light exposure. Another option for short-term suppression is the induction of ovulation, which leads to pseudopregnancy. Mechanical vaginal stimulation and/or teaser male (vasectomized or even neutered tomcats), as well as medical induction of ovulation by hCG or GnRH agonists will cause ovulation, and the high levels of progesterone will last for around 45 days (range 35–76 days) (Wildt *et al.*, 1980).

3.3.1 Progestins

Progestins are the most commonly used medical drugs for prevention or suppression of estrus in cats (Jackson 1984; Romagnoli and Concannon, 2003; Kutzler and Wood, 2006; Romagnoli and Sontas, 2010; Goericke-Pesch *et al.*, 2014). There are several available progestins to control fertility in small animals, the most common are: megestrol acetate (MA), medroxyprogesterone (MPA) and proligestone (PROL).

The mechanism of estrus suppression with synthetic analogs of progesterone remains controversial. One of the pathways of progestins proposed is the negative feedback to suppress GnRH from the hypothalamus and FSH and LH from the pituitary, blocking follicular growth and ovulation (Munson, 2006). However, there is evidence that this mechanism is not the most important one. Progestins likely have a contraceptive effect because they seem to prevent the transportation of spermatozoa and oocytes impairing fertilization by altering uterine motility (Munson, 2006; Goericke-Pesch, 2010; Goericke-Pesch *et al.*, 2014) and interfering with implantation through alteration of the endometrial receptivity (Attardi, 1984; Brache *et al.*, 1985).

The major limitations of the use of progestins are the variety and gravity of the side effects (Table 3.3). The adverse reactions to progestins are related to the affinity of the drug to bind and mimic the progesterone effect and to bind to other receptors of steroid hormones as androgens and glucocorticoids (Duncan *et al.*, 1964; Fekete and Szebere´nyi, 1965; Kloosterboer *et al.*, 1988). Therefore, cases of masculinization, insulin resistance, abnormal growth, and suppression of immune system function have been described (Middleton *et al.*, 1987; Johnston *et al.*, 2001; Munson, 2006). Moreover, a direct effect on the reproductive system leading to uterine pathology, mammary hyperplasia, and tumor development has been suspected (Hernandez *et al.*, 1975; Concannon and Meyers-Wallen, 1991; MacDougall, 2003; Loretti *et al.*, 2004, 2005; Payan-Carreira, 2013). The mechanism of the mammary gland pathology, although still controversial, concerns mainly the proliferation of parenchyma, potentially leading to the development of benign or malignant mammary tumors after repeated administration. The secretion of growth hormone (GH) can be stimulated by progestins in bitches (Romagnoli and Concannon, 2003) and most likely also occurs in the queen. High levels of GH can cause the development of mammary nodules (Romagnoli and Concannon, 2003). Therefore, one explanation for the increase in the incidence of mammary tumors in queens under progestin treatment is through GH along with the direct effect on the mammary gland leading to hyperplasia and neoplasia (Romagnoli and Concannon, 2003). Pyometra may also develop, especially when progestins are administered during the secretory phases of the cycle. Domestic female cats under progestin treatment can have a high blood glucose concentration. Hyperglycemia seems to have little impact on the health of young females. The most likely pathway for the diabetes mellitus observed during progestin treatment is related to increased secretion of GH, leading to insulin resistance, or due to a direct action of progestin (Findik *et al.*, 1999). Even in normal cycles, during diestrus, high levels of endogenous progesterone have been associated with insulin resistance.

Progestins can also induce subclinical adrenocortical suppression most likely due to the glucocorticoid-like negative feedback to the corticotrophin secretion by the pituitary. However, the clinical impact in the response of stress is unknown. Local injection reactions may include discoloration, alopecia, calcinosis, and skin atrophia. Queens treated with progestins often show increased food consumption leading to weight gain and polydipsia (Romagnoli and Concannon, 2003).

Side effects of progestins can lead to infertility and can sometimes also be life threatening (Keskin *et al.*, 2009). Due to the side effects, the use of progestins should be considered case by case (dose, frequency

Table 3.3. Overview of the list of side effects and risks of the use of progestins to prevent estrus in the queen. (Author's own table.)

Degree of severity	Side effects	Risk	References
Serious	Mucometra and CEH-pyometra complex	Higher with MPA > MA > PROL	Agudelo (2005) Johnston *et al.* (2001)
	Mammary fibroepithelial hyperplasia	Higher with high doses	Munson (2006)
	Fibroadenomatosis	Higher in long duration suppression	Greenberg *et al.* (2013) Wehrend *et al.* (2001)
	Mammary tumors	Higher in older animals	Loretti *et al.* (2005)
	Insulin resistance Hyperglycemia and glycosuria – diabetes mellitus	Higher is animals with prior conditions	Keskin *et al.* (2009) Hayden *et al.* (1989)
Mild/general	Lethargy Depression Hair discoloration Increased appetite and weight gain		Henik *et al.* (1985)
Uncommon	Epidermal atrophy and alopecia Cutaneous xanthomatosis Uterine tumor		Henik *et al.* (1985) Sapierzynski *et al.* (2009)

Side effects based on the severity and frequency of progestin treatment in queens.

and duration of treatment) and be avoided in non-pubertal females, potentially pregnant queens and/or in any female with clinical signs of hepatic, mammary, or uterine pathology (Romagnoli and Concannon, 2003; Goericke-Pesch, 2010). It is also important to emphasize that the misuse of progestins is the cause of some of the observed side effects. Therefore, the secondary effects can be minimized by adapting the dose (Romagnoli, 2015) and by treating only during the anestrus or interestrous period (Romagnoli and Sontas, 2010).

Medroxyprogesterone acetate (MPA)

Medroxyprogesterone acetate (17α-hydroxy-6α-methylprogesterone acetate) is the most potent synthetic progesterone and widely used progestin. MPA has a high progesterone receptor affinity and could explain the mammary development and increasing risk of tumor development. In addition, its progestagenic effect increases the risk of uterine pathology and metabolic disease. Although its affinity for androgen and glucocorticoid receptors is not strong, its long-acting characteristics are responsible for the side effects. Therefore, the use of MPA, in general, is under serious scrutiny and in some countries its use is forbidden in small animals.

Side effects associated with MPA are highly dose dependent. The dose of 5 mg/day orally or 25–100 mg for the injectable form achieves suppression of estrus for 2–4 months. Injections are usually repeated every 6 months, as reviewed by Munson (2006) and Romagnoli (2015). Other doses have been proposed as 2 mg/kg with injections every 3-4 months and 3-5 mg/kg every 5-6 months (Romagnoli and Concannon, 2003), or 2 mg/kg intramuscularly every 5 months (Romagnoli and Sontas, 2010),

As cited by Romagnoli (2015), a study in 1963 from Harris and Wolchuk, one of the first publications on MPA in cats, mentioned low oral doses of 0.01 and 0.05 mg/kg q24h for 12 months with 100% efficacy with the latest dosage. Nowadays, with third-generation progestins, it is recommended to avoid the use of MPA in queens (Munson, 2006; Kutzler and Wood, 2006).

Megestrol acetate

Megestrol acetate is a synthetic progestin with a short half-life and slight glucocorticoid and very slight mineralocorticoid activity. Therefore, the side effects are less noticeable than after administration of MPA. Due to these characteristics, MA is more suitable as a progesterone supplementation for domestic cats (Romagnoli and Concannon, 2003; Max *et al.*, 2014). Ideally the treatment should start during anestrus and the most common dose proposed is 2.5–5 mg/day for 3 to 5 days, followed by the same dose for maintenance once a week (Burke, 1982; Henik *et al.*, 1985; Munson, 2006). Other dosing options are 5 mg/queen every two weeks, 2.5 mg/queen every week, or divide the dose in half and give every 3 to 4 days (Romagnoli and Sontas, 2010).

There is a higher risk of mammary cancer, glucocorticoid suppression, and weight gain in cats treated with MA. The side effects appear to be dose dependent. MA at the dose of >0.625 mg/kg q24h for 1 week or q48h for up to 2 weeks was used in the past for dermatological or behavioral issues, leading to some short-term side effects such as adrenocortical suppression (Chastain *et al.*, 1981; Middleton *et al.*, 1987) and diabetes mellitus (Middleton and Watson, 1985; Mansfield *et al.*, 1986). MA may be used more safely with lower dosages repeated more frequently (0.625 mg/kg/week for up to 30 weeks) with the main side effect being increased appetite in one-third of treated queens (Romagnoli, 2015).

Although not recommended due to increasing risk of side effects (mainly pyometra), treatment can start during estrus to prevent estrus continuation. In this case, the dose described is 5 mg/cat/day until estrus stops (treatment for 3–4 days at least), and then the dose should be decreased to 2.5 mg/cat/week or 5 mg/cat every 2 weeks (Munson, 2006; Romagnoli and Sontas, 2010). A very low dose (0.01–0.03 mg/kg q24h) MA is now available in Italy (Estropill, MSD) to suppress estrus (Romagnoli, 2015) but needs further investigation on efficacy and safety.

While MA is considered safer than MPA, irregular, prolonged treatment can lead to similar side effects as MPA (Table 3.3). Due to the concern of potential side effects, it is no longer recommended to repeat administrations throughout the life of queens as long-term estrus suppression.

Proligestone (PROL)

Proligestone has more anti-gonadotrophic action and less gestational and anti-estrogenic effects than MPA and MA (Kutzler and Wood, 2006; Max *et al.*, 2014). Therefore, it is considered a safer drug and reported to have marginal side effects (Kutzler and Wood, 2006; Romagnoli and Sontas, 2010; Goericke-Pesch *et al.*, 2014; Max *et al.*, 2014) compared to the other compounds. Proligestone at a minimal dose of 10 mg/kg up to 30 mg/kg (Findik *et al.*, 1999) was developed to be contraceptive with only minor effects on the uterus, the mammary gland, and the endocrine system. The duration of suppression varies from 4.5 to 10 months (Findik *et al.*, 1999). The most common recommendation is to repeat the injection after 3 months, then 4 months later, and then every 5 months.

Other progestins

Other progestins like levonorgestrel, delmadinone, chlormadinone, and altrenogest are being evaluated experimentally. Levonorgestrel (LEV) is a subcutaneous implant (16 mg) used to suppress cyclicity for 12 months, but there is no immediate effect. Subsequent fertility was proven although some uterine problems have been reported after treatment (Baldwin *et al.*, 1994). A dose response of levonorgestrel implants was determined in the cat indicating that a threshold concentration of six implants (36 mg, Norplant®) was necessary to induce ovarian suppression (Pelican *et al.*, 2008).

Chlormadinone acetate (CMA) is available in oral or implant formulation in Europe. The main observed side effect is weight gain. When treatment was maintained for longer time (6 years or more), the mammary gland and uterus developed some pathologies (Murakoshi *et al.*, 1996, 2000; Tamada *et al.*, 2003). Little is known about delmadinone acetate as a contraceptive in queens. Altrenogest (ALG) has been used successfully to suppress estrus in queens (Stewart *et al.*, 2010) without noticeable short-term side effects.

Conclusion

The authors of this chapter do not endorse the use of long-acting progestin as contraception in queens at the current recommended dose. Depot or long-acting progestins should be avoided in immature queens, since treated young animals might develop a form of mammary hypertrophy that potentially could be a life-threatening condition (Romagnoli and Concannon, 2003).

The duration of treatment should be adapted to the needs of the pet owner, age of cat, and safety of treatment. Young post-pubertal queens without health problems could be treated for 12 to 24 months (Romagnoli and Concannon, 2003). In cases of long-term estrus suppression with progestins (over 12 months), it is recommended to withdraw the treatment for a couple of months to reduce the impact of the drug over time. Starting with a short duration of treatment (up to 6 months) followed by a clinical evaluation and blood analysis (cell count, liver and renal function, glucose profile) during the resting time can allow early diagnosis of any possible side effects. Long-term treatment of progestins should be prescribed with caution. There is no scientific indication on what length of treatment can be considered safe. Any progestin treatment should be started during anestrus or interestrus since the combination of high estrogen and progesterone-like product could increase the risk of pyometra (Romagnoli and Concannon, 2003) and feline mammary fibroadenomatous hyperplasia (Payan-Carreira, 2013). A vaginal cytology and progesterone concentration should be performed to determine the queen's stage of cycle. If the queen presents in estrus, she should be evaluated a week later to restage the time of the cycle. If the queen is in interestrus, the treatment can be started, and if in diestrus, another evaluation should be done around 30 days later. Although induction of ovulation using GnRH has been suggested (Romagnoli and Concannon, 2003), it is not a common practice in our clinical setting.

3.3.2 Induction of ovulation and pseudopregnancy for short-term suppression

Estrus in the queen can also been interrupted by inducing ovulation. In natural breeding, the intensity and frequency of the LH surge (Concannon *et al.*, 1980) depend on the number of days in estrus and the frequency of matings. Ovulation without fertilization incites a prolonged state of luteal activity known as pseudopregnancy. The duration of pseudopregnancy is variable from 35 to 76 days (average 45 days; Wildt *et al.*, 1980) and can be obtained by mechanical stimulation of the vagina, sterile teaser tomcat, or by hormonal treatment (hCG or GnRH agonist). Vaginal stimulation with a cotton swab can be used to mimic the stimulus caused by penile spines during copulation and therefore induce the LH surge. The procedure needs to be repeated to achieve the goal of inducing ovulation. There are two limitations to this method of contraception. First, the technique is not always well tolerated by the female cat. Second, the use of the procedure repeatedly can increase the risk of pathologies related to prolonged progesterone treatment. This is more used as a short-term solution for estrus suppression.

3.3.3 Light protocols and social interactions

Since the queen is very sensitive to the photoperiod, cyclicity ceased immediately when the length of light was decreased from 14 hours to 8 hours per day and queens entered anestrus phase (Leyva *et al.*, 1989a). Under 8 hours of light and 16 hours of darkness, estrus was never observed (Michel, 1993). Reducing the exposure to light induces the secretion of high levels of endogenous melatonin, leading to a decrease in sexual activity.

3.3.4 Melatonin (N-acetyl-5-methoxytryptamine)

Melatonin (N-acetyl-5-methoxytryptamine) is a hormone secreted by the pineal gland during periods of dark. The presence of melatonin will suppress the hypothalamus secretion of GnRH. In female domestic cats, melatonin will suppress GnRH and lead to low levels of FSH, LH, and inhibition of estrous cycle (Leyva *et al.*, 1984). The impact of the presence or absence of light is very expressive in the queens and a difference of 15-fold in melatonin secretion has been demonstrated during the dark phase (Graham *et al.*, 2004).

Injectable melatonin is not a viable option since the administration is difficult and very impractical in this species. However, Leyva *et al.*, (1989b) demonstrated that the use of SQ injections of 5 mg melatonin every other day would suppress estrus for 60 days, even under 24 hours of light exposure, and that the treatment was completely reversible. At the return to estrus after treatment, higher values of estradiol-17 β, longer follicle growth patterns, and longer duration of estrus were noted, showing that queens perceived the photoperiod of 24 hours light regardless of the melatonin treatment. Melatonin administration delayed or prevented the post-coital LH surge needed for ovulation induction and increased the refractory period between coitus. Even though melatonin could reduce LH release, 67% of cats showed estrus and ovulated (Leyva *et al.*, 1989b). No side effects were reported and females that were bred afterwards became pregnant (Gimenez *et al.*, 2009; Faya *et al.*, 2011). All research testing the use of melatonin has been done during periods of cyclicity for the queen (either during natural breeding season with long days or under light regimen). All the studies using oral preparations show the reversibility of the treatment.

For the oral preparation, treatment needs to be given every day and it is not so easy to give a cat oral medication. Exogenous melatonin supplementation administered at 30 mg/cat/day 3 hours before lights-off for 35 days to six female cats effectively suppressed ovarian activity (Graham *et al.*, 2004). The circulating levels of melatonin were above the endogenous night-time concentrations for the 8-hour blood sampling period. None of the queens showed signs of estrus during treatment and they returned to normal ovarian activity 21–40 days after the end of treatment. The effect of oral melatonin was not immediate in all queens with elevated fecal estrogens during the first 3 weeks of treatment (Graham *et al.*, 2004). A lower oral dose of 4 mg melatonin tablets/cat/day (Melatol; Elisium) given 2 hours prior to lights-off resulted in similar results (Faya *et al.*, 2011) with estrous suppression averaging 50 days from the beginning of treatment. However, the effect was immediate since none of the queens showed estrus at onset of treatment. The authors stress the necessity to follow the cycle of the queen precisely in order to start the treatment during interestrus to obtain an immediate effect. For the 12 queens included in the trial with 19 interestrus intervals observed, ovulation and pseudopregnancy were observed in seven of those cycles and could be a co-factor of the estrus prevention.

Our group assessed the efficacy of oral supplementation for 2 months by comparing three doses of melatonin 0.9 mg, 5 mg and 10 mg/cat/day given 2–3 hours before sunset on privately owned purebred cats (Furthner *et al.*, 2019). In the first group with the lowest amount of melatonin, 7/10 queens showed estrus behavior within the first week of treatment, which stopped the follow-up in the study. For the two other groups, 5/24 females were excluded because of ovulation at onset of treatment. Another 5/24 cats showed estrus signs within 10 days of inclusion in the study. The breeds of these cats (Oriental, Sphynx and Devon Rex) were known to have short interestrus intervals before treatment. In 3/24 queens, the treatment was discontinued due to the reluctance of the patient to receive oral tablets every day. In 7/24 females, estrus suppression was successful. Therefore, the use of low dosage of melatonin orally is questionable.

The pharmacokinetics of melatonin implants (Melovine, CEVA Santé Animale, Libourne, France) were not studied in queens and their use is strictly off-label (Table 3.4).

The effect of the melatonin implant is not always immediate. It seems that a minimum time of at least 11 days is needed to suppress follicular activity (Gimenez *et al.*, 2009). Therefore, it is highly recommended to separate treated females from a tomcat for at least 2 weeks, since the estrus right after onset of melatonin treatment can be fertile (Schäfer-Somi, 2017). It seems important to initiate melatonin treatment at the end of estrus until early interestrus (Faya *et al.*, 2011) since the length of suppression seemed to depend on the stage of the estrous cycle when animals are treated. When the subcutaneous implant of 18 mg was placed during interestrus as compared to during estrus, the inhibition was twice as long (113.3 ± 6.1 days versus 61.1±6.8 days; Gimenez *et al.*, 2009) However, in the study by Faya *et al.* (2011), all the queens were implanted in early interestrus and were suppressed for 63.8 ± 5.4 days. One explanation suggested for this observation is that high concentrations of estrogens downregulate the expression of melatonin receptors in ovaries of rats and humans (Kutzler, 2015), but this has not been proven in cats. Duration of estrus suppression also seems to

Table 3.4. Overview of publications using melatonin implants to prevent estrus in queens. (Author's own table.)

	Griffin *et al.* (2001)	Gulyuz *et al.* (2009)	Gimenez *et al.* (2009)	Faya *et al.* (2011)	Schäfer-Somi (2017)
Control (placebo)	4	6	5	12	
Single implant	4	6	9	17	27
Five implants	4				
Concentration	12 mg to 60mg (5 × 12)	18 mg	18 mg	18 mg	18 mg
Stage of estrous cycle	Not evaluated	Not evaluated	9 during interestrus 9 during estrus	Interestrus	Interestrus
Results	Duration of suppression unknown. Successful in 75% of cases	When daylight was 10.5 h Control – all animals showed estrous signs Treated – only one female in estrus	Implantation during estrus – suppression of estrus for 61.1 days	Suppression of estrus for 63.8 days	No estrus occurred for an average of 103.9 days in 22 queens 6 queens in estrus from 1 to 10 days after implantation with one queen getting pregnant
Side effects	Uterine pathologies	None	None	None	None
Conclusion		Melatonin implant can prolong seasonal anestrus			Effectiveness in puerperal cats has not been well investigated
Particularities			Presence of superficial cells on vaginal cytology after 2 days - implants interestrus With estrous signs 2 and 2–3 days after implantation (interestrus vs estrus)	Ovulation and pseudopregnancy in 43.3%. No signs of estrus post-implantation. Results were highly individual	Significant differences between British Shorthair and Norwegian Forest Cats ($p < 0.05$)

Concentration of implant, timing, results and side effects of melatonin implants administered for estrus suppression in queens.

be influenced by the season at which treatment is started (Schäfer-Somi, 2017). Using this implant to prolong the natural anestrus period may be possible (Gulyuz *et al.*, 2009). There were no side effects from the implants and queens that were bred after the treatment, 6/8 (Gimenez *et al.*, 2009) and 12/17 (Furthner *et al.*, 2020) became pregnant. Implanting prepuberal queens of 1.5–2.0 kg of body weight at time of treatment with the 18 mg (Melovine) did not postpone puberty. Treatment did not alter growth as all animals of the study reached puberty when expected (at 75% of adult body weight) (Faya *et al.*, 2011). The difference in action between pre- and post-pubertal cats is unclear. The use of melatonin implants could be optimized with an applicator better adapted to cats. As they are commercialized for ewes to induce estrus, the implants are packaged in two rods of 25 implants with a single application gun and one single sterile needle. The use of a single sterile applicator easy to manipulate with a 12-gauge needle would be ideal.

Conclusion

High individual variation to the response of melatonin treatment is observed. A breed effect appears to have an impact on the response but, due to lack of sufficient numbers of animals of each specific breed, cannot be confirmed. Since the implant seems to be more effective in breeds more susceptible to seasonality, a duration of estrus suppression of 6–9 months after implantation would be optimal, but further studies are needed to see if this goal can be reached.

3.4 GnRH agonists

3.4.1 Use in adult queens

Slow-release GnRH agonist implants, such as Suprelorin®, are suitable for long-term suppression of the feline estrous cycle. The implant is placed under the skin near the umbilicus with the cat restrained in dorsal recumbency. The hair over the implant area should be clipped and the skin cleaned with antibacterial scrub. The skin is grasped in the operator's hand and the needle of the implant device is inserted under the skin and the implant is delivered (Fig. 3.1). It is important to check the placement of the implant and preferably to compress the skin for a about a minute after implant insertion to avoid implant loss. Placement in this area allows easy removal if necessary. Following treatment with a GnRH agonist-containing slow-release implant, an initial flare-up resulting in induction of a fertile estrus is observed in adult queens (Munson *et al.*, 2001; Rubion and Driancourt, 2009; Ackermann *et al.*, 2012; Toydemir *et al.*, 2012; Goericke-Pesch *et al.*, 2013a; Zambelli *et al.*, 2015). The subsequent increase of progesterone concentrations indicates that ovulation occurs (Rubion and Driancourt, 2009; Goericke-Pesch *et al.*, 2013a). The duration of efficacy of the deslorelin slow-release implant is quite variable: the described mean duration of efficacy of a 4.7 mg deslorelin implant is 22.7 ± 2.1 months (range: 16.1–36.7 months, $n = 20$) in a research population (Goericke-Pesch *et al.*, 2013a) and 16.0 ± 5.7 months (range: 8–38 months, $n = 26$) in breeder-owned cats (Furthner *et al.*, 2020). For the 9.4 mg deslorelin implant, a duration of efficacy of >18.5 months is described (Toydemir *et al.*, 2012). Whereas no side effects were reported in one study ($n = 20$; Goericke-Pesch *et al.*, 2013a), side effects (6/26), such as persistent estrus ($n = 2/26$), lactation ($n = 2/26$), fibroadenomatosis ($n = 1/26$), cystic endometrial hyperplasia ($n = 1/26$) (Furthner *et al.* 2020), and reduced activity and weight gain were observed in others (Munson *et al.*, 2001; Furthner *et al.*, 2020). Delayed onset of efficacy (Goericke-Pesch *et al.*, 2013a), estrus signs, and estradiol increase (Goericke-Pesch *et al.*, 2013a; Munson

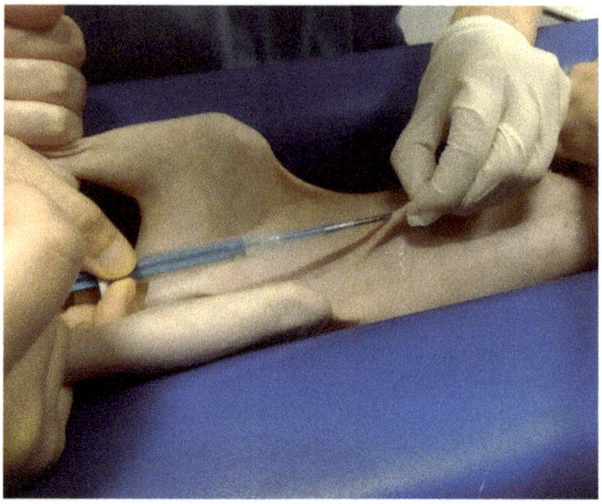

Fig. 3.1. Placement of a GnRH implant near the umbilicus on a Sphinx queen. The cat is gently restrained in dorsal recumbency and the implant is inserted just under the skin. Placing the implant in this area allows easy removal when needed. (Image: author's own.)

et al., 2001) and non-responders (Toydemir *et al.*, 2012) have been observed. The individual onset and termination of efficacy require detailed observations and care of the owner to avoid unwanted mating. Treatment effects are reversible with cats returning to seasonal estrus after the end of efficacy (Goericke-Pesch *et al.*, 2013b) or estrus is inducible with eCG and hCG (Ackermann *et al.*, 2012). Cats conceive (n = 9/9, Goericke-Pesch *et al.*, 2013a; n = 12/unknown number of mated queens, Furthner *et al.*, 2020) and give birth to normal litters. Litter size did not differ significantly from untreated animals and queens show normal lactation and maternal care (Goericke-Pesch *et al.*, 2013a). Treatment in early pregnancy must be avoided as lack of maternal behavior after delivery was described in a case report (Goericke-Pesch *et al.*, 2013b).

3.4.2 Pre-pubertal use

Application of one-third of a 4.7 mg Suprelorin® (approximately 1.6 mg deslorelin) in neonatal and pre-pubertal animals younger than 114.4 ± 12.7 days and 50% of body weight of adult animals did not result in estrus induction, but significantly postponed puberty (Risso *et al.*, 2012; Carranza *et al.*, 2014). Induced effects were fully reversible after the end of efficacy which was in mean 281.2 ± 21.6 days (range: 180–428 days) compared to 177.8 ± 10.8 days in controls (Risso *et al.*, 2012; Carranza *et al.*, 2014, 2015). Administration of a (full) 4.7 mg deslorelin implant was described to be safe in 3- to 9-month old queens with estrus induction observed clinically in one, and subclinically (full vaginal keratinization) in another cat. Puberty was postponed significantly and at the end of the observation period, animals aged 21 to 36 months (n = 4) were still pre-pubertal (Cecchetto *et al.*, 2017).

3.5 Conclusion

Stimulation of estrus is a clinical option for practitioners to pursue in cases of female cats with reproductive problems. The best treatment is the one with less risk. Therefore, in cases of anestrus (primary or secondary), the first option should be light management and social stimulation before using hormonal treatment. Trying to diagnose the cause of the reproductive problems is the first clue to better address the problem.

Alternative methods of estrus suppression in domestic cats are a common request for owned pets and animal control associations. Although the ideal non-surgical method for population control and estrus suppression has not yet been developed, there are some possibilities for pet animals. The benefits and inconveniences for each drug should be openly discussed with the owner. Even medications with high possibilities of side effects could be an option if it is done as a target drug for the right patient. Before choosing the approach for estrus suppression, one must consider the reason, the duration desired, age, breed, overall health and reproductive status of the animal, financial constraints, the involvement of the owner, and, finally, the schedule and simplicity of the administration of the treatment. As aforementioned, different drugs can give a safe and predicable result if correctly chosen and administrated. Although some protocols are safer, each case for estrus suppression treatment should be evaluated closely and cautiously. The search for new drugs and safer protocols for estrus suppression are a constant challenge for the veterinary medicine in all species, but especially for domestic cats.

3.6 References

Ackermann, C. L., Volpato, R., Destro, F. C., Trevisol, E., Sousa, N. R., *et al.* (2012) Ovarian activity reversibility after the use of deslorelin acetate as a short-term contraceptive in domestic queens. *Theriogenology* 78(4), 817–822. doi: 10.1016/j.theriogenology.2012.03.030

Agudelo, C. F. (2005) Cystic endometrial hyperplasia-pyometra complex in cats. *A review. Veterinary Quarterly* 27(4), 173–182.

Attardi, B. (1984) Progesterone modulation of the luteinizing hormone surge: regulation of hypothalamic and pituitary progestin receptors. *Endocrinology* 115(6), 2113–2122. doi: 10.1210/endo-115-6-2113

Baldwin, C. J, Peter, A. T., and Bosu, W. T. (1994) The contraceptive effects of levonorgestrel in the domestic cat. *Laboratory Animal Science* 44(3), 261–269.

Brache, V., Faundes, A., and Johansson, E. (1985) Anovulation, inadequate luteal phase and poor sperm penetration in cervical mucus during prolonged use of Norplant implants. *Contraception* 31(3), 261–273. doi: 10.1016/0010-7824(85)90096-4

Burke, T.J. (1982) Pharmacologic control of estrus in bitch and queen. *Veterinary Clinics North America Small Animal Practice* 12(1), 79– 84. doi: 10.1016/s0195-5616(82)50007-1

Carranza, A., Faya, M., Merlo, M. L., Batista, P., and Gobello, C. (2014) Effect of GnRH analogs in postnatal domestic cats. *Theriogenology* 82(1), 138–143. doi: 10.1016/j.theriogenology.2014.03.012

Carranza, A., Faya, M., Fernandez, P., Barbeito, C., and Gobello, C. (2015) Histologic effect of a postnatal slow-release GnRH agonist on feline gonads. *Theriogenology* 83(8), 1368–1372. doi: 10.1016/j.theriogenology.2015.01.027

Cecchetto, M., Salata, P., Baldan, A., Milani, C., Mollo, A., *et al.* (2017) Postponement of puberty in queens treated with deslorelin. *Journal of Feline Medicine and Surgery* 19(12), 1224–1230. doi: 10.1177/1098612X16688406

Chastain, C. B., Graham, C. L., and Nichols, C. E. (1981) Adrenocortical suppression in cats given megestrol acetate. *American Journal of Veterinary Research* 42(12), 2029–2035.

Cline, E. M., Jennings, L. L., Sojka, N. J. (1980) Breeding laboratory cats during artificially induced estrus. *Laboratory Animal Science* 30(6), 1003–1005.

Concannon, P. W. and Meyers-Wallen, V. N. (1991) Current and proposed methods for contraception and termination of pregnancy in dogs and cats. *Journal of the American Veterinary Medical Association* 198(7), 1214–1225.

Concannon, P., Hodgson, B., and Lein, D. (1980) Reflex LH release in estrous cats following single and multiple copulations. *Biology of Reproduction* 23(1), 111–117.

Corrada, Y. A. and Gobello, M. C. (2000) Reproducción felina: características del gato doméstico. *Buenos Aires: Asociación Argentina de Medicina Felina.* Available at: https://aamefe.org/ (accessed 8 November 2020).

da Silva, T. F. P., da Silva, L. D. M., Uchoa, D. C., Monteiro, C. L. B., and Thomaz, L. A. (2006) Sexual characteristics of domestic Queen kept in a natural equatorial photoperiod. *Theriogenology* 66, 1476–1481. doi: 10.1016/j.theriogenology.2006.02.008

Dawson, A. B. (1941). Early estrus in cat following increased illumination. *Endocrinology* 28(6), 907–991. doi: 10.1210/endo-28-6-907

Donoghue, M., Johnston, L. A., Munson, L., Brown, J. L., and Wildt, D.E. (1992) Influence of gonadotropin treatment interval on follicular maturation, in vitro fertilization, circulating steroid concentrations, and subsequent luteal function in the domestic cat. *Biology of Reproduction* 46(5), 972–980. doi: 10.1095/biolreprod46.5.972

Dresser, B. L., Sehlhorset, C. S., Wachs, K. B., Keller, G. L., Gelwicks, E. J., *et al.* (1987) Hormonal stimulation and embryo collection in the domestic cat (*Felis catus*). *Theriogenology*, 28(6), 915–927. doi: 10.1016/0093-691X(87)90042-2

Duncan, G. L., Lyster, S. C., Hendrix, J. W., Clark, J. J., and Webster, H. D. (1964) Biologic effects of melengestrol acetate. *Fertility and Sterility* 15, 419–432.

Faya, M., Carranza, A., Priotto, M., Graiff, D., Zurbriggen, G., *et al.* (2011) Long-term melatonin treatment prolongs interestrus, but does not delay puberty, in domestic cats. *Theriogenology* 75(9), 1750–1754. doi: 10.1016/j.theriogenology.2011.01.015

Fekete, G. and Szebere´nyi, S. (1965) Data on the mechanism of adrenal suppression by medroxyprogesterone acetate. *Steroids* 6(2), 159–166. doi: 10.1016/0039-128x(65)90044-9

Feldman, E. C. and Nelson, R.W. (1996) Feline reproduction. In: Feldman, E. C. and Nelson, R. W. (eds), *Canine and Feline Endocrinology and Reproduction*. W.B. Saunders, Philadelphia, Pennsylvania, pp. 741–767.

Findik, M., Maral, N. E., and Aslan, S. (1999) The use of proligestone, megestrol acetate and GnRH on queens with the aim of hormonal contraception. *Turkish Journal of Veterinary and Animal Sciences* 23, 455–459.

Furthner, E., Maenhoudt, C., Amiriantz, S., Priam, J., and Fontbonne, A. (2019) Oral melatonin supplementation in female domestic cats, a double blinded prospective study [abstract]. In: *Proceedings of the 22nd EVSSAR Congress*. Berlin, Germany. European Veterinary Society for Small Animal Reproduction (EVSSAR), p 103–104.

Furthner, E., Roos, J., Niewiadomska, Z., Maenhoudt, C., and Fontbonne, A. (2020) Contraceptive implants used by cat breeders in France: a study of 140 purebred cats. *Journal of Feline Medicine and Surgery* 22(10), 984–992. doi: 10.1177/1098612X19901023

Gimenez, F., Stornelli, M.C., and Tittarelli, C.M. (2009) Suppression of estrus in cats with melatonin implants. *Theriogenology* 72(4), 493–499. doi: 10.1016/j.theriogenology.2009.04.004

Goericke-Pesch, S. (2010) Reproduction control in cats: new developments in non-surgical methods. *Journal of Feline Medicine and Surgery* 12(7), 539–546. doi: 10.1016/j.jfms.2010.05.005

Goericke-Pesch, S., Georgiev, P., Atanasov, A., Albouy, M., Navarro, C., *et al.* (2013a) Treatment of queens in estrus and after estrus with a GnRH-agonist implant containing 4.7 mg deslorelin; hormonal response, duration of efficacy, and reversibility. *Theriogenology* 79, 640–646. doi:10.1016/j.theriogenology.2012.11.018

Goericke-Pesch, S., Georgiev, P., Atanasov, A., and Wehrend, A. (2013b) Treatment with Suprelorin in a pregnant cat. *Journal of Feline Medicine and Surgery* 15, 357–360. doi: 10.1177/1098612X12468837

Goericke-Pesch, S., Wehrend, A., and Georgiev, P. (2014) Suppression of fertility in adult cats. *Reproduction in Domestic Animals* 49(2), 33–40. doi:10.1111/rda.12301

Goodrowe, K. L., Howard, J. G., and Wildt, D. E. (1986) Embryo recovery and quality in the domestic cat: natural versus induced oestrus. *Theriogenology* 25, 156.

Graham, L. H., Swanson, W. F., Wildt, D. E., and Brown, J. L. (2004) Influence of oral melatonin on natural and gonadotropin-induced ovarian function in the domestic cat. *Theriogenology* 61(6), 1061–1076. doi: 10.1016/j.theriogenology.2003.05.004

Greenberg, M., Lawler, D., Zawistowski, S., and Jöchle, W. (2013) Low-dose megestrol acetate revisited: a viable adjunct to surgical sterilization in free roaming cats? *Veterinary Journal* 196, 304–308. doi: 10.1016/j.tvjl.2013.01.038

Griffin, B., Heath, A. M., and Young, D. W. (2001) Effects of melatonin implants on ovarian function in the domestic cat [abstract]. In: *Proceedings of the 19th American College of Veterinary Internal Medicine*. Lakewood, CO: American College of Veterinary Internal Medicine (ACVIM), Denver, Colorado, p 843.

Gulyuz, F., Tasal, I., and Uslu, B. A. (2009) Effects of melatonin on the onset of ovarian activity in Turkish van cats. *Journal of Animal and Veterinary Advances* 8, 2033–2037.

Harris, T. W. and Wolchuk, N. (1963) The suppression of oestrus in the dog and cat with long term administration of synthetic progestational steroids. *American Journal of Veterinary Research* 24, 1003–1006.

Hayden, D. W., Barnes, D. M., Johnson, K. H. (1989) Morphologic changes in the mammary gland of megestrol acetate-treated and untreated cats: a retrospective study. *Veterinary Pathology* 26, 104–113.

Henik, R. A., Olson, P. N., and Rosychuk, R. A. (1985) Progestagen therapy in cats. *Compendium on Continuing Education for the Practising Veterinarian* 7, 132–141.

Hernandez, F. J., Fernandez, B. B., Chertack, M., and Gage, P. A. (1975) Feline mammary carcinoma and progestogens. *Feline Practice.* 5, 45–48.

Hurni, H. (1981) Daylength and breeding in the domestic cats. *Laboratory Animal* 15, 229–233.

Jackson, E. K. M. (1984) Contraception in the dog and cat. *British Veterinary Journal* 140, 132–137. doi: 10.1016/0007-1935(84)90073-3

Jemmet, J. E. and Evans, J. M. (1977) A survey of sexual behaviour and reproduction of female cats. *Journal of Small Animal Practice* 18, 31–37. doi: 10.1111/j.1748-5827.1977.tb05821.x

Johnston, S. D., Root, M. V., and Olson, P. N. S. (1996) Ovarian and testicular function in the domestic cat: clinical management of spontaneous reproductive disease. *Animal Reproduction Science* 42, 261–274.

Johnston, S. D., Kustritz, M. V. R., and Olson, P. S. (2001) The Feline Estrous Cycle. In: Johnston, S. D., Kustritz, M. V. R., and Olson, P. S. (eds) *Canine and Feline Theriogenology*. Elsevier Health Sciences, Philadelphia, Pennsylvania, pp. 396–403.

Keskin, A., Yilmazbas, G., Yilmaz, R., Musa, O., and Gumen, A. (2009) Pathological abnormalities after long-term administration of medroxyprogesterone acetate in a queen. *Journal of Feline Medicine and Surgery* 11, 518–521. doi: 10.1016/j.jfms.2008.10.006

Kloosterboer, H. J., Vonk-Noordegraaf, C. A., and Turpijn, E. W. (1988) Selectivity in progesterone and androgen receptor binding of progestagens used in oral contraceptives. *Contraception* 38, 325–332. doi: 10.1016/0010-7824(88)90104-7

Kutzler, M. A. (2007) Estrus induction and synchronization in canids and felids. *Theriogenology* 68, 354–374. doi: 10.1016/j.theriogenology.2007.04.014

Kutzler, M. A. (2015) Alternative methods for feline fertility control: Use of melatonin to suppress reproduction. *Journal of Feline Medicine and Surgery* 17, 753–757. doi: 10.1177/1098612X15594988

Kutzler, M. and Wood, A. (2006) Non-surgical methods of contraception and sterilization. *Theriogenology* 66, 514–525. doi: 10.1016/j.theriogenology.2006.04.014

Kutzler, M., Lamb, S. V., and Volkmann, D. (2009) Comparison between vestibular and subcutaneous insertion of deslorelin implants for oestrus induction in bitches. *Reproduction in Domestic Animals* 44, 83–86. doi: 10.1111/j.1439-0531.2009.01384

Leyva, H., Addiego, L., and Stabenfeldt, G. (1984) The effect of different photoperiods on plasma concentrations of melatonin, prolactin and cortisol in the domestic cat. *Endocrinology* 115, 1729–1736. doi: 10.1210/endo-115-5-1729

Leyva, H., Madley, T., and Stabenfeldt, G. H. (1989a) Effect of light manipulation on ovarian activity and melatonin and prolactin secretion in the domestic cat. *Journal of Reproduction and Fertility* Supplement 39, 125–133.

Leyva, H., Madley, T., and Stabenfeldt, G. H. (1989b) Effect of melatonin on photoperiod responses, ovarian secretion of oestrogen, and coital responses in the domestic cat. *Journal of Reproduction and Fertility* Supplement 39, 155–142.

Little, S.E. (2012) Female reproduction. *The Cat*, 1195–1227. doi:10.1016/B978-1-4377-0660-4.00040-5

Loretti, A., Ilha, M., Breitsameter, I., and Faraco, C. (2004) Clinical and pathological study of feline mammary fibroadenomatous changes associated with depot medroxyprogesterone acetate therapy. *Arquivo Brasileiro de Medicina Veterinária e Zootecnia* 56, 270–274. doi: 10.1590/S0102-09352004000200020

Loretti, A., Ilha, M., Ordás, J., and de las Mulas, J. M. (2005) Clinical, pathological and immunohistochemical study of feline mammary fibroepithelial hyperplasia following a single injection of depot medroxyprogesterone acetate. *Journal of Feline Medicine and Surgery* 7, 43–52. doi: 10.1016/j.jfms.2004.05.002

MacDougall, L. (2003). Mammary fibroadenomatous hyperplasia in a young cat attributed to treatment with megestrol acetate. *Canadian Veterinary Journal* 44, 227–229.

Maenhoudt, C., Santos, N. R., Fontaine, E., Mir, F., Reynaud, K., *et al.* (2012) Results of GnRH agonist implants in oestrous induction and oestrous suppression in bitches and queens. *Reproduction in Domestic Animals* 47, 393–397. doi: 10.1111/rda.12041

Maenhoudt, C., Santos, N. R., and Fontbonne, A. (2018) Manipulation of the oestrous cycle of the bitch-what works… for now. *Reproduction in Domestic Animals* 53, 44–52. doi: 10.1111/rda.13364

Mansfield, P. D., Kemppainen, R. J., and Sartin, J. L. (1986) The effects of megestrol acetate treatment on plasma glucose concentration and insulin response to glucose administration in cats. *Journal of the American Animal Hospital Association* 22, 515–518.

Mattos, M. R. F., da Silva, T. F. P., Pereira, B. S., Uchoa, D. C., Cardoso, R. C. S., *et al.* (2001) Embryo transfer in the cat: first success in Latin America. In: *Proceedings from Memorias de II Congresso Internacional de Medicina Felina [on CD-ROM]*. Rio de Janeiro, Brazil, June 2001.

Max, A., Jurka, P., Dobrzyński, A., and Rijsselaere, T. (2014) Non-surgical contraception in female dogs and cats. *Acta Scientiarum Polonorum Zootechnica*, 13, 3–18.

Michel, C. (1993) Induction of oestrus in cats by photoperiodic manipulations and social stimuli. *Laboratory Animal* 27, 278–280. doi:10.1258/002367793780745381

Middleton, D. J. and Watson, A. D. (1985) Glucose intolerance in cats given short-term therapies of prednisolone and megestrol acetate. *American Journal of Veterinary Research* 46, 2623–2625.

Middleton, D. J., Watson, A., Howe, C., and Caterson, I. D. (1987) Suppression of cortisol responses to exogenous adrenocorticotrophic hormone, and the occurrence of side effects attributable to glucocorticoid excess, in cats during therapy with megestrol acetate and prednisolone. *Canadian Journal of Veterinary Research* 51, 60–65.

Munson, L. (2006) Contraception in felids. *Theriogenology* 66, 126–134. doi: 10.1016/j.theriogenology.2006.03.016

Munson, L., Bauman, J. E., Asa, C. S., Jochle, W., and Trigg, T. E. (2001) Efficacy of the GnRH analogue deslorelin for suppression of oestrous cycles in cats. *Journal of Reproduction and Fertility* 57, 269–273.

Murakoshi, M., Tagawa, M., Ikeda, R., Hoshin, T., Suzuki, M., *et al.* (1996) The effect of subcutaneous implantation of chlormadinone acetate for preventing estrus in queens. *Journal of Toxicologic Pathology* 9, 185–190. doi: 10.1293/tox.9.185

Murakoshi, M., Tagawa, M. and Ikeda, R. (2000) Histopathological studies of subcutaneous implantation of chlormadinone acetate (CMA) for preventing estrus in queens. *Tokai Journal of Experimental and Clinical Medicine* 25, 7–10.

Orosz, S. E., Morris, P. J., Doody, M. C., Niemeyer, G. P., Cortelyou Lee, J., *et al.* (1992) Stimulation of folliculogenesis in domestic cats with human FSH and LH. *Theriogenology* 37, 993–1004. doi: 10.1016/0093-691x(92)90098-c

Payan-Carreira, R. (2013) feline mammary fibroepithelial hyperplasia: a clinical approach. In: Payan-Carreira, R. (ed.) *Insights from Veterinary Medicine, InTech*, London. doi: 10.5772/55550

Pelican, K. M., Wildt, D. E., Pukazhenthi, B., and Howard, J. (2006) Ovarian control for assisted reproduction in the domestic cat and wild felids. *Theriogenology* 66, 37—48. doi: 10.1016/j.theriogenology.2006.03.013

Pelican, K. M., Wildt, D. E., Ottinger, M. A., and Howard, J. (2008) Priming with progestin, but not GnRH antagonist, induces a consistent endocrine response to exogenous gonadotropins in induced and spontaneously ovulating cats. *Domestic Animal Endocrinology* 3, 160-175. doi: 10.1016/j.domaniend.2007.01.002

Pope, C. E., Keller, G. L. and Dresser, B. L. (1993) In vitro fertilization in domestic and non-domestic cats including sequences of early nuclear events, development in vitro, cryopreservation and successful intra- and interspecies embryo transfer. *Journal of Reproduction and Fertility* 47, 189–201.

Pope, C. E. (2000) Embryo technology in conservation efforts for endangered felids. *Theriogenology* 53, 163–174. doi: 10.1016/S0093-691X(99)00249-6

Risso, A., Corrada, Y., Barbeito, C., Diaz, J., and Gobello, C. (2012) Long-term-release GnRH agonists postpone puberty in domestic cats. *Reproduction in Domestic Animals* 47, 936–938. doi:10.1111/j.1439-0531.2012.01994.x

Romagnoli, S. (2003) Clinical approach to infertility in the queen. *Journal of Feline Medicine and Surgery* 5, 143–146. doi: 10.1016/S1098-612X(02)00131-6

Romagnoli, S. (2006) Recent Advances in Feline Reproduction. In: *World Small Animal Veterinary Association World Congress Proceedings*, Prague, Czech Republic, pp. 2006696–2006700.

Romagnoli, S. (2015) Progestins to control feline reproduction: Historical abuse of high doses and potentially safe use of low doses. *Journal of Feline Medicine and Surgery* 17, 743–752. doi: 10.1177/1098612X15594987

Romagnoli, S. and Concannon, P.W. (2003) Clinical use of progestins in bitches and queens: a review. In: Concannon, P. W., England, G., Verstegen, J., and Linde Forsberg, C. (eds) *Recent Advances in Small Animals Reproduction*. International Veterinary Information Service, USA.

Romagnoli, S. and Sontas, B.H. (2010) Prevention of breeding in the female. In: England, G. and von Heimendahl, A. (eds), *BSAVA Manual of Canine and Feline Reproduction and Neonatology*. British Small Animal Veterinary Association, Gloucester, UK, pp. 23–33.

Romagnoli, S., Bensaia, C., Ferré-Dolcet, L., Sontas, H., and Stelletta, C. (2019) Fertility parameters and reproductive management of Norwegian Forest Cats, Maine Coon, Persian and Bengal cats raised in Italy: a questionnaire-based study. *Journal of Feline Medicine and Surgery* 21, 1188–1198. doi: 10.1177/1098612X18824181

Rubion, S. and Driancourt, M. A. (2009) Controlled delivery of a GnRH agonist by a silastic implant (Gonazon) results in long-term contraception in queens. *Reproduction in Domestic Animals* 44, 79–82. doi: 10.1111/j.1439-0531.2009.01415.x

Santana, M. L., Paula, T. A. R., Costa, E. P., Costa, D.S. (2012). Exogenous induction of ovarian activity and ovulation and transfer of fresh embryos of domestic cat (*Felis catus*). *Revista Ceres* 59, 499–505. doi:10.1590/S0034-737X2012000400010

Sapierzynski, R. A., Dolka, I., and Cywinska, A. (2009) Multiple pathologies of the feline uterus: a case report. *Veterinari Medicina* 52, 345–350. doi: 10.17221/101/2009-VETMED

Schäfer-Somi, S. (2017) Effect of melatonin on the reproductive cycle in female cats: a review of clinical experiences and previous studies. *Journal of Feline Medicine and Surgery* 19, 5–12. doi: 10.1177/1098612X15610369

Schmidt, P. M. (1986) Feline breeding management. *Veterinary Clinics of North America Small Animal Practice* 16, 435–451. doi: 10.1016/S0195-5616(86)50052-8

Scott, P. P. and Lloyd-Jacob, M. A. (1959) Reduction in the anestous period of laboratory cats by increased illumination. *Nature* 184, 2022. doi: 10.1038/1842022a0

Stewart, R. A., Pelican, K. M., Brown, J. L., Wildt, D. E., Ottinger, M. A., *et al.* (2010) Oral progestin induces rapid, reversible suppression of ovarian activity in the cat. *General and Comparative Endocrinology* 166, 409–416. doi:10.1016/j.ygcen.2009.12.016

Swanson, W. F., Roth, T. L., Graham, K., Horohov, D. W., and Godke, R. A. (1996) Kinetics of the humoral immune response to multiple treatments with exogenous gonadotropins and relation to ovarian responsiveness in domestic cats. *American Journal of Veterinary Research* 57, 302–307.

Swanson, W. F., Wolfe, B. A., Brown, J. L., Martin-Jimenez, T., Riviere, J. E., *et al.* (1997) Pharmokinetics and ovarian-stimulatory effects of equine and human chorionic gonadotropins administered singly and in combination in the domestic cat. *Biology of Reproduction* 57, 295–302. doi: 10.1095/biolreprod57.2.295

Tamada, H., Kawate, N., and Inaba, T. (2003) Long-term prevention of estrus in the bitch and queen using chlormadinone acetate. *Canadian Veterinary Journal* 44, 416–417.

Toydemir, T. S., Kılıçarslan, M. R., and Olgaç, V. (2012) Effects of the GnRH analogue deslorelin implants on reproduction in female domestic cats. *Theriogenology* 77, 662–674. doi: 10.1016/j.theriogenology.2011.07.046

Tsutsui, T. and Stabenfeldt, G. H. (1993) Biology of ovarian cycles, pregnancy and pseudopregnancy in the domestic cat. *Journal of Reproduction and Fertility*, Supplement, 47, 29–35.

Tsutsui, T., Sato, M., and Kurosawa, N., *et al.* (1989) Embryo transfer in the cat during the non-breeding season. Nihon Juigaku zasshi. *The Japanese Journal of Veterinary Science* 51, 871–877. doi: 10.1292/jvms1939.51.871

Tsutsui, T., Yamane, I., Hattori, I., Kurosawa, N., Matsunaga, H., *et al.* (2000) Feline embryo transfer during the non-breeding season. *Journal of Veterinary Medical Science* 62(11), 1169–1175. doi: 10.1292/jvms.62.1169

Verstegen, J. P., Onclin, K., da Silva, L. D. M., Donnay, I., Mettens, P., *et al.* (1993) Superovulation and embryo in vitro culture following treatment with ultra-pure follicle-stimulating hormone in cats. *Journal of Reproduction and Fertility* Supplement 47, 209–218.

Wehrend, A., Hospes, R., and Gruber, A. D. (2001) Treatment of feline mammary fibroadenomatous hyperplasia with a progesterone-antagonist. *Veterinary Record.* 148, 346–347. doi: 10.1136/vr.148.11.346

Wildt, D. E., Seager, S. W. J., and Chakraborty, P. K. (1980) Effect of copulatory stimuli on incidence of ovulation and on serum luteinizing hormone in the cat. *Endocrinology* 107, 1212–1217. doi: 10.1210/endo-107-4-1212

Zambelli, D., Bini, C., Küster, D. G., Molari, V., and Cunto, M. (2015) First deliveries after estrus induction using deslorelin and endoscopic transcervical insemination in the queen. *Theriogenology* 84, 773–778. doi: 10.1016/j.theriogenology.2015.05.010

4 Breeding and Cattery Management

Aime K. Johnson

Auburn University College of Veterinary Medicine, Department of Clinical Sciences, Auburn, Alabama, USA

4.1 Introduction

Appropriate breeding management is the key to good fertility in a cattery. Minor changes in procedures may have a significant impact on pregnancy rate and litter size. Cattery management may differ between a private breeding operation, a research colony, or a single cat in a household. A detailed history and onsite visit to the cattery will help the veterinarian and owner identify management problems that could affect feline health and fertility.

4.2 Overall Management

The vaccination records of all the animals should be reviewed as well as the procedures used for vaccine handling and storage to ensure adequate disease control. Current recommended core feline vaccinations can be found at: https://www.aaha.org/aaha-guidelines/2020-aahaaafp-feline-vaccination-guidelines/feline-vaccination-home/ (accessed 17 January 2022) (*Stone et al.*, 2020).

While a closed cattery with no new animals entering is preferable to eliminate new disease introduction, such a strategy does not allow for genetic diversity and resilience. A quarantine period of at least 2 weeks in a separate location away from resident animals, along with strict testing procedures, should be mandatory for all new additions. Any individuals returning after leaving for veterinary care, breeding, exhibition, etc. should also go through a quarantine process. Cats that show clinical signs of disease should be kept in an isolation area away from all other cats until they have either tested negative or have been without symptoms for 2 weeks. Owners should be instructed to care for quarantined animals after healthy animals in order to prevent fomite spread on their clothes, hands, or other items.

In catteries, strict sanitation and adequate ventilation is essential to reduce or eliminate disease. Poor sanitation often leads to clinical signs of disease and neonatal mortality from sepsis. Standard operating procedures (SOPs) should be followed to prevent hygiene errors. Litter boxes, bedding, toys, and food and water bowls should be cleaned and disinfected regularly. Frequency will depend on the density of the cattery, but in general, cleaning should be performed daily, with complete disinfectant used weekly. Caution should be taken to ensure the disinfectant used is at an appropriate concentration, is sufficient for the major pathogens, and is safe for cats (see Fig. 4.1) (Stull *et al.*, 2018).

Catteries can vary in design depending on the number of animals and purpose. Many production catteries house animals in group kennels or runs with easily disinfected floors, walls, litterboxes, and toys (Fig. 4.2). This is ideal for catteries that require constant sanitation such as catteries that house animals used for research. Although sanitation and disease prevention are best in these situations, this type of housing involves less interaction with people and everyday objects than would occur in a home setting. The home setting is more ideal for socialization of kittens that will be sold as pets (Fig. 4.3). Figure 4.4 shows a cattery that is located in a converted horse stall and Fig. 4.5 shows a queening area made from a converted chicken coup. Alternatively, cats can be group housed in rooms according to age or breeding status. Special attention to water quality, food, and sanitation is of utmost importance regardless of the facility. A good quality, balanced, commercial cat food is best. Raw food diets are risky in breeding animals and may not provide the correct nutrients needed and may introduce harmful bacteria that can lead to uterine infections or neonatal septicemia.

Asking specific questions concerning the cattery and individual animals are important in gaining a baseline knowledge of each situation. An example questionnaire for obtaining a detailed history for a cattery is included here (Fig. 4.6). An additional questionnaire for each breeding animal should also be obtained

 Feline Reproduction (eds. A.K. Johnson and M.A. Kutzler)
DOI: 10.1079/9781789247107.0004

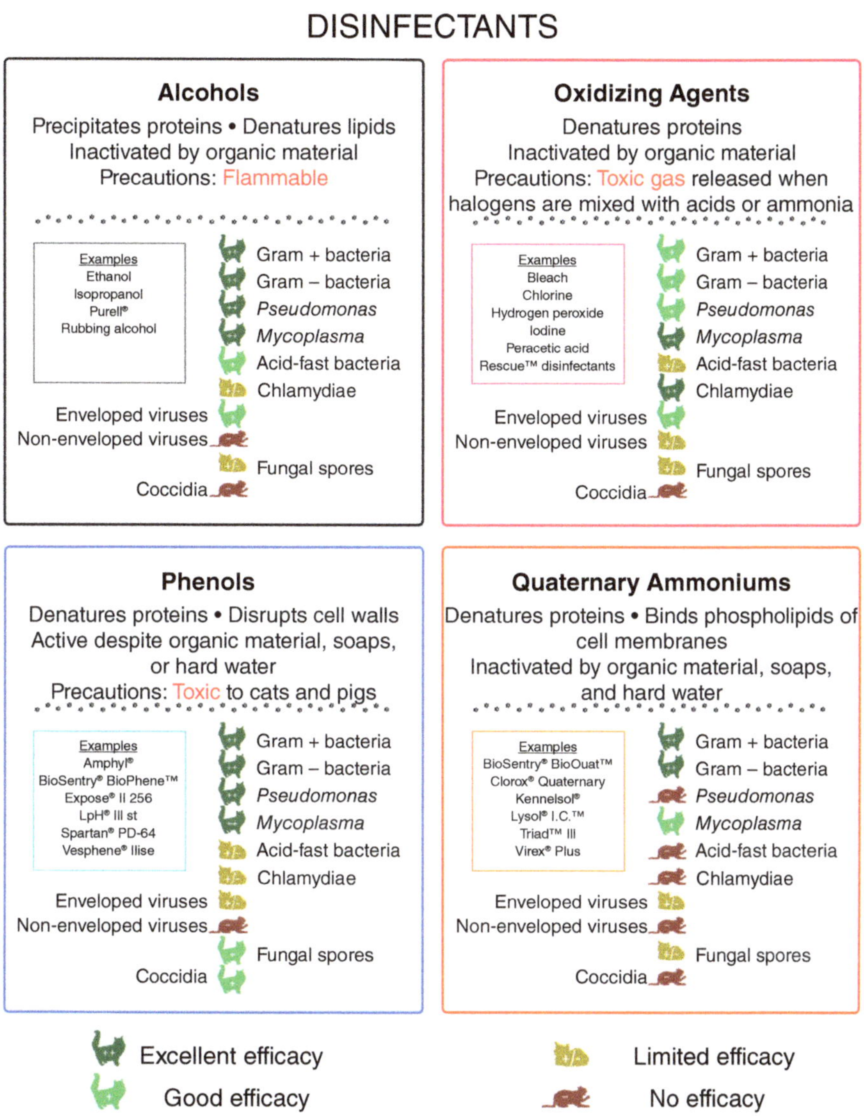

Fig. 4.1. A table of disinfectants and the properties they contain. It is important to choose the best disinfectant that causes the least potential harm to the animals, but will still eliminate the desired contaminants (Stull *et al.*, 2018). (Image: author's own with Dr Jamie Douglas.)

(Fig 4.7). These questionnaires allow the veterinarian to have useful information about the animals, but also lets the veterinarian know how organized a cattery is by their ability to provide needed information.

4.3 Lighting

Because the queen is a long-day breeder, maintaining the animals under artificial lighting for at least 14 hours per day reduces seasonal variation. However, in this author's experience, even cats maintained under this lighting system may experience a slight decrease in pregnancy rates during the shorter days of the year. A queen will typically show estrus within 1–2 months after initiating an artificial lighting period. Providing lighting for 24 hours a day will maintain cyclicity, but the number of heat cycles has been shown to reduce from two per month to only one (Leyva *et al.*, 1989).

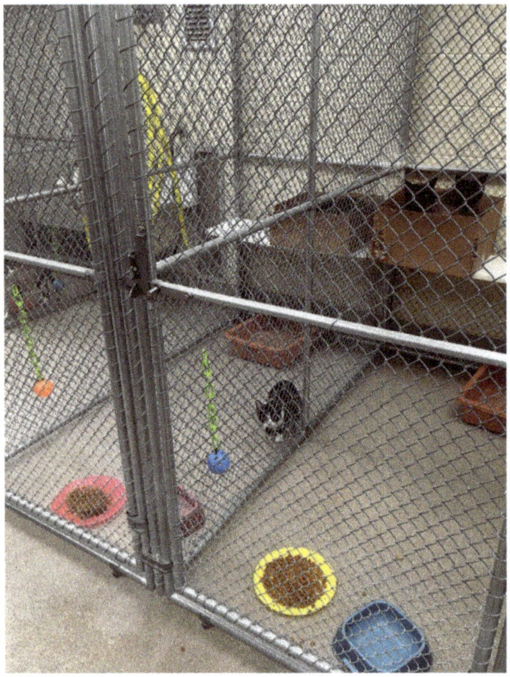

Fig. 4.2. Cattery with strict biosecurity and sanitation. All surfaces can be disinfected readily and sleeping boxes can be changed. Cats have visual access to other cats in the room. Kennels include a resting board allowing cats to climb. Kennels are enclosed on all sides including the top. (Image: author's own.)

If the queen has been maintained under long-term artificial lighting (years) and the overall fertility has declined, allowing the queen to experience a season of anestrus by shortening the lighting period (8 hours of light) for 2 to 3 months may be beneficial before restarting the extended day lighting. Queens housed in a home setting are often exposed to a combination of natural and artificial light. However, the queens have the freedom to hide under objects or in dark rooms so the light they are exposed to is variable. Because of this, queens in a house setting will often display seasonality and not show cyclicity during the short daylight period.

4.4 Breeding Management

Before beginning the breeding process, ensure that the queen's vaccinations are current. When breeding naturally in a cattery, the queen should be taken to the tom's location as establishment of a territory is important for the male. The queen should be exposed to the tom when she is showing signs of estrus (heat). Signs include vocalization, rubbing on walls, and rolling on the floor. Estrus can also be confirmed using vaginal cytology. If heat detection is not possible in a natural mating situation, the queen can be placed with the male for an extended period (usually at least 2 weeks). The pair should be monitored

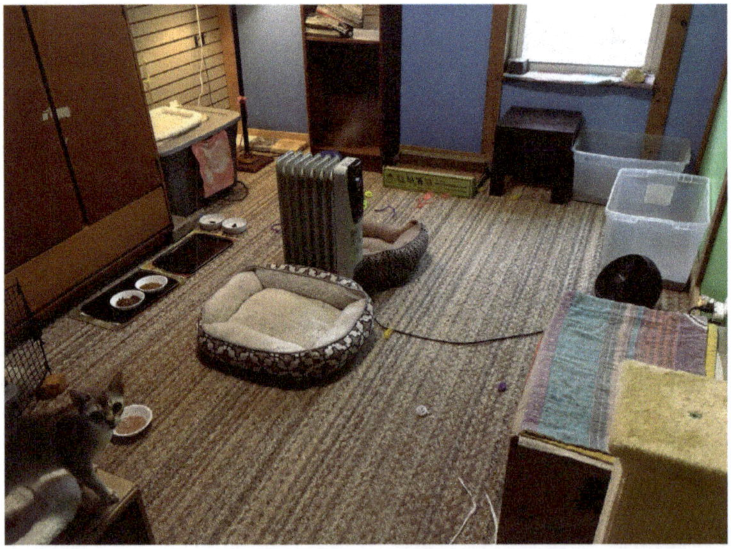

Fig. 4.3. A home cattery queening room with resting areas and hiding boxes. The various surfaces provide enrichment for the cats, but can also harbor diseases or parasites if not cleaned regularly. (Image: author's own.)

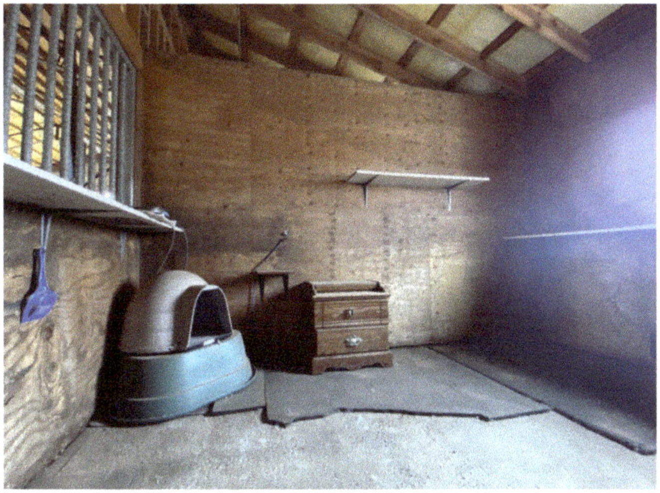

Fig. 4.4. A cattery that is located in a modified horse barn. Stalls are converted into rooms for groups of cats. Resting boards and hiding places provide enrichment. (Image: author's own.)

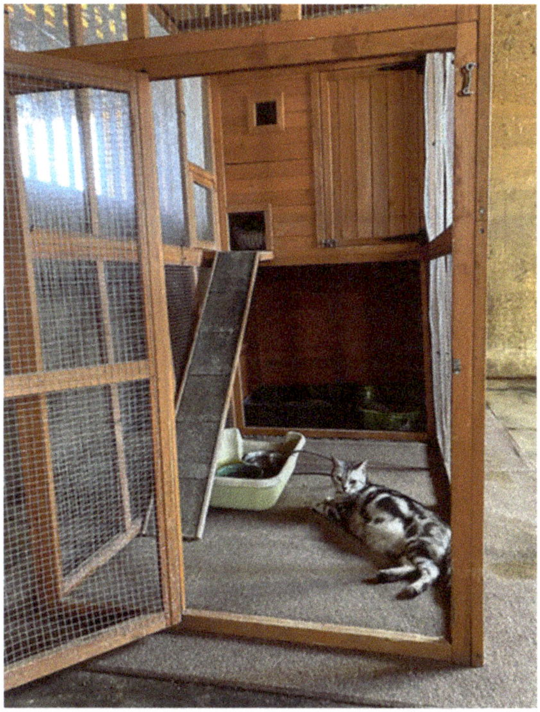

Fig. 4.5. A queening room made from a converted chicken coup. It allows the queen to hide and have privacy as well as allowing growing kittens a place to play that is confined. (Image: author's own.)

closely for breeding activity or fighting (if the queen is not in estrus). If fighting occurs, the pair should be separated for a few days before retrying, or until the vaginal cytology indicates estrus. Once the pair has been together for at least 2 weeks, serum progesterone concentration can be used to confirm ovulation (greater than 2 ng/ml). After ovulation is confirmed, the queen may be returned to her housing. If the progesterone is less than 2 ng/ml, mating has not occurred, or sufficient mating has not occurred to induce the luteinizing hormone surge and ovulation. The queen should be returned to the male and monitored for breeding activity.

Housing the queen with the tom for shorter periods (several hours instead of days) and observing for mating behavior is another method of breeding management. Time together can be repeated daily until the queen refuses to be mated. Serum progesterone can be sampled 1–2 weeks after observed matings. A value greater than 2 ng/ml confirms there is luteal tissue, and the queen has ovulated. This method allows a more accurate determination of gestational age and delivery date. Observation of breeding episodes is helpful to determine the number of times the tom attempts to copulate, and evaluating the female for the classic 'after reaction' to confirm copulation took place. The 'after reaction' is when the queen separates from the tom and rubs her face and body on the floor or walls, rolls onto her back, and licks her perineum. If the 'after reaction'

Cattery History Questionnaire

Please use additional paper as needed

Name of cattery ____________________ Breed ____________________

Total number of animals ____________________

Queens ____________ Toms ____________ Kittens under 1 year ____________

List diet and water source for colony ____________________

What is your preventative health plan (vaccines, deworming, etc) ____________________

What is your current lighting program? ____________________

What is your current disinfection policy? What do you use, how often, etc. ____________________

How are queens and toms housed? ____________________

What bedding or boxes are provided for each stage (breeding, gestation, queening, lactation) ____________________

What is your procedure for introducing male and female for breeding? ____________________

Is breeding observed? ____________ What method? ____________

Is queening observed? ____________ What method? ____________

Where are pregnant queens housed during gestation, queening, and lactation? ____________________

How many litters are born each year? ____________________

What is the average litter size? ____________ What age are queens first bred? ____________

How are kittens handled from birth to weaning? ____________________

What are the specific issues the cattery is experiencing? ____________________

Fig. 4.6. Cattery history questionnaire.

does not occur, penetration of the penis into the vagina was unlikely. Cameras provide the ability to monitor breeding activity without disrupting behavior.

If the queen is shy or becomes overly stressed in new situations, placing the tom in her environment, placing the pair in a neutral location, or pairing her and another more experienced queen that she is comfortable with may help her feel more at ease when exposed to the male. Alternatively, artificial insemination with ovulation induction can be used when natural breeding methods are unsuccessful.

4.5 Breeding Records

Records for each queen should be as detailed as possible and include all dates of breeding, observed matings, observations when with male, pregnancy diagnosis, queening date, litter size, and any other details that may be significant. Records should also include illness, injury, or breeding problems. Detailed records for the tom should include dates exposed to queens, behavior, documented breedings, pregnancy rate, and litter size for every queen

Individual Cat Information Form

Fill out form for each breeding animal in colony

Name ______________________ Breed __________ Age ______

QUEENS

Number of litters ______________ Average litter size ______

List each breeding episode starting with her first. Include the following for each breeding attempt:

- Queen age at the time of breeding
- Tom used
- Breeding method
- How long queen was with tom
- If she became pregnant or not pregnant
- C-Section or natural birth
- Litter size
- # live kittens
- # stillborn kittens
- # kittens that died before 2 weeks of age

TOMS

Number of litters produced ______________ Average litter size ______________

Number of queens serviced ______________________________

How often is the male used for breeding? ______________________________

Number of missed breedings ______________________________

BOTH

Past health issues ______________________________

Fever, illness, injury, etc within last 2 months ______________________________

Date of last vaccination and deworming ______________________________

Any additional information ______________________________

____

Fig. 4.7. Individual cat information form.

bred. Because fertility declines as the queen ages, the ages of the queens should be monitored closely as part of overall management. In this author's experience, fertility begins to decline as early as 4 years of age and can be severely affected by 5 years. However, many queens can continue to produce litters at older ages (7–9 years). Analyzing records of previous fertility and litter size will allow management decisions to be made as to when a queen should be retired from breeding.

Current recommendations for registered cats from the Governing Council of the Cat Fancy (GCCF) advise a minimum of 26 weeks between litters and no more than three litters over 2 years. This organization also recommends that if a queen has had three or more litters in her lifetime, one litter per year is advised. Further considerations should be made as to the condition of the queen following pregnancy and lactation, overall health of the queen and her kittens, and any extenuating circumstances surrounding the queen, pregnancy and delivery, and lactation/weaning. Exceptions to this rule can be made in cases where the health of the female would benefit from breeding such as post pyometra treatment or loss of body condition due to continuous estrus. Such exceptions should be supported by a letter from the primary veterinarian. Queens should be registered as an active breeder which states they are fit to be used as a breeding animal and are free from medical and genetic conditions.

4.6 Management of the Pregnant Queen

Examination for pregnancy should be performed about 25–30 days after exposure to the tom. Ultrasound can detect kittens as early as 16–20 days, but kittens with a heartbeat are easier to see between 25–30 days. Early pregnancy confirmation is vital to allow management decisions to be made concerning the queen. Pregnant queens should be placed in a quiet area, alone if possible and with a covered box for nesting and queening. A stressed queen is more likely to cannibalize her young so every attempt should be made to reduce stress around the time of queening. A dedicated queening room that is quiet and warm, where the queen can be alone is best. This also allows the queens to be isolated from other animals to prevent disease transmission. If the queen shows increased stress when completely alone, other pregnant queens can be housed within visual contact to decrease her anxiety.

4.7 References

Leyva, H., Madley, T., and Stabenfeldt, G. H. (1989) Effect of light manipulation on ovarian activity and melatonin and prolactin secretion in the domestic cat. *Journal of Reproduction and Fertility,* Supplement 39, 125–133.

Stone, A. E., Brummet, G. O., Carozza, E. M., Kass, P. H., Petersen, E. P., *et al.* (2020) 2020 AAHA/AAFP Feline Vaccination Guidelines. *Journal of Feline Medicine and Surgery* 22, 813–830. doi: 10.1177/1098612X20941784

Stull, J. W., Bjorvik, E., Bub, J., Dvorak, G., Petersen, C., *et al.* (2018) 2018 AAHA Infection Control, Prevention, and Biosecurity Guidelines. *Journal of the American Animal Hospital Association* 54, 297–326. doi: 10.5326/JAAHA-MS-6903

5 Causes of Infertility in the Queen

ALAIN FONTBONNE AND ZUZANNA NIEWIADOMSKA

Centre d'Etudes en Reproduction des Carnivores, Ecole Nationale Vétérinaire d'Alfort, Maisons-Alfort Cedex, France

5.1 Introduction

It is a common statement to say that the cat is the top companion animal of the 21st century. Indeed, cat breeding is rapidly growing all over the Western world, and cat breeders and owners are seeking the help of their veterinarian when they are faced with reproductive problems. Infertility, which is defined as the inability to conceive and produce viable offspring, is one of the most common presenting complaints. It is a disaster when infertility stops a breeding line that has been carefully and patiently selected during several successive generations. Unfortunately, in domestic animal theriogenology, the cat remains under studied. As an indication, we analyzed the scientific abstracts printed in the proceeding books of the successive congresses of the European Veterinary Society for Small Animal Reproduction (EVSSAR) between 1998 – date of the first EVSSAR congress – and 2015, and we found that around 85% of the abstracts concerned dog reproduction and less than 15% were specifically devoted to cats (Robin and Fontbonne, 2019). Even during the last EVSSAR congress in 2019, among 166 submitted presentations that were selected by the scientific committee, only 24 (14.5%) were devoted to cat reproduction. All this to say that there is a clear and urgent need to improve the knowledge in the field of feline theriogenology, especially infertility. Fortunately, some founding publications have opened the door to a better understanding about the causes of infertility in the queen (Romagnoli, 2003, 2005; Axnér *et al.*, 2008).

5.2 Infertility Among Pedigree Queens

In purebred queens, infertility has been poorly studied and remains an enigma. Fortunately, some recently published data about the performances of pedigree cats in different countries is now available. In Sweden, Ström-Holst and Frössling analyzed the results of a questionnaire and found that 32% of breeders claimed that some queens did not conceive after mating, and around 10% of presumably pregnant queens (showing some degree of abdominal development and mammary enlargement around one month of pregnancy) did not deliver kittens (Ström-Holst and Frössling, 2009). In an analysis of the reproductive performances of 5203 pedigree queens in France, Fournier *et al.* found that around 15% of mated queens were not pregnant, and cat breeders reported that 8.2% of apparently pregnant queens did not give birth to kittens, potentially due to a pregnancy arrest (Fournier *et al.*, 2017). This study reported important differences in the pregnancy rate between different breeds, with extreme values varying from 58.1% (117 matings) in Oriental queens to up to 100% (15 matings) in Burmese cats. These studies show that feline infertility is not a myth and that there may be differences depending on the breed.

5.3 Lack of puberty

Lack of or delayed puberty, also called primary anestrous, may be due to lack of social contact with other cats, low luminosity within the breeding facility, a body weight below 2.3 kg (except in giant breeds) or excessive stress. The influence of the season may vary depending on the latitude. In Italy, which is a sunny country with stronger light stimulation, Romagnoli *et al.* (2019) found that the season of birth had no effect on the age of puberty. In northern countries, reduced lighting is often stated as being a cause of lack of puberty in young queens reaching adult development in winter (Johnston *et al.*, 2001). Nowadays, this seasonal effect is decreased in breeding catteries, as most of them are exposed to 14 hours of artificial lighting all year round. A queen presented for delayed puberty should be carefully examined to detect any anatomical malformations or intersexual state, often

 Feline Reproduction (eds. A.K. Johnson and M.A. Kutzler)
DOI: 10.1079/9781789247107.0005

linked with chromosomal defects (see Section 5.10). It may be useful to submit a karyotype to fully evaluate chromosomes. Iatrogenic causes of delayed puberty should also be evaluated. It is important to know if the young queen has been treated with progestins or antifungal drugs, often used for treating dermatological problems such as pruritus or ringworm which interferes with the hormonal balance and may postpone puberty. Lastly, as more early neutering of purebred queens is performed before the sale of kittens, it may be useful to detect the potential absence of ovaries. Luteinizing hormone (LH) (Rohlertz *et al.* 2012) and/or anti-Mullerian hormone (AMH) assays (Axnér and Ström-Holst, 2015) may help diagnosing the absence of ovaries in a queen presenting for delayed puberty. Promising studies are also showing that assaying AMH may even help to detect if a queen is still at a pre-pubertal stage (Flock *et al.*, 2019).

5.4 Lack of Cyclicity in an Adult Queen

Lack of cyclicity in an adult queen who had cycled before, often called secondary anestrous, is a common cause of consultation, especially in long-haired breeds such as Maine Coons, Norwegians or Persians. These breeds also seem to be more sensitive to light stimulation. A study in UK found that a non-breeding season (short days) existed for 90% of long-haired cats versus 39.2% of short-haired cats (Jemmett and Evans, 1977). However, the effect of the season of the year may play a role in the absence of cyclicity in any breed. In Italy, the study of 128 queens from four different breeds showed that only 20% of the queens were cyclic in November versus more than 70% in March and April (Romagnoli *et al.*, 2019).

Lack of estrous in an adult queen may also be due to a spontaneous ovulation without pregnancy. In such a case, cyclicity will stop for around 40–45 days while progesterone is elevated. Ovarian luteinized cysts or ovarian tumors producing progesterone may also stop cyclicity (Johnston *et al.*, 2001).

Apart from the true absence of estrus, some females may experience ‘silent heats.’ These are heat periods without clinical signs such as vocalizing or lordosis. It is especially a problem in breeding facilities when no male is present to detect when the females are in heat. Maine Coons and Persians seem to be predisposed to silent heats (Fontbonne, 2014).

5.5 Problems Related to Mating

In the dog, an appropriate timing of mating within the heat period is essential for pregnancy. This is also important in the feline species. Concannon *et al.* demonstrated that 100% (36/36) of the queens ovulate when mated on the third day of estrus (Concannon *et al.*, 1980). Another study found that more than 85% of queens ovulated in response to multiple matings on the second or third day of estrus (Swanson *et al.*, 1994). In Domestic Shorthair cats, Donoghue *et al.* (1993) found that follicular oocytes that ovulated after matings performed on the first day of estrus were immature and of poor quality. Therefore, it is recommended to allow queens to be mated longer than just the first day of estrus. If owners remove their queens from the male as soon as matings have been observed, sufficient matings may not have occurred or not occurred on the appropriate day to result in pregnancy.

Even if the partners are put together, there may be a lack of effective mating, where no coitus occurs (Fig. 5.1). Mating may not occur simply because a queen in estrus and the tom cat are put together in the same place, and the owners are often unaware. In a study in Sweden, it was found that the owners are present in the same room to observe the mating in only 35% of cases (Ström-Holst and Frössling, 2009). A missed mating may be due to behavioral incompatibility. An aggressive or an abnormally stressed female may not accept the male. Some shy females lie on their back to avoid being penetrated. There may also be partner preferences, as, in an observational study, queens accepted to be mated in only 15/38 (39.5%) attempts despite a confirmed estrus (Root *et al.*, 1995). Missed matings could occur also when too immature or inexperienced partners are put together, or in breeds that are well known for having many males that present a low libido, such as Persians or Maine Coons (personal data). Anatomical problems may prevent the penetration to occur, such as a vaginal or a vulvar atresia in females or, in males, the presence a preputial hair ring in long-haired cats or a phimosis.

Even if apparently successful matings occur, there may be a failure to ovulate. In the cat, it is well known that if the number or frequency of male penetrations are too low, the vagina may not be stimulated enough, and the magnitude of the reflex LH surge may be insufficient to induce ovulation.

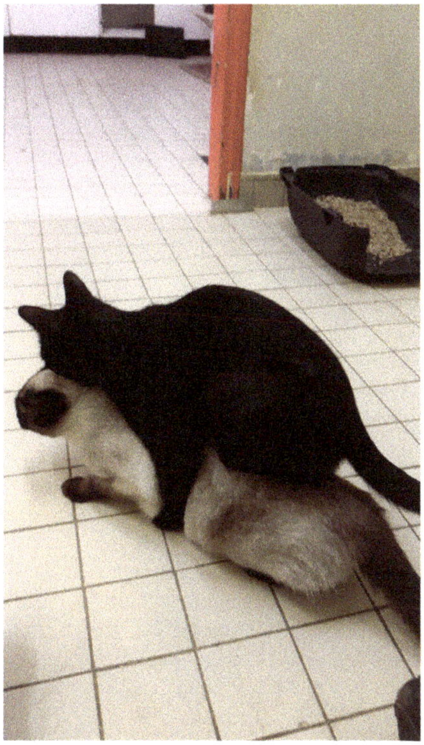

Fig. 5.1. Mating failure is common, especially with an inexperienced tom. Pain (hind limbs or back) may also be a cause for inability to mate properly. (Image: author's own.)

Only approximately 50% of queens ovulate after a single mating. The optimal LH release to stimulate ovulation appears to be when four or more matings occur within a 2- to 4-hour window of time (England, 2010). This may be a problem when trying to mate inexperienced or young partners, an aggressive queen, or a male with a poor libido. The method to detect an ovulation failure is measuring progesterone concentrations and is discussed fully in Chapter 25.

5.6 Spontaneous Ovulation

Spontaneous ovulation is an ovulation that occurs without any coitus and can be detected by an elevated progesterone in a non-mated queen. In most books and academic reviews, the queen is presented as an induced ovulator, and LH release from the pituitary gland and subsequent ovulation is said to be induced by copulation. However, since the early nineties some authors have reported cases of spontaneous ovulation in groups of queens housed together (Lawler *et al.*, 1993). In Domestic Shorthair queens living in groups of females, the occurrence of spontaneous ovulations may be as high as 87% (Gudermuth *et al.*, 1997). In wild felids, such as lions, clouded leopards, leopards, pallas' cats, fishing cats, or margays may show alternatively induced or spontaneous ovulations (Brown, 2011). Moreover, it is well known that some non-mated queens may develop pyometra during their life, and that this disease, apart from treatment with exogenous progestins, is often linked to progesterone influence that follows ovulation. Although a study conducted on the demand of an insurance company in Sweden (Hagman *et al.*, 2014) showed that the overall incidence rate (IR) of pyometra appeared low (17 cats per 10,000), a significant breed effect was observed. The breed with the highest IR (433 cats per 10,000) was the Sphynx, and other breeds with IR over 60 cats per 10,000 were the Siberian cat, Ocicat, Korat, Siamese, Ragdoll, Maine Coon and Bengal. Of course, we cannot be sure that the frequency of pyometra within a specific breed is directly linked with the frequency of spontaneous ovulation, but it is a possibility. Although just a hypothesis, spontaneous ovulation may represent a real problem in pedigree queens as many of them are living with other females and may have already ovulated when they are brought to the male for the mating. To know to what extent premature spontaneous ovulation leads to infertility, and if some breeds are more concerned than others, further studies have to be carefully conducted.

5.7 Uterine Pathology

In a study of seven cases of infertile purebred queens belonging to six different breeds, Axnér *et al.* (2008) found that in 4/7 cases, uterine pathology was diagnosed: two cases of cystic endometrial hyperplasia (CEH), one case of pyometra with acute endometritis and one case of suspected mild endometritis.

In breeding bitches, sub-clinical endometritis is now recognized as a major factor leading to infertility or subfertility (Mir *et al.*, 2013; Gifford *et al.*, 2014). In the latter study, performed after analyzing 399 incisional endometrial biopsies taken from subfertile bitches, the most prevalent lesion was endometritis (170/399: 42.6%). Among them, 89 bitches (52.4%) presented with lymphocytic or lymphoplasmatic infiltrates in the endometrium, and 30 bitches (17.6%) suffered from an acute endometritis with neutrophils. In cats, mild endometritis is difficult to diagnose. As in bitches, surgical incisional biopsies remain the gold standard, preferentially performed at the time of diagnosis (by ultrasound) of lack of pregnancy or embryonic resorption (Gifford *et al.*, 2014) (Fig. 5.2). The procedure allows histological, bacteriological and even molecular examination of samples; the latter for the detection of microbial antigens by means of PCR. However, in Europe cat breeders are often reluctant to accept this invasive procedure. Trans-cervical uterine flushing with a sterile saline solution appears as a potential diagnostic tool since it has been demonstrated that trans-cervical catheterization with endoscopic guidance is possible in the queen (Zambelli *et al.*, 2015). Preliminary unpublished trials in our laboratory with a 1.9 mm diameter rigid endoscope (ref. 67030BA, Karl Storz, Germany) and a 3 Fr flushing catheter revealed that it is a useful tool and deserves further investigation (Fig. 5.3). The pathogenicity of sub-clinical endometritis is still unclear. Above all, the presence and the exact role of bacteria remain unclear. In an observation, among seven infertile purebred queens, vaginal bacteria were isolated in some of these queens and two queens treated with antibiotics became pregnant later (Axnér *et al.*, 2008). In a preliminary study performed in our laboratory (Niewiadomska and Fontbonne, unpublished data), nine post-pubertal adult queens were presented to our hospital for several fertility problems such as repetitive matings with fertile males without pregnancy ($n = 4$), abnormally small litter size ($n = 2$), and embryonic resorption and abortion ($n = 3$). Animals were aged 1–6 years. Among other complementary tests, we performed surgical uterine biopsies (3/9) and ovariohysterectomies (6/9) under general anesthesia. The samples were sent for histopathological examination. During laparotomy, a sterile swab was inserted into the lumen of one uterine horn for further aerobic and anaerobic bacteriological analysis. Histological analysis revealed the presence of CEH in 4/9 animals. Among them, 2/4 queens showed a neutrophilic and lymphoplasmocytic inflammation of the endometrium, compatible with sub-clinical endometritis. Another queen (1/9) showed a slight neutrophilic and macrophagic endometritis with the presence of chronic hemorrhage. No intra-uterine bacteria were cultivated in any of the samples. In conclusion, the presence of endometritis in 33% (3/9) of these

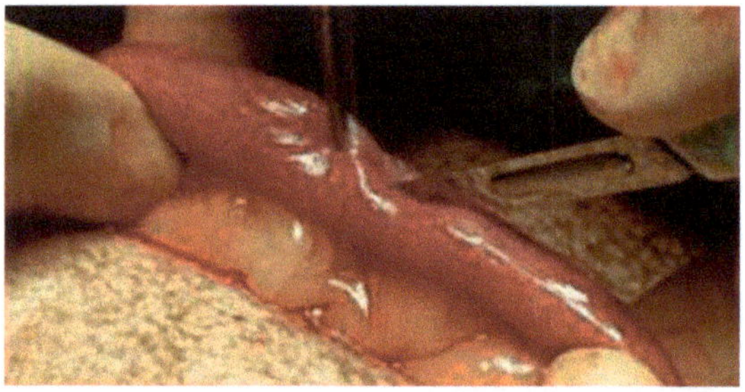

Fig. 5.2. As in the dog, an incisional uterine biopsy is a good method to investigate the cause of infertility in a queen. These require general anesthesia and an incision into the abdomen. (Image: author's own.)

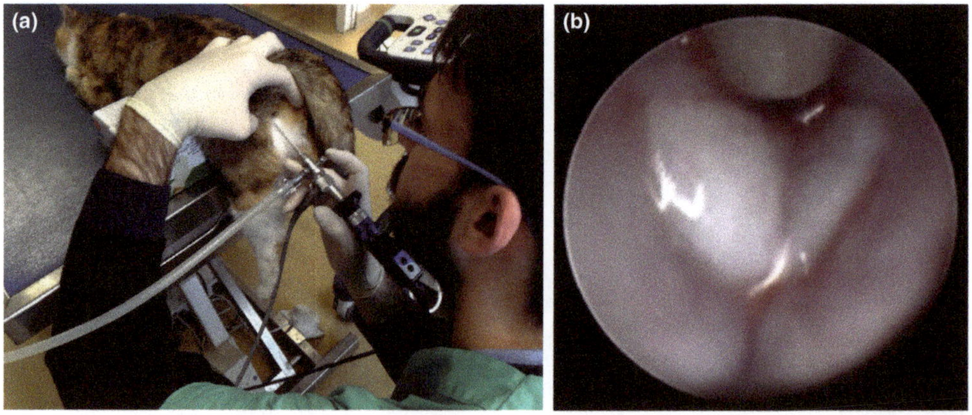

Fig. 5.3 **(a)** Vaginoscopy procedure in a queen. **(b)** A transcervical catheterization in a queen. Note the catheter entering the cervix at the top of the image. Once the catheter is within the uterus, fluid can be infused and then aspirated to analyze for endometritis. (Images: author's own.)

infertile queens reveals that this problem may well be a cause of infertility, as it appears to be in the bitch.

As it is shown in the study from Axnér *et al.* (2008) where it affected 2/7 infertile queens, and also in our preliminary study in which it was diagnosed in 4/9 incisional biopsies, CEH may also be a potential cause of feline infertility, especially since the incidence of CEH increases with age (Axnér, 2010; Binder *et al.*, 2019). Cystic endometrial hyperplasia may occur following the use of exogenous progestins (Chatdarong *et al.*, 2005) or in aged queens having presented with several episodes of spontaneous ovulations with subsequent progesterone secretion leading to endometrial development without pregnancy. It may of course be a cause of infertility due to the incapacity of embryos to survive in such a hostile environment.

Other uterine troubles may lead to fertility problems in breeding queens. In subfertile bitches, endometrial fibrosis was common (101/399: 25.3% of the cases; Gifford *et al.*, 2014). There are not enough studies to know if this also represents a significant problem in the breeding queen.

A mucometra, or mucous filling the lumen of the uterus, is sometimes found in infertile young queens without any clinical signs and is often diagnosed by ultrasound (Fig. 5.4). The exact cause is often impossible to determine (Verstegen *et al.*, 2008). In our preliminary study described above, one (of 9) queen presented with a unilateral partial uterine horn aplasia associated with fluid retention and mucometra (Fig. 5.5) (Niewiadomska and Fontbonne, unpublished). Finally, other cases of uterine problems have been recently described in bitches, and may also exist in infertile queens, such as the lack of endometrial progesterone receptors (Dockweiler *et al.*, 2017). In our study, one queen showed very scarce endometrial glands which could evocate a lack of progesterone stimulation on the endometrium and affect the support of a pregnancy to term.

5.8 Hormonal Problems

Hormonal problems are also often stated as a potential cause of infertility. Hyperestrogenism may exert a negative effect either on ovulation, or on the early embryonic migration toward the uterus, or on the endometrium leading to infertility or pregnancy arrest. Follicular cysts or granulosa cell tumors may be the source of increased estrogen (Johnston *et al.*, 2001). Some queens, frequently Oriental or Siamese breeds (personal observations), show abnormally frequent estrus which can be so close to each other that the successive follicular waves overlap creating prolonged heats (Axnér, 2010). If a queen is suffering from hyperestrogenism and ovulates spontaneously,

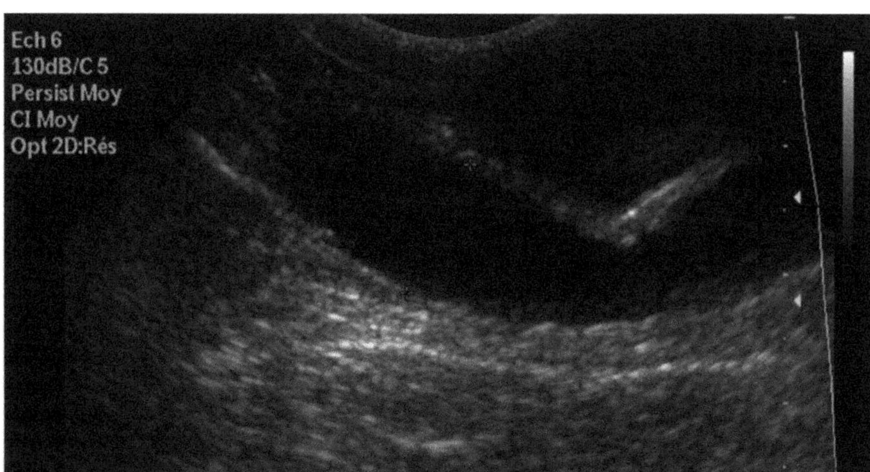

Fig. 5.4. Ultrasound image of a mucometra in an infertile 2-year-old Siamese cat. See the anechoic content of the uterus. The queen exhibited no symptom except infertility. (Image: author's own.)

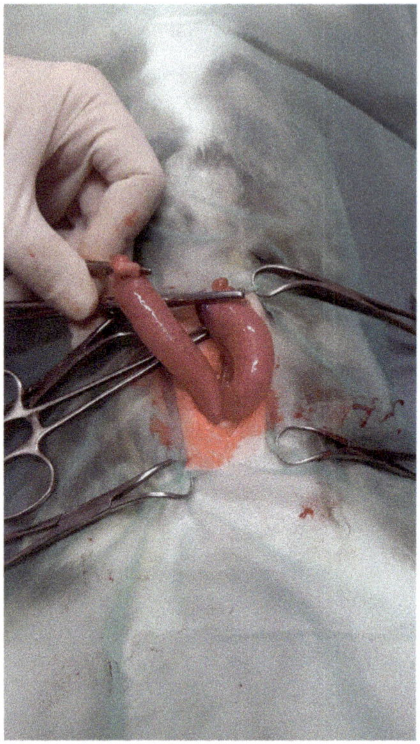

Fig. 5.5. Surgical removal of a mucometra in a 3-year-old Maine Coon queen. (Image: author's own.)

the hormonally presensitized uterus is at a high risk of developing pyometra. Such abnormal cycles need to be diagnosed and treated without delay, as they may lead to further development of a non-regenerative anemia due to bone marrow toxicity of estrogens (personal observations). Hypoluteoidism or lack of progesterone to maintain the pregnancy has been suspected to occur occasionally in the queen (Verstegen *et al.*, 2008), although not confirmed. In a survey, the Maine Coon was the most frequent breed to be cited by veterinarians as suspected to suffer from hypoluteoidism (Fontbonne, 2014). The role of other hormones is unclear. Hypothyroidism has been suspected to be a cause of fertility problems in the dog, but naturally-occurring hypothyroidism is rare in the cat (Peterson *et al.*, 2018).

5.9 Infectious Problems

The risk of infection is potentially higher in breeding facilities, especially when some matings are performed with males living elsewhere or when the cats are taken to cat shows. A study conducted in Sweden has shown that, when returning from a show, 10.4% of breeders reported conjunctivitis in their cats, and 14.6% reported upper respiratory tract diseases (Ström-Holst and Frössling, 2009). The role of shows in the existence of reproductive problems, including infertility, has not been studied but cannot be excluded. There are few reviews about the role of infectious agents causing feline infertility (Decaro *et al.*, 2012; Graham and Taylor, 2012). These agents may prevent implantation and/or embryonic development or induce pregnancy loss, which may not be diagnosed if the embryos are resorbed *in utero* and therefore appear as 'infertility.'

Among viral diseases, only retroviruses (FeLV, FIV) and the parvovirus have been confirmed as 'aborting' agents. The role of Feline Herpesvirus (FHV) or Calicivirus remains unclear and not fully demonstrated in the field, but more studies should be done on this aspect, as these two diseases are of major concern in most catteries. After an experimental inoculation with FHV a pregnancy loss may occur (Hoover and Griesemer, 1971). However, its exact role effect on reproduction in breeding catteries is still unclear and controversial. Resorption or abortion due to Calicivirus may occur in unvaccinated queens due to fetal contamination (Van Vuuren *et al.*, 1999), and there is no full protection from vaccination. Furthermore, asymptomatic carriers exist. Feline Coronavirus is considered as an uncommon cause of reproductive problems (Ström-Holst, 2002).

Among bacterial diseases, the main concern is about *Chlamydophila felis* (previously *Chlamydia psittaci,* variety *felis*). It is not clear if this agent can cause reproductive disturbances, but it has been suggested as a causative agent of abortions or pregnancy arrest in cats (Sykes *et al.*, 1999). For some authors, there is circumstantial evidence that *C. felis* may cause abortion (Gruffydd-Jones *et al.*, 2009). Other publications report a potential negative effect on fertility of *Coxiella burnetii* (Shapiro *et al.*, 2015), *Leptospira* spp., or *Bartonella henselae* (Guptill *et al.*, 1998). A report indicated also that cats may be sensitive to *Brucella* spp., as *Brucella abortus* may induce pyometra in queens (Wareth *et al.*, 2017), but it is unknown if it induces infertility, embryonic resorption, or late abortion in this species.

The role of the imbalance of the vaginal flora is probably underestimated. Very few studies have been done on the genital flora in cats, and pure growth of bacteria within the vagina seems to be a normal finding in many queens without any reproductive failure (Clemetson and Ward, 1990; Ström-Holst *et al.*, 2003). Overgrowth of *Escherichia coli* or other potentially pathogenic strains of bacteria may play a role in the development of vaginitis and further endometritis, but to the best of our knowledge this remains to be proven.

Feline reproduction may also be impaired by parasitic infection. There is a special concern about *Toxoplama gondii*, because cats are both definitive and intermediate hosts, although a detrimental effect on reproduction is probably quite rare. Experimentally, trans-placental contamination and even abortion may occur (Sakamoto *et al.*, 2009). If a pregnant queen is seronegative, she should not be allowed to hunt or eat raw meat around the time of breeding, gestation, or lactation. *Cytauxzoon felis*, a tick-transmitted protozoal parasite, has also been mentioned in a case report of a queen with a history of aborting three kittens, although it remains unclear whether the organism crossed the placenta and led to the abortion (Weisman *et al.*, 2007).

5.10 Chromosomal or Genetic Problems

Chromosomal problems are not uncommon in cats. Abnormal chromosomic formulas may be found, such as a monosomy 37X0, trisomies (39XXY, 39XXX, 39XYY) chimerism or mosaicism (Szczerbal *et al.*, 2018). This may lead to primary anestrous, infertility in females that seem to cycle normally, or abortion of fetuses with an abnormal karyotype.

Inbreeding, which is often cited as a cause of low reproductive performances, can be quantified by calculating a coefficient of inbreeding (COI). A study among Polish purebred cats evaluated the degree of inbreeding at around 3% (Mucha *et al.*, 2011). Only Siberian cats were slightly more inbred (more than 5%). A low COI in well-maintained breeding colonies may be due to the fact the large majority of breeders use their reproducers with moderation. In research colonies and wild felid populations, the COI is often higher due to limited genetic variability. In these cases, infertility is observed in both male and female cats.

5.11 Nutrition

Nutrition may have an effect on reproductive performances. In particular, essential nutrients such as taurine, arachidonic acid, polyunsaturated fatty acids, and copper have to be provided in sufficient amounts within the cat food. Due to the growing interest of purebred cat breeders for raw-food diets, concerns are raised about the microbiological content exerting potential bad effects on reproduction and general health. Organisms such as *Salmonella* spp., *Campylobacter* spp., *Listeria* spp., *E. coli*, etc., may be isolated if the preservation of the food has not been done correctly (Davies *et al.*, 2019). The contamination of industrial food by mycotoxins has been put forward as a potential problem affecting reproduction (Koerich de Souza and Scussel, 2012). In South Africa, a recent publication found a high content of mycotoxins in pelleted cat food (Singh *et al.*, 2017).

5.12 Environmental Pollutants

Compounds such as bisphenol A, a common chemical in plastics, are being cited more often as negative agents on reproductive processes in humans. Bisphenol A has been recently demonstrated to have a suppressive effect on uterine contractions in queens that may potentially lead to infertility (Kabakci *et al.*, 2019). There is more concern about the effect of environment on reproduction, and we could expect more research on this topic in the coming years.

5.13 Conclusion

Although there is much less published data about cat infertility than there is for dogs, it appears to be a reality in pedigree queens. Some potentially predominant causes, such as uterine pathology or the role of infectious diseases, deserve more dedicated research in order to understand how these factors act on fertility or subfertility. The clinical approach of the infertile queen is presented in Chapter 25. Also, male infertility should not be forgotten, and is discussed in Chapter 19.

5.14 References

Axnér, E. (2010) Clinical approach to conditions of the non-pregnant and neutered queen. In: England, G. and Van Heimendahl, A. *BSAVA Manual of Canine and Feline Reproduction and Neonatology*. British Small Animal Veterinary Association, Gloucester, UK, pp. 185–190.

Axnér, E., and Ström-Holst, B. (2015) Concentrations of anti-Müllerian hormone in the domestic cat. Relation with spay or neuter status and serum estradiol. *Theriogenology.* 83, 817–821.

Axnér, E., Agren, E., Båverud, V., and Holst, B. S. (2008) Infertility in the cycling queen: seven cases. *Journal of Feline Medicine and Surgery* 10, 566–576. doi: 10.1016/j.jfms.2008.04.005

Binder, C., Aurich, C., Reifinger, M., and Aurich, J. (2019) Spontaneous ovulation in cats – uterine findings and correlations with animal weight and age. *Animal Reproduction Science* 51, 177–184. doi: 10.1016/j.anireprosci.2019.106167

Brown, J. L. (2011) Female reproductive cycles of wild female felids. *Animal Reproduction Science* 124, 155–162. doi: 10.1016/j.anireprosci.2010.08.024

Chatdarong, K., Rungsipipat, A., Axnér, E., and Linde-Forsberg, C. (2005) Hysterographic appearance and uterine histology at different stages of the reproductive cycle and after progestagen treatment in the domestic cat. *Theriogenology* 64, 12–29. doi: 10.1016/j.theriogenology.2004.10.018

Clemetson, L. L. and Ward, A. C. (1990) Bacterial flora of the vagina and uterus of healthy cats. *Journal of the American Veterinary Medical Association* 196, 902–906.

Concannon, P., Hodgson, B., and Lein, D. (1980) Reflex LH release in estrous cats following single and multiple copulations. *Biology of Reproduction* 23, 111–117. doi: 10.1095/biolreprod23.1.111

Davies, R. H., Lawes, J. R., and Wales, A. D. (2019) Raw diets for dogs and cats: A review, with particular reference to microbiological hazards. *Journal of Small Animal Practice* 60, 329–339. doi: 10.1111/jsap.13000

Decaro, N., Carmichael, L. E., and Buonavoglia, C. (2012) Viral reproductive pathogens of dogs and cats. *Veterinary Clinics of North America – Small Animal Practice* 42, 583–598. doi: 10.1016/j.cvsm.2012.01.006

Dockweiler, J. C., Cossic, B., Donnelly, C. G., Gilbert, R. O., Buckles, E., *et al.* (2017) Infertility associated with the absence of endometrial progesterone receptors in a bitch. *Reproduction in Domestic Animals* 52, 174–178. doi: 10.1111/rda.12874

Donoghue, A. M., Johnston, L. A., Goodrowe, K. L., O'Brien, S. J., and Wildt, D. E. (1993) Influence of day of oestrus on egg viability and comparative efficiency of in vitro fertilization in domestic cats in natural or gonadotrophin-induced oestrus. *Journal of Reproduction and Fertility* 98, 85–90. doi: 10.1530/jrf.0.0980085

England, G. (2010) Physiology and endocrinology of the female. In: England, G. C. W., and von Heimendahl, A. (eds). *BSAVA Manual of Canine and Feline Reproduction and Neonatology*. British Small Animal Veterinary Association, Gloucester, UK, pp. 1–12.

Flock, U., Reese, S., Leykam, C., Otzdorff, C., Klein, R., *et al.* (2019) Changes in anti-Müllerian hormone concentrations in queens throughout the oestrous cycle. *Reproduction in Domestic Animals* 54: 91.

Fontbonne, A. (2014) Potential causes of infertility in purebred cats: a survey of data collected from different countries. In: *Proceedings of 17th EVSSAR Congress*. Wroclaw, Poland, pp. 81–85.

Fournier, A., Masson, M., Corbière, F., Mila, H., Mariani, C., *et al.* (2017) Epidemiological analysis of reproductive performances and kitten mortality rates in 5,303 purebred queens of 45 different breeds and 28,065 kittens in France. *Reproduction in Domestic Animals* 52, 153–157. doi: 10.1111/rda.12844

Gifford, A. T., Scarlett, J. M., and Schlafer, D. H. (2014) Histopathologic findings in uterine biopsy samples from subfertile bitches: 399 cases (1990-2005). *Journal of the American Veterinary Medical Association* 244, 180–186. doi: 10.2460/javma.244.2.180

Graham, E. M. and Taylor, D. J. (2012) Bacterial reproductive pathogens of cats and dogs. *Veterinary Clinics of North America – Small Animal Practice* 42, 561–582. doi: 10.1016/j.cvsm.2012.01.013

Gruffydd-Jones, T., Addie, D., Belák, S., Boucraut-Baralon, C., Egberink, H., *et al.* (2009) *Chlamydophila felis* infection. ABCD guidelines on prevention and management. *Journal of Feline Medicine and Surgery* 11, 605–609. doi: 10.1016/j.jfms.2009.05.009

Gudermuth, D. F., Newton, L., Daels, P., and Concannon, P. (1997) Incidence of spontaneous ovulation in young, group-housed cats based on serum and faecal concentrations of progesterone. *Journal of Reproduction and Fertility* Supplement 51, 177–184.

Guptill, L., Slater, L. N., Wu, C. C., Lin, T. L., Glickman, L. T., *et al.* (1998) Evidence of reproductive failure and lack of perinatal transmission of Bartonella henselae in experimentally infected cats. *Veterinary Immunology and Immunopathology* 65, 177–189. doi: 10.1016/s0165-2427(98)00153-6

Hagman, R., Ström Holst, B., Möller, L., and Egenvall, A. (2014) Incidence of pyometra in Swedish insured cats. *Theriogenology* 82, 114–120. doi: 10.1016/j.theriogenology.2014.03.007

Hoover, E. A. and Griesemer, R. A. (1971) Experimental feline herpesvirus infection in the pregnant cat. *American Journal of Pathology* 65, 173–188.

Jemmett, J. E. and Evans, J. M. (1977) A survey of sexual behaviour and reproduction of female cats. *Journal of Small Animal Practice* 18, 31–37. doi: 10.1111/j.1748-5827.1977.tb05821.x

Johnston, S. D., Root Kustritz, M. V., and Olson, P. N. S. (2001) *Canine and Feline Theriogenology*. W.B. Saunders Company, Philadelphia, Pennsylvania.

Kabakci, R., Macun, H. C., Polat, I. M., and Yildirim, E. (2019) Inhibitory effect of Bisphenol A on in vitro feline uterine contractions. *Animal Reproduction Science* 205, 27–33. doi: 10.1016/j.anireprosci.2019.03.017

Koerich de Souza, K. and Scussel, V. M. (2012) Occurrence of dogs and cats diseases records in the veterinary clinics routine in South Brazil and its relationship to mycotoxins. *International Journal of Applied Science and Technology* 2, 129–134.

Lawler, D. F., Johnston, S. D., Hegstad, R. L., Keltner, D. G., and Owens, S. F. (1993) Ovulation without cervical stimulation in domestic cats. *Journal of Reproduction and Fertility* Supplement 47, 57–61.

Mir, F., Fontaine, E., Albaric, O., Greer, M., Vannier, F., *et al.* (2013) Findings in uterine biopsies obtained by laparotomy from bitches with unexplained infertility or pregnancy loss: an observational study. *Theriogenology* 79, 312–322. doi: 10.1016/j.theriogenology.2012.09.005

Mucha, S., Wolc, A., Gradowska, A., and Szwaczkowski, T. (2011) Inbreeding rate and genetic structure of cat populations in Poland. *Journal of Applied Genetics* 52, 101–110. doi: 10.1007/s13353-010-0018-9

Peterson, M. E., Carothers, M. A., Gamble, D. A., and Rishniw, M. (2018) Spontaneous primary hypothyroidism in 7 adult cats. *Journal of Veterinary Internal Medicine* 32, 1864-1873. doi: 10.1111/jvim.15239

Robin, T. and Fontbonne, A. (2019) Descriptive analysis of the abstracts printed in the successive proceeding books of the EVSSAR congresses from 1998 to 2015, which have not been published in international peer-reviewed journals. *Reproduction in Domestic Animals* 54, 77.

Rohlertz, M., Ström Holst, B., and Axnér, E. (2012) Comparison of the GnRH-stimulation test and a semi-quantitative quick test for LH to diagnose presence of ovaries in the female domestic cat. *Theriogenology* 78, 1901–1906. doi: 10.1016/j.theriogenology.2012.06.027

Romagnoli, S. (2003) Clinical approach to infertility in the queen. *Journal of Feline Medicine and Surgery* 5, 143–146. doi: 10.1016/S1098-612X(02)00131-6

Romagnoli, S. (2005) Failure to conceive in the queen. *Journal of Feline Medicine and Surgery* 7, 59–63. doi: 10.1016/j.jfms.2004.04.006

Romagnoli, S., Bensaia, C., Ferré-Dolcet, L., Sontas, H. B., and Stelletta, C. (2019) Fertility parameters and reproductive management of Norwegian Forest Cats, Maine Coon, Persian and Bengal cats raised in Italy: A questionnaire-based study. *Journal of Feline Medicine and Surgery* 21, 1188–1197. doi: 10.1177/1098612X18824181

Root, M. V., Johnston, S. D., and Olson, P. N. (1995) Estrous length, pregnancy rate, gestation and parturition lengths, litter size, and juvenile mortality in the domestic cat. *Journal of the American Animal Hospital Association* 31, 429–433. doi: 10.5326/15473317-31-5-429

Sakamoto, C. A. M., da Costa, A. J., Gennari, S. M., Pena, H. F. J., Toniollo, G. H., *et al.* (2009) Experimental infection of pregnant queens with two major Brazilian clonal lineages of *Toxoplasma gondii*. *Parasitology Research* 105, 1311–1316. doi: 10.1007/s00436-009-1558-y

Shapiro, A. J., Bosward, K. L., Heller, J., and Norris, J. M. (2015) Seroprevalence of Coxiella burnetiid in domesticated and feral cats in eastern Australia. *Veterinary Microbiology* 177, 154–161. doi: 10.1016/j.vetmic.2015.02.011

Singh, S. D., Baijnath, S., and Chuturgoon, A. A. (2017) A comparison of mycotoxin contamination of premium and grocery brands of pelleted cat food in South Africa. *Journal of the South African Veterinary Association* 88, e1–e4. doi: 10.4102/jsava.v88i0.1480

Ström-Holst, B. (2002) Disease transmission by mating or artificial insemination in the cat: Concerns and prophylaxis. In: Concannon, P. W., England, G., Verstegen, J., and Linde Forsberg, C. (eds) *Recent Advances in Small Animal Reproduction.* International Veterinary Information Service, Ithaca, New York.

Ström-Holst, B. and Frössling, J. (2009) The Swedish breeding cat: population description, infectious diseases and reproductive performance evaluated by a questionnaire. *Journal of Feline Medicine and Surgery* 11, 793–802. doi: 10.1016/j.jfms.2009.01.008

Ström-Holst, B., Bergström, A., Lagerstedt, A.-S., Karlstam, E., Englund, L., *et al.* (2003) Characterization of the bacterial population of the genital tract of adult cats. *American Journal of Veterinary Research* 64, 963–968. doi: 10.2460/ajvr.2003.64.963

Swanson, W. F., Roth, T. L., and Wildt, D. E. (1994) In vivo embryogenesis, embryo migration, and embryonic mortality in the domestic cat. *Biology of Reproduction* 51, 452–64. doi: 10.1095/biolreprod51.3.452

Sykes, J. E., Anderson, G. A., Studdert, V. P., and Browning, G. F. (1999) Prevalence of feline Chlamydia psittaci and feline herpesvirus 1 in cats with upper respiratory tract disease. *Journal of Veterinary Internal Medicine* 13, 153–162. doi: 10.1892/0891-6640(1999)013<0153:pofpaf>2.3.co;2

Szczerbal, I., Krzeminska, P., Dzimira, S., Tamminen, T. M., Saari, S., *et al.* (2018) Disorders of sex development in cats with different complements of sex chromosomes. *Reproduction in Domestic Animals* 53, 1317–1322. doi: 10.1111/rda.13263

van Vuuren, M., Geissler, K., Gerber, D., Nöthling, J. O., and Truyen, U. (1999) Characterisation of a potentially abortigenic strain of feline calicivirus isolated from a domestic cat. *Veterinary Record* 144, 636–638. doi: 10.1136/vr.144.23.636

Verstegen, J., Dhaliwal, G., and Verstegen-Onclin, K. (2008) Mucometra cystic endometrial hyperplasia, and pyometra in the bitch: advances in treatment and assessment of future reproductive success. *Theriogenology* 70, 364–374. doi: 10.1016/j.theriogenology.2008.04.036

Wareth, G., Melzer, F., El-Diasty, M., Schmoock, G., Elbauomy, E., *et al.* (2017) Isolation of Brucella abortus from a dog and a cat confirms their biological role in re-emergence and dissemination of bovine brucellosis on dairy farms. *Transboundary and Emerging Diseases* 64, 27–30. doi: 10.1111/tbed.12535

Weisman, J. L., Woldemeskel, M., Smith, K. D., Merrill, A., and Miller, D. (2007) Blood smear from a pregnant cat that died shortly after partial abortion. *Veterinary Clinical Pathology* 36, 209–211. doi: 10.1111/j.1939-165X.2007.tb00212.x

Zambelli, D., Bini, C., and Cunto, M. (2015) Endoscopic transcervical catheterization in the domestic cat. *Reproduction in Domestic Animals* 50(1), 13–16. doi: 10.1111/rda.12442

6 Pregnancy Diagnosis and Management

JULIETTE ROOS AND ALAIN FONTBONNE

Centre d'Etudes en Reproduction des Carnivores, Ecole Nationale Vétérinaire d'Alfort, Maisons-Alfort Cedex, France

6.1 Introduction

As well as in all other species, pregnancy needs to be closely followed and pregnant females need special care and management. Thus, the first step is to identify pregnant animals. In a large-scale study conducted in a French population of purebred cats (45 breeds), the average pregnancy rate, all breeds together, was estimated to be at 85.2% with 8.4% of presumably pregnant queens failing to maintain pregnancy (Fournier *et al.*, 2017).

In this chapter, we will first go through the steps of embryonic and fetal development during pregnancy. Then we will describe the different techniques to diagnose and follow pregnancy in cats and to predict the time of parturition. Finally, we will present the key factors in the management of the pregnant queen (housing is discussed in Chapter 4).

6.2 Embryonic and Fetal Development in Cats and the Hormonal Control of Pregnancy

6.2.1 Embryonic, fetal, and placental development

Like many other aspects of feline reproduction, the embryonic and fetal developments have been only minimally studied. However, histological studies from Miglino *et al.* in 2006 and Pieri *et al.* in 2015 provide new insights on this subject (Miglino *et al.*, 2006; Pieri *et al.*, 2015).

After ovulation, fertilization occurs in the oviducts and the morulae enter the uterine horns 4 to 5 days after ovulation. From then on, the free-floating embryos migrate through both horns and develop until day 10 to 12 when implantation occurs (Johnston *et al.*, 2001). Free-floating embryos are sustained by the 'uterine milk' produced by the endometrial glands (Concannon *et al.*, 2001). After implantation, the placenta starts to develop.

According to Miglino *et al.* (2006), the choriovitelline placenta (formed by the yolk sac and the chorion) remains until day 20 of pregnancy. At that time, the yolk sac is prominent and fully vascularized (vessels originating from the umbilical cord). At day 24, the yolk sac is three times as long as the embryo. The amnion totally encloses the embryo. It is avascular and will stay poorly vascularized throughout pregnancy. It is connected to the yolk sac by the vitelline duct. The allantoic sac measures twice that of the yolk sac. The placental contact with the endometrium takes place at the central part of the allantoic sac and is endotheliochorial. In dogs, this part encircles the embryo totally. In cats, this zonary placenta is incomplete in around 62% of embryos and the empty space (or just reduced thickness of the placenta in 10% of embryos observed histologically) is called the placental fissure. It is located distally to the insertion of the umbilical cord. The two peripheral parts of the placenta are formed by hematomas that are macroscopically brown in cats and only microscopically detectable. The materno-fetal contact in the placenta is lamellar. The cats' feto-maternal blood flow is a simple crosscurrent type. Branches of the blood vessels of the umbilical cord supplying the yolk sac and the placental girdle can be observed from the 25th to 30th day of pregnancy. Up to day 45, the fetus does not exceed the dimensions of the yolk sac. At day 53, the fetus is already almost completely developed inside the amnion which is totally covered by the allantois (Miglino *et al.*, 2006).

Amniotic and allantoic fluids reach an average peak volume of 26 and 24 mL, respectively, and the placenta

DOI: 10.1079/9781789247107.0006

weight goes from 5.7 g on day 24 to 15.0 g at day 39 when it reaches a plateau (Johnston *et al.*, 2001).

The amniotic fluid is the result of the secretions from the fetal respiratory tract, oral cavity, gastrointestinal tract and skin. It provides mechanical protection and essential nutrients to the fetus. The allantoic fluid comes from the mesonephros, metanephros, and kidney secretions, and is very similar to the fetal urine composition. A study from Fresno *et al.* in 2012 reveals that feline fetal fluids composition does not result from a simple filtration from the maternal blood. The fetus seems to play a role in their biochemical composition. Moreover, a diffusion from amniotic to allantoic fluid is possible which explains their similar biochemical composition. This composition changes throughout pregnancy but will not be discussed in more detail here (Fresno *et al.*, 2012).

Size of the embryo throughout the pregnancy and formation of the organs is described in Table 6.1, according to a study by Pieri *et al.* (2015). The embryo life ends at the time when organogenesis is over with organs and systems established. It is followed by the fetal life. In cats, the transition from embryo to fetus occurs at 28 days of pregnancy (Knospe, 2002).

6.2.2 Hormonal control of pregnancy

After ovulation, plasma estradiol (E2) shows a sharp decrease within the first five days reaching basal values. Progesterone plasma values (P4) increase similarly in pregnant and pseudopregnant (which is a diestrus without pregnancy) queens until day 10–12 corresponding to the implantation period. Progesterone profiles and concentrations are similar in pregnant and non-pregnant queens in the early luteal phase (England, 2010). P4 reaches a peak at 21 days of pregnancy (with values reported after mating reaching between 11 ng/mL and 60 ng/mL) (Root Kustritz, 2006). In pregnant queens, P4 remained elevated until day 47 of pregnancy. P4 declines progressively after that period (García Mitacek *et al.*, 2015). It is important to notice that in pseudopregnant queens, P4 reaches basal values between days 40 and 45 meaning that pseudopregnancy is shorter than pregnancy which is not the case in canine pseudopregnancy (Johnston *et al.*, 2001; Zschockelt *et al.*, 2014).

In cats, the capacity of the placenta to produce P4 by conversion of pregnenolone and to produce steroidogenic metabolites is highly suspected (Siemieniuch

Table 6.1. Time of ultrasound appearance of fetal and extra-fetal structures, according to Zambelli *et al.* (2002a) and Pieri *et al.* (2015).

		Days after mating	
		Mean	Range
Gestational vesicle	Spherical shape	10	10–11
	Lemon shape	20	19–21
Place of the embryo	On the wall of the gestational chamber	14	13–16
	In the center of the gestational chamber	20	19–21
Size of embryo/fetus	7 mm	21–22	
	12–14 mm	24–25	
	20 mm	26	
	22–30 mm	28–32	
	30–50 mm	35	
Heart	Heartbeat	16–17	16–18
	Cardiac chambers	50	48–50
Embryo with a C-form (head and trunk)		18	17–19
Early development of forelimbs and hindlimbs		22–25	
Primitive gut		21	
Stomach	Punctiform	30	29–39
	Caudal to the liver	49	48–50
Brain vesicles		22–25	
Tail and head		27	
Pelvic members		28–32	
Bladder		29–30	29–32
Respiratory system first noted		28–32	
Hyperechoic lung versus liver		30	29–32
Umbilical cord		30	30–32
Urogenital system		28–32	
Optic pigmented, retina		32	
Skeleton	Hyperechoic skeleton (long bones, thoracic limb and head)	30	30–33
	Ossification: long bone diaphysis	50	48–50
Fetal movements (laterally)		30	30–34
Intestines	Appearance	40	38–42
	Layered structured	54	52–56
Eyes		35	35–39
Kidneys (cortex and medulla visible)		50	48–50
Diaphragm		50	50–56

et al., 2012). Indeed, ovariectomy of pregnant queens may induce abortion in many cases – but not all (even though a sharp decrease of P4 is observed) – especially when performed after 45 days of pregnancy (Tsutsui *et al.*, 2009). The role of the placenta as a source of progesterone to maintain pregnancy is, however, still controversial (Verstegen *et al.*, 1993b). Nevertheless, there is a consensus to consider ovaries as the main source of P4 during pregnancy.

Compared with the bitch, progesterone is not always basal at the time of parturition and can even be over 6 ng/mL on the day of parturition (Johnston *et al.*, 2001; Root Kustritz, 2006; García Mitacek *et al.*, 2015; Keiser *et al.*, 2017). For example, in the study by García Mitacek *et al.* in 2015 in a group of 16 mixed-breeds queens, the mean P4 value in the 24 hours before parturition was 2.99 ±1.29 ng/mL (García Mitacek *et al.*, 2015).

Relaxin is, as in the bitch, a pregnancy-specific peptide hormone produced by the feto-maternal unit (Braun *et al.*, 2012). It is first detected at day 20 of pregnancy then increases and reaches a maximum level at day 30 to 35. A decrease is observed within the last 10 to 15 days of pregnancy and relaxin then seems to be rapidly undetectable after parturition (Stewart and Stabenfeldt, 1985; Johnston *et al.*, 2001).

Finally, prolactin is also an essential hormone for the cat pregnancy as a luteotropic hormone after 30 to 40 days of pregnancy. Indeed, it has been shown that the use of cabergoline, an anti-prolactinic agent, at 30 days of pregnancy may induce abortion in queens (Verstegen *et al.*, 1993a,b). In this species, prolactin starts to increase from the 20th day of pregnancy. A sharp increase is then observed just before parturition and its production is stimulated by neonates suckling. It returns to basal levels one to two weeks after weaning (Johnston *et al.*, 2001; Root Kustritz, 2006).

Figure 6.1 shows a schematic evolution of the different hormones during the pregnant or not pregnant diestrus in queens.

6.3 Pregnancy Diagnosis

6.3.1 Macroscopical Changes in the Pregnant Queen

Physical development of the pregnant queen

The queen is very different from the bitch concerning the external signs of pregnancy. Indeed, the pregnant cat shows a linear increase in body weight starting 14 days after mating. This may be considered as one of the first signs of pregnancy if

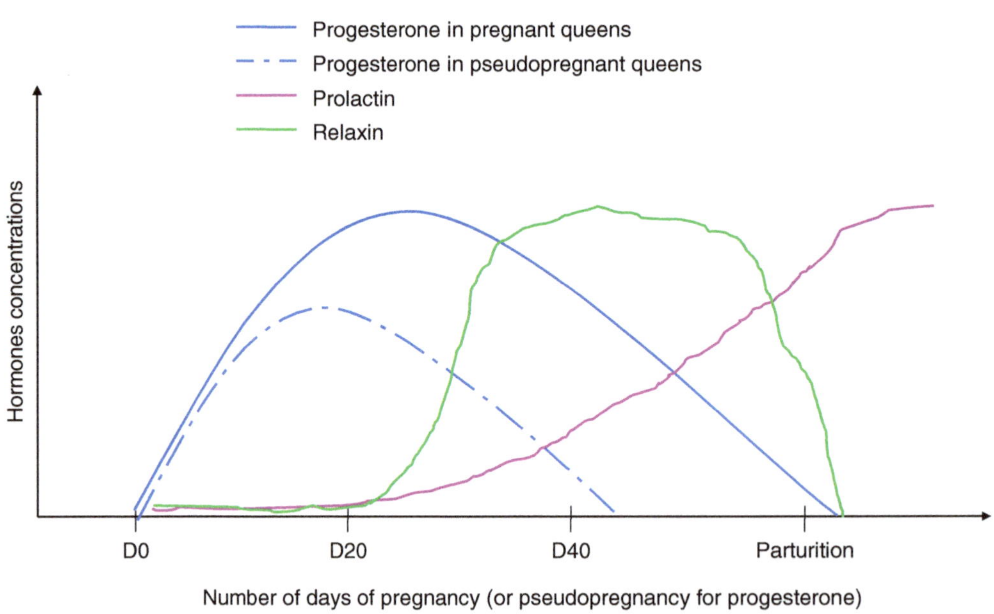

Fig. 6.1. Schematic evolution of the different hormones during diestrus in the queen. (Image: author's own.)

the queens are weighed regularly after mating. Another particular sign in the pregnant queen is the reddening of the nipples associated with an increased size that can be observed from the 21st day of pregnancy onward (Levy and England, 2010).

Later, the mammary gland enlarges (i.e. mammogenesis) and the colostral secretions can be observed in some queens during the last week of pregnancy. Lactation is rarely observed during pseudopregnancy but is possible in pseudopregnant cats (Levy and England, 2010).

On the other hand, as in the bitch, behavioral changes are not reliable signs of pregnancy. Usual modifications include excessive grooming of the perineal and mammary gland area and increased docility and nesting behavior. They are more often observed during late pregnancy or during the first stage of parturition (Levy and England, 2010).

Finally, the absence of return to estrus within 21 days after mating is not a good sign of pregnancy in queens since spontaneous ovulation or an infertile mating will lead to a state of pseudopregnancy which will postpone the next estrus to 40 to 45 days. However, estrus signs one and a half months after mating are quite often reliable signs of pseudopregnancy.

Abdominal palpation

Gentle abdominal palpation is an easy and reliable method to detect pregnancy in the queen if performed at the right period. The best time to easily diagnose the pregnancy by palpation is between 20 to 35 days after mating when the vesicles are round and tense (with the best period for early diagnosis between 20 and 25 days when the vesicles are tense and around 2.5 cm in diameter, with an accuracy of nearly 90% for an experienced clinician) and after 55 days when the fetuses are sufficiently ossified to easily palpate the heads. Experienced clinicians and breeders can palpate smaller vesicles as early as 15 to 17 days of pregnancy. Between 35 and 55 days after mating, conceptuses become elongated, enlarged and they lose their tenseness, making them hard to palpate (Johnston *et al.*, 2001; Levy and England, 2010).

Abdominal palpation is not a precise technique for counting the number of embryos and should only be used to classify a queen as pregnant or not pregnant. In addition, it does not give any idea of the embryo/fetus vitality.

6.3.2 Hormonal assays

Blood progesterone concentration is not a good tool for early pregnancy diagnosis in cats. As mentioned before, P4 values are not significantly different in pregnant and pseudopregnant queens. However, this measurement can be used after 45 days of pregnancy which is the end of pseudopregnancy. Hence, progesterone assays only allow a late diagnosis and do not give any information on the embryo/fetus vitality (Levy and England, 2010).

Relaxin is a peptide produced by the feto-placental unit. As such, it is a pregnancy-specific hormone in the queen. Relaxin assays for veterinary clinics (ELISA) have been developed for pregnancy diagnosis in both the bitch and the queen. Plasma concentration of relaxin can also be detected in queens from day 20 of pregnancy onward (DiGangi *et al.*, 2010). Relaxin can also be detected in urine from 21 to 28 days of pregnancy (van Dorsser *et al.*, 2007). However, relaxin does not give any information on the litter vitality either.

6.3.3 Imaging

Ultrasound

The use of ultrasonography to diagnose a pregnancy in queens is the best method to simultaneously offer an early diagnosis, a litter count (if done at early stages) and assess the vitality of embryo/fetuses.

If B-mode ultrasonography is started from the third week post-mating to see the vesicles, some publications show that first signs of pregnancy could be observed as soon as 10 to 11 days post-mating (Zambelli *et al.*, 2002a; Topie *et al.*, 2015). However, being able to give a reliable answer at this stage needs a trained clinician and a powerful ultrasound scanner. Moreover, if signs of pregnancy can effectively be observed, it may be difficult to estimate the number of embryonic vesicles at this early stage. At the 14th day of pregnancy, diagnosis seems easier because gestational vesicles are more visible and are surrounded by a circular hyperechoic wall. Until day 20, vesicles are circular before taking on a 'lemon' shape. The embryos will be easy to observe from the 17th day of pregnancy onward. To assess their viability, the shape of the gestational vesicle is important to note. The presence of heartbeat is also a good indication of pregnancy and can be observed from the 16th day of pregnancy onward (Zambelli *et al.*, 2002a).

The vitality of fetuses is also important to assess by ultrasound. Evaluation of the heart rate (HR, possible to observe from day 16 of pregnancy onward) is essential during pregnancy examination. Most authors generally consider that the HR should be above 190 bpm. A normal fetal HR is usually two to three times greater than the mother's HR. A sustained decrease in HR reveals a fetal stress. Temporary decrease (lasting less than 1 to 2 minutes) is possibly due to uterine contractions at the time of evaluation (Lopate, 2018). However, there are few studies about threshold values of fetal HR in queens.

Triplex Doppler ultrasonography is also used to follow pregnancy through the analysis of uterine and fetal vessels. It allows the clinician the ability to measure the pulsatility (PI) and resistivity (RI) indexes in those vessels and to observe the flow waveforms (see Fig. 6.2). Those criteria reflect the perfusion of the uterus and its contents. During normal pregnancy, uterine arteries, fetal aorta, and caudal cava vein and umbilical cord show a decrease in those two indexes (except the PI of the fetal aorta) (Scotti *et al.*, 2008). Moreover, Pereira *et al.* in 2012 observed that the RI and PI of the major uterine horn (the horn with a higher number of fetuses) were lower than the other one. The values were also different before mating which may allow one to identify the future major horn (Pereira *et al.*, 2012).

In the case of medical abortion, the resistivity index of the uterine arteries increases (Blanco *et al.*, 2016). Moreover, the presence of a diastolic notch (characterized on the waveforms by a protodiastolic incisure) has been associated with negative outcome in canine and human pregnancies. In studies in queens, the presence of an end diastolic notch was normal before the end of organogenesis and should disappear during the second half of pregnancy (Brito *et al.*, 2010; Pereira *et al.*, 2012). Its persistency, as well as an abnormal increase in uterine arteries' RI, could be a predictor of a negative outcome.

Radiology

Giving a reliable pregnancy diagnosis using radiographs is challenging before the calcification of the fetuses' skeletons has happened. This starts around day 39 of pregnancy. However, uterine spherical swellings may be visible as soft tissue opacities from day 21 onward (and even from day 17 in some queens) (Lopate, 2018).

This technique is not recommended for early pregnancy diagnosis. Moreover, it does not give any information about embryo/fetal vitality except when specific signs of fetal death are present such as disjunction or deformation of the skull's bones (Fig. 6.3), presence of gas in the uterus or in/around the fetuses (which is a sign of putrefaction), abnormal flexion of the fetus, or hyperextension of the hindlimbs (Lopate, 2018). However, it is a very good indicator for counting kittens

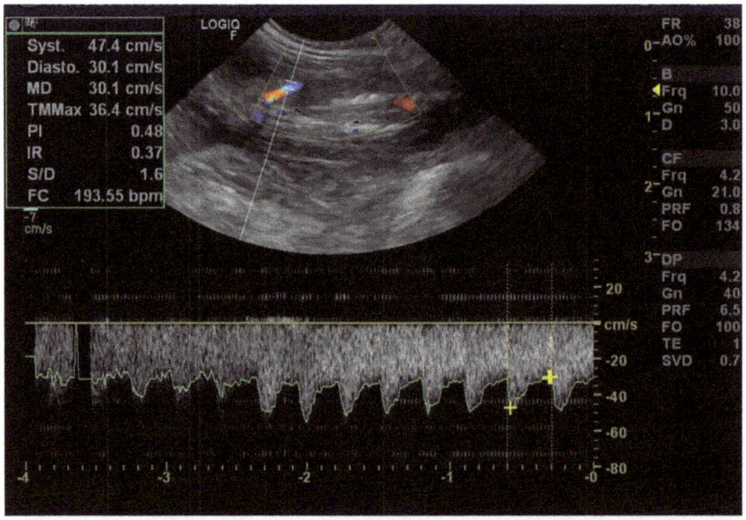

Fig. 6.2. Triplex Doppler ultrasonography of the right uterine artery of a pregnant queen. (Image from the CERCA.)

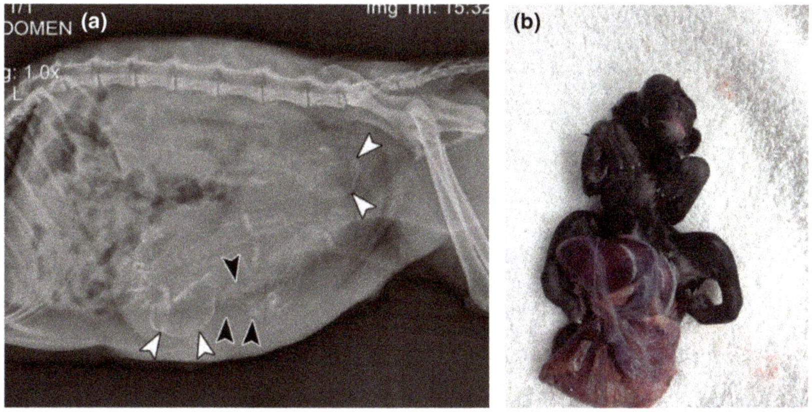

Fig. 6.3 **(a)** Radiograph of a late term pregnant queen. One fetus in the caudal abdomen has a deformed head (black arrowheads) and limbs. Two other normal fetal heads and bodies can be seen (white arrowheads). **(b)** The deceased fetus was naturally delivered with live littermates. (Reproduced with permission from John Wiley & Sons, Inc.)

before parturition when performed the final week before the due date.

6.4 Pregnancy Aging

6.4.1 Precise timing of the matings

A study showed that 100% of queens ovulated after multiple copulations on the 3rd day of the heat (Concannon *et al.*, 1980). Allowing cats to mate during a short period (2 to 3 days) around the third day of estrus without letting cats together uncontrolled during the whole estrus period permits the breeder to have a more precise date of ovulation and to date pregnancy. Follicular growth monitoring via ultrasound can allow the veterinarian to choose that ideal period. The female should be in contact with the male in the days following the moment when follicles reach at least 3 mm in diameter or at least on the third day of estrus and mating should be observed by the owner to confirm the typical behavior of the female following a successful mating(Malandain *et al.*, 2011).

When matings are not observed or the cats have been together for a long period, other techniques using ultrasonography or radiography can be used to date pregnancy.

6.4.2 Ultrasound diagnosis

Evolution of the conceptus and organs

The organogenesis takes place at a specific time during pregnancy. The development of the embryo and fetus can be followed, and it allows one to date the pregnancy. However, the evaluations will depend on the precision of the ultrasound scanner (Topie *et al.*, 2015).

One study gives good insight of pregnancy timing using the development of the conceptus (Zambelli *et al.*, 2002a). Table 6.1 sums up the main dates in correlation with the development of fetal and extra-fetal structures.

Determining the gender is also possible by ultrasound from 38 to 43 days post-mating. Male fetuses are characterized by a building of the scrotum appearing dorsally to a ventral prepuce that is visible under the tail on a midsagittal view. In females, a single triangular bulge of the vulvar lips distant to the tail base is observable under the tail in the same view (Zambelli *et al.*, 2004; Lopate, 2018).

Fetometry

Fetometry is the use of fetal and extra-fetal structure measurements to date pregnancy using different formulas.

Extra-fetal structures are represented by the inner chorionic circumference (ICC) and the outer uterine diameter (OUD). It should only be used until the 30th day of pregnancy when vesicles are still well defined and round or slightly oval (Zambelli *et al.*, 2002a). It is important to measure at least three embryonic vesicles and, for each of them, take two perpendicular measures through the middle of the sac. Even though the average will be used to get rid of the difference in measurements associated with the ovoid shape of some vesicles, it is important not to deform those vesicles with an excessive pressure of the probe. Figure 6.4 shows an example. Formulas are as follows (Zambelli *et al.*, 2002b):

- Gestational age = 1.368 × ICC – 11.566 where the ICC is in mm.
- Gestational age = 1.602 × OUD – 12.13 where the OUD is in mm.

The study of Socha and Janowski (2019) gives a specific formula using ICC for Maine Coon cats (which are bigger than other breeds):

- Date before parturition in Maine Coon cats = (–0.79 × ICC) + 57.9 where the ICC is in mm

Fetal parameters that may be used to determine pregnancy age are as follows:

- Crown–rump length (CRL, shown in Fig. 6.5) = measured in a sagittal plane from the most

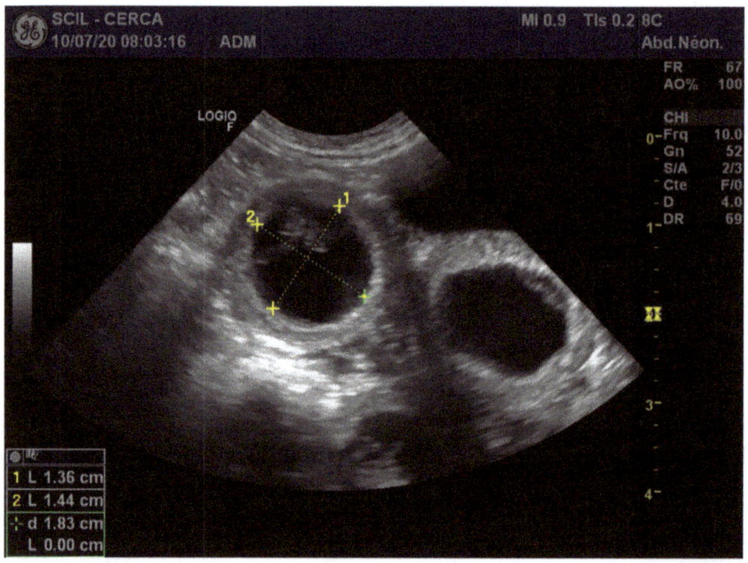

Fig. 6.4. Measurement of the gestational chamber by two perpendicular measures. The average between measures 1 and 2 will be calculated and several gestational sacs will be measured to date pregnancy. (Images from the CERCA.)

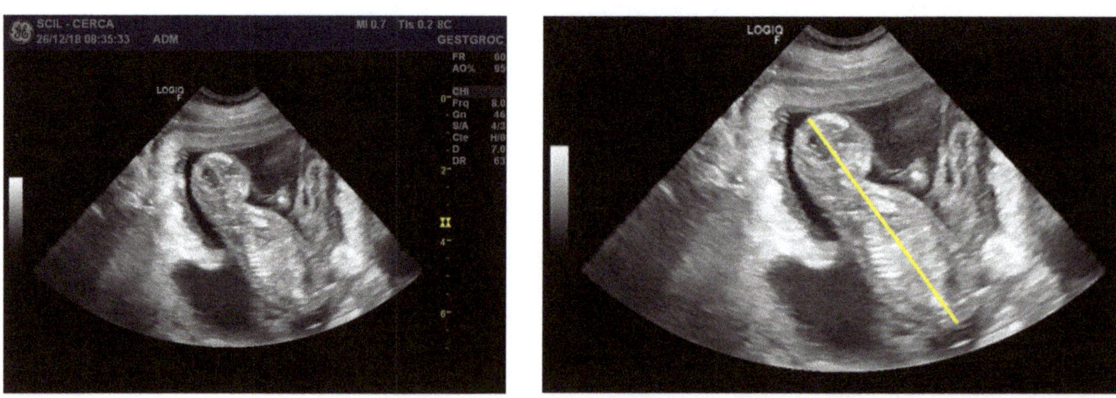

Fig. 6.5. Measurement of the crown–rump length. The yellow line on the right figure shows how to take the measure from the most rostral part of the head to the base of the tail. (Images from the CERCA.)

rostral part of the head to the base of the tail (Lopate, 2018).

- Biparietal diameter (BPD, shown in Fig. 6.6) = measured at the widest point on the skull in a frontal or dorsal view, at the central location of the echogenic line produced by the falx cerebri (Lopate, 2018).
- Body diameter (BD, shown in Fig. 6.7) = taken by two transverse measurements at the widest point of the abdomen, which occurs at the level of the stomach and liver (Lopate, 2018).
- Deep portion of the fetal diencephalo-telencephalic vesicle (DPTV, shown in Fig. 6.8) = observed as asymmetric anechoic area viewed on sagittal midline in the fetal skull, it represents the fetal thalamus and the primordial basal nuclei (Lopate, 2018).
- Femur length (FL).
- Gastric diameter (GD).

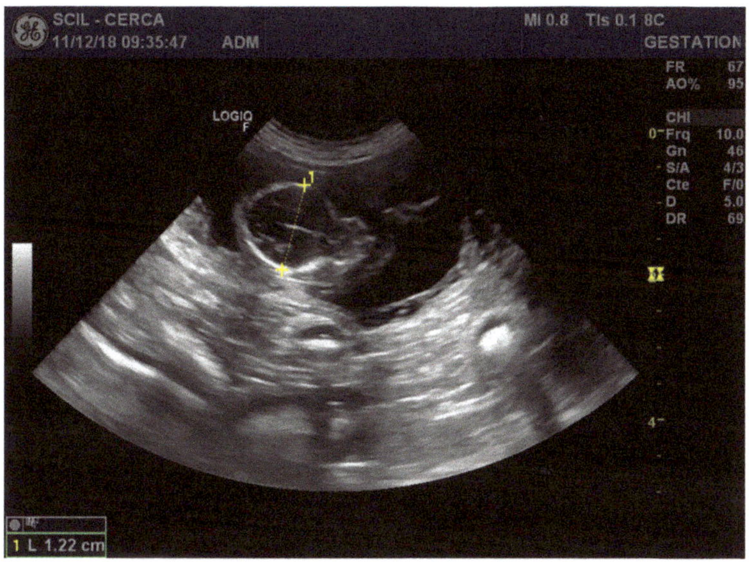

Fig. 6.6. Measurement of the biparietal diameter at the widest point on the skull in dorsal view, at the central location of the echogenic line (white line). (Images from the CERCA.)

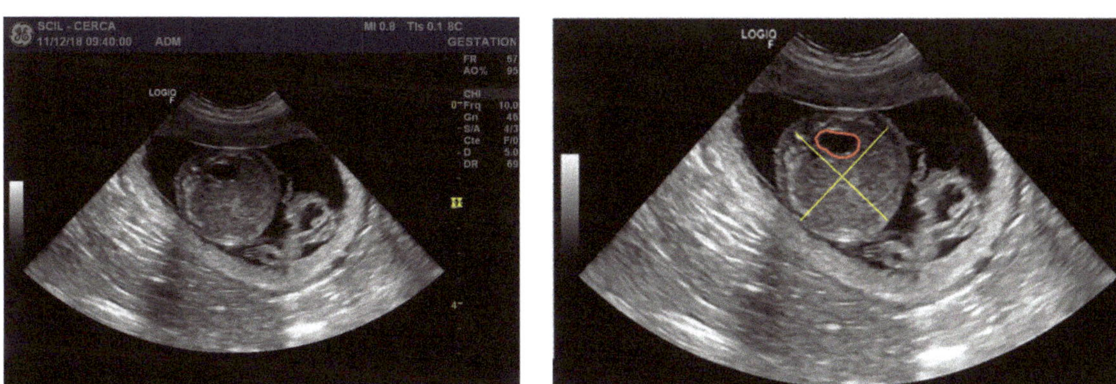

Fig. 6.7. Measurement of the body diameter: the right figure shows the two transverse measurements at the widest point of the abdomen, which occurs at the level of the stomach (circled by the red mark) and liver. (Images from the CERCA.)

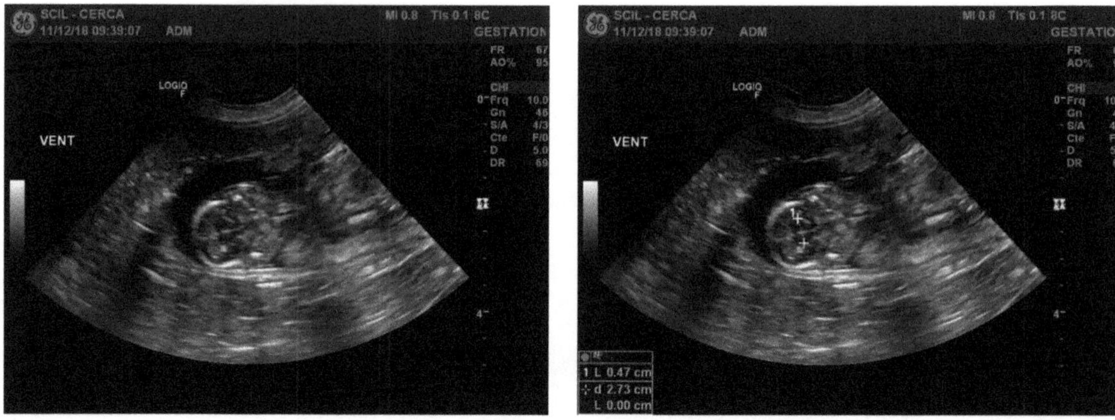

Fig. 6.8. Measurement of the deep portion of the fetal diencephalo-telencephalic vesicle. The right-hand figure shows the DPTV measure. (Images from the CERCA.)

Table 6.2. Different formulas to assess gestational age using fetal structures.

Parameter	Formula	Reference
CRL	GA = 2.0087 × CRL − 31.43 where the CRL is in mm	Zambelli *et al.* (2002b)
BPD	GA = Log(BPD(mm)/0.483873)/0.02756	Zambelli *et al.* (2004)
	DBP = (BPD (mm) − 23.39)/0.47	Beccaglia *et al.* (2008a)
BPD in Maine Coon cats	DBP = −1.86 × + 49.3 where the BPD is in mm	Socha and Janowski (2019)
DPTV	DBP = (DPTV (mm) − 10.74)/0.22	Beccaglia *et al.* (2008b)
BD	GA = Log(BD(mm)/0.405565)/0.0372141	Zambelli *et al.* (2004)
GD	GA = Log(GD(mm)/0.115113)/0.0388901	Zambelli *et al.* (2004)
FL	DBP = 37.864 − 0.193 × FL(mm) + 1.227 × weight (kg) − 0.615 × litter size − 0.832 × age(years)	Gatel *et al.* (2015)

GA, gestational age; DBP, date before parturition; CRL, crown–rump length; BPD, biparietal diameter; BD, body diameter; GD, gastric diameter; FL, femur length.

All measurements should be taken on multiple fetuses and the average should be used in the formulas. All parameters can be used after 30 days of pregnancy. Different formulas have been published. They are recorded in Table 6.2.

BPD in queens is the most accurate parameter to date pregnancy in latter stages. Its accuracy is of 64.3% within 1 day and 85.7% within 2 days. The use of DPTV seems less accurate than the BPD, with only 38.5% of queens beginning parturition within 1 day and 61.5% within 2 days (Beccaglia *et al.*, 2008a). However, BPD does not reliably predict a parturition that should start within 24 to 72 hours. Indeed the accuracy of parturition day prediction using BPD is 27–53% (and using the BD the accuracy is 17–35%) (Keiser *et al.*, 2017).

In another study, Gatel *et al.* (2015) used the femur length to predict parturition. They found a correlation with this parameter, age and weight of the queen, and the litter. This formula has an accuracy of 70% within 1.6 days (Gatel *et al.*, 2015).

Finally, the study by García Mitacek *et al.* in 2015 gives formulas to predict the size of the gestational sacs and fetal parameters (CRL, BPD, and BD) according to the number of days from mating. This may be a new criteria to monitor the accurate development of conceptuses (García Mitacek *et al.*, 2015).

6.4.3 Radiographic diagnosis

Mineralization of the fetuses takes place progressively. It is possible to approximately age a pregnancy according to the different bones that can be observed.

In a study conducted on 17 queens that were radiographed three times per week starting around

3 weeks (when diagnosis could be done by abdominal palpation) until parturition, the time of mineralization of the different bones were recorded and associated with the number of days before parturition (Haney *et al.*, 2003). Results of this study are presented in Table 6.3. The first detection of mineralization is possible 25 to 29 days before parturition without being able to identify the different bones (Haney *et al.*, 2003).

In the same study, 32 pregnant queens were used to assess the accuracy of this method. One X-ray was taken per animal and the parturition date was estimated. Actual parturition occurred within 3 days of the estimated date in 75% of queens and in 100% of queens within 7 days with no association with the litter size (Haney *et al.*, 2003).

If radiography is not the best way for dating pregnancy, it would appear to be the most exact method to estimate the number of fetuses.

Ultrasound and radiography are very good tools to make a pregnancy diagnosis, follow pregnancy, and predict the parturition date. However, it is always very important to take into account the quality of the machine used and the experience of the clinician. The accuracy of the images and their interpretation can be quite variable, especially with the introduction of digital radiography, and this is the reason why those techniques should never be used alone to plan a cesarean section.

Table 6.3. Mineralization of the different fetal bones in relation to the number of days before parturition according to the study by Haney *et al.* (2003).

	Number of days before parturition	
	Mean ± SD	Range
General mineralization	26 ±1	25–29
Vertebral column	24 ± 1	22–27
Skull	22 ± 1	21–27
Ribs	22 ± 2	22–25
Scapula	20 ± 2	17–24
Humerus	20 ± 1	20–24
Femur	21 ± 1	19–23
Radius	19 ± 2	15–22
Tibia	19 ± 1	15–21
Ulna	17 ± 2	5–21
Pelvis	19 ± 1	8–20
Fibula	13 ± 3	0–17
Tail	15 ± 2	8–16
Metacarpals and metatarsals	8 ± 3	3–14
Phalanges	6 ± 3	0–11
Calcaneus	6 ± 3	0–10
Teeth	2 ± 1	1–6

6.5 Management Of The Pregnant Queen

6.5.1 Nutrition

One specific aspect of the queen's pregnancy is the linear increase of the body weight starting from the second week of pregnancy onward (Wichert *et al.*, 2009; Hand *et al.*, 2010). In other species of carnivores, the body weight has a rapid increase only during the last third of pregnancy and just slight modifications before. This early increase seems to allow the formation of energy reserve to prepare and sustain the lactation needs rather than to participate in the pregnancy development (Hand *et al.*, 2010). Mean weight gain at the end of pregnancy is about 40% of the pre-mating weight. Another specific aspect of the pregnant queen is the loss of only 40% of its pregnancy-gained weight immediately after queening (Hand *et al.*, 2010).

Poor queen nutrition during pregnancy may lead to different adverse effects: failure to conceive, fetal death, fetal malformation, underweight kittens, and kittens with poor immunocompetence. Moreover, overweight has negative consequences too: stillbirth, dystocia, and cesarian sections are more often observed with increased body condition. An ideal body condition score at mating should be 3/5 (Hand *et al.*, 2010).

About the change in nutrition during pregnancy, one of the most important things to consider is the increased demand in energy supply which will be the most limiting nutrient. If the needs linearly increase throughout pregnancy from the second week onward, the food intake, however, changes slightly and even decreases around two weeks after mating, corresponding to the embryos' implantation. Another decline is observed the last week of pregnancy. The energy allowance during pregnancy should be 25–50% above maintenance level (and can reach 70%, especially in large litter pregnancies) corresponding to 90–110 kcal/kg body weight/day (376–460 kJ/kg body weight/day). A free-choice feeding allows queens to adjust their food intake to correspond to their own energy demand (Hand *et al.*, 2010).

The second essential nutrient to adapt to the pregnant status is the protein intake. A food containing 35–50% DM (dry matter) of good quality, mainly animal based proteins should be used (Hand *et al.*, 2010).

Taurine is an essential nutrient to the cat physiology. Taurine deficiency is known to induce fetal death near the 25th day of pregnancy, abortion, fetal deformities, and delayed growth and development. However, taurine demand of the pregnant queen is similar to the maintenance stage (Hand *et al.*, 2010).

Finally, recommended levels of calcium and phosphorus for food during gestation and lactation should be between ranges of 1.1 and 1.6 for calcium and 0.8 and 1.4 for phosphorus DM. Moreover, the calcium:phosphorus ratio should be between 1:1 and 1.5:1. Although eclampsia is uncommon in cats and its etiology still unknown, it is not recommended to increase calcium intake above the previously cited ratios (Hand *et al.*, 2010).

The transition from regular food to pregnancy-specific diet should be done at or just before mating. Dry food may be more desirable, especially for queens with a decreased appetite since this form is more nutrient dense. On the other hand, moist food will have the advantage of containing higher amounts of fat and water (especially needed for lactation). Therefore, it is ideal to mix diets, giving dry food free choice and multiple moist food meals daily (Hand *et al.*, 2010). During this very specific period of pregnancy, it is not recommended to give bones or raw food diet since the risk of misbalance and infectious diseases is increased with this kind of nutrition, which can be dramatic especially during pregnancy.

Finally, to assess the good nutrition plan, pregnant queens should be weighed once a week to observe their linear weight gain.

6.5.2 Parasite prevention and vaccination

Before mating, both cats should be correctly vaccinated and treated against ectoparasites and endoparasites. Moreover, the blood group of each animal should be known to avoid any risk of neonatal isoerythrolysis (which can take place when a b-group queen is mated with an A or A/b male) (Bücheler, 1999).

A good vaccination status of the queen is essential to provide a high-quality colostrum (to ensure a good level of antibodies) and protect the neonates during their first weeks of life before their own immunity can react appropriately. It is essential for the queen to be fully vaccinated before mating without needing any vaccine administration during pregnancy. Indeed, even if most killed vaccines (except for the feline panleukopenia (FPL) live virus vaccine) are not known to be directly harmful to the embryos and fetuses, the post-vaccination reaction (like a transient hyperthermia) may increase the risk of pregnancy arrest. The FPL vaccine is usually composed of a modified live virus that can induce the same adverse effect in fetuses as the virus itself. Indeed, vaccination of pregnant queens can induce a cerebellar hypoplasia in fetuses (Root Kustritz, 2006; Zambelli, 2012). Vaccination with this kind of vaccine is strictly forbidden during pregnancy in cats.

Control of both endoparasites and ectoparasites is essential during pregnancy, and especially before queening to avoid any transmission to the kittens. However, no official guidelines have been given in the literature for pregnant queens. It is common to deworm queens following the same protocol as in bitches: use fenbendazole (50 mg/kg over 3 to 5 days) starting 40 to 45 days of pregnancy and at 2 weeks of lactation. Concerning external parasites, all cats should be treated before mating and treatment during pregnancy should be done only in case of heavy contamination with ectoparasites (Smith, 2011).

6.5.3 Good practice in the use of usual drugs during pregnancy

Unfortunately, research about drug toxicity during pregnancy in cats is quite scarce. Little data is available. The metabolism of the queen changes during pregnancy. As such, pharmacokinetics of the usual drugs (antibiotics, analgesics, etc.) are modified. It is therefore necessary to adapt different formulations (doses and dosage intervals). The increase of progesterone plasma levels during diestrus/pregnancy induces a reduced gastrointestinal motility and an increased gastrointestinal blood flow which may affect the oral absorption and bioavailability of drugs (Rebuelto and Loza, 2010). Moreover, an extensive maternal cardiovascular adaptation is observed to sustain the development of the fetus: blood volume and cardiac output increase, and the blood flow to the different organs is redistributed (Carlin and Alfirevic, 2008). Consequently, a marked increase in the glomerular filtration rate is observed. According to Smith (2011), hematological parameters are modified as shown in Table 6.4 and include a gradual decline in hematocrit that is associated with an increased plasma volume. Finally, changes in inflammation factors (increase in acute phase proteins post-implantation, in fibrinogens, C-reactive protein and haptoglobin from

Table 6.4. Effects of pregnancy on hematological parameters (according to Smith, 2011)

Pregnancy duration	1st day	2 weeks	4 weeks	6 weeks	8 weeks	Term
Red blood cells (million/µL)	8.0	7.9	7.1	6.7	6.2	6.2
Packed cell volume (%)	36.1	37.0	33.0	32.0	28.0	29.0
Hemoglobin (gm/dL)	12.5	12.0	11.0	10.8	9.5	10.0
Reticulocytes (%, includes punctate)	9	11	99	10	20	15

mid-gestation, and also increase in the white blood cells post-implantation) are described in dogs and suspected in queens although not confirmed in this species (Verstegen-Onclin and Verstegen, 2008). All parameters have to be taken into account even though pharmacokinetics in the pregnant queen has not been studied specifically. Moreover, for each drug prescribed, two main aspects have to be taken into account: the drug toxicity for the fetuses and the stage of pregnancy. The feline placenta is endotheliochorial. This barrier allows high lipid solubility drugs to reach the fetuses. Drugs that are polar, ionized and protein bound, or water soluble are less likely to penetrate (Mathews, 2008).

Concerning anti-parasitic drugs, fenbendazole (50 mg/kg over 3 to 5 days) is often chosen for deworming during pregnancy. The use of avermectin is possible. It is important to choose an approved medication for pregnant queens to treat ectoparasites since some drugs like carbaryl may be teratogenic and causes dystocia in the bitch (see next paragraph). The use of fipronil appears safe during pregnancy and lactation.

Appendix 6.1 sums up the drugs currently used in veterinary practice and their safety when used during pregnancy (Papich and Davis, 1986; Mathews, 2008; Rebuelto and Loza, 2010).

6.6 Conclusion

In conclusion, pregnancy diagnosis is easy to perform in the queen and should be done as soon as possible. Ultrasound examination seems to be the most accurate tool since it allows not only to make the diagnosis but also to follow the pregnancy (vitality and growth of the conceptuses) and to estimate the parturition date. Radiography stays essential in order to count the fetuses before parturition. Those two examinations are complementary. Management of the pregnant queen is also essential. A balanced nutrition adapted to the pregnant status, an updated vaccination status, and a good deworming program are necessary to ensure a normal pregnancy, a normal lactation, and the good health of the neonates.

6.7 References

Beccaglia, M., Anastasi, P., Grimaldi, E., Rota, A., Faustini, M., *et al.* (2008a) Accuracy of the prediction of parturition date through ultrasonographic measurement of fetal parameters in the queen. *Veterinary Research Communications* 32, 99–101. doi: 10.1007/s11259-008-9107-1

Beccaglia, M., Faustini, M., and Luvoni, G. C. (2008b) Ultrasonographic study of deep portion of diencephalo-telencephalic vesicle for the determination of gestational age of the canine foetus. *Reproduction in Domestic Animals* 43, 367–370. doi: 10.1111/j.1439-0531.2007.00916.x

Blanco, P. G., Vercellini, R., Rube, A., Rodríguez, R., Arias, D. O., *et al.* (2016) Evaluation of feline uterine and umbilical arteries blood flow in a pharmacologically induced abnormal gestation model. *Theriogenology* 86, 2323–2327. doi: 10.1016/j.theriogenology.2016.07.028

Braun, B. C., Vargas, A., and Jewgenow, K. (2012) The molecular detection of relaxin and its receptor RXFP1 in reproductive tissue of *Felis catus* and *Lynx pardinus* during pregnancy. *Reproduction* 143, 399–410. doi: 10.1530/REP-11-0316

Brito, A.B., Miranda, S.A., Ruas, M.R., Santos, R.R., and Domingues, S.F.S. (2010) Assessment of feline fetal viability by conceptus echobiometry and triplex Doppler ultrasonography of uterine and umbilical arteries. *Animal Reproduction Science* 122, 276–281. doi: 10.1016/j.anireprosci.2010.09.003

Bücheler, J. (1999) Fading kitten syndrome and neonatal isoerythrolysis. *Veterinary Clinics of North American Small Animal Practice* 29, 853–870.

Carlin, A. and Alfirevic, Z. (2008) Physiological changes of pregnancy and monitoring. *Best Practice and Research Clinical Obstetrics and Gynaecology* 22, 801–823. doi: 10.1016/j.bpobgyn.2008.06.005

Concannon, P., Hodgson, B., and Lein, D. (1980) Reflex LH release in estrous cats following single and multiple copulations. *Biology of Reproduction* 23, 111–117. doi: 10.1095/biolreprod23.1.111

Concannon, P., Tsutsui, T., and Shille, V. (2001) Embryo development, hormonal requirements and maternal responses during canine pregnancy. *Journal of Reproduction and Fertility* Supplement 57, 169–179.

DiGangi, B. A., Griffin, B., Levy, J. K., Smith, B. F., and Baker, H. J. (2010) Use of a commercially available relaxin test for detection of pregnancy in cats. *Journal of the American Veterinary Medical Association* 237, 1267–1274. doi: 10.2460/javma.237.11.1267

England, G. C. W. (2010) Physiology and endocrinology of the female. In: England, G. C. W. and Heimendahl, A. (eds) *BSAVA Manual of Canine and Feline Reproduction and Neonatology*. British Small Animal Veterinary Association, Gloucester, UK, pp. 1–12.

Fournier, A., Masson, M., Corbière, F., Mila, H., Mariani, C., *et al.* (2017) Epidemiological analysis of reproductive performances and kitten mortality rates in 5,303 purebred queens of 45 different breeds and 28,065 kittens in France. *Reproduction in Domestic Animals* 52, 153–157. doi: 10.1111/rda.12844

Fresno, L., Rodriguez-Gil, J. E., Rigau, T., Pastor, J., and Rivera del Alamo, M.M. (2012) Modulation of the biochemical composition of amniotic and allantoic fluids as a control mechanism of feline foetal development. *Placenta* 33, 522–527. doi: 10.1016/j.placenta.2012.03.002

García Mitacek, M. C., Stornelli, M. C., Praderio, R. G., de la Sota, R. L., and Stornelli, M. A. (2015) Ultrasonographic and progesterone changes during Days 21 to 63 of pregnancy in queens. *Theriogenology* 84, 1131–1141. doi: 10.1016/j.theriogenology.2015.06.014

Gatel, L., Rault, D., Chalvet-Monfray, K., Saunders, J., and Buff, S. (2015) Prediction of parturition time in queens using radiography and ultrasonography. *Anatomia, Histologia, Embryologia* 44, 241–246. doi: 10.1111/ahe.12130

Hand, M. S., Thatcher, C. D., Remillard, R. L., Roudebush, P., and Novotny, B. (2010) Feeding reproducing cats. In: Hand, M. S., Thatcher, C. D., Remillard, R. L., Roudebush, P., and Novotny, B. (eds) *Small Animal Clinical Nutrition*. Mark Morris Institute, Topeka, Kansas, pp. 401–413.

Haney, D. R., Levy, J. K., Newell, S. M., Graham, J. P., and Gorman, S. P. (2003) Use of fetal skeletal mineralization for prediction of parturition date in cats. *Journal of the American Veterinary Medical Association* 223, 1614–1616. doi: 10.2460/javma.2003.223.1614

Johnston, S. D., Root Kustritz, M. V., and Olson, P. N. S. (2001) Feline pregnancy. In: Johnston, S. D., Root Kutritz, M. V. and Olson, P. N. S. (eds) *Canine and Feline Theriogenology*. Saunders, London, pp. 414–430.

Keiser, R., Reichler, I. M., and Balogh, O. (2017) Are foetal ultrasonographic and maternal blood progesterone measurements near parturition reliable predictors of the time of birth in the domestic cat? *Reproduction in Domestic Animals* 52, 487–494. doi: 10.1111/rda.12939

Knospe, C. (2002) Periods and stages of the prenatal development of the domestic cat. *Anatomia, Histologia, Embryologia* 31, 37–51. doi: 10.1046/j.1439-0264.2002.00360.x

Levy, X. and England, C.W. (2010) Pregnancy diagnosis, normal pregnancy and parturition in the queen. In: England, G. C. W. and Heimendahl, A. (eds) *BSAVA Manual of Canine and Feline Reproduction and Neonatalogy*. British Small Animal Veterinary Association, Gloucester, UK, pp. 98–105.

Lopate, C. (2018) Gestational aging and determination of parturition date in the bitch and queen using ultrasonography and radiography. *Veterinary Clinics of North America Small Animal Practices* 48, 617–638. doi: 10.1016/j.cvsm.2018.02.008

Malandain, E., Rault, D., Froment, E., Baudon, S., Desquilbet, L., *et al.* (2011) Follicular growth monitoring in the female cat during estrus. *Theriogenology* 76, 1337–1346. doi: 10.1016/j.theriogenology.2011.06.002

Mathews, K. A. (2008) Pain management for the pregnant, lactating, and neonatal to pediatric cat and dog. *Veterinary Clinics of North America Small Animal Practice* 38, 1291–1308. doi: 10.1016/j.cvsm.2008.07.001

Miglino, M. A., Ambrósio, C. E., Martins, D. dos S., Wenceslau, C. V., Pfarrer, C., *et al.* (2006) The carnivore pregnancy: The development of the embryo and fetal membranes. *Theriogenology* 66, 1699–1702. doi: 10.1016/j.theriogenology.2006.02.027

Papich, M. G. and Davis, L. E., 1986. Drug therapy during pregnancy and in the neonate. *Veterinary Clinics of North America Small Animal Practice* 16, 525–538. doi: 10.1016/S0195-5616(86)50058-9

Pereira, B. S., Freire, L. M. P., Pinto, J. N., Domingues, S. F. S., and Silva, L. D. M. (2012) Triplex Doppler evaluation of uterine arteries in cyclic and pregnant domestic cats. *Animal Reproduction Science* 130, 99–104. doi: 10.1016/j.anireprosci.2011.12.019

Pieri, N., Souza, A., Casals, J., Roballo, K., Ambrósio, C., *et al.* (2015) Comparative development of embryonic age by organogenesis in domestic dogs and cats. *Reproduction in Domestic Animals* 50, 625–631. doi: 10.1111/rda.12539

Rebuelto, M. and Loza, M. E. (2010) Antibiotic treatment of dogs and cats during pregnancy. *Veterinary Medicine International* 2010:385640. doi: 10.4061/2010/385640

Root Kustritz, M. V. (2006) Clinical management of pregnancy in cats. *Theriogenology* 66, 145–150. doi: 10.1016/j.theriogenology.2006.03.018

Scotti, L., Di Salvo, P., Bocci, F., Pieramati, C., and Polisca, A. (2008) Doppler evaluation of maternal and foetal vessels during normal gestation in queen. *Theriogenology* 69, 1111–1119. doi: 10.1016/j.theriogenology.2008.01.025

Siemieniuch, M. J., Jursza, E., Szostek, A. Z., Skarzynski, D. J., Boos, A., *et al.* (2012) Steroidogenic capacity of the placenta as a supplemental source of progesterone during pregnancy in domestic cats. *Reproductive*

Biology and Endocrinology 10, 89. doi: 10.1186/1477-7827-10-89

Smith, F. O. (2011) Prenatal care of the bitch and queen, In: Peterson, M. E. and Kutzler, M. A. (eds) *Small Animals Pediatrics: The First 12 Months of Life*. Elsevier, St. Louis, Missouri, pp. 1–10.

Socha, P. and Janowski, T. (2019) Development of specific fetometric formulas of ICC and BP for predicting the parturition date in Maine Coon queens. *Reproduction in Domestic Animals* 54, 622–626. doi: 10.1111/rda.13404

Stewart, D. R. and Stabenfeldt, G. H. (1985) Relaxin activity in the pregnant cat. *Biology of Reproduction* 32, 848–854. doi: 10.1095/biolreprod32.4.848

Topie, E., Bencharif, D., Briand, L., and Tainturier, D. (2015) Early pregnancy diagnosis and monitoring in the queen using ultrasonography with a 12.5 MHz probe. *Journal of Feline Medicine and Surgery* 17, 87–93. doi: 10.1177/1098612X14532088

Tsutsui, T., Suzuki, Y., Toyonaga, M., Oba, H., Mizutani, T., *et al.* (2009) The role of the ovary for the maintenance of pregnancy in cats. *Reproduction in Domestic Animals* 44, 120–124. doi: 10.1111/j.1439-0531.2009.01452.x

van Dorsser, F. D. H., Lasano, S., and Steinetz, B. G. (2007) Pregnancy diagnosis in cats using a rapid, bench-top kit to detect relaxin in urine. *Reproduction in Domestic Animals* 42, 111–112. doi: 10.1111/j.1439-0531.2006.00736.x

Verstegen, J. P., Onclin, K., Silva, L. D., and Donnay, I. (1993a) Abortion induction in the cat using prostaglandin F2 alpha and a new anti-prolactinic agent, cabergoline. *Journal of Reproduction and Fertility* Supplement 47, 411–417.

Verstegen, J. P., Onclin, K., Silva, L. D., Wouters-Ballman, P., Delahaut, P., *et al.* (1993b) Regulation of progesterone during pregnancy in the cat: Studies on the roles of corpora lutea, placenta and prolactin secretion. *Journal of Reproduction and Fertility* Supplement 47, 165–173.

Verstegen-Onclin, K. and Verstegen, J. (2008) Endocrinology of pregnancy in the dog: A review. *Theriogenology* 70, 291–299. doi: 10.1016/j.theriogenology.2008.04.038

Wichert, B., Schade, L., Gebert, S., Bucher, B., Zottmaier, B., *et al.* (2009) Energy and protein needs of cats for maintenance, gestation and lactation. *Journal of Feline Medicine and Surgery* 11, 808–815. doi: 10.1016/j.jfms.2009.02.006

Zambelli, D. (2012) Feline neonatal physiology, behavior, and socialization. In: Lopate, C. (ed.) *Management of Pregnant and Neonatal Dogs, Cats, and Exotic Pets*. John Wiley & Sons, Ames, Iowa, pp. 147–158.

Zambelli, D., Caneppele, B., Bassi, S., and Paladini, C. (2002a) Ultrasound aspects of fetal and extrafetal structures in pregnant cats. *Journal of Feline Medicine and Surgery* 4, 95–106. doi: 10.1053/jfms.2001.0153

Zambelli, D., Castagnetti, C., Belluzzi, S., and Bassi, S. (2002b) Correlation between the age of the conceptus and various ultrasonographic measurements during the first 30 days of pregnancy in domestic cats (*Felis catus*). *Theriogenology* 57, 1981–1987. doi: 10.1016/s0093-691x(01)00686-0

Zambelli, D., Castagnetti, C., Belluzzi, S., and Paladini, C. (2004) Correlation between fetal age and ultrasonographic measurements during the second half of pregnancy in domestic cats (*Felis catus*). *Theriogenology* 62, 1430–1437. doi: 10.1016/j.theriogenology.2004.02.009

Zschockelt, L., Amelkina, O., Siemieniuch, M. J., Koster, S., Jewgenow, K., *et al.* (2014) Corpora lutea of pregnant and pseudopregnant domestic cats reveal similar steroidogenic capacities during the luteal life span. *Journal of Steroid Biochemistry and Molecular Biology* 144, 373–381. doi: 10.1016/j.jsbmb.2014.08.010

Appendix 6.1

Usual drugs used in carnivores and their use during pregnancy according to Papich and Davis (1986). Classification:

A: Probably safe. Although specific studies may not have proved the safety of all drugs in dogs and cats, there are no reports of adverse effects in laboratory animals or in women.

B: Safe for use if used cautiously. Studies in laboratory animals may have uncovered some risk, but these drugs appear to be safe in dogs and cats or these drugs are safe if they are not administered when the animal is near term.

C: These drugs may have potential risks. Studies in people or laboratory animals have uncovered risks, and these drugs should be used cautiously, as a last resort when the benefit of therapy clearly outweighs the risks.

0: Contraindicated. These drugs have been shown to cause congenital malformations or embryotoxicity.

Drug categories	Molecule	Classification	Known side effects in different species	Forbidden period during pregnancy	Specificities
Antimicrobial drugs	Betalactams Cephalosporins Lincosamides Macrolides	A	N/A or information not known		
	Specific Macrolide: Tylosin	B	No information	No information	N/A or information not known
	Sulfonamides		Mice/Rat: congenital malformations, Women: neonatal icterus	Avoid long-acting drugs	N/A or information not known
	Trimethoprim-sulfadiazine		Trimethoprim is teratogenic in rat but probably safe in other species	N/A or information not known	N/A or information not known
	Aminoglycosides	C	Neurotoxic and nephrotoxic in fetuses	N/A or information not known	Gentamicin can be used cautiously if necessary
	Metronidazole		Congenital malformation and embryotoxicity	First 3 weeks	N/A or information not known
	Chloramphenicol		Decrease protein synthesis in fetuses, particularly in bone marrow	N/A or information not known	
	Fluoroquinolones	D	Articular, cartilage defects in fetuses	After 10 days post-ovulation	N/A or information not known
	Tetracycline		Bone and teeth malformations in fetus and toxicity in mother	N/A or information not known	
	Specific aminoglycoside: Streptomycin		Neurotoxic and nephrotoxic in fetuses		

Continued

Continued.

Drug categories	Molecule	Classification	Known side effects in different species	Forbidden period during pregnancy	Specificities
	Specific aminoglycoside: Neomycin	A	N/A or information not known		
Anti-parasitic drugs	Praziquantel Piperazine Fenbendazole Ivermectin	A	N/A or information not known		
	Amitraz	D	WARNING Lethal in cats		
Antifungal drugs	Miconazole	A	N/A or information not known	N/A or information not known	
	Ketoconazole	B	Teratogenic and embryotoxic in rats, antiandrogenic, stillbirth in dogs		
	Amphotericin B	C	Congenital anomalies		
	Griseofulvin	D	Teratogenic in rats, skeleton and brain malformation in cats		
Anticancer	Doxorubicin Azathioprine Chlorambucil Cisplatin Cyclophosphamide Methotrexate Vincristine	C	Teratogenic and embryotoxic Congenital malformation but used in women Teratogenic and embryotoxic Teratogenic, embryotoxic and nephrotoxic Congenital malformation, embryotoxic and nephrotoxic Malformation in newborn and embryotoxicity	N/A or information not known	
Analgesic	Acetaminophen Aspirin, salicylate	C	WARNING Toxic in cats Embryotoxic in laboratory animals	Late in pregnancy: pulmonary hypertension and bleeding	N/A or information not known
	Flunixin meglumine Indomethacin		No information N/A or information not known	Late in pregnancy: premature closure of ductus arteriosus	Toxic in **DOGS**
	Phenylbutazone		No information (possible bone marrow suppression used in a long period)		

Continued

Continued.

Drug categories	Molecule	Classification	Known side effects in different species	Forbidden period during pregnancy	Specificities
Anesthetic	Lidocaine	A	Safe as all local anesthetic agents for local nerve block and epidural	N/A or information not known	
	Naloxone		Safe in newborns within a few minutes after birth		
	Morphine	B	Neonatal sedation and respiratory depression => REVERSIBLE with naloxone in newborns after cesarean sections		
	Fentanyl, Butorphanol, Codeine, Oxymorphone		Safe for short-term use. Neonatal sedation and respiratory depression => REVERSIBLE with naloxone		
	Acepromazine		Neonatal central nervous system depression	Avoid near term	N/A or information not known
	Atropine		May cause fetal tachycardia but seem safe	N/A or information not known	
	Glycopyrrolate		Safe in laboratory animals, does not cross the placenta as readily as atropine		
	Isoflurane/ sevoflurane		N/A or information not known		
	Ketamine		Safe but may produce premature labor		
	Xylazine, Methoxyflurane	C	Neonatal depression in cesarean section use		
Gastrointestinal	Anti-acids Sucralfate	A	Safe	Safety of ranitidine and cimetidine not established	
	Anti-emetics	B	Probably safe in short-term use	No information in dogs and cats, metoclopramide safe in laboratory animals	
	Laxative			N/A or information not known	
	Loperamide	C	Adverse effects in laboratory animals but not reported in dogs, cats, and humans		
	Misoprostol	D	Pregnancy termination	From 2d half of pregnancy: abortion	

Continued

Continued.

Drug categories	Molecule	Classification	Known side effects in different species	Forbidden period during pregnancy	Specificities
Cardiovascular	Digitalis	A	Probably safe	N/A or information not known	
	Furosemide	B	Probably safe		
	Dopamine		Probably safe at therapeutic dose but pregnancy termination at high doses	N/A or information not known	
	Heparin		Does not cross placenta	N/A or information not known	
	Theophylline		No reports of adverse effect		
	Quinidine		Probably safe but may cause fetal bradycardia		
	Propranolol	C	Fetal bradycardia, respiratory depression, neonatal hypoglycemia	Avoid near term	N/A or information not known
Anti-convulsant	Phenobarbital	B	Rare congenital defects and bleeding tendency in newborn but may be the best option that others	N/A or information not known	
	Diazepam	C	Congenital malformations in laboratory animals and Human		
Myorelaxants	Dantrolene	C	Safety not established		
Endocrine	Thyroxine	B	Does not cross the placenta	N/A or information not known	
	Betamethasone, Cortisone, Dexamethasone, Flumethasone	C	Increased incidence of cleft palates, and other congenital malformations and can induce premature labor and abortion	N/A or information not known	Abortion in dogs
	Estradiol cypronate	D	Malformation of male and female genital tract + bone marrow aplasia		
	Androgens		Masculinization of fetuses		
	Mitotane		Adrenocortical necrosis	N/A or information not known	Forbidden

7 Causes of Abortion

Jamie M. Douglas and Aime K. Johnson

Auburn University College of Veterinary Medicine, Department of Clinical Sciences, Auburn, Alabama, USA

7.1 Introduction

Pregnancy loss, and the many ways in which it occurs, is a common cause of infertility in the breeding queen (Johnston, 2001; Little, 2012). Pregnancy loss occurs early in gestation via fetal resorption. At term, fetuses may be stillborn. When fetal death occurs, retention of a fetus *in utero* can lead to maceration or mummification (Fig. 7.1). Pregnancy loss can even be medically induced by veterinary professionals through use of pharmacologic agents.

Abortion describes a state in which fetuses are prematurely expelled prior to the natural end of gestation. Abortion is further defined as delivery of one or more fetuses that cannot survive outside of the uterus (Verstegen *et al.*, 2008). An entire litter may be aborted or, less commonly, just a few individuals with the remaining litter being carried to term. In the event that abortion does occur, effort must be made to investigate its etiology. At a minimum, investigating the etiology of abortion should include acquisition of a detailed history, a thorough physical examination of the queen, and necropsy of aborted fetuses. Other modalities useful to abortion investigation include bloodwork and imaging modalities like ultrasound and radiographs. Investigation should occur swiftly to improve chances of a diagnosis.

Etiology of abortion in the queen can be divided into two general categories: noninfectious or infectious. The remainder of this chapter aims to familiarize the reader with common causes in both categories.

7.2 Noninfectious Abortion

Noninfectious causes of abortion, by definition, are those that cannot be communicated via pathogens. When it comes to noninfectious abortion in cats, both maternal and fetal factors play a role in their development. Maternal factors include underlying uterine pathology, disease burden, drug exposure, toxin exposure, and nutritional imbalance. Fetal factors often include toxin and teratogen exposure, chromosomal defect, and congenital defect.

A common disease encountered in the uterus of aging queens is cystic endometrial hyperplasia (CEH) (Johnston, 2001; Agudelo, 2005; Schlafer and Gifford, 2008). Cystic endometrial hyperplasia is believed to be an underreported cause of noninfectious abortion and pregnancy loss in the queen, likely due to the need for advanced imaging for identification and characterization of the disease. Hyperplastic changes within the endometrium cater to the formation of endometrial cysts, which vary in size, number, and distribution (Agudelo, 2005; Schlafer and Gifford, 2008). The number, size, and distribution of cysts is prone to increase in the endometrium as queens age. Over time, the queen's endometrium may become inhospitable to maintenance of offspring. This can manifest as implantation failure, early embryonic death, and abortion, as influenced by degree of uterine disease. In queens with CEH, definitive diagnosis is often difficult to obtain prior to spay; however, advanced ultrasonographic study can aid in reaching diagnosis of CEH. Unfortunately, not only are the cystic changes of CEH irreversible, but they also predispose affected queens to development of pyometra (Agudelo, 2005). Alongside pregnancy loss and abortion, cessation of fertility is a likely sequela of CEH, and ovariohysterectomy of the queen is treatment of choice for the condition.

The availability of commercial cat diets has greatly reduced the incidence of noninfectious abortion as a result of nutritional imbalance (Verstegen, 2008). However, as the popularity of feeding home-prepared or raw diets increases, unintentional reproductive consequences are likely. A general threat of the non-commercial cat diet is

DOI: 10.1079/9781789247107.0007

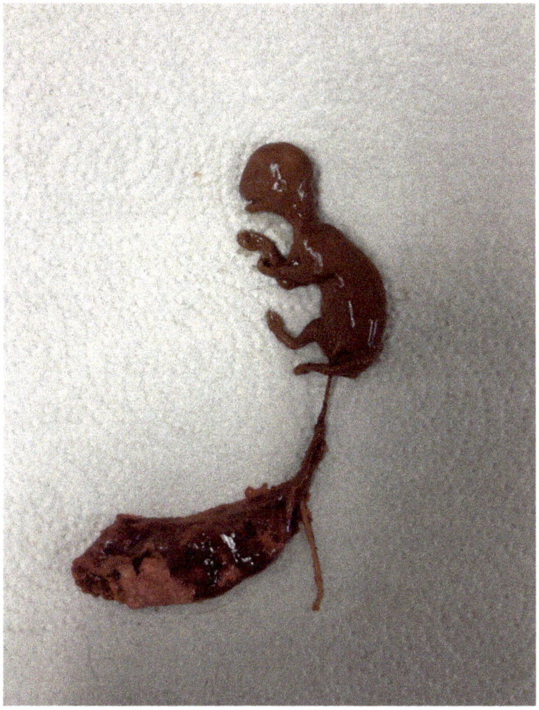

Fig. 7.1. Image of a mummified fetus, placenta attached, aborted by a queen. (Image: author's own.)

improper or insufficient caloric intake. The diet of the gestating queen must meet the energy demands of the queen herself, the growing embryos or fetuses, and the remodeling of her body and mammary chains. When the queen's diet cannot efficiently meet all of these demands on her energy reserves, reproductive investment can be sacrificed. This sacrifice often results in early termination of pregnancy via fetal resorption, early embryonic death, and abortion.

An additional threat of the non-commercial cat diet is absent or inadequate concentrations of taurine. Taurine is an essential amino acid in cats, which are obligate carnivores (Hayes, 1982; Herrick *et al.*, 2018). Essential amino acids are those that cannot be made by the body and must be acquired through the diet. Discovery that taurine was essential in the cat was made in 1975 (Hayes and Trautwein, 1989). For the wild felid catching and consuming prey to meet this requirement, taurine deficiency is uncommon due to the amino acid's abundance in animal tissues. For the domestic housecat, which moved inside the home to receive scheduled feedings of commercial cat chows, taurine deficiency became a problem. Since discovery of the health threats posed by taurine deficiency, commercial cat diets are now commonly fortified with taurine (Sturman, 1992). In households creating home-cooked, raw, or vegetarian diets, risk of taurine deficiency poses imminent threat. Reproductive consequences of taurine deficiency in the gravid queen include reduced litter size, stillbirth, fetal resorption, and abortion (Herrick *et al.*, 2018). Additional clinical signs in cats and kittens include growth retardation, gait abnormality, central retinal degeneration, blindness, dilated cardiomyopathy, hepatic lipidosis, and neurologic deficit (Sturman *et al.*, 1986; Ferasin *et al.*, 2003; Rothuizen, 2020). Perinatal consequences include nursing kittens with poor thriftiness, a consequence of poor milk and poor colostral quality. If taurine deficiency is suspected, plasma, whole blood, or urine samples can be assessed for taurine concentrations via high performance liquid chromatography or amino acid analyzer (Heinze *et al.*, 2009). It is vitally important that the diet of a breeding queen meets her nutritional demands at all stages.

Another fact that cannot be understated is that administration of medications poses risks during feline pregnancy. The majority of medications, including those employed in both human and veterinary medicine, cross into and can accumulate in the placenta (Al-Enazy *et al.*, 2017). While the effects of many medications on developing fetuses are unknown, it is known that many medications can reach significant concentrations in the fetal tissues. Drugs that are considered teratogens are those that cause direct or indirect structural or functional changes in the fetus (Wiebe and Howard, 2009). A working list of teratogenic drugs to avoid administering to the gravid queens has been previously compiled and is summarized in Table 7.1 (Papich and Davis, 1986; Mathews and Sinclair, 2018). As to the extent to which these drugs cause abortion, that information is largely unknown. It is safe to assume that teratogenic drugs that affect placental blood supply, target developing tissues, or negatively affect viability could lead to abortion. In general, drug administration should be avoided in the pregnant queen. If drugs must be administered, review of published data regarding reproductive threat should be performed.

Ingestion of toxins, plants, even human medications, pose risk to the pregnant queen. Hazardous substances commonly found in and around the household, the list is non-exhaustive, include

Table 7.1. Drug use in pregnant cats and potential effects on the fetus. Modified from: Mathews and Sinclair, (2018); Papich and Davis (1986); and Romm (2010).

Drug class	Drug	Effect on fetus
Antimicrobials	Chloraphenicol	Fetal death
	Nitrofurantoin	Fetal Hemolysis
	Streptomycin	Ototoxicity, congenital anomalies
	Gentamicin	Nephrotoxicity, ototoxicity
	Amikacin	Ototoxicity
	Tetracycline	Altered bone and tooth development
	Trimethoprim	Teratogenic
	Sulfonamides	Liver dysfunction, hyperbilirubinemia
	Amphotericin B	Congenital anomalies
	Griseofulvin	Congenital anomalies
	Fluocytosine	Congenital anomalies
	Erythromycin estolate	Liver disease in dam
	Metronidazole	Mutagenesis in lab animals
Anti-inflammatory drugs	NSAID (aspirin, phenylbutazone, indomethacin)	Premature closure of the ductus arteriosus, neonatal bleeding, nephrosis, pulmonary hypertension, prolongs onset of labor
	Ketamine	Can increase uterine tone and cause abortion. Doses up 0.25 mg/kg appear to be safe
	Glucocorticoids	Cleft Palate
	Alpha$_2$ adrenoceptor agonists	No reported studies showing it as safe, so use should be avoided
	Dimethyl sulfoxide	Congenital anomalies
	Gabapentin	Appears to be safe for use
	Pregabalin	Associated with increased risk of birth defects in first trimester exposure
	Amantadine	Not recommended for use
	Local Anesthetics	Considered safe and non-teratogenic
Anticonvulsants	Phenytoin	Congenital anomalies
	Diazepam	Neonatal depression
	Phenobarbital	Hemorrhage in newborn
	Primidone	Hemorrhage in newborn
Miscellaneous drugs	Androgens	Masculinization of female fetus
	Acetazolamide	Fetal anomalies
	Amitriptyline	Limb deformities and developmental delays have been reported in humans along with neonatal withdrawal symptoms
	Chlorpromazine	Hepatic necrosis, fetal tachycardia
	Cholinesterase inhibitors	Neonatal myasthenia
	Cyclizine	Congenital anomalies
	EDTA	Congenital anomalies
	Estrogens	Feminization of male fetus, abortion
	Gold Salts	Congenital anomalies
	Iodides	Fetal goiter
	Isoproterenol	Fetal tachycardia
	Lithium Salts	Fetal goiter
	Meclizine	Congenital anomalies
	Methoxamine	Fetal hypoxia
	Meperidine	Patent ductus arteriosus
	Prochlorperazine	Congenital anomalies
	Propranolol	Hypoglycemia, fetal bradycardia
	Phenylephrine	Fetal Hypoxia

Continued

Table 7.1. Continued.

Drug class	Drug	Effect on fetus
	Quinine	Thrombocytopenia
	Reserpine	Respiratory obstruction
	Thiazides	Fetal death
	Tolbutamide	Hypoglycemia
Nutraceuticals	Vitamin A	Large doses can cause fetal anomalies
	Vitamin D	Large doses can cause CNS dysfunction
	Vitamin K	Hyperbilirubinemia
	Scotch broom	Can cause abortion
	Mugwort	Can cause abortion
	Yarrow	Can cause abortion
Opioids	Methadone	Parenteral and oral transmucosal routes have been reported safe in cats
	Fentanyl	High doses throughout pregnancy have caused withdrawal symptoms in newborn humans
	Hydromorphone	Caused fetal tachycardia in humans
	Morphine	Therapeutic use during pregnancy can cause neonatal withdrawal symptoms
	Buprenorphine	Can reportedly cause neonatal withdrawal symptoms
	Butorphanol	No reported effects
Anesthesia	Nitrous oxide	Teratogenic in humans
	Bensodiazepines	Repeated uses are teratogenic in humans

acetaminophen, birth control pills, blood pressure medication, topical steroid creams, chocolate, xylitol, onions, garlic, raisins, grapes, alcohol, bleach, disinfectants, fertilizers, insecticides, rodenticides, and antifreeze. While most cats are discriminate eaters, ingestion of these hazardous substances when not properly stored and secured is possible. The myriad of ways in which ingestion of any of these hazardous substances causes disease is vast. Recall that the dose of the poison often dictates severity of illness. Abortion can result if the dose is high enough and the dam's overall health can no longer support pregnancy.

Other fetal factors in cases of feline pregnancy loss include congenital and chromosomal abnormalities. Congenital abnormalities may include gastroschisis (Fig. 7.2), cleft palate, or other fetal monster. Some may be carried to full term, while others are aborted during pregnancy. Chromosomal abnormalities account for 15% of pregnancy loss in domestic animals (Berepubo and Long, 1983). Monogenic (or single-gene) traits, observed in the cat include Manx syndrome, where inheritance of two mutant tailless Manx (*M*) genes disrupt central nervous system development in the early embryo, which can later cause abortion (Deforest and Basrur, 1979; Robinson, 1993). Chromosomal errors of developing fetuses reported to cause pregnancy loss in the cat include trisomy of autosome D-2, reported to be responsible for *in utero* maceration, and X-chromosome monosomy (37,XO), contributing to stillbirth (Long and Berepubo, 1980; Johnston *et al.*, 1983; Mayr *et al.*, 1994; Balogh *et al.*, 2015). Data regarding distinct chromosomal abnormalities that cause abortion are greatly lacking in the cat. Diagnosis can be made by submitting fetal tissue and blood for karyotyping, but this is rarely performed due to expense.

7.3 Infectious Abortion

7.3.1 Viral pathogens

Of the infectious pathogens that contribute to feline abortion, viral pathogens are among the most important. First for discussion is feline herpesvirus-1 (FeHV-1) infection in the queen (Hoover and Griesemer, 1971; Johnston, 2001; Gaskell *et al.*, 2007). Feline herpesvirus-1 is a member of the *Alphaherpesvirinae* subfamily of family *Herpesviridae* (Davison *et al.*, 2009). Domestic cats are the primary host for FeHV-1, though lions and cheetahs are also susceptible (Gaskell *et al.*, 2007).

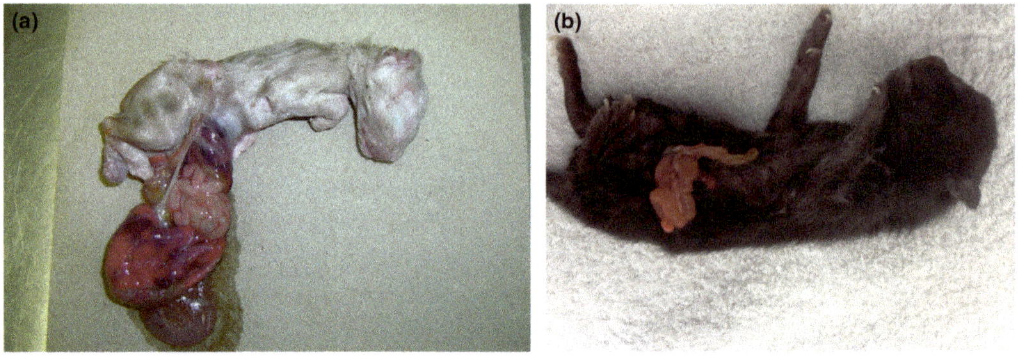

Fig. 7.2. Two feline fetuses aborted late gestation with varying severity of gastroschisis: **(a)** is severe, **(b)** is mild. Both were delivered dead. (Image: author's own.)

The incubation period of FeHV-1 is typically between 2 and 6 days, though it can be longer (Gaskell and Povey, 1979). Acutely infected cats transmit FeHV-1 via direct contact with infected oronasal and ocular secretions, though viral transmission can reactivate after a period of latency in historically infected cats (Gaskell *et al.*, 2007; Verstegen *et al.*, 2008; Maes, 2012). Vertical transmission of the virus *in utero* has not been shown outside of experimental conditions (Verstegen *et al.*, 2008).

Of the host of symptoms that result from FeHV-1 infection, viral rhinotracheitis and ocular lesions are most common. Clinical signs include fever, nasal and ocular discharge, ptyalism, paroxysmal sneezing, dyspnea, anorexia, dehydration, and weight loss (Hoover and Griesemer, 1971; Maes, 2012). For the gravid queen, exposure to FeHV-1 is classically documented to cause late-stage abortion, though controlled experiments assessing consequences of FeHV-1 inoculation during early and mid-stage gestation are lacking. Research performed in 1971 reported experimental FeHV-1 infection of queens between day 42 and day 50 of gestation with abortion occurring in all queens. However, the authors of this article felt that abortion was a nonspecific reaction secondary to severe, debilitating upper respiratory disease (Hoover and Griesemer, 1971). Record of partial abortion of one fetus 3-weeks prepartum in a queen experimentally inoculated with FeHV-1 followed by delivery of two healthy kittens at term is also reported (Hoover and Griesemer, 1971; Verstegen *et al.*, 2008). Current general consensus is that FeHV-1 as a cause of abortion in the cat is uncommon (Gaskell *et al.*, 2007).

Grossly, significant lesions are not typically reported in placentas or fetuses following FeHV-1 abortion, though edema, congestion, and placental site hemorrhage are reported to occur in the queen's uterus (Hoover and Griesemer, 1971). Atypically, fetal autolysis and partial maceration has been observed. Of interest, young kittens that acquire FeHV-1 infection can show skeletal deformity alongside previously described clinical signs, a consequence of viral predilection for regions of skeletal growth (Gaskell *et al.*, 2007). Diagnosis of FeHV-1 is made after assessment of discharge or tissue homogenates via direct fluorescent antibody (FA) test, virus isolation (VI), or polymerase chain reaction (PCR) (Gaskell *et al.*, 2007; Gould, 2011; Maes, 2012).

Treatment of FeHV-1 is largely supportive, ideally emphasizing restoration of fluids, appetite, and appropriate treatment of symptoms. Vaccination is recommended for prevention of FeHV-1 infection in cats, consisting of an initial two-dose vaccination regimen with first vaccine administered no sooner than 6 weeks of age and then every 3-4 weeks until the kitten reaches 20 weeks of age. Revaccination is then recommended at 6 months of age to decrease window of susceptibility if maternally-derived antibodies were present at last booster, after which booster vaccination can occur every 3 years (Stone *et al.*, 2020). In the United States, both modified-live and inactivated vaccines are available for use. In the pregnant queen, safety concerns dictate that the inactivated vaccine is preferred.

Feline immunodeficiency virus (FIV) causes an acquired immunodeficiency syndrome in cats (Elder *et al.*, 2010). Feline immunodeficiency virus is a member of the *Orthoretrovirinae* subfamily of family *Retroviridae* (Elder *et al.*, 2010; Kenyon and Lever, 2011). The virus is a single-stranded RNA (ssRNA) lentivirus, a genus of viruses characterized by extensive incubation periods, persisting throughout life, and possessing high mutation rates. Feline immunodeficiency virus infects both domestic and wild felid species and will also infect hyenas (Troyer *et al.*, 2005). The mode of transmission of FIV is primarily via bite and associated saliva, though transplacental, lactational, and venereal transmission also occur. Once FIV has been transmitted, the virus persists in the host's blood supply and lymphoid tissues (Kolenda-Roberts *et al.*, 2007). There are three stages of FIV infection: acute, subclinical, and terminal (Hartmann, 2011).

On average, the acute stage of FIV infection occurs within the first 3 months of exposure (Kolenda-Roberts *et al.*, 2007). While rare, transplacental FIV infection is reported in naturally-infected cats. In experimentally-infected cats, vertical transmission of FIV is common in gravid queens (O'Neil *et al.*, 1996; Kolenda-Roberts *et al.*, 2007; Medeiros *et al.*, 2012). Semen collected from infected toms has been shown to transmit FIV to uninfected queens (Coats, 2005). *In utero* transmission of FIV can cause fetal and neonatal death via abortion, stillbirth, or failure-to-thrive in kittens born alive. Neonates are more severely affected by FIV infection due to severe immunologic deficit (Kolenda-Roberts *et al.*, 2007). Additional symptoms observed in FIV-infected queens include fever, gingivitis-stomatitis, lymphadenopathy, neutropenia, and cachexia (Elder *et al.*, 2010; Kenyon and Lever, 2011). Gross lesions are largely dependent on the stage of FIV infection. On histology, lymphoid lesions have progressive hyperplastic change, evidenced by increased number and/or size of lymphoid follicles (Orandle and Baldwin, 1995).

In breeding catteries, rigid quarantine protocols and rigorous screening for FIV is essential. If infected cats are identified, they should be immediately removed from the cattery to limit spread of the virus, all cats should be tested, and no new cats should be introduced pending results and management decisions following subsequent testing 3–6 months later (Little, 2012; Scherk *et al.*, 2013). Cats that acquire FIV infection are persistently infected throughout life (Hosie *et al.*, 2009). Diagnosis of FIV infection is confirmed via VI, PCR, or indirect FA following positive in-practice ELISA result. Treatment of FIV-positive cats is largely symptomatic and supportive care, emphasizing frequent health screening, aggressive resolution of clinical signs, and may incorporate antibiotics, corticosteroids, and antiviral therapy (O'Neil *et al.*, 1996; Hosie *et al.*, 2009; Hartmann, 2011). An inactivated, whole-virus vaccine is available for prevention. The vaccine is only recommended for use in high-risk cats, due to diagnostic test interference, uncertain efficacy, and risk of vaccine-associated sarcomas (Scherk *et al.*, 2013; Day *et al.*, 2016). It is important to note that existing serologic assays cannot differentiate between natural infection and vaccination. Breeding of FIV-positive cats is not recommended.

Feline leukemia virus (FeLV) is also a member of the *Orthoretrovirinae* subfamily of family *Retroviridae*; however, FeLV is a ssRNA gammaretrovirus (Hartmann, 2011). Compared to FIV, FeLV has higher pathogenicity and has a greater impact on fetal mortality (Hartmann, 2011). Feline leukemia virus affects domestic and small wild felids, and its mode of transmission is via direct contact with saliva, nasal secretions, and milk from infected host. Viremia manifests once bone marrow becomes infected, typically within 2–3 weeks (Hartmann, 2011; Sykes and Hartmann, 2014). Cats become latently infected with FeLV once acquired, and infected queens can pass FeLV transplacentally to their offspring (Hartmann, 2011). Reproductive failures include fetal resorption, abortion, and neonatal death, known as 'fading kitten syndrome' (Hartmann, 2011). Abortions typically occur in late gestation, with expelled fetuses having a normal appearance. Loss of pregnancy is associated with direct fetal infection (Verstegen *et al.*, 2008).

Similar to protocols for managing FIV-infected cats in catteries, FeLV-infected cats should be immediately removed from the cattery to limit spread. Diagnosis of FeLV in blood is performed first using ELISA; samples testing positive on ELISA should be followed by confirmation of infection via indirect FA, VI, or PCR methodologies (Lutz *et al.*, 2009). Further research is needed to define what histologic lesions develop from FeLV infection at the fetus and placenta. The FeLV vaccine is considered a core annual vaccine in kittens and cats less than 1 year of age, while the FeLV vaccine is considered non-core in low-risk adult cats (Stone *et al.*, 2020). For cats in high-risk settings, where risk of infection can be as high as 33%, the FeLV vaccine is recommended (Scherk *et al.*, 2013; Day *et al.*, 2016). Similar to previously discussed diseases, treatment is largely symptomatic and supportive and may incorporate corticosteroids, pain management, appetite stimulants, and antiviral therapies (Lutz *et al.*, 2009). Vaccines against FeLV include one that uses an inactivated virus and another using a vectored recombinant virus (Stuke *et al.*, 2014). Inactivated vaccination is recommended for kittens. Vaccination of the queen is recommended via inactivated vaccine prior to breeding (Day *et al.*, 2016).

Feline panleukopenia virus (FPLV) causes a variety of outcomes in the pregnant queen. Early in gestation, fetal death and resorption occur as the virus invades rapidly-dividing fetal cells. Abortion with expulsion of fetuses is seen when infection occurs mid-gestation. In late gestation, stillbirth or the birth of live kittens affected with cerebellar hypoplasia, retinal dysplasia, and optic neuropathy occurs (Verstegen *et al.*, 2008; Bergmann *et al.*, 2018). Feline panleukopenia virus is a member of the *Parvovirinae* subfamily of family *Parvoviridae* (Franzo *et al.*, 2017; Bergmann *et al.*, 2018). All members of family Felidae are susceptible to infection with FPLV, the virus considered ubiquitous and highly contagious among unvaccinated cats (Parrish, 2017; Bergmann *et al.*, 2018). Transmission of FPLV occurs via the fecal–oral route, with FPLV stable in the environment and highly shed in the saliva, vomit, feces, and urine of acutely infected cats (Decaro *et al.*, 2012; Parrish, 2017).

Clinical signs of illness and subsequent treatment depend on age of the cat, reproductive status, viral load, and robustness of the immune system. Clinical signs of infection in prenatally infected neonates include ataxia, tremors, seizure, retinal degeneration, and blindness. Signs in postnatally infected kittens include fever, vomiting, inappetence, dehydration, depression, and hemorrhagic diarrhea (Decaro *et al.*, 2012). Gross lesions of FPLV also depend on time of FPLV infection. Prenatally infected neonates can develop hydrocephaly, hydranencephaly, cerebellar aplasia, cerebellar hypoplasia, optic nerve atrophy, and retinopathy (Greene *et al.*, 1982; Sharp *et al.*, 1999; Sykes, 2014). On histology, disruption of cerebellar architecture is evidenced by reduction in granular and Purkinje cell layers, vacuolation of parenchyma, astrocytosis, and disorganization of ependymal cells (Decaro *et al.*, 2012). Gross pathology in postnatally infected kittens includes hemorrhagic enteritis and lymphadenopathy. Histologically, hemorrhagic enteritis presents with intestinal crypt necrosis, crypt dilation, and shortening of intestinal villi, while lymphadenopathy is characterized by lymph nodes depleted of lymphocytes (Decaro *et al.*, 2012). Abortion may be the sole clinical sign of FPLV infection in the queen, as FPLV infection in young adult to adult cats is typically subclinical if immunocompetent (Sykes, 2014).

Diagnosis of FPLV is complicated by the fact that the virus is widespread. When needed, FPLV may be detected in fecal and fetal tissue samples via ELISA tests used for diagnosis of canine parvovirus and can be detected using fecal electron microscopy, VI, or PCR (Decaro *et al.*, 2012; Sykes, 2014). Alternatively, documented seroconversion in the dam can also be diagnostic in cases of high suspicion (Verstegen *et al.*, 2008). Treatment of symptomatic cats, particularly neonates and kittens, relies on aggressive supportive care, focusing on fluid resuscitation, parenteral nutrition, parenteral antimicrobials, antiemetics, and support of glucose. Young cats that survive the first 5 days of treatment usually recover and have a traditional lifespan (Sykes, 2014). Due to its pathogenicity, vaccination against FPLV is considered core and is recommended for all cats. Vaccination schedule is similar to that of FeHV and consists of an initial two-dose vaccination regimen, initial vaccine received no sooner than 6 weeks of age and then every 3-4 weeks until the kitten reaches 20 weeks of age. Revaccination is then recommended at 6 months of age to decrease window of susceptibility if maternally derived antibodies were present at last booster. Booster vaccination can then be scheduled every 3 years thereafter (Stone *et al.*, 2020). Two types of vaccination are available, inactivated and modified-live. In breeding queens, vaccination should occur prior to pregnancy; however, when vaccinating a pregnant queen, the inactivated vaccine is believed to be the safer choice (Stone *et al.*, 2020). Because naturally-infected cats can shed high amounts of virus in all body secretions, adhering to strict biosecurity and quarantine protocol should limit unintended exposure in catteries (Ikeda *et al.*, 2002; Meli *et al.*, 2004).

7.3.2 Bacterial

The remaining pathogens that cause abortion in cats include bacteria and protozoa (Johnston, 2001; Root Kustritz, 2006; Verstegen *et al.*, 2008; Little, 2012). Bacterial abortion is an uncommon finding in the queen and is poorly understood. In instances of bacterial abortion, it is presumed that pathogens ascend into the uterus via the vagina and cervix. While *Brucella canis* is a common cause of abortion in the bitch, *B. canis* does not appear to be an important cause of abortion in the gravid queen (Pretzer, 2008). The common bacterial species with potential to cause feline abortions include *Streptococcus* spp., *Staphylococcus* spp., and *Escherichia coli* (Verstegen *et al.*, 2008). Common clinical signs accompanying bacterial infection of the female reproductive tract include vaginitis, metritis, mastitis, pyometra, and associated signs of malaise such as fever, anorexia, and lethargy; importantly, abortion as an outcome is considered a rare event in the queen (Graham and Taylor, 2012). *Mycoplasma* spp. and *Ureaplasma* spp. are urogenital and respiratory pathogens and are among the smallest free-living cells. Both have also been historically suggested to be abortifacient in queens, though suspicion was based on experimental inoculation (Tan and Miles, 1974; Prezter, 2008; Tatarinova *et al.*, 2016). Reproductive signs that accompanied experimental *Mycoplasma* infection in a 1971 experiment were abortion and kitten death (Tatarinova *et al.*, 2016).

7.3.3 Protozoa

The protozoal pathogen *Toxoplasma gondii* has also been reported to cause abortion in cats (Pretzer, 2008; Sakamoto *et al.*, 2009). Cats are the definitive host for *T. gondii*. Despite repeated attempts, experimental induction of transplacental infection and subsequent abortion via *T. gondii* infection in queens has had mixed results (Dubey and Hoover, 1977; Dubey and Carpenter, 1993; Dubey *et al.*, 1996). Similar to FeHV-1, researchers suspect that abortion occurs secondary to the stress that results from debilitation and systemic illness.

7.4 Case Management

For clinicians attending to a case of feline abortion, acquisition of thorough history is paramount. Important information to obtain include vaccine, travel, medical, and reproductive history, implemented biosecurity measures (if present), antiparasitic schedule (if present), changes in the queen's diet and environment, and breeding dates (to gauge day in gestation). Additional details that would be helpful include health problems encountered in previous litters (if multiparous) and any information on the tom's previous litters (if proven). Consider ascertaining current hygiene in the queen's environment, health of housemates, and potential for accidental ingestion of any medications, toxins, or plants that may cause severe systemic illness. Given the growing popularity of holistic approach, authors recommend investigating use of nutraceuticals, probiotics, and commercially available food additives, making special effort to acquire brand name, date of purchase, and retail venue to better understand if the product was produced/sold via trusted sources. Additionally, inquiring about the use of cannabidiol (CBD) treats is also encouraged, as ingredients in CBD treats vary greatly and can incorporate high amounts of phytoestrogens, which can result in reproductive abnormality and abortion in some species (Patisaul and Jefferson, 2010).

Physical examination and sample collection should follow, results from complete blood count, serum chemistry, and urinalysis are all valuable. Collecting a blood sample for evaluation of progesterone concentration should also be considered. In the event that the queen has vaginal discharge (Fig. 7.3), collecting vaginal swab(s) in a sterile manner will allow practitioners to submit for bacterial and fungal culture and/or viral isolation. Using a double guarded swab made for obtaining

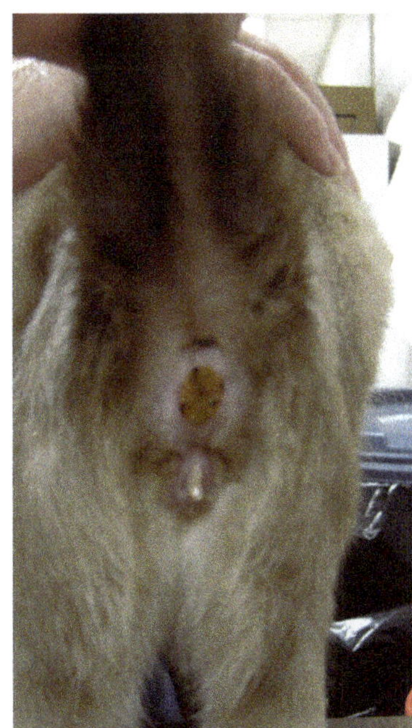

Fig. 7.3. Purulent discharge present at the vulva of an otherwise apparently healthy queen who presented with pyometra. (Image: author's own.)

uterine samples from the mare will provide a clean sample from the cranial vagina. A swab for vaginal cytology should also be taken to characterize cell type(s) present in discharge. Dependent upon suspected day of gestation, acquiring abdominal radiographs (e.g. to diagnose retained fetuses, pyometra) and abdominal ultrasound will provide the clinician a better understanding of uterine and ovarian health. Make sure clients bring any aborted fetuses and placentas with the queen. Due to the multitude of causative agents in cases of feline abortion, submitting fetuses for necropsy at a large diagnostic lab improves chances that a pathoetiologic agent is identified if infectious causes are suspected; however, etiologic diagnosis is never guaranteed in cases of abortion.

7.5 References

Agudelo, C. F. (2005) Cystic endometrial hyperplasia-pyometra complex in cats. A review. *Veterinary Quarterly* 27, 173–182.

Al-Enazy, S., Ali, S., Albekairi, N., El-Tawil, M., and Rytting, E. (2017) Placental control of drug delivery. *Advanced Drug Delivery Reviews* 116, 63–72. doi: 10.1016/j.addr.2016.08.002

Balogh, O., Berger, A., Pieńkowska-Schelling, A., Willmitzer, F., Grest, P., *et al.* (2015) 37,X/38,XY mosaicism in a cryptorchid Bengal cat with Müllerian duct remnants. *Sexual Development* 9, 327–332. doi: 10.1159/000443233

Berepubo, N. A. and Long, S. E. (1983) A study of the relationship between chromosome anomalies and reproductive wastage in domestic animals. *Theriogenology* 20, 177–190. doi: 10.1016/0093-691X(83)90213-3

Bergmann, M., Schwertler, S., Reese, S., Speck, S., Truyen, U., *et al.* (2018) Antibody response to feline panleukopenia virus vaccination in healthy adult cats. *Journal of Feline Medicine and Surgery* 20, 1087–1093. doi: 10.1177/1098612X17747740

Coats, K. S. (2005) The feline immunodeficiency virus-infected cat: a model for lentivirus-induced placental immunopathology and reproductive failure (mini-review). *American Journal of Reproductive Immunology* 54, 169–185. doi: 10.1111/j.1600-0897.2005.00296.x

Davison, A. J., Eberle, R., Ehlers, B., Hayward, G. S., McGeoch, D. J., *et al.* (2009) The order Herpesvirales. *Archives of Virology* 154, 171–177. doi: 10.1007/s00705-008-0278-4

Day, M. J., Horzinek, M. C., Schultz, R. D., and Squires, R. A. (2016) WSAVA Guidelines for the vaccination of dogs and cats. *Journal of Small Animal Practice* 57, E1–E45.doi: 10.1111/jsap.2_12431

Decaro, N., Carmichael, L. E., and Buonavoglia, C. (2012) Viral reproductive pathogens of dogs and cats. *Veterinary Clinics: Small Animal Practice* 42, 583–598. doi: 10.1016/j.cvsm.2012.01.006

Deforest, M. E. and Basrur, P. K. (1979) Malformations and the Manx syndrome in cats. *Canadian Veterinary Journal* 20, 304–314.

Dubey, J. P. and Carpenter, J. L. (1993) Neonatal toxoplasmosis in littermate cats. *Journal of the American Veterinary Medical Association* 203(11), 1546–1549.

Dubey, J. P. and Hoover, E. A. (1977) Attempted transmission of *Toxoplasma gondii* infection from pregnant cats to their kittens. *Journal of the American Veterinary Medical Association* 170(5), 538–540.

Dubey, J. P., Mattix, M. E., and Lipscomb, T. P. (1996) Lesions of neonatally induced toxoplasmosis in cats. *Veterinary Pathology* 33, 290–295. doi.org/10.1177/030098589603300305

Elder, J. H., Lin, Y-C., Fink, E., and Grant, C. K. (2010) Feline immunodeficiency virus (FIV) as a model for study of lentivirus infections: parallels with HIV. *Current HIV Research* 8, 73–80.

Ferasin, L., Sturgess, C. P., Cannon, M. J., Caney, S. M. A., Gruffydd-Jones, T. J., *et al.* (2003) Feline idiopathic cardiomyopathy: a retrospective study of 106 cats (1994–2001). *Journal of Feline Medicine and Surgery* 5, 151–159. doi: 10.1016/S1098-612X(02)00133-X

Franzo, G., Tucciarone, C. M., Cecchinato, M., and Drigo, M. (2017) Canine parvovirus type 2 (CPV-2) and feline panleukopenia virus (FPV) codon bias analysis reveals a progressive adaptation to the new niche after the host jump. *Molecular Phylogenetics and Evolution* 114, 82–92. doi: 10.1016/j.ympev.2017.05.019

Gaskell, R.M. and Povey, R.C. (1979) The dose response of cats to experimental infection with feline viral rhinotracheitis virus. *Journal of Comparative Pathology* 89, 179–191. doi: 10.1016/0021-9975(79)90057-4

Gaskell, R., Dawson, S., Radford, A., and Thiry, E. (2007) Feline herpesvirus. *Veterinary Research* 38, 337–354. doi: 10.1051/vetres:2006063

Gould, D. (2011) Feline herpesvirus-1: ocular manifestations, diagnosis and treatment options. *Journal of Feline Medicine & Surgery* 13, 333–346. doi: 10.1016/j.jfms.2011.03.010

Graham, E. M. and Taylor, D. J. (2012) Bacterial reproductive pathogens of cats and dogs. *Veterinary Clinics of North America: Small Animal Practice* 42, 561–582. doi: 10.1016/j.cvsm.2012.01.013

Greene, C. E., Gorgasz, E. J., and Martin, C. L. (1982) Hydranencephaly associated with feline panleukopenia. *Journal of the American Veterinary Medical Association* 180, 767–768.

Hartmann, K. (2011) Clinical aspects of feline immunodeficiency and feline leukemia virus infection. *Veterinary Immunology and Immunopathology* 143, 190–201. doi: 10.1016/j.vetimm.2011.06.003

Hayes, K.C. (1982) Nutritional problems in cats: taurine deficiency and vitamin A excess. *Canadian Veterinary Journal* 23, 2–5.

Hayes, K. C. and Trautwein, E. A. (1989) Taurine deficiency syndrome in cats. *Veterinary Clinics of North America: Small Animal Practice* 19, 403–413. doi: 10.1016/s0195-5616(89)50052-4

Heinze, C. R., Larsen, J. A., Kass, P. H., and Fascetti, A. J. (2009) Plasma amino acid and whole blood taurine concentrations in cats eating commercially prepared diets. *American Journal of Veterinary Research* 70, 1374–1382. doi: 10.2460/ajvr.70.11.1374

Herrick, J. R., Lyons, S. M., Greene-Ermisch, A. F., Broeckling, C. D., Schoolcraft, W. B., *et al.* (2018) A carnivore embryo's perspective on essential amino acids and ammonium in culture medium: effects on the development of feline embryos. *Biology of Reproduction* 99, 1070–1081. doi: 10.1093/biolre/ioy122

Hoover, E. A. and Griesemer, R. A. (1971) Experimental feline herpesvirus infection in the pregnant cat. *American Journal of Pathology* 65, 173–188.

Hosie, M. J., Addie, D., Belák, S., Boucraut-Baralon, C., Egberink, H., *et al.* (2009) Feline immunodeficiency. ABCD guidelines on prevention and management. *Journal of Feline Medicine & Surgery* 11, 575–584. doi: 10.1016/j.jfms.2009.05.006

Ikeda, Y., Nakamura, K., Miyazawa, T., Tohya, Y. Takahashi, E., *et al.* (2002) Feline host range of canine parvovirus: recent emergence of new antigenic types in cats. *Emerging Infectious Diseases* 8, 341–346. doi: 10.3201/eid0804.010228

Johnston, S. (2001) Canine pregnancy. In: Johnston, S. D., Root Kustritz, M. V., and Olson, P. N. S. (eds) *Canine and Feline Theriogenology*. W.B. Saunders Company, Philadelphia, Pennsylvania, pp. 66–104.

Johnston, S. D., Buoen, L. C., Madl, J. E., Weber, A. F., and Smith, F. O. (1983) X-Chromosome monosomy (37, XO) in a Burmese cat with gonadal dysgenesis. *Journal of the American Veterinary Medical Association* 182, 986.

Kenyon, J. C. and Lever, A. M. L. (2011) The molecular biology of feline immunodeficiency virus (FIV). *Viruses* 3, 2192–2213. doi: 10.3390/v3112192

Kolenda-Roberts, H. M., Kuhnt, L. A., Jennings, R. N., Mergia, A., Gengozian, N., *et al.* (2007) Immunopathogenesis of feline immunodeficiency virus infection in the fetal and neonatal cat. *Frontiers in Bioscience: a Journal and Virtual Library* 12, 3668. doi: 10.2741/2343

Little, S. E. (2012) Female reproduction. In: Little S. E. (ed.) *The Cat*. W.B. Saunders, St. Louis, Missouri, pp. 1195–1227.

Long S. E. and Berepubo, N. A. (1980) A 37XO chromosome complement in a kitten. *Journal of Small Animal Practice* 21, 627–631. doi: 10.1111/j.1748-5827.1980.tb01366.x

Lutz, H., Addie, D., Belák, S., Boucraut-Baralon, C., Egberink, H., *et al.* (2009) Feline leukaemia. ABCD guidelines on prevention and management. *Journal of Feline Medicine & Surgery* 11, 565–574. doi: 10.1016/j.jfms.2009.05.005

Maes, R. (2012) Felid herpesvirus type 1 infection in cats: a natural host model for alphaherpesvirus pathogenesis. *International Scholarly Research Notices* 2012. doi: 10.5402/2012/495830

Mathews, K. and Sinclair, M. (2018) Analgesia and anesthesia for pregnant cats and dogs. In: Kathews, K. A., Sinclair, M., Steele, A. M., and Grubb, T. (eds) *Analgesia and Anesthesia for the Ill or Injured Dog and Cat*. Wiley-Blackwell, Hoboken, New Jersey, pp. 279–293.

Mayr, B., Hofstadler, E., Schleger, W., Reifinger, M., and Eisenmenger, E. (1994) Trisomy D1, marker F1: new cytogenetic findings in two cases of feline fibrosarcoma. *Zentralblatt Fur Veterinarmedizin Reihe A* 41, 197–201. doi: 10.1111/j.1439-0442.1994.tb00086.x

Medeiros, S. de O., Martins, A. N., Dias, C. G. A., Tanuri, A., and Brindeiro, R. de M. (2012) Natural transmission of feline immunodeficiency virus from infected queen to kitten. *Virology Journal* 9, 99. doi: 10.1186/1743-422X-9-99

Meli, M., Kipar, A., Müller, C., Jenal, K., Gönczi, E., *et al.* (2004) High viral loads despite absence of clinical and pathological findings in cats experimentally infected with feline coronavirus (FCoV) type I and in naturally FCoV-infected cats. *Journal of Feline Medicine and Surgery* 6, 69–81. doi: 10.1016/j.jfms.2003.08.007

O'Neil, L. L., Burkhard, M. J., and Hoover, E. A. (1996) Frequent perinatal transmission of feline immunodeficiency virus by chronically infected cats. *Journal of Virology* 70, 2894–2901.

Orandle, M. S. and Baldwin, C. J. (1995) Clinical and pathological features associated with feline immunodeficiency virus infection in cats. *Iowa State University Veterinarian* 57, 5.

Papich, M. G. and Davis, L. E. (1986) Drug therapy during pregnancy and in the neonate. *Veterinary Clinics of North America: Small Animal Practice* 16, 525–538. doi: 10.1016/S0195-5616(86)50058-9

Parrish, C. R. (2017) Parvoviridae. In: MacLachlan, N. J. and Dubovi, E. J. (eds) *Fenner's Veterinary Virology*, 5th edn. Academic Press, Boston, Massachussetts, pp. 245–257.

Patisaul, H. B. and Jefferson, W. (2010) The pros and cons of phytoestrogens. *Front Neuroendocrinol* 31, 400–419. doi: 10.1016/j.yfrne.2010.03.003

Pretzer, S. D. (2008) Bacterial and protozoal causes of pregnancy loss in the bitch and queen. *Theriogenology* 70, 320–326. doi: 10.1016/j.theriogenology.2008.04.035

Robinson, R. (1993) Expressivity of the Manx gene in cats. *Journal of Heredity* 84, 170–172. doi: 10.1093/oxfordjournals.jhered.a111311

Romm, A. (2010) Pregnancy and botanical medicine use and safety. In: Romm, A., Hardy, M. L., and Mills, S. (eds) *Botanical Medicine for Women's Health.* Elsevier, St. Louis, Missouri, pp. 321–333.

Root Kustritz, M. V. (2006) Clinical management of pregnancy in cats. *Theriogenology* 66, 145–150. doi: 10.1016/j.theriogenology.2006.03.018

Rothuizen, J. (2020) Metabolic, toxic, and neoplastic diseases of the liver. *Clinical Small Animal Internal Medicine* 62, 677–686. doi: 10.1002/9781119501237.ch62

Sakamoto, C. A. M., da Costa, A. J., Gennari, S. M., Pena, H. F. J., Toniollo, G. H., *et al.* (2009) Experimental infection of pregnant queens with two major Brazilian clonal lineages of Toxoplasma gondii. *Parasitology Research* 105, 1311. doi: 10.1007/s00436-009-1558-y

Scherk, M. A., Ford, R. B., Gaskell, R. M., Hartmann, K., Hurley, K. F., *et al.* (2013) 2013 AAFP feline vaccination advisory panel report. *Journal of Feline Medicine and Surgery* 15, 785–808. doi: 10.1177/1098612X13500429

Schlafer, D. H. and Gifford, A. T. (2008) Cystic endometrial hyperplasia, pseudo-placentational endometrial hyperplasia, and other cystic conditions of the canine and feline uterus. *Theriogenology* 70, 349–358. doi: 10.1016/j.theriogenology.2008.04.041

Sharp, N. J., Davis, B. J., Guy, J. S., Cullen, J. M., Steingold, S. F., *et al.* (1999) Hydranencephaly and cerebellar hypoplasia in two kittens attributed to intrauterine parvovirus infection. *Journal of Comparative Pathology* 121, 39–53. doi: 10.1053/jcpa.1998.0298

Stone, A. E. S., Brummet, G. O., Carozza, E. M., Kass, P. H., Petersen, E. P., *et al.* (2020) 2020 AAHA/AAFP Feline Vaccination Guidelines. *Journal of Feline Medicine and Surgery* 22, 813–830. doi.org/10.1177/1098612X20941784

Stuke, K., King, V., Southwick, K., Stoeva, M. I. Thomas, A., *et al.* (2014) Efficacy of an inactivated FeLV vaccine compared to a recombinant FeLV vaccine in minimum age cats following virulent FeLV challenge. *Vaccine* 32, 2599–2603. doi: 10.1016/j.vaccine.2014.03.016

Sturman, J. A. (1992) Review: Taurine deficiency and the cat. In: Lombardini, J. B., Schaffer, S. W., and Azuma, J. (eds) *Taurine: Nutritional Value and Mechanisms of Action*. Springer US, Boston, Massachussetts, pp. 1–5.

Sturman, J. A., Gargano, A. D., Messing, J. M., and Imaki, H. (1986) Feline maternal taurine deficiency: effect on mother and offspring. *The Journal of Nutrition* 116, 655–667. doi: 10.1093/jn/116.4.655

Sykes, J. E. (2014) Feline panleukopenia virus infection and other viral enteritides. In: Sykes, J. E. (ed.) *Canine and Feline Infectious Diseases*. Elsevier, St. Louis, Missouri, pp. 187–194. doi: 10.1016/B978-1-4377-0795-3.00019-3

Sykes, J. E. and Hartmann, K. (2014) Feline leukemia virus infection. In: Sykes, J. E. (ed.) *Canine and Feline Infectious Diseases*. Elsevier, St. Loius, Missouri, pp. 224-238. doi: 10.1016/B978-1-4377-0795-3.00022-3

Tan, R. J. and Miles, J. A. (1974) Possible role of feline T-strain mycoplasmas in cat abortion. *Australian Veterinary Journal* 50, 142–145. doi: 10.1111/j.1751-0813.1974.tb06877.x

Tatarinova, T. V., Lysnyansky, I., Nikolsky, Y. V., and Bolshoy, A. (2016) The mysterious orphans of Mycoplasmataceae. *Biology Direct* 11, 2. doi: 10.1186/s13062-015-0104-3

Troyer, J. L., Pecon-Slattery, J., Roelke, M. E., Johnson, W., VandeWoude, S., *et al.* (2005) Seroprevalence and genomic divergence of circulating strains of feline immunodeficiency virus among Felidae and Hyaenidae species. *Journal of Virology* 79, 8282–8294. doi: 10.1128/JVI.79.13.8282-8294.2005

Verstegen, J., Dhaliwal, G., and Verstegen-Onclin, K. (2008) Canine and feline pregnancy loss due to viral and non-infectious causes: a review. *Theriogenology* 70, 304–319. doi: 10.1016/j.theriogenology.2008.05.035

Wiebe, V.J. and Howard, J.P. (2009) Pharmacologic advances in canine and feline reproduction. *Topics in Companion Animal Medicine* 24, 71–99. doi: 1.1053/j.tcam.2008.12.004

8 Periparturient Disease in the Queen

NATALIE S. MATICKA

Guide Dogs Queensland, Bald Hills, Australia

In the vast majority of cats, pregnancy progresses without complication and queening is uneventful. There are some diseases and disorders of pregnancy and the postpartum period that clinicians should be aware of and prepared to manage as needed.

8.1 Prepartum and Peripartum Disorders

8.1.1 Uterine torsion

Uterine torsion is defined as the twisting of a uterine horn or the uterine body along its long axis. There are multiple case reports on this condition in cats (Biller and Haibel, 1987; Young *et al.*, 1991; Ridyard *et al.*, 2000; Thilagar *et al.*, 2005; Stanley and Pacchiana, 2008; Kuroda *et al.*, 2017). The etiology of this condition is unknown, but hypothesized to be secondary to broad ligament stretching in multiparous queens, fetal movement, or increased physical activity (Kuroda *et al.*, 2017). There are reports of fetal survival in uterine torsion cases, particularly if only one horn is affected. Torsion has also been reported in nonpregnant queens (De La Puerta *et al.*, 2008). Preoperative diagnosis of uterine torsion can be difficult as clinical signs such as anemia, lethargy, anorexia, and abdominal pain are fairly non-specific in nature. Therefore, uterine torsion should be included as a differential diagnosis in pregnant cats, particularly those in late gestation, with non-specific signs of illness and when signs of fetal distress or demise are present. A presumptive diagnosis can be made in pregnant queens with signs of acute abdomen such as shock, circulatory collapse, and abdominal pain.

In larger animals, such as cows and mares, where torsion occurs more frequently, it is possible to correct the torsion by trapping the uterus in place and rolling the animal. In queens, this technique is not practical due to the difference in anatomy of the uterus, multiple fetuses in each horn, and the incidence of a single horn torsion. Also, it is impossible to determine if the uterus has been returned to its normal position. The treatment of choice is surgical exploration and ovariohysterectomy (OHE) especially given the difficulty in making a definitive diagnosis preoperatively (Kuroda *et al.*, 2017). With the relatively delayed diagnosis in queens compared to other species, congestion and necrosis of the affected horn(s) are common. Therefore, detorsion to correct the condition is not recommended, as the tissue is typically devitalized necessitating ovariohysterectomy (Ridyard *et al.*, 2000). Detorsion may also result in the release of endotoxins and inflammatory mediators into the systemic circulation, increasing the risk of further complications (Ridyard *et al.*, 2000). Queens should be provided with supportive care as needed postoperatively, and survival rate for the queen after surgery is reported as approximately 80% (Freeman, 1988). Due to the degree of fetal hypoxia present, kittens that survive delivery may be severely compromised and die in the early neonatal period.

8.1.2 Extrauterine fetuses

The presence of fetuses outside of the uterus has been reported many times in the literature, often mistakenly as 'ectopic pregnancy'. There is no evidence that ectopic pregnancy, where the developing embryo forms a placental attachment to an organ other than the uterus, occurs in queens. Often the fetuses are identified incidentally at the time of OHE as bacteriologically sterile mummified fetuses. Some cases had a historical association of trauma, which may have led to uterine rupture. Fetuses can be found within uterine tissue, omentum, or free floating in the abdomen (McKeating, 1979). Treatment is surgical removal via ventral midline celiotomy.

 Feline Reproduction (eds. A.K. Johnson and M.A. Kutzler)
DOI: 10.1079/9781789247107.0008

8.1.3 Vaginal prolapse

A single case of vaginal prolapse has been reported in a pregnant queen (McKelvey *et al.*, 2015), although the condition occurs commonly in ruminants and canines. Prior to queening, the prolapse was reduced and maintained with a retention suture. The litter was delivered via elective cesarean section, and ovariohysterectomy was performed at that time. Postoperatively, the retention suture was maintained for 2 weeks and prolapse did not reoccur. Since vaginal prolapse is so rarely reported in queens, it is difficult to ascertain if this is a typical progression for this disease process in felids.

8.1.4 Uterine prolapse

Uterine prolapse is a relatively uncommon complication associated with parturition in queens, and typically occurs in the immediate postpartum period up to 48 hours after delivery of the kittens (Deroy *et al.*, 2015). Uterine prolapse occurs when the uterus everts through the cervix, into the vaginal vault, and out the vulvar lips (Fig. 8.1). The diagnosis is straightforward and made by observation. The prolapse can be complete, involving both uterine horns and the body of the uterus, or can be limited to the uterine body and a single horn. The etiology of uterine prolapse in queens is unknown.

Uterine prolapse is a medical emergency that must be attended to rapidly. Depending on the time to presentation at the clinic, the queen's clinical condition can vary. The exposed tissue should be gently cleaned with saline. In most cases, reduction of the prolapse will be easier if the queen is heavily sedated or anesthetized. The exposed tissue will be edematous, congested, and may be necrotic depending on the length of time the prolapsed tissue is exposed to the external environment. If no necrosis is present and the queen is desired for breeding, the uterus can be manually replaced, either through gentle manipulation externally through the vaginal vault, or through a celiotomy incision (Deroy *et al.*, 2015). The author has used a clean glass blood tube to act as a probang for replacement and extension of the uterine horns into a normal anatomical position without the need for an abdominal incision. Gentle compression of the tissue, along with the application of osmotic agents such as hypertonic saline, can help reduce edema prior to replacement. Sugar can also be used but is a medium for bacterial growth so careful rinsing

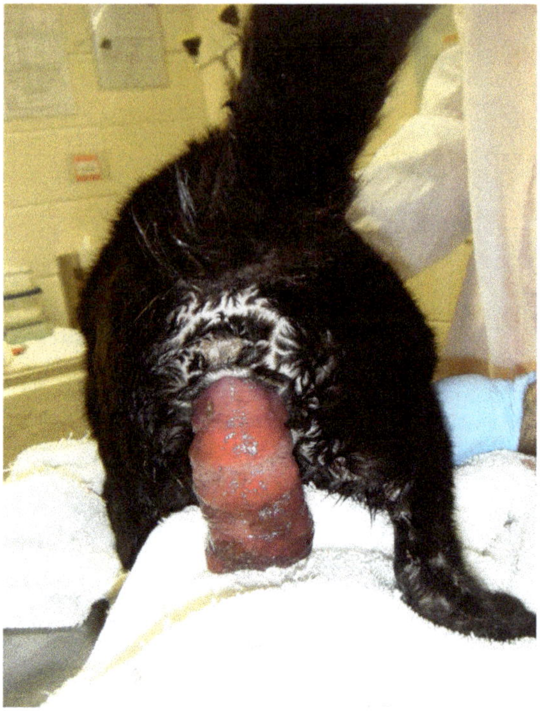

Fig. 8.1. Prolapse of one uterine horn in a postpartum queen. This cat delivered a normal litter 24 hours before. (Image courtesy of Dr Aime Johnson.)

prior to replacement is ideal. Care should be taken that the uterus is completely replaced within the abdomen or blood flow to the uterus or oviducts will continue to be compromised. This may be difficult to ascertain without an abdominal incision.

If the uterus cannot be replaced externally, surgery is warranted (Fig. 8.2). In queens desired for breeding, gentle traction can be placed on the affected horn(s) while an assistant helps push the uterine tissue back into place through the vaginal vault. Colposuspension, where the uterus is attached to the abdominal wall, can be performed in patients where recurrence has occurred (Hopper, 2007). If the uterus is necrotic, or the queen is not desired for future breeding, ovariohysterectomy can be performed. Generally, this is easier to perform in two stages: first performing bilateral ovariectomy, and then amputation of the uterus. Care must be taken to identify the urethral tubercle prior to ligation of the uterine vessels and transection of the uterine body; a hysterotomy incision will make it easier to expose the vessels for ligation. The uterus should be removed as far

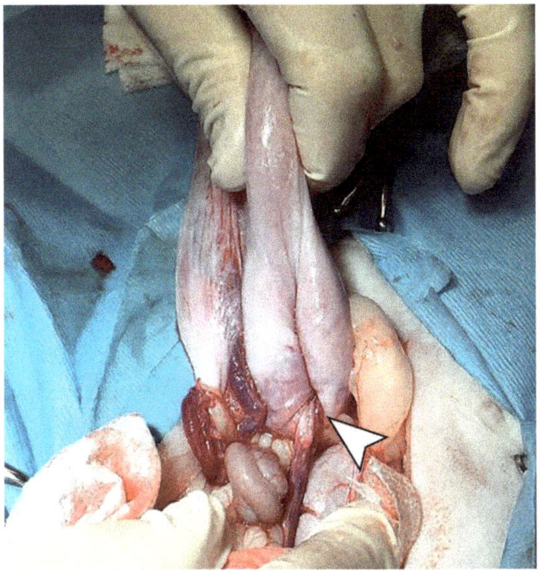

Fig. 8.2. The same cat as Fig. 8.1 in surgery. The affected horn is inverted and prolapsed. The ovarian vessels can be seen leading into the prolapsed horn (arrow). The prolapsed horn was corrected, and a routine ovariohysterectomy was performed. (Image courtesy of Dr Aime Johnson.)

caudally as possible, and the uterine stump should be oversewn after transecting through the body. If only one uterine horn is affected, it may be possible to perform a hemi-ovariohysterectomy (hemi-OHE) where the affected uterine horn and ovary are removed. The affected horn is resected at the bifurcation of the uterus, and the resultant incision closed as per routine hysterotomy closure. Queens that undergo hemi-OHE will have reduced litter sizes secondary to reduced uterine capacity.

8.2 Postpartum Disorders

8.2.1 Retained fetal membranes

Retained placenta occurs infrequently in queens. Queens will often ingest the placentas during queening, so it can be difficult for the owner to determine if a placenta was passed for every kitten, and occasionally twin kittens will share a single placenta. Presence of retained placenta can be confirmed with ultrasonography (Fig. 8.3). Abdominal palpation and radiography may reveal a mass effect within the uterus in queens with retained fetal membranes. Ecbolic therapy with oxytocin (0.25–2 IU per queen) will usually result in expulsion of the membranes, but uterine responsiveness to oxytocin will diminish in the first few days postpartum (Wiebe and Howard, 2009). Queens that fail to respond to multiple doses of oxytocin should be treated with prostaglandin $F_{2\alpha}$ (0.25–0.5 mg/kg, IM) (Wiebe and Howard, 2009). Prostaglandin administration is associated with side effects such as vomiting, diarrhea, hypersalivation, and abdominal cramping. In some cases, queens may experience signs of hypotensive shock. Ideally, prostaglandin should be administered while the queen is hospitalized to allow monitoring of any side effects. Adverse effects typically subside in 60 minutes and may become less severe with repeated dosing. In the vast majority of queens that are systemically well and nursing kittens, exogenous oxytocin release will allow release and passage of the placentas without development of systemic illness or metritis. Queens that develop systemic illness should be treated for metritis.

8.2.2 Metritis

Metritis in the queen occurs in the postpartum period secondary to ascending bacteria. Inciting causes can include uterine trauma, protracted delivery, retained fetal or placental tissue, or unhygienic attempts at fetal manipulation and delivery. Queens with metritis typically present with lethargy, anorexia, fever, poor mothering, and fetid vaginal discharge early in the postpartum period. Abdominal ultrasonography typically reveals a flaccid, fluid-filled uterus, and complete blood cell count is generally consistent with leukocytosis. Fetid vulvar discharge is generally present that can be sanguineous to purulent in appearance.

Queens should receive supportive care, appropriate antimicrobial therapy, and ecbolic therapy to aid in uterine evacuation. Queens that are febrile and anorexic may benefit from intravenous fluid therapy. In the author's experience, judicious use of non-steroidal anti-inflammatories (NSAID) can be hugely beneficial in resolving fever and generally helping the queen feel better, allowing resolution of anorexia. Care should be taken to ensure the queen is fully hydrated prior to receiving an NSAID. Uterine evacuation can be achieved with repeated doses of oxytocin, or ideally prostaglandin F2a for a more prolonged treatment effect. Antimicrobials should ideally be selected on the basis of culture and susceptibility testing; augmented penicillins, such as amoxicillin-clavulonic acid, are a good first choice for empirical therapy pending culture results

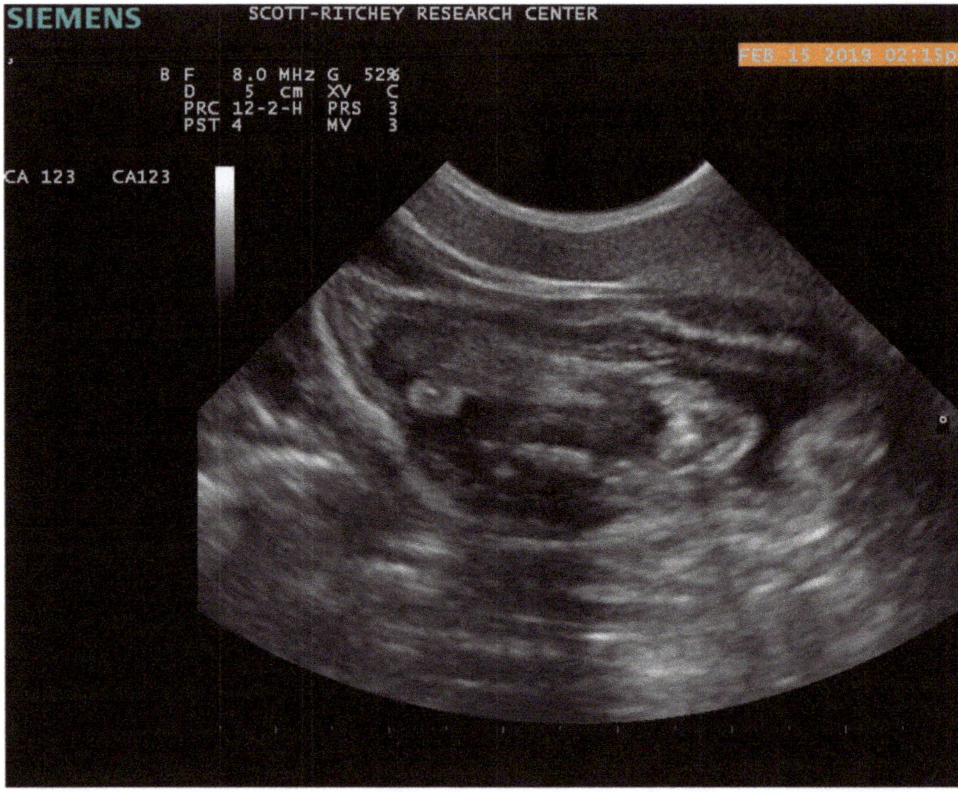

Fig. 8.3. Ultrasound image of a postpartum queen with a retained placenta. All kittens were delivered uneventfully. Following delivery, a single placenta was visualized within the uterus. This queen was treated with oxytocin and delivered the placenta without complications within 24 hours after queening. (Image courtesy of Dr Aime Johnson.)

and is relatively safe for the queen and her nursing kittens (Rebuelto and Loza, 2010). The majority of queens will respond to medical therapy, but if the uterus appears particularly friable and risk of uterine rupture is high, ovariohysterectomy may be warranted. Uterine rupture can occur if the wall of the uterus is thin and friable, which may result in sudden decompensation and increase the risk of death. Generally, the prognosis for survival is good. There are no scientific studies regarding the prognosis for future fertility in queens with metritis, but in the author's experience if the queen responds to medical management and predisposing conditions (i.e. dystocia) are managed in subsequent pregnancies the prognosis for fertility is favorable.

8.2.3 Eclampsia (puerperal tetany)

Eclampsia, or puerperal tetany, is an acute, life-threatening hypocalcemia that occurs in the periparturient period. This condition occurs less commonly in queens compared to bitches, and has also been reported to occur in late gestation prepartum (Davidson, 2012). Clinical signs include muscle fasciculation and tetany. Clients may confuse this behavior with seizures, but mentation and consciousness are maintained in the initial stages of the disease. Other clinical signs include facial pruritus, panting, limb pain, trembling, weakness, and ataxia. Clinical signs can rapidly progress to tonic-clonic spasms, opsithotonos, and death. Hypocalcemia occurs when total serum calcium concentration is less than 8 mg/dL in adult queens, or the serum ionized calcium concentration is less than 1.0 mmol/L (Fascetti and Hickman, 1999). Hypocalcemia occurs when ionized calcium is depleted in the extracellular compartment. During lactation, there are several mechanisms that support calcium homeostasis despite the amount of calcium secreted in mammary secretions. These mechanisms include increased absorption of calcium from the gastrointestinal tract, decreased renal excretion, and increased osteolysis (Davidson, 2012). When these mechanisms cannot compensate for the increased lactational demand of calcium, clinical hypocalcemia can develop.

In lactating queens presented with clinical signs consistent with eclampsia, treatment should be instituted immediately prior to final laboratory confirmation of results. If practical, a blood sample should be collected prior to administration of calcium, but in severe cases, treatment should not be delayed in order to obtain and process laboratory samples. Queens should be treated with 10% calcium gluconate as a slow intravenous infusion (2–5 mL over 5–10 minutes), given to effect. An electrocardiogram can be placed to allow for continuous cardiac monitoring during administration to ensure that bradycardia or arrhythmias do not occur; if any cardiac abnormalities are detected, the calcium infusion should be temporarily discontinued until the arrhythmia resolves, then continuation of treatment at a slower rate. The calcium can be diluted with sterile fluids and loaded into a syringe pump for administration to reduce the likelihood of cardiac side effects. Response to treatment is typically rapid and profound, occurring while the initial calcium bolus is administered. If cerebral edema has developed secondary to seizure activity, diazepam, barbiturates, or mannitol can be used to reduce seizures and edema/inflammation, respectively (Davidson, 2012). Administration of corticosteroids is not advised due to adverse effects on calcium metabolism such as decreased intestinal absorption, calciuria, and impairment of osteoclastia.

After initial cessation of clinical signs, queens should be transitioned to subcutaneous boluses of calcium gluconate. An equal volume to the initial dose needed to control clinical signs should be diluted 1:1 volume/volume with saline and administered subcutaneously every 6–8 hours until oral medication can be administered. Oral supplementation with calcium gluconate or carbonate, 10–30 mg/kg every 8 hours should be instituted as soon as the queen is stable and able to consume oral medications. Nursing kittens can be resumed gradually until the neonates can be safely weaned, and efforts should be made to improve the queen's nutritional plane. If eclampsia reoccurs after the kittens are reintroduced, they should be weaned from the dam to diminish lactational demands and supplement fed as appropriate for their age.

Eclampsia is best prevented with proper nutrition. Queens should be fed an AAFCO-approved diet appropriate for gestation and lactation; most commercially available kitten foods will meet the appropriate calcium requirements. Target calcium levels should be between 1.0% and 1.8% calcium, and 0.8% to 1.6% phosphorous. Postpartum, the diet should contain at least 1.4% calcium with a calcium:phosphorous ratio of 1:1. Clients should be advised to avoid supplementation of calcium during gestation as this may impair normal release of parathyroid hormone, predisposing the queen to the development of eclampsia. Diets that are high in muscle meats and organs, such as many raw diets, are excessively high in phosphorous and should be avoided. In queens with a history of eclampsia, supplementation of calcium during lactation as a preventive measure can be considered.

8.2.4 Mastitis

See Chapter 16 (Disorders of the Mammary Gland).

8.2.5 Lactation failure/agalactia

Lactation failure is poorly understood in queens, but failure of mammary development and milk production can account for neonatal losses due to inadequate colostral intake or starvation. Agalactia can be primary or secondary, with most cases of agalactia occurring secondary to failure of prolactin release from the anterior pituitary from physiologic stress (Jensen *et al.*, 2016). Risk factors for secondary agalactia include systemic disease, genetic factors, poor nutritional status or body condition, or environmental stressors. Primary agalactia is a diagnosis of exclusion when all causes of secondary agalactia have been ruled out and may occur from failure of endocrine mechanisms regarding mammary development and lactation.

Treatment of agalactia in queens is directed at managing any underlying or inciting causes, providing nutritional support to the kittens, and simultaneously encouraging kittens to suckle to stimulate lactation and milk let-down. The antidopaminergic drug, domperidone, has been reported to be successful in the treatment of primary agalactia in queens (Jensen *et al.*, 2016). Domperidone antagonizes D2-dopaminergic receptors and 5HT3 serotonergic receptors. As it is indicated for use in mares for the treatment of agalactia related to fescue toxicosis, its use in queens is considered extra label. Recommended dosing is 2.2 mg/kg orally every 12–24 hours. If a queen has a history of agalactia from previous litters, treatment can be instituted 5–7 days prior to queening. In bitches, metoclopramide has been demonstrated to cause a transient increase in prolactin (0.2 mg/kg, orally every 6 h), and has been used anecdotally as a galactologue in queens (Keller *et al.*, 2018). Acepromazine also increases plasma prolactin concentration, as demonstrated in sheep (Bryant *et al.*, 1968) and the sedative effect of acepromazine may be beneficial in queens that appear nervous or unsettled mothering their kittens. Acupuncture, although lacking in rigorous scientific studies, may be a beneficial adjunctive therapy. Reported acupuncture points in bitches include SI11 and LI4; other points may be useful depending on the queen's specific traditional diagnosis.

8.3 References

Biller, D. S. and Haibel, G. K. (1987) Torsion of the uterus in a cat. *Journal of the American Veterinary Medical Association* 191, 1128–1129.

Bryant, G. D., Connan, R., and Greenwood, F. (1968) Changes in plasma prolactin induced by acepromazine in sheep. *Journal of Endocrinology* 41, 613–614. doi: 10.1677/joe.0.0410613

Davidson, A. P. (2012) Reproductive causes of hypocalcemia. *Topics in Companion Animal Medicine* 27, 165–166. doi: 10.1053/j.tcam.2012.09.002

De La Puerta, B., McMahon, L. A., and Moores, A. (2008) Uterine horn torsion in a non-gravid cat. *Journal of Feline Medicine and Surgery* 10, 395–397. doi: 10.1016/j.jfms.2008.01.004

Deroy, C., Bismuth, C., and Carozzo, C. (2015) Management of a complete uterine prolapse in a cat. *Journal of Feline Medicine and Surgery Open Reports* 1, 1. doi: 10.1177/2055116915579681

Fascetti, A. J. and Hickman, M. A. (1999.) Preparturient hypocalcemia in four cats. *Journal of the American Veterinary Medical Association* 215, 1127–1129.

Freeman, L. (1988) Feline uterine torsion. *The Compendium on Continuing Education for the Practicing Veterinarian* 10, 1078–1082.

Hopper, R. M. (2007) Surgical correction of abnormalities of genital organs of cows. In: Youngquist, R. S. and Threlfall, W. R. (eds) *Current Therapy in Large Animal Theriogenology*. Elsevier, St. Louis, Missouri, pp. 463–472.

Jensen, R. L., Johnson, A. K., Wilborn, R. R., and Fraser, N. S. (2016) A case report on the use of domperidone for management of agalactia in a queen. *Clinical Theriogenology* 8, 121–128.

Keller, S. R., Abonyi-Tóth, Z., Sprenger, N., Austin, S. C., Wichert, B. A., *et al.* (2018) Effect of metoclopramide treatment of bitches during the first week of lactation on serum prolactin concentration, milk composition, and milk yield and on weight gain of their puppies. *American Journal of Veterinary Research* 79, 233–241. doi: 10.2460/ajvr.79.2.233

Kuroda, K., Osaki, T., Harada, K., Yamashita, M., Murahata, Y., *et al.* (2017) Uterine torsion in a full-term pregnant cat. *Journal of Feline Medicine and Surgery Open Reports* 3. doi: 10.1177/2055116917726228

McKeating, F. J. (1979) Ectopic pregnancy in a cat. *Veterinary Record*, 104, 240–241.

McKelvey, K., Beachler, T., Ferris, K., Diaw, M., Vasgaard, J., *et al.* (2015) Vaginal prolapse in a pregnant Maine coon cat: a case report. *Journal of Small Animal Practice* 56, 473–475. doi: 10.1111/jsap.12310

Rebuelto, M. and Loza, M. E. (2010) Antibiotic treatment of dogs and cats during pregnancy. *Veterinary Medicine International* 2010, 385640. doi: 10.4061/2010/385640

Ridyard, A. E., Welsh, E. A., and Gunn-Moore, D. A. (2000) Successful treatment of uterine torsion in a cat with severe metabolic and haemostatic complications. *Journal of Feline Medicine and Surgery* 2, 115–119. doi: 10.1053/jfms.2000.0082

Stanley, S. W. and Pacchiana, P. D. (2008) Uterine torsion and metabolic abnormalities in a cat with a pyometra. *Canadian Veterinary Journal* 49, 398–400.

Thilagar, S., Yew, Y. C., Dhaliwal, G. K., Toh, I., and Tong, L. L. (2005) Uterine horn torsion in a pregnant cat. *Veterinary Record* 157, 558–560. doi: 10.1136/vr.157.18.558

Wiebe, V. J. and Howard, J. P. (2009) Pharmacologic advances in canine and feline reproduction. *Topics in Companion Animal Medicine* 24, 71–99. doi: 10.1053/j.tcam.2008.12.004

Young, J. D., Hillis, G. P., and McKibbin, M. L. (1991) Uterine torsion in a cat. *Canadian Veterinary Journal*, 32, 479.

9 Management of Parturition

Natalie S. Maticka

Guide Dogs Queensland, Bald Hills, Australia

9.1 Background/Introduction

Normal gestation in queens is reported to last between 52 and 74 days from the time of breeding, with a mean reported gestation length of 65 days (Root Kustritz, 2006). Normal queening occurs in three stages. In the first stage of labor, which is typically the longest, cervical dilation occurs. Queens in stage I may appear restless or show nesting behavior, isolate themselves, pant, or vomit. Queens will often pace, interspersed with bouts of purring during stage I and II of labor. Stage II is active expulsion of the fetuses and begins with the rupture of the first chorioallantoic membrane. A small volume of clear to blood-tinged fluid is passed prior to delivery of the first kitten. Once stage II begins, the first kitten should be delivered within 4 hours. Queens with constant, active contractions should deliver a kitten within 30 minutes. Queens will often adopt a squatting position to deliver the kitten, and it may take several minutes from the time when a portion of the kitten is visible at the vulva until it is completely expelled (Fig. 9.1). Unlike bitches, active queening may be prolonged with reports of live kittens being born over several days (Root Kustritz *et al.*, 1995). Some queens, when disturbed, will pause stage II of parturition, which can complicate the diagnosis of dystocia in this species. A conservative guideline would expect no longer than a 4-hour timespan between the birth of individual kittens. As each kitten is delivered, the queen usually cleans the kitten by vigorously licking and removing the allantoic membrane with her tongue and teeth. During the cleaning process, the queen will rupture the umbilical cord. Stage III of parturition is passage of the placenta (Fig. 9.2). Placentas should be passed within 15 minutes after the birth of the kitten, and it is normal for stage II and stage III to alternate until the entire litter is delivered. Many queens will ingest the placentas during parturition.

In general, parturition is fairly straightforward and easy in this species. Queens that are progressing normally in labor, with no evidence of fetal death/distress may benefit from being left alone in a dark place. A hidden area (for example, a cardboard box) can provide the necessary privacy for the queen to continue progressing labor normally. Most queens will give birth at night without assistance, and overzealous owners may actually prolong the process by interrupting the queen repeatedly.

9.2 Differentiating Eutocia from Dystocia

Dystocia in cats is less common than in dogs, with a reported incidence of 3–6%, and occurs with greater incidence in purebred cats than mixed breeds (Holst *et al.*, 2015). Brachycephalic and dolicocephalic breeds are reported to have a higher incidence of dystocia than mesocephalic breeds (Holst *et al.*, 2015). Dystocia can be due to maternal or fetal causes. Maternal causes include primary or secondary uterine inertia, inadequate pelvic diameter, or abnormalities of the pregnancy. Abnormalities of pregnancy can include conditions like uterine prolapse, torsion, or rupture; there is also a case reported in the literature of an ectopic artery causing a stricture over a uterine horn resulting in obstructive dystocia (Stedile *et al.*, 2011). Primary uterine inertia occurs when there are no active uterine contractions, and is the most common reported cause of dystocia in queens (Ekstrand and Linde-Forsberg, 1994). Given the broad range of normal gestation length in this species, a diagnosis of primary uterine inertia must be interpreted with caution, as it is possible that the queen simply has not initiated parturition at the time of diagnosis. Secondary uterine inertia occurs when there is myometrial fatigue due to repeated, non-productive contractions. Secondary uterine inertia typically occurs secondary to obstructive dystocia, where

 Feline Reproduction (eds. A.K. Johnson and M.A. Kutzler)

DOI: 10.1079/9781789247107.0009

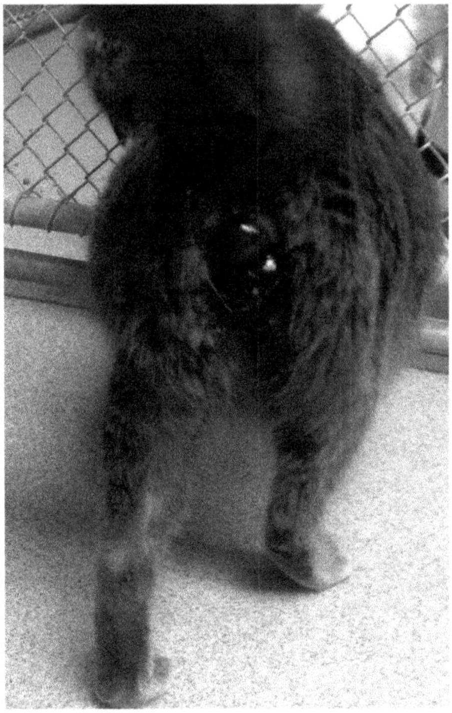

Fig. 9.1. Normal queen during parturition. Note the presence of the amnionic sac, intact, at the vulvar lips. (Photo courtesy of Dr Aime Johnson.)

something is prohibiting the passage of a kitten through the birth canal.

Fetal causes of dystocia include fetal oversize and abnormalities of fetal presentation, posture, and position. Fetal oversize may be absolute, such as in single kitten litters, where the kitten has grown overly large in utero and cannot pass vaginally, or relative, where a portion of the kitten (for example, the head) cannot enter the birth canal. Fetal deformities or fetal monsters may also result in obstructive dystocia (Figs 9.3 and 9.4). Absolute fetal oversize may also be seen in young primigravida queens where the queen has not yet reached full body size or pelvic diameter. Normal presentation can be either anterior or posterior, and posterior presentation does not predispose to dystocia. The absolute shape of fetal kittens makes abnormalities of position less common relative to other species, as the majority of the fetal mass is the head, neck, and body with relatively short limbs. However, displacement or flexure of the head and neck can result in abnormalities of position resulting in dystocia. Fetal postural abnormalities occur when the fetal and maternal spinal columns are not in alignment. Normal posture for kittens is dorsosacral, where the dorsum of the kitten is against the sacrum of the queen. An example of postural abnormality would be dorsopubic posture (kitten is upside down in the birth canal with fetal limbs and abdomen pointed to the maternal spine).

Diagnosis of dystocia can be achieved by compiling information from several diagnostic aids. A careful history should be taken, including information about previous pregnancies and gestation lengths, breeding dates for the current pregnancy, time of labor onset, and the time of delivery of any previous kittens in the litter. Serum progesterone in the pregnant queen does not decrease to baseline prior to parturition as it does in the dog. Keiser reported that on the day of delivery, serum progesterone in the queen averaged 2.99 ng/mL in one report and 3.18 ng/mL in a second (Keiser *et al.*, 2017) Therefore, unlike in the dog, daily progesterone testing to detect a decrease to baseline that indicates parturition is imminent is not useful in the queen. Queens with prolonged duration of stage I or II labor should be at high suspicion for dystocia. If the duration of stage I exceeds 24 hours, the queen should be evaluated further. Queens exhibiting strong contractions for 30 minutes or more without producing a kitten should also be evaluated for dystocia. Clinical assessment becomes more difficult in queens with a prolonged lag between the delivery of kittens. Although 2–4 hours is considered a benchmark for intervention, there have been reports of queens delivering normal kittens over a much more prolonged period of time (days). Diagnosis of feline dystocia can be based on failure to initiate labor (primary inertia), failure of normal progression of labor, or intrapartum maternal compromise such as secondary to shock or dehydration.

A clinical examination, including digital vaginal exam, should be performed on all queens presenting for suspected dystocia. Abdominal radiographs can be very helpful to determine fetal number, approximate size, and presentation relative to the birth canal. If a kitten is identified in transverse presentation, for example, the clinician can rapidly proceed to delivery via cesarean section without wasting further time on medical management that has no possibility of being successful. Measurement of ionized calcium can be beneficial in detecting queens that may benefit from treatment with calcium. Anecdotally, the author uses a benchmark of

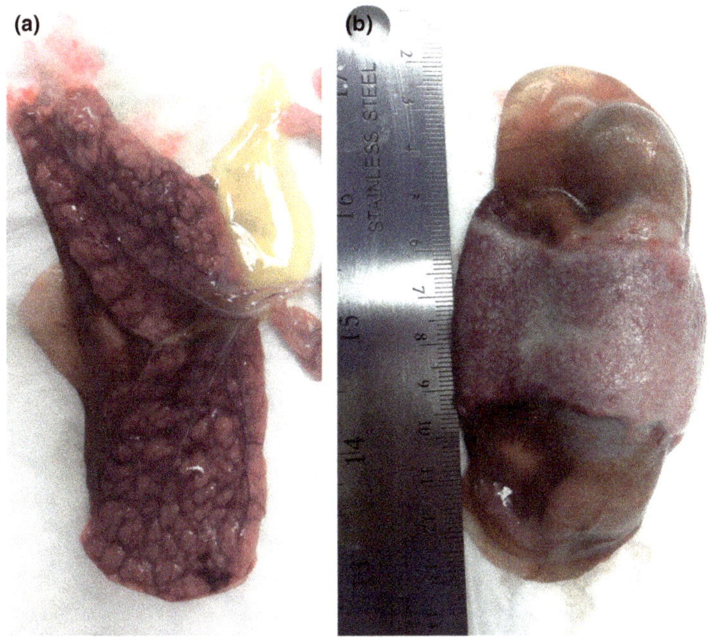

Fig. 9.2 **(a)** A normal placenta removed from a delivered fetus showing the surface that would be in contact with the amnion. **(b)** A late term fetus within its placenta. The visible surface of the zonary area of the placenta surrounding the middle of the fetus would be in contact with the uterus. (Photos courtesy of Dr Aime Johnson.)

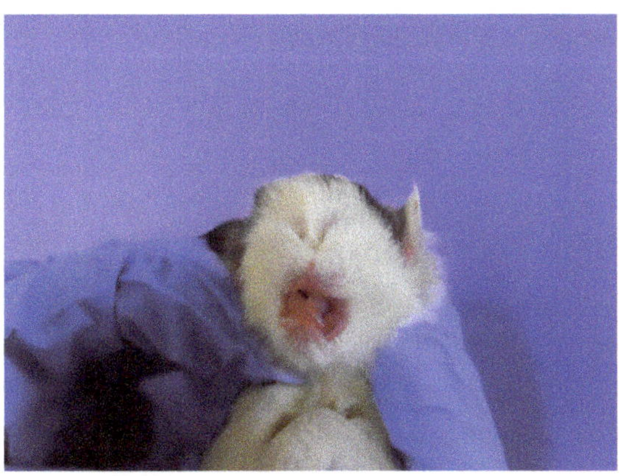

Fig. 9.3. This fetal malformation resulted in a dystocia. The fetal head is misshaped with a lack of eyes and nose. (Photo courtesy of Dr Aime Johnson.)

<1.3 mmol/L for administration of supplemental calcium. Abdominal ultrasonography is extremely useful for evaluating fetuses for signs of distress. Fetal heart rate is easy to measure; fetuses with <180 bpm should be considered in distress (Fig. 9.5). Normal fetal heart rates are approximately twice that of the queen and are typically over 200 bpm.

9.3 Medical Management of Dystocia

If radiographs and ultrasound demonstrate that the fetuses are not in distress and are of appropriate size and presentation to be delivered vaginally, oxytocin and/or calcium can be administered to augment uterine contractions and aid in expulsion of the fetuses. Calcium will improve the strength of contractions, whereas oxytocin will increase the frequency. In the author's experience, the efficacy of oxytocin therapy is dramatically improved if the queen's calcium is normalized first. Reported dosing is 0.5–1.0 mL 10% calcium gluconate solution per queen (Jutkowitz, 2005), which equates to approximately 1–2 mg elemental calcium/kg. Calcium gluconate can be administered slowly IV or subcutaneously but may result in local tissue reaction and necrosis when given subcutaneously. The likelihood of tissue reaction can be reduced by diluting calcium gluconate with sterile fluids. Queens treated with IV calcium should be monitored during administration to ensure bradycardia or arrhythmias do not develop during treatment. A syringe pump can be utilized to deliver IV calcium at a slow, predictable rate to reduce the likelihood of adverse events. Appropriate oxytocin doses for

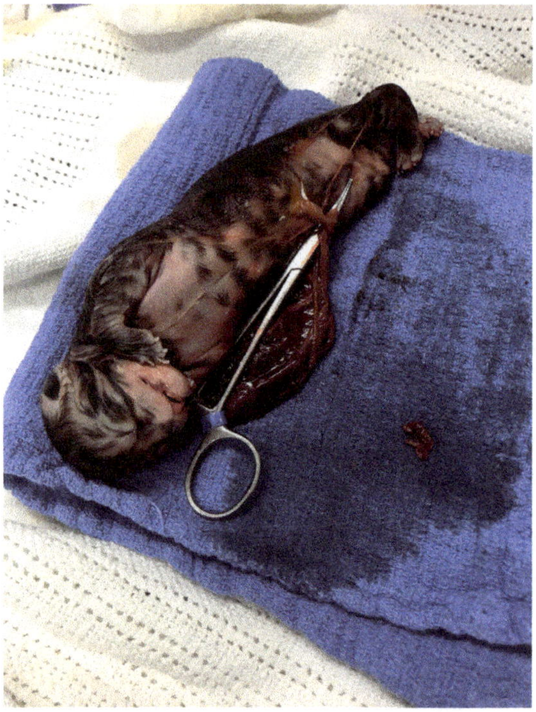

Fig. 9.4. This kitten was delivered during a cesarean section. This kitten was deceased and edematous and lodged in the pelvic canal causing an obstructive dystocia. (Photo courtesy of Dr Jamie Douglas.)

queens are 0.25–2 IU at 20- to 30-minute intervals. Oxytocin is rapidly absorbed by multiple routes and can be administered SQ, IM, or IV. When used carelessly, high doses of oxytocin can actually inhibit fetal progression and delivery by causing contractions that effectively trap the fetus or disrupt blood flow to the fetal placental unit (Pretzer, 2008). If oxytocin is administered in the face of an obstructive dystocia, the force of contractions can result in uterine rupture. When used at reasonable doses with appropriate case selection, complications from the use of oxytocin are rare. As oxytocin receptors in the myometrium become saturated, subsequent dosing will become less effective (Phaneuf *et al.*, 2000). Thus, a maximum of two to three doses should be administered, and if no progress is made, consideration should be given to cesarean section. Surgical intervention is required in approximately 60–80% of dystocia cases in queens (Traas, 2008).

Queens showing evidence of maternal compromise are poor candidates for medical management of dystocia, excluding stabilization and supportive care prior to progressing to surgical resolution. Intrapartum maternal compromise is associated with conditions such as uterine rupture or torsion. Clinical signs associated with maternal compromise include depression, anorexia, weak vocalizations, delayed capillary refill time, weak/thready pulses, tachycardia, and possibly collapse. Abdominal ultrasonography can be helpful in these cases to determine the presence of large amounts of free abdominal fluid and/or abnormal blood flow patterns to the uterus. Additional diagnostics, such as complete blood count, serum biochemistry, and blood gas analysis can aid in stabilization of the queen prior to surgery.

Vaginal manipulation of fetuses is difficult in queens due to small body size. Simple abnormalities of posture, such as rotation from dorsopubic to dorsosacral, can be accomplished with gentle manipulation. However, correction of position or presentation is much more challenging, if not impossible, due to the relatively small diameter of the vaginal canal. Aggressive attempts at delivery can result in removal of limbs or dislocation of the cervical spine and head. A red rubber catheter attached to a syringe of sterile lubricant can be used to apply additional lubrication to the vaginal canal to aid in expulsion of fetuses.

9.4 Cesarean Section

The goal of cesarean section is to progress to delivery of the kittens as rapidly as possible while minimizing total anesthetic time. Most queens can have surgical preparation performed prior to anesthetic induction, such as clipping the hair from the abdomen, a 'rough scrub' with either chlorhexidine or povidone iodine, or placement of an intravenous catheter. If tolerated by the queen, oxygen can be provided via mask during surgical preparation.

There are a variety of anesthetic techniques reported for use in feline cesarean section. The author prefers premedication with an opioid, rapid induction with propofol or alfaxalone IV, and maintenance via endotracheal intubation with oxygen and isofluorane or sevofluorane. In the author's experience, adverse effects on the neonates from administration of opioids as a premedication are minimal and offset by the improvement of rapid, safe anesthetic induction of the queen. Further discussion of anesthesia for cesarian sections is discussed in Chapter 10. If necessary, any respiratory

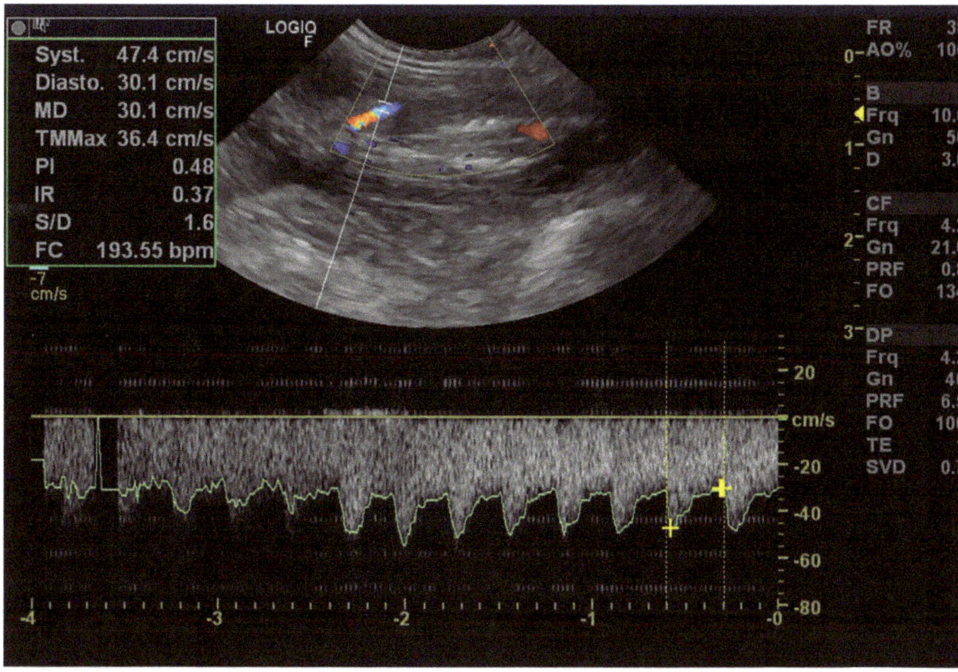

Fig. 9.5. Ultrasonic measurement of feline fetal heart rates using M-mode ultrasonography. As fetal heart rates are typically >200 bpm, using M-mode to calculate the heart rate is more accurate than attempting a manual count. (Image: author's own.)

depression in neonates can be totally or partially reversed with the administration of naloxone via the umbilical vessels, dependent on the particular opiate administered to the queen. In cats, opioid use can be associated with postoperative hyperthermia (Posner *et al.*, 2010). Although many of these cases are self-limiting, body temperature should be closely monitored during the anesthetic episode. There appears to be an inverse relationship between body temperature at extubation and degree of post anesthetic hyperthermia (Posner *et al.*, 2010); patient warming to prevent heat loss may aid in mitigating this side effect.

Routine surgical technique for cesarean section in queens includes a ventral midline celiotomy, extended large enough to easily expose the uterine horns and exteriorize them from the abdomen. The exteriorized horn(s) should be packed off from the rest of the abdomen with moistened laparoptomy sponges. The entire uterus can also be reflected caudally in some cases, allowing the uterus to be completely packed off from the abdominal cavity preventing contamination. An incision is made into an avascular portion of the uterine horn, typically along the greater curvature, with kittens subsequently 'milked' down the horns toward the incision for delivery. It is at the preference and jurisdiction of the surgeon whether one or multiple incisions (i.e. one in each horn) are made. If it is difficult to milk the kittens from one horn toward the hysterotomy incision, it may be preferable to make a second incision to facilitate more rapid delivery of the kittens rather than continuing to struggle with the delivery. In term fetuses, gentle traction against the umbilical cord will typically result in placental release from the uterine wall (Fig. 9.6). If the placentas are firmly adhered, or if significant hemorrhage occurs during their removal, the placentas may be left in situ to detach on their own. Although retained fetal membranes can be an inciting cause of metritis in queens, in the author's experience these typically pass without complication. Oxytocin and/or prostaglandin can be administered to aid in placental expulsion (Jutkowitz, 2005).

The delivered kitten is then passed to a non-sterile assistant, using care not to contaminate the surgeon or sterile field. The assistant may hold a sterile towel stretched out, and the kitten is gently

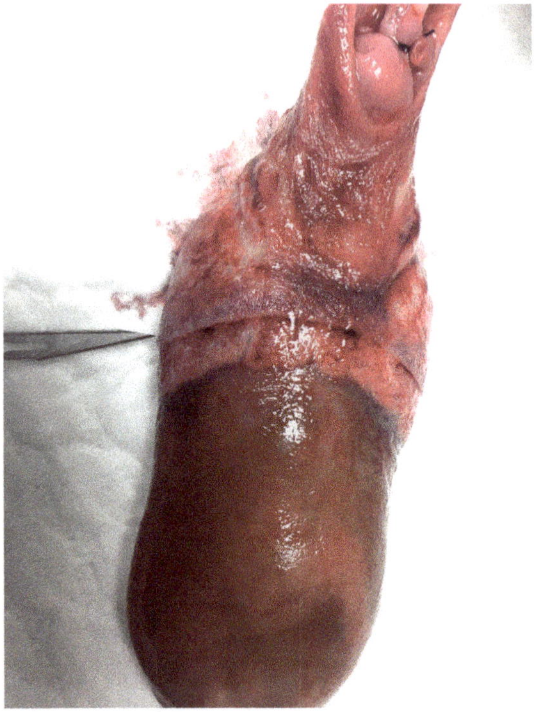

Fig. 9.6. Manual separation of the placenta from the uterus. The surgical blade on the left is placed at the junction between the uterus and the releasing placenta. Gentle traction can be placed on the placenta to 'unzip' it from the uterus. (Photo courtesy of Dr Aime Johnson.)

dropped into the towel to allow the assistant to begin resuscitation. If the umbilical cord and placenta are delivered with the kitten, the team performing neonatal resuscitation can utilize these vessels for drug administration in the neonate if required. If the umbilicus is ligated by the surgeon upon removal of the kitten, a longer umbilicus (2.5–5 cm) should be left to allow access to the umbilical veins for medication administration if needed. The umbilicus can be shortened later using sterile suture. The membranes should be rapidly removed from the kitten's head/muzzle and the kitten should be rubbed vigorously to stimulate respiration. It is important to have adequate assistance available such that the surgeon can solely focus on continued delivery of the entire litter, without trying to simultaneously resuscitate kittens as they are delivered. Additionally, a dedicated anesthetist should be monitoring the queen as the removal of the kittens can cause hypotension and other anesthetic complications.

The uterus should be examined until the tip of the horn and ovary is visualized to ensure no kittens are accidentally left in the uterus at surgery. Likewise, a finger can be used to sweep the body of the uterus into the pelvic canal to find any kittens that may have moved caudally during induction or the start of surgery. Once delivery of the litter is complete, the hysterotomy incision can be closed with an appositional or inverting pattern. Traditionally, an inverting pattern such as an Utrecht is used to close hysterotomy incisions as this provides a rapid and secure closure (Fig. 9.7). A second layer of closure can be performed over the first if there are any concerns about the integrity of the incision.

In queens not desired for further reproduction, ovariohysterectomy can be performed at the same time as cesarean section. In cases of fetal demise, autolyzed fetuses, or pyometra, en bloc removal of the uterus is the preferred technique as it reduces the risk of abdominal contamination with material from the uterus. The uterine body and both ovarian pedicles are isolated and ligated, and the uterus is removed without a hysterotomy incision. If this technique is utilized with live kittens, the progression from interruption of uterine blood flow to delivery of the kittens must be extremely rapid (within 60 seconds) to prevent hypoxia and subsequent neonatal mortality (Robbins and Mullen, 1994; Traas, 2008). Alternatively, routine ovariohysterectomy can be performed after delivery of the last kitten with or without hysterotomy closure. The decision to perform ovariohysterectomy in queens at the time of cesarean section should be made on individual consultation regarding the patient's condition and owner's needs. In the gravid queen, the risk of surgical complications such as postoperative hemorrhage must be balanced against performing the procedure concurrently or at a later date.

Queens should be provided with postoperative analgesia following cesarean section. Analgesic options include nonsteroidal anti-inflammatory drugs and opioids. Given the unique physiology of feline metabolism of NSAIDs, a single dose can be administered perioperative, and opioids such as buprenorphine (0.01–0.04 mg/kg, IM, IV, or transmucosally) or methadone (0.25–0.5 mg/kg, SC, IM, slow IV) can be administered for post-operative analgesia. Anecdotally, queens with good post-operative pain control appear to mother their kittens more readily.

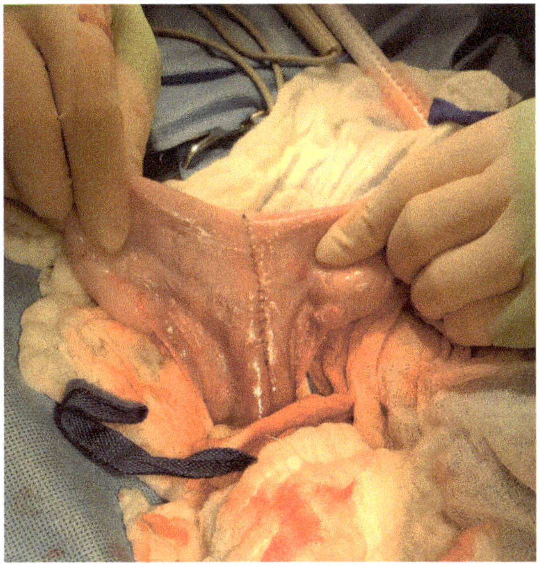

Fig. 9.7. An Utrecht closure pattern on a feline cesarean section. (Photo courtesy of Dr Aime Johnson.)

9.5 References

Ekstrand, C. and Linde-Forsberg, C. J. (1994) Dystocia in the cat: A retrospective study of 155 cases. *Journal of Small Animal Practice* 35, 459–464. doi: 10.1111/j.1748-5827.1994.tb03951.x

Holst, B. S., Axnér, E., Öhlund, M., Möller, L., and Egenvall, A. (2015) Dystocia in the cat evaluated using an insurance database. *Journal of Feline Medicine and Surgery* 8, 1–6 doi: 10.1177/1098612X15600482

Jutkowitz, L. A. (2005) Reproductive emergencies. *Veterinary Clinics North America: Small Animal Practice* 35, 397–420. doi: 10.1016/j.cvsm.2004.10.006

Keiser, R., Reichler, I. M., and Balogh, O. (2017) Are foetal ultrasonographic and maternal blood progesterone measurements near parturition reliable predictors of the time of birth in the domestic cat? *Reproduction in Domestic Animals* 52, 487–494. doi: 10.1111/rda.12939

Phaneuf, S., Rodíguez Liñares, B., TambyRaja, R. L., MacKenzie, I. Z., and López Bernal, A. (2000) Loss of myometrial oxytocin receptors during oxytocin-induced and oxytocin-augmented labour. *Journal of Reproduction and Fertility* 120, 91–97. doi: 10.1530/jrf.0.1200091

Posner, L. P., Pavuk, A. A., Rokshar, J. L., Carter, J. E., and Levine, J. F. (2010) Effects of opioids and anesthetic drugs on body temperature in cats. *Veterinary Anaesthesia and Analgesia* 37, 35–43. doi: 10.1111/j.1467-2995.2009.00508.x

Pretzer, S. D. (2008) Medical management of canine and feline dystocia. *Theriogenology* 70, 332–336. doi: 10.1016/j.theriogenology.2008.04.031

Robbins, M. A. and Mullen, H. S. (1994) En bloc ovario-hysterectomy as a treatment for dystocia in dogs and cats. *Veterinary Surgery* 23, 48–52. doi: 10.1111/j.1532-950x.1994.tb00442.x

Root Kustritz, M. V. (2006) Clinical management of pregnancy in cats. *Theriogenology* 66, 145–150. doi: 10.1016/j.theriogenology.2006.03.018

Root Kustritz, M. V., Johnston, S. D., and Olson, P. N. (1995) Estrous length, pregnancy rate, gestation and parturition lengths, litter size, and juvenile mortality in the domestic cat. *Journal of the American Animal Hospital Association* 31, 429–433. doi: 10.5326/15473317-31-5-429

Stedile, R., Oliveira, S. T., Muccillo Mde, S., Contesini, E. A., and Beck, C. A. (2011) Dystocia in a cat due to an ectopic artery. *Veterinary Record* 169, 556. doi: 10.1136/vr.d5516

Traas, A. M. (2008) Surgical management of canine and feline dystocia. *Theriogenology* 70, 337–342. doi: 10.1016/j.theriogenology.2008.04.014

10 Neonatal Resuscitation and Care

AIME K. JOHNSON AND JACOB A. JOHNSON

Auburn University College of Veterinary Medicine, Department of Clinical Sciences, Auburn, Alabama, USA

10.1 Introduction

The neonatal period is a critical time for kitten growth and development. Major milestones that occur in the neonatal period include establishing passive immunity through ingestion of colostrum, rapid gain in bone and tissue density, and opening of the eyes. For the neonate, self-regulation of body temperature is not yet autonomous, with kitten thermoregulation developing over the first 45 days. Threats to the health of the neonatal kitten are of utmost importance and include improper nutrition, exposure to pathogens, inherited disease, and savaging by the dam or other adult cats. The neonatal period is defined as the first 2 weeks of life followed by the pediatric period from 2–6 weeks and the juvenile period that lasts until 12 weeks. Overall, kitten mortality rates during the neonatal period have appeared to decline over time, from as high as 28% in 1978 to 13% in 2020 in kittens less than 8 weeks of age (Scott and Geissinger, 1978; Dolan *et al.*, 2020). Factors that negatively correlate with survival are low birthweight (13 times greater chance of death) and weight loss over the first week of life (nine times greater risk) (Dolan *et al.*, 2020). For further information on disease processes leading to neonatal illness and death, see Chapter 11. In a pathogen-free facility, the rate of neonatal death was about 15% (Young, 1973). Causes of neonatal death in this colony were not due to diseases as is common in shelter medicine or catteries. Neonatal loss was due to direct maternal neglect (19%), cannibalism (12.5%), coliform infection (10.5%), congenital abnormalities (19%), undetermined stillborn (21%), and undetermined cause when kitten was born alive (18%). One study also showed a correlation between increasing litter size and higher likelihood of still births (Sparkes *et al.*, 2006). Careful monitoring and support of kittens during the neonatal period is essential to maximize survival.

10.2 Preparing for Birth

Signs of readiness for parturition in the queen begins with increasing mammary development up to 1 week before their due date. Within a few days of birth, the queen will often seek a hiding place. On transabdominal ultrasound, the fetal heart rates should be over 200 beats per minute. Fetal kidney definition can be observed within a few days of birth, where the cortex and medulla become distinguishable (Fig. 10.1). One of the last developments in the fetus is intestinal lumen (Fig. 10.2) and peristalsis. If this is observed, most likely the fetus is ready for delivery or cesarean section. Typically, this author detects good intestinal development around 64–66 days from breeding.

In most cases, the queen will deliver the kittens unassisted. Distant observation is the best practice during the delivery process unless a complication arises. For further information on delivery of kittens, see Chapter 9. Once kittens are born, the queen will remove the amnion from each kitten and lick them until they are stimulated. The queen will also move them toward her abdomen for nursing. It is best to allow the queen and kittens to bond during this time and not disturb them. If the queen becomes stressed around the delivery process, she is more likely to cannibalize the kittens. Once the bonding has occurred, the kitten can be removed to be weighed, marked for identification, and examined before returning it to the queen. An easy way to identify kittens in a litter is to clip a small patch of hair in different locations for each kitten (back of the neck, back by the tail, either shoulder, either hip, etc.).

DOI: 10.1079/9781789247107.0010

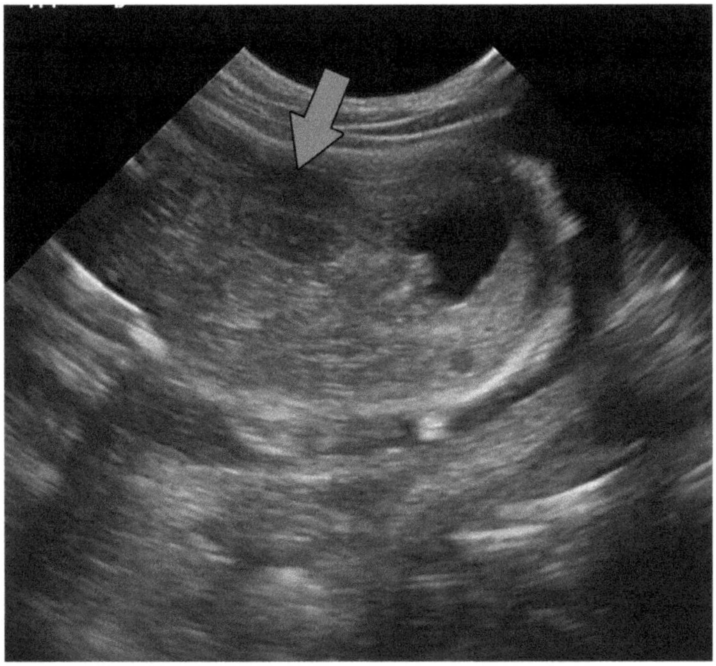

Fig. 10.1. Ultrasound image in a late term fetus where the kidney definition is evident within the fetal abdomen. The fetal kidney is marked with the arrow. The fetal stomach can also be visualized as the hypoechoic structure to the right of the kidney. (Image: author's own.)

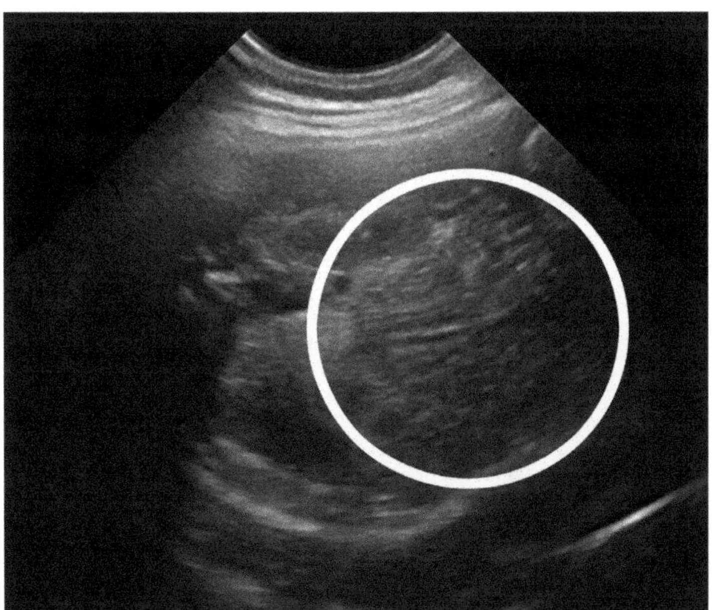

Fig. 10.2. Ultrasound image of the fetal abdomen in a late term fetus. The intestinal development and visible intestinal lumen are seen. This can be visualized when the kitten reaches maturity and birth typically occurs within 1–2 days. (Image: author's own.)

10.3 Anesthesia for Cesarean Section

If assistance is necessary, the delivery process can determine the fate of the neonates. If delivery is prolonged, or a dystocia is present, fetal survival decreases. Additionally, if a cesarean section is needed, the process also contributes to the health and survival of the neonates. The optimum anesthetic plan for feline C-sections is rarely described (Dodman, 1979; Benson and Thurmon, 1984; Tranquilli, 1992). The general principles have been extrapolated from canine and human information (Robertson and Moon, 2003; Kraus, 2016; Robertson, 2016; Mathews and Sinclair, 2018). Preoperative work-up should begin with a history and physical examination. Unless any unexpected findings are discovered, then no additional work-up is necessary. Any abnormal findings could warrant additional diagnostics such as a packed cell volume/total solids, complete blood cell count, biochemistry profile, and/or radiographs.

Non-steroidal anti-inflammatory drugs are beneficial for the control of postoperative inflammatory pain (Shih *et al.*, 2008). Robenacoxib (2 mg/kg, SQ) is approved for preoperative and multi-day use, making it most suitable for short-term use in a cesarean section. Meloxicam (0.3 mg/kg, SQ) is also approved for preoperative administration.

Preoperative sedatives have the advantage of reducing induction and maintenance requirements and reducing stress in a fractious queen. However, these drugs will also impact fetal resuscitation efforts (Moon *et al.*, 1998). Place an intravenous catheter without a sedative if the queen is compliant. Otherwise, administer dexmedetomidine (5–20 mcg/kg, IM) and allow time for sedation prior to catheter placement.

Preoperative opioids provide analgesia and sedation, lowering induction and maintenance requirements. Shorter acting and/or reversible mu agonists, such as hydromorphone, are most appropriate. Butorphanol may not provide sufficient analgesia for the surgical procedure. Buprenorphine provides long-acting analgesia, but cannot be reversed and may limit the ability to provide additional analgesia intraoperatively. Opioids can be combined with dexmedetomidine for sedation or given intravenously prior to induction.

In order to limit anesthesia time, it is advantageous to clip and perform initial surgical prep on a compliant or sedated queen prior to induction. Preoxygenation for 3–5 minutes prior to induction will overcome some of the respiratory changes present in gravid females. This should only be performed in the compliant patient. A balanced, replacement intravenous fluid, such as Lactated Ringer's Solution, should be started at 3-5 mL/kg/h prior to induction.

Because of increased risk of regurgitation in pregnant females, a rapid induction with a hypnotic agent is preferred. Alfaxalone (1–2 mg/kg, IV) has been shown to improve fetal vigor during cesarean section when compared to propofol (2–6 mg/kg, IV) (Doebeli *et al.*, 2013). Dissociative agents, such as ketamine and tiletamine and zolazepam (Telazol^{R}), have been shown to reduce fetal vigor (Moon-Massat and Erb, 2002). Inhalant inductions should be avoided due to the lack of airway control and high concentrations needed to induce anesthesia.

Once the patient is induced, endotracheal intubation is performed, and the queen is maintained on inhalant with the balance of oxygen. Sevoflurane is less soluble than isoflurane, which should promote a more rapid recovery for the queen and kittens. Late-term pregnancy reduces inhalant requirements by up to 40%, so anesthetic depth should be monitored closely, and inhalant levels reduced to the lowest possible to maintain unconsciousness (Palahniuk *et al.*, 1974). Consideration should be given to administering atipamezole (ten times the dose of dexmedetomidine given, IM) to ensure a minimal effect on fetal vigor.

An epidural injection of preservative-free morphine (0.1 mg/kg at 1 mg/mL) and equivolume of preservative-free 2% lidocaine provides ideal intraoperative and postoperative analgesia (DeRossi *et al.*, 2016). If an epidural is not feasible, then additional doses of the same opioid used in premedication can be used to control surgical stimulation. Monitoring techniques and parameters should be the same as for other surgical procedures. If an epidural was not performed, consideration should be given to performing a line block along the incision site after closure with bupivacaine (not to exceed 4 mg/kg, SQ).

10.4 Neonatal Resuscitation

Once the kittens are delivered and passed from the surgeon to the attendant, the kitten should be placed sternal with the head tilted slightly downward. The kitten is rubbed vigorously with a warm clean towel and gently pinched at the scruff to stimulate the kitten to breathe and help remove mucus from the airway. The mouth and nose are then cleared using a neonatal bulb syringe (Fig. 10.3) and/or a DeLee mucous trap (Fig. 10.4). Supplemental heat is required as kittens that are cold will be slow to resuscitate. An external heat source such as a Bair Hugger Warming Blanket™ (3M), Hot Dog™ Patient Warming System (Augustine Surgical, Inc), or a well-padded heating pad to protect against burns is sufficient. If none of these are available, rubber gloves filled with warm water and tied closed can be used to provide external heat. Care must be taken not to get the gloves too hot which will burn the kittens or allow water to leak as the kittens will become wet and cold.

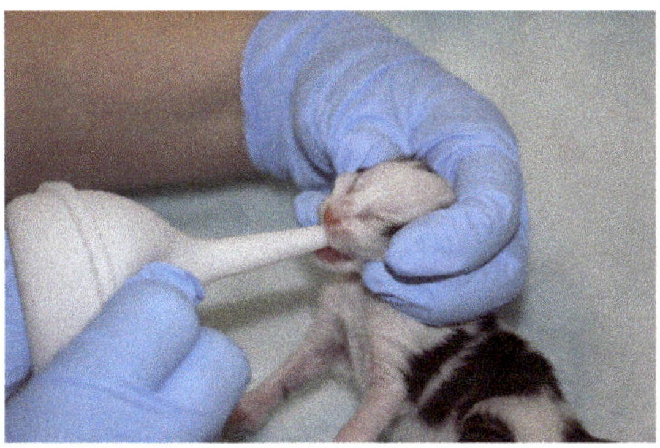

Fig. 10.3. Using a bulb syringe can clear mucous and fluid from the airway during resuscitation. (Image: author's own.)

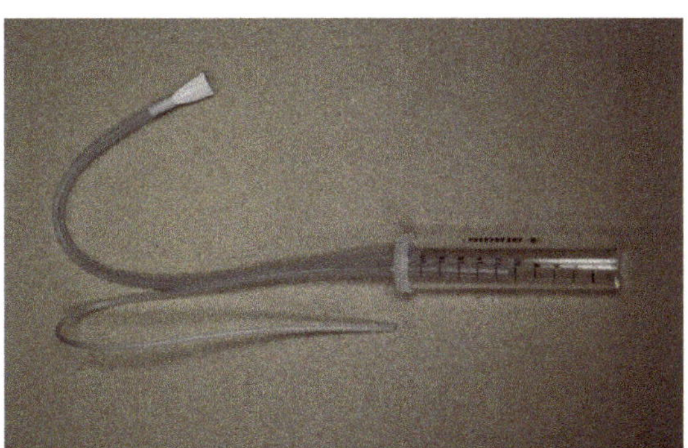

Fig. 10.4. A DeLee mucous trap for clearing the airway of the neonate. One end is inserted into the clinician's mouth, the other is inserted into the kitten's mouth/airway. The mucous enters the collection device. (Image: author's own.)

If the kitten is not breathing on its own and vocalizing within 3 minutes, oxygen supplementation should be initiated via a face mask. A neonatal oxygen mask is preferred and should be placed over the kitten's muzzle (Fig. 10.5). If a neonatal mask is not available, an adult mask can be used. If using a larger mask, the diaphragm should be blocked with a towel to concentrate the oxygen within the mask. While receiving oxygen, the presence of a heartbeat should be determined. This can be performed by digital palpation but is easier if a Doppler probe is placed over the heart (Fig. 10.5). Using the Doppler, the kitten's heart rate can be audibly heard and monitored continuously. If the kitten is not breathing, bradycardia is likely also present. Gentle, quick chest squeezes using the thumb and forefinger can be performed while the kitten is receiving oxygen. This allows oxygen to enter the lungs and encourages further clearance of the airway of fluid and mucous. Once oxygen enters the lungs, the heart rate will often increase. This process (clearing the airway, simulating the

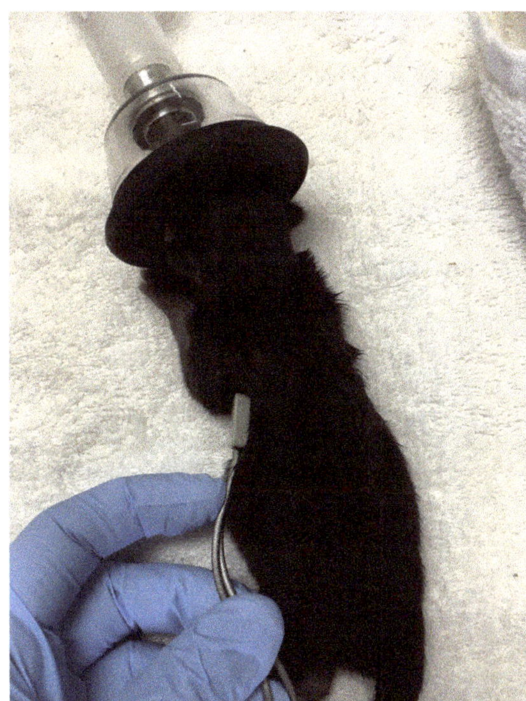

Fig. 10.5. A neonatal mask placed over the nose of a neonate to deliver supplemental oxygen. A Doppler probe is placed over the heart to assess heartrate. (Image: author's own.)

kittens by vigorous rubbing, then continuing oxygen) should be repeated until the kitten is actively breathing on its own and fully resuscitated.

If the kitten is still not breathing, the acupuncture point, GV26 can be used by placing a 22–25-gauge needle between the upper lip and nose into the philtrum (Fig. 10.6). If an opioid premedication was administered, 0.05–0.1 mL of naloxone can be administered to the kitten to reverse any potential effect. This is only needed if the kitten is slow to recover and prolonged effects of the opioid is suspected. The best route of administration is intravenously. However, gaining venous access in a small kitten is technically challenging. The umbilical vein is ideal for drug administration in the immediate postpartum period. During the cesarean section, the umbilical cord should be ligated approximately 6–8 cm from the body wall (Fig. 10.7). This allows easy access to the umbilical vessels. The umbilicus can be shortened after the kitten is fully resuscitated. In this author's hands, supplemental oxygen, supplemental heat, and stimulation are sufficient for most resuscitation. Epinephrine can be used at 0.05–0.1 mL into the umbilical vein if no heartbeat is detected via Doppler or auscultation. Atropine is not currently recommended due to its effects of increased cardiac workload in an already hypoxic patient. Slinging kittens by swinging them downward to remove mucus is no longer a recommended process due to the damage incurred when the organs and brain are also placed under that force. Administration of doxapram to stimulate breathing is also no longer recommended in domestic species as it has been shown in human neonates to increase the brain's need for oxygen in a time when the neonate may already be hypoxic (Roll and Horsch, 2004). Intubation may be performed in kittens that are not wanting to breathe independently. Intubation in small kittens is challenging but may be accomplished using small uncuffed endotracheal tubes, large intravenous catheters (needle stylet removed), or red rubber catheters. This tends to be a treatment of last resort due to the risk of damaging the airway by intubating or over insufflating the lungs when administering breaths. In this author's opinion, oxygen provided by a face mask with or without

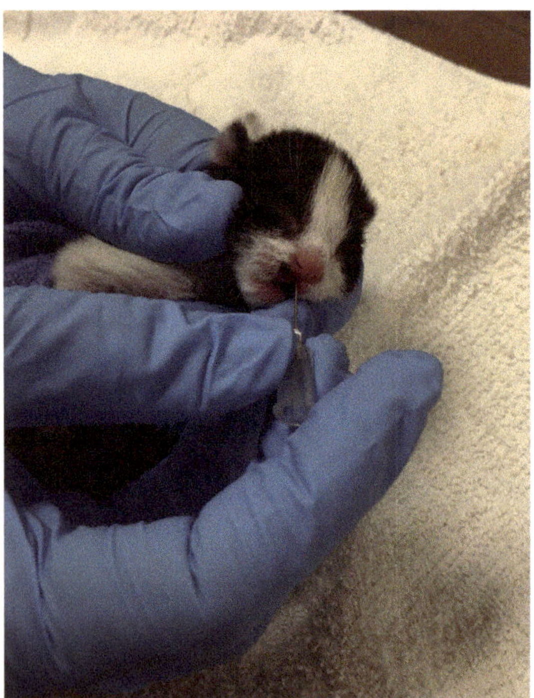

Fig. 10.6. Placement of a needle at GV 26 to stimulate respiration. (Image: author's own.)

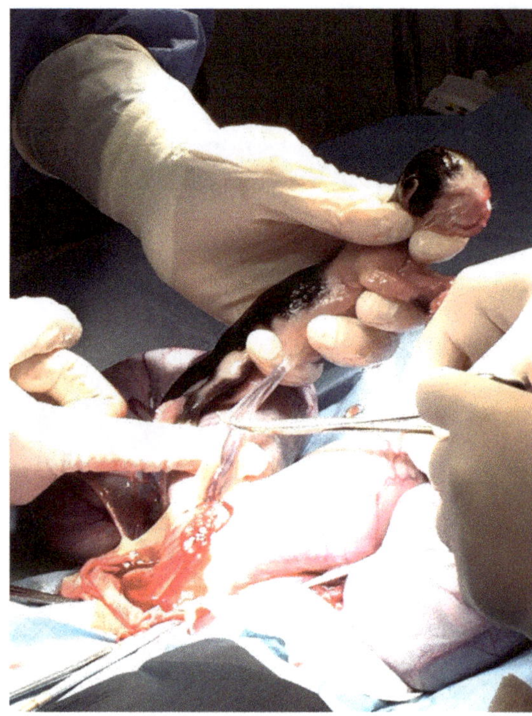

Fig. 10.7. When delivering kittens during cesarian section, the umbilicus should be tied at least 6–8 cm from the body to allow access to the umbilical vein for medication administration. (Image: author's own.)

positive pressure ventilation (through a tight-fitting mask) is superior to intubation.

Once fully resuscitated (breathing well, vocalizing, wiggling, and warm), the kittens should be placed into a pre-warmed incubator or covered box to keep them warm until they can be returned to the queen. A list of suggested items for a neonatal resuscitation kit is listed in Box 10.1.

Physical examinations should be performed on all kittens once they are resuscitated. Although small, a general physical examination can be performed to check for any abnormalities such as a heart murmur, cleft palate (Fig. 10.8), and fetal deformities. Congenital defects are common in purebred litters or litters with a high coefficient of inbreeding. Examples of common congenital defects that may have the potential to be corrected or survivable include umbilical hernia, syndactyly, eyelid coloboma or dermoids (may require the removal of one eye), and flat chest syndrome. Life-threatening conditions that can be seen at birth that often are not survivable include cleft palate, gastroschisis, imperforate rectum (Fig. 10.9), and pectus excavatum. Other conditions that may not be readily visible at birth but can cause significant kitten mortality within the neonatal period include intestinal atresia, hydrocephalus, lysosomal storage diseases, hyperchylomicroanemia, polycystic kidneys, portosystemic shunt, and organ dysgenesis.

Box 10.1. Neonatal resuscitation kit

- 1 mL syringes
- 25–22 gauge needles
- Neonatal oxygen mask
- Non-rebreathing anesthesia tubing
- Pediatric bulb syringe
- DeLee mucous trap
- Heat source for working area
- Oxygen source
- Small towels (up to 10)
- Kitten box with heat source
- Suture for umbilicus
- Mosquito hemostats (2–3)
- Small scissors
- Doppler and gel
- Pediatric stethoscope
- Naloxone
- Epinephrine
- Atropine
- Clippers or neck collars to mark kittens

10.5 After Care

Some kittens will be pushed away by the queen a few days after birth, or there may be weaker, smaller kittens within a litter that cannot compete for resources. If this occurs, removing them from their mother and either raising them as an orphan or cross fostering them may help survival. Cross-fostering kittens is also beneficial if a queen is not a good mother, has health issues such as mastitis or metritis, or if a litter is especially large. When cross-fostering the kitten to another queen, it is helpful to remove one of the queen's own kittens, place her kitten with the new one long enough to exchange scent, and place the new kitten with the original kitten back together. Most queens will accept cross-fosters readily as long as the kittens are within a few days of each other. It is not ideal to attempt cross-fostering a newborn to a litter that is more than a week ahead. The older kittens are much stronger and can push the smaller kitten away. Once placed with the new queen, she should be monitored very closely to ensure there is no aggression toward the fostered kitten. Queens can kill kittens quickly with a single bite, so the first few hours are critical. The queen will show signs of acceptance by licking the new kitten, moving it toward her mammary glands, and not showing more attention to it than she does the other kittens in her litter. Signs of aggression/non-acceptance include moving the kitten around excessively, sniffing it but then ignoring it, hissing toward it, and general agitation that continues more than a few minutes.

Because kitten mortality is much higher in kittens that are low birthweight or fail to gain appropriately, weight is extremely important to monitor for overall kitten growth. Kittens should be weighed twice daily on a gram scale (Fig. 10.10) to monitor weight gain. Kittens may lose a few grams the first 24 hours after birth but should gain steadily after that. Typical weight gain depends on litter size and breed but should be 2–10 grams over a 24-hour period. If after the first 24 hours, a kitten fails to gain weight (weight stays the same for more than 24 hours) or loses weight, supplemental feeding is recommended. Bottle feeding is risky and can lead to aspiration of milk into the lungs. It is also relying on the kitten's suckle and appetite to intake nutrients, both of which may be decreased in weak kittens that fail to thrive. Tube feeding assures that the appropriate amount of nutrients is delivered, is overall safer for the kitten, and is less time consuming

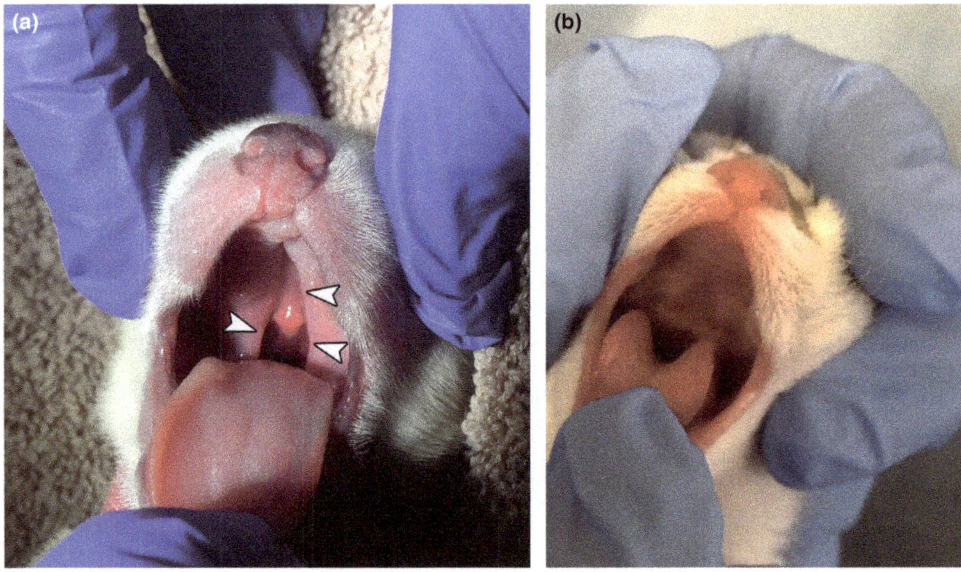

Fig. 10.8 **(a)** Severe cleft palate in a newborn kitten (white arrows). **(b)** Normal palate in a kitten for comparison. (Image: author's own.)

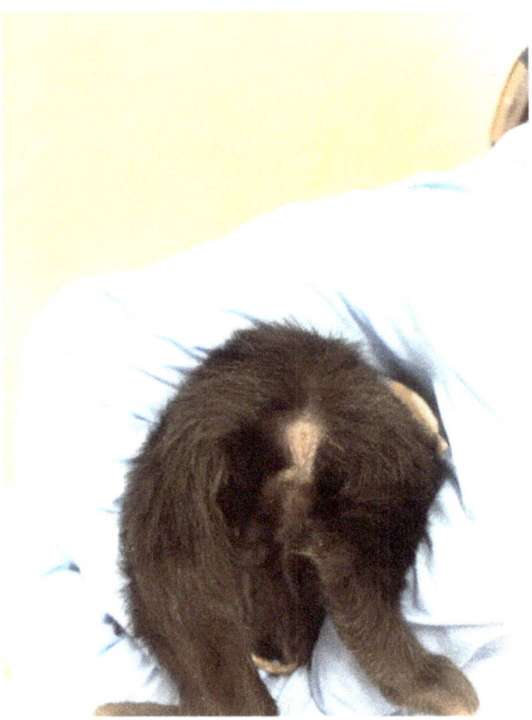

Fig. 10.9. A kitten born without a tail or rectal opening. This kitten was born alive but was euthanized due to this defect. (Image: author's own.)

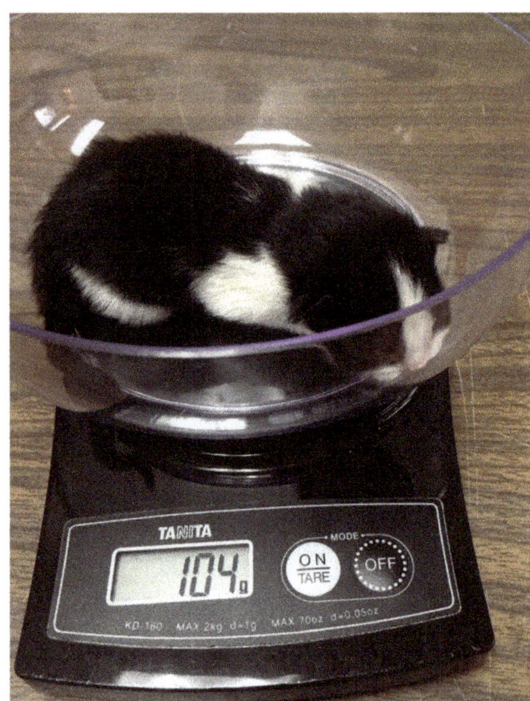

Fig. 10.10. A bowl gram scale to contain kitten while obtaining an accurate weight. (Image: author's own.)

than bottle feeding. Using a 5 French red rubber catheter as the tube, place the tip of the tube at the level of the last rib in the kitten, then mark the point of the tube that touches the nose (Fig. 10.11). This will ensure the tube is placed into the stomach and not the trachea. The kitten should be held upright (sternal and with front end elevated). This can be easily accomplished by a scruff of the kitten's neck. Once the kitten is restrained in the correct position, the tube can be passed through the open mouth and placed into the stomach using gentle pressure. The kitten should be able to cry when the tube is inserted, ensuring that the tube is not in the trachea. Once the tube is inserted to the mark, the correct amount of warmed milk replacer can be administered over 1–2 minutes and the tube removed in a steady pulling motion. The kitten should be watched closely as the milk is administered for any regurgitation. If this occurs, stop the feeding, remove the tube, place the kitten in a head down position, and suction the mouth with a bulb syringe to decrease risk of aspiration. The tube should be rinsed with water and left to dry.

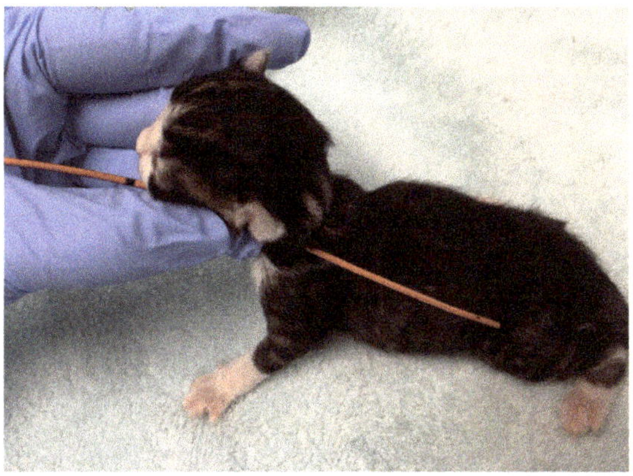

Fig. 10.11. Measurement of a feeding tube from the last rib to the muzzle. Note the mark on the feeding tube at the muzzle to indicate how far to place the tube within the esophagus and stomach. (Image: author's own.)

For kittens that are not nursing at all (orphaned or rejected kittens), the amount of supplementation must meet all nutritional needs and is based on weight of the kitten (Table 10.1). Feedings for a 24-hour period should be divided into every 2-hours for the first week to provide adequate nutrition without overextending the stomach. If weight gain is adequate after the kittens are a week

Table 10.1. Frequency and volume of feedings should be increased or decreased as needed to provide adequate weight gain for the kittens. The stomach capacity for kittens is 0.045 mL/g (45 mL/kg). When initiating feeding, begin with half to two-thirds the amount required and increase the amount over four to five feedings to allow the kitten to adjust to the milk replacer. (Author's own table, adapted from Lawler (2008).)

Weight in ounces	Weight in grams	Amount to feed in 24 hours (mL)	Amount per feeding (mL)	Number of feedings per day	Amount to supplement while nursing (mL)[a]	Number of feedings per day[a]
2	57	14	2	8–9	1–2	6–7
3	85	23	3	8–9	1–2	6–7
4	113	30	5	8–9	2	6
5	142	38	6	7	3–4	6
6	170	46	7	7	4	4–5
7	198	54	8	7	5	4
8	227	61	9	7		
9	255	70	10	6–7		
10	283	77	11	6–7		
11	312	85	12	6–7		
12	340	92	14	5–6		
13	680	100	15	5–6		
14	397	107	16	4–5		
15	425	115	17	4–5		
16 (1 lb)	454	123	18	4–5		

[a]Amount to supplement kittens if losing weight while still nursing. This is based on author's experience and should be adjusted (increased volume or frequency) as needed to provide adequate weight gain.

old, the volume of each feeding can be increased, and the frequency decreased slowly (drop one feeding at a time). Ideally, kittens can be fed every 2–3 hours during the daytime hours and then every 5–6 hours at night to allow the caretaker some rest. If the kittens are nursing, but are simply not gaining weight on their own, tube feeding can be used to 'boost' the kitten's nutritional intake and prevent it from becoming hypoglycemic or weak, further affecting the nursing. In this author's experience, supplementing one-third to one-half the total daily nutritional requirement over three to four feedings has been sufficient to provide adequate weight gain. As the kittens start to gain, the frequency or amount can be decreased until the feedings can be stopped (usually within a few days). If the kitten fails to gain, the frequency should be increased (from three to four times a day to every 2–3 hours) until the kitten begins to show weight gain. Commercially available kitten/puppy-specific formula should be used as a milk replacer.

If the mother is not stimulating the kittens to urinate or defecate, they can be stimulated by applying a warm moistened cotton ball to the genitalia and rubbing in a circular direction. This should be done following any supplemental feedings and should be performed gently as the genitalia can become irritated with excessive rubbing.

10.6 Neonatal Isoerythrolysis

One cause of neonatal death within the first few days of life is neonatal isoerythrolosis (NI). Neonatal isoerythrolysis is one of the most common causes of noninfectious neonatal morbidity and mortality in kittens (Cave *et al.*, 2002). Clinical signs include icterus, hemoglobinuria, hematuria (Fig. 10.12), tachypnea, and tachycardia in the perinatal period (Silvestre-Ferreira and Pastor, 2010). The clinical signs of NI occur as a result of ingestion of alloantibodies present in the queen's colostrum. This leads to immune-mediated destruction of red blood cells and life-threatening hemolytic anemia. Immediate intervention is needed to improve outcomes in cases of NI. Mortality is common in kittens, likely due to the smaller size of the neonate and the difficulty to diagnose this condition prior to severe clinical signs and death because the queen often keeps the kittens hidden or in an enclosed box.

The feline AB blood group system is the most described feline antigen system and characterizes cats with one of three main blood types: type A, type B, and type AB. Inheritance of blood type occurs by simple autosomal Mendelian genetics in cats. The *A* allele is dominant to the *B* allele, therefore the *A* allele is also dominant over *AB*, and *AB* is dominant over *B*. Type AB in cats is rare and is separately inherited, with the a^c allele (co-) dominant to *b* and recessive to the *A* allele (Giger, 2014). A sole genotype, *b/b*, exists for cats phenotypic for type B blood. Type AB cats are cats with genotype a^c/a^c or a^c/b. Both type A and type B cats produce naturally-occurring anti-B or anti-A alloantibodies, respectively. Type AB cats produce neither anti-A nor anti-B alloantibodies. In all type B cats, anti-A alloantibodies are present by 3 months of age. These anti-A alloantibodies possess strong hemolyzing activity. Examples of cat breeds in North America possessing high prevalence of type B blood include British Shorthair, Cornish and Devon Rex, and Turkish Angora/van, though this list is not exhaustive. Frequency of cats with type B blood is influenced geographically (Giger, 2014). In contrast, type A cats possess a less robust presence of anti-B alloantibodies at 3 months, with these antibodies characterized by a weaker hemolyzing ability. For those in clinical practice, it is important to note that type A blood has the highest prevalence in domestic short- and medium-haired cats (Silvestre-Ferreira and Pastor, 2010; Giger, 2014; Kehl *et al.*, 2018).

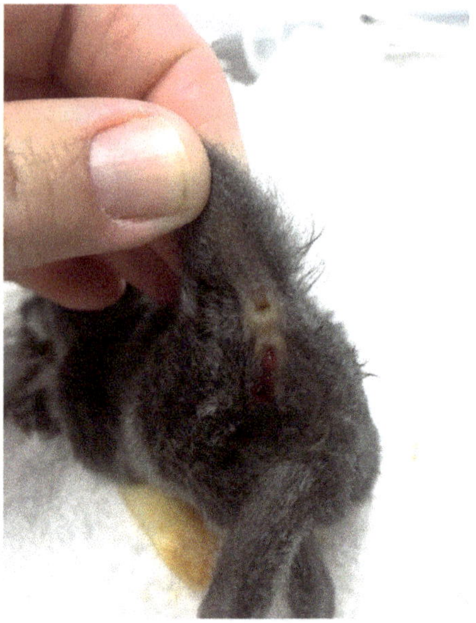

Fig. 10.12. Hematuria in a 1-day old kitten diagnosed with neonatal isoerythrolysis (NI). (Image: author's own.)

Primiparous queens bred to toms of differing blood type can develop NI. Disease is most commonly observed in a type B queen bred to a type A tom. To confirm suspicions of NI in the kittens, whole blood should be collected from the litter's sire and dam and a blood-typing agglutination assay can be performed (Fig. 10.13). Consideration of genotype is important when assessing NI in a queen bred to an *A/b* or a^c/b tom. Because the tom is a carrier of the B allele, his mating to the type B queen can result in the absence of NI at their first mating and its presentation following future matings.

Treatment of NI should be aggressive and is largely focused on supportive care (Silvestre-Ferreira and Pastor, 2010; Giger, 2014). Further ingestion of colostrum by neonates must be prevented. Thermal and nutritional support are mandated as clinical manifestation of NI progresses. Dependent on severity of clinical symptoms, blood transfusion and fluid therapy should be considered. Fluid therapy is important for neonates being treated for NI to prevent pigment-induced renal and hepatic disease.

If NI-affected kittens are less than 72 hours old and if banked, typed blood is unavailable, use of the queen's blood for transfusion is recommended (Silvestre-Ferreira and Pastor, 2010). Recall that NI is the direct result of ingestion of anti-A alloantibodies from the type B queen's colostrum. Transfusing kittens with type A blood while anti-A alloantibodies are still at great concentration in the kittens' circulation contributes to ongoing hemolysis. Because the type B queen does not sequester anti-B alloantibodies in her colostrum, she makes the ideal blood donor for kittens in the acute stages of NI. Feline maternal alloantibodies are reported to have a short life span, 1.9 and 4.4 days for IgA and IgG, respectively (Casal *et al.*, 1996). If continued transfusion support is needed after kittens reach 72 hours of age, a cross-matched donor can be used as anti-*A* alloantibodies wane.

Neonatal isoerythrolysis is best managed by prevention. Understanding the blood type of the sire and dam allows insight into the likelihood of NI following breeding. For queens with type B blood, breeding to a type B tom selects for type B kittens and eliminates risk of NI in the produced litter. If breeding to a type A or type AB tom is desirable, effort must be made to prevent colostral intake by kittens. Supplemental nutrition can be offered via tube feeding and milk replacer until blood typing of kittens has been performed, or until gut closure has occurred. Gut closure in kittens is reported to occur between 12- and 24-hours of birth (Casal *et al.*, 1996; Silvestre-Ferreira and Pastor, 2010). Kittens with foreign blood type to the queen can be cross fostered if a lactating queen with the tom's blood type is available.

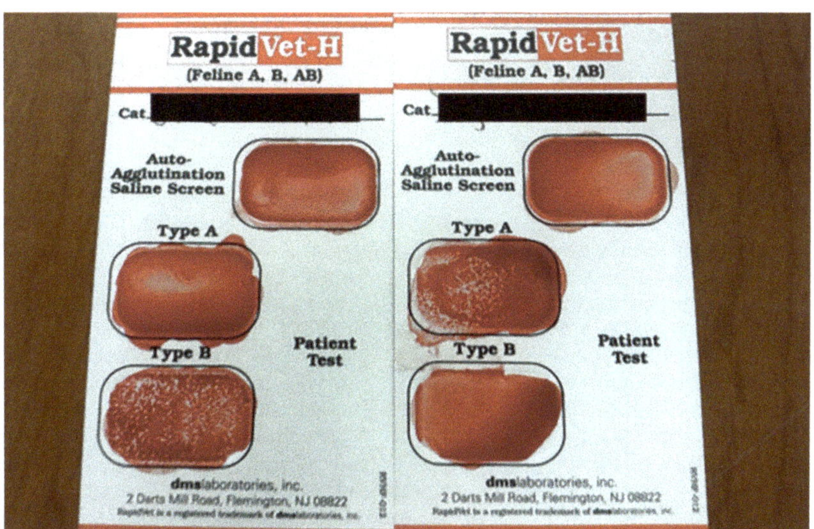

Fig. 10.13. A blood-typing agglutination assay showing blood typing. The card on the left is the queen whose blood type is B (note the agglutination in the 'Type B' area). The card on the right is the tom who has type A (note the agglutination in the 'Type A' area). The kittens from this litter were affected by NI. This test can be performed rapidly and is available for clinic use. (Image: author's own.)

10.7 Conclusion

An important consideration for at-risk neonates is establishing passive immunity in absence of colostrum. Oral or intravenous delivery of plasma or serum collected from donors sharing the same environment can achieve this goal. Oral plasma or serum should be delivered within 12–24 hours of birth so that immunoglobins can be absorbed prior to gut closure.

Nursing care within the neonatal period is essential for survival. Although intensive, appropriate resuscitation and nursing care can increase survival rates of the kittens.

10.8 References

Benson, G. J. and Thurmon, J. C. (1984) Anesthesia for cesarean section in the dog and cat. *Modern Veterinary Practice* 65, 29–32.

Casal, M. L., Jezyk, P. F., and Giger, U. (1996) Transfer of colostral antibodies from queens to their kittens. *American Journal of Veterinary Research* 57, 1653–1658.

Cave, T. A., Thompson, H., Reid, S. W. J., Hodgson, D. R., and Addie, D. D. (2002) Kitten mortality in the United Kingdom: a retrospective analysis of 274 histopathological examinations (1986 to 2000). *Veterinary Record* 151, 497–501. doi: 10.1136/vr.151.17.497

DeRossi, R., Hermeto, L. C., Jardim, P. H. A., Bicudo, N. de A., and de Assis, K. T. (2016) Postoperative pain control in cats: clinical trials with pre-emptive lidocaine epidural co-administered with morphine or methadone. *Journal of Feline Medicine and Surgery* 18, 882–888. doi: 10.1177/1098612X15602738

Dodman, N. H. (1979) Anesthesia for Cesarean-section in the dog and cat - review. *Journal of Small Animal Practice* 20, 449–460. doi: 10.1111/j.1748-5827.1979.tb06750.x

Doebeli, A., Michel, E., Bettschart, R., Hartnack, S., and Reichler, I. M. (2013) Apgar score after induction of anesthesia for canine cesarean section with alfaxalone versus propofol. *Theriogenology* 80, 850–854. doi: 10.1016/j.theriogenology.2013.07.006

Dolan, E. D., Doyle, E., Tran, H. R., and Slater, M. R. (2020) Pre-mortem risk factors for mortality in kittens less than 8 weeks old at a dedicated kitten nursery. *Journal of Feline Medicine and Surgery* doi: 10.1177/1098612X20974960

Giger, U. (2014) Blood-typing and crossmatching to ensure blood compatability. In: Bonagura, J. D. and Twedt, D. C. (eds) *Kirk's Current Veterinary Thepary XV.* Elsevier, St. Louis, Missouri, pp. 143–148.

Kehl, A., Heimberger, K., Langbein-Detsch, I., Boehmer, S., Raj, K., *et al.* (2018) Molecular characterization of blood type A, B, and C (AB) in domestic cats and a CMAH genotyping scheme. *PLoS One* 13. doi: 10.1371/journal.pone.0204287

Kraus, B. H. (2016) Anesthesia for cesarean section in the dog. *Veterinary Focus* 26, 24–31.

Lawler, D.F. (2008) Neonatal and pediatric care of the puppy and kitten. *Theriogenology* 70, 384–392.

Mathews, K. and Sinclair, M. (2018) Analgesia and anesthesia for pregnant cats and dogs. In: Mathews, K., Sinclair, M., Steele, A. M., and Grubb, T. *Analgesia and Anesthesia for the Ill or Injured Dog and Cat.* Wiley, Hoboken, New Jersey, pp. 279–293.

Moon, P. F., Erb, H. N., Ludders, J. W., Gleed, R. D., and Pascoe, P. J. (1998) Perioperative management and mortality rates of dogs undergoing cesarean section in the United States and Canada. *Journal of the American Veterinary Medical Association* 213, 365–369.

Moon-Massat, P. F. and Erb, H. N. (2002) Perioperative factors associated with puppy vigor after delivery by cesarean section. *Journal of the American Animal Hospital Association* 38, 90–96. doi: 10.5326/0380090

Palahniuk, R. J., Shnider, S.M., and Eger II, E. I. (1974) Pregnancy decreases the requirement for inhaled anesthetic agents. *Anesthesiology,* 41, 82–83. doi: 10.1097/00000542-197407000-00021

Robertson, S. (2016) Anaesthetic management for caesarean sections in dogs and cats. *In Practice* 38, 327–339 doi: 10.1136/inp.i3201

Robertson, S. A. and Moon, P. F. (2003) Anesthetic management for cesarean section in bitches. *Veterinary Medicine* 98, 675–694.

Roll, C. and Horsch, S. (2004) Effect of doxapram on cerebral blood flow velocity in preterm infants. *Neuropediatrics* 35, 126–129. doi: 10.1055/s-2004-817904

Scott, F. W. and Geissinger, C. (1978) Kitten mortality survey. *Feline Practice* 8, 31–34.

Shih, A. C., Robertson, S., Isaza, N., Pablo, L., and Davies, W. (2008) Comparison between analgesic effects of buprenorphine, carprofen, and buprenorphine with carprofen for canine ovariohysterectomy. *Veterinary Anaesthesia and Analgesia* 35, 69–79. doi: 10.1111/j.1467-2995.2007.00352.x

Silvestre-Ferreira, A. C. and Pastor, J. (2010) Feline neonatal isoerythrolysis and the importance of feline blood types. *Veterinary Medicine International* 2010, 753726. doi: 10.4061/2010/753726

Sparkes, A. H., Rogers, K., Henley, W. E., Genn-Moore, D. A., May, J. M. *et al.* (2006) A questionnaire-based study of gestation, parturition and neonatal mortality in pedigree breeding cats in the UK. *Journal of Feline Medicine and Surgery* 8, 145–157. doi: 10.1016/j.jfms.2005.10.003

Tranquilli, W. J. (1992) Anesthesia for cesarean section in the cat. *Veterinary Clinics of North America Small Animal Practice* 22, 484–486. doi: 10.1016/s0195-5616(92)50679-9

Young, C. (1973) Preweaning mortality in specific pathogen free kittens. *Journal of Small Animal Practice* 14, 391–397. doi: 10.1111/j.1748-5827.1973.tb06476.x

11 Neonatal Diseases

Aime K. Johnson

Auburn University College of Veterinary Medicine, Department of Clinical Sciences, Auburn, Alabama, USA

11.1 Introduction

Although proper breeding management and veterinary intervention can prevent some newborn kitten losses, overall kitten mortality rates remain high. As many as 9.7% of kittens may be stillborn and up to 16% of kittens may die before weaning (Holst and Frössling, 2009; Fournier *et al.*, 2017). However, other reports of kitten mortality are lower, with as few as 7.2% of kittens being stillborn and only 8.3% of kittens dying in the first 12 weeks of life (Sparkes *et al.*, 2006; Holst and Frössling, 2009). Kittens are most vulnerable when they are newborn with over half of all kitten deaths occurring in the first two weeks of life (Casal, 1996; Holst and Frössling, 2009; Sparkes *et al.*, 2006). Kittens that are born with a low birth weight are much more likely to die than heavier kittens, even within the same litter. Single kitten litters had a lower survival rate than litters of five or more. Obese queens had a lower kitten survival than normal weight queens. Smaller queens tended to have smaller litters, but survival of these kittens was higher (Lawler *et al.*, 1984). Kittens must nurse within 2 hours of birth. Frequent nursing over the first 18-24 hours of life is vital to absorb maternally-derived antibodies from the colostrum.

11.2 General Clinical Signs

Normal kittens will sleep together to help regulate their temperature. They nurse regularly, sleep well between feedings, and gain weight each day. Sick kittens tend to separate themselves from the litter (or the mother pushes them away), do not nurse or nurse weakly, and are restless and vocal. This leads to hypothermia, hypoglycemia, and dehydration. One of the first signs that a kitten is sick is weight loss and failure to thrive. Kittens should be weighed twice daily for the first 2–3 weeks of life to monitor weight gain. Kittens that fail to gain weight are nine times more likely to die than those that continue to gain, and the smallest kittens are 13 times more likely to die than heavier kittens (Dolan *et al.*, 2020). If a kitten fails to gain, examination for clinical disease and supportive care should be initiated immediately. Clinical signs related to the affected system may be apparent such as diarrhea, tachypnea, or nasal or ocular discharge. However, signs may be nonspecific and are often classified by the broad terminology of 'fading kitten syndrome' (Bucheler 1999). During an evaluation of 59 Persian and Devon Rex purebred kittens, maternal neglect (kitten found isolated, kitten not groomed, etc.) and hypothermia (normal body temperature 97–98°F) were reported as common signs before death (Omoto, 2019). Clinical signs related to respiratory tract disease were reported with dyspnea being the most common abnormal clinical sign reported before death in thirteen kittens from ten litters. Failure to gain weight, abnormal feces, and failure to nurse were observed before death in several kittens from different litters. In a recent study, risk factors associated with increased mortality in a neonatal nursery were low weight at intake, weight loss, anorexia, diarrhea, and upper respiratory signs (Dolan *et al.*, 2020).

11.3 Etiology

Causes of kitten mortality can be broken down into infectious and noninfectious etiologies. Noninfectious causes of kitten mortality include trauma, congenital defects, nutritional imbalances, immune-mediated diseases, degenerative disorders, and poor husbandry. Infectious causes include viruses, bacteria, and parasites. It has been estimated that of kittens that die within the first 2 weeks of age, 50% succumb to infectious causes, 19% from idiopathic causes, 12% from immune-mediated causes (such as neonatal isoerythrolysis), 9.5% from congenital causes, 4.8% from nutritional causes, and 4.8%

DOI: 10.1079/9781789247107.0011

from traumatic causes (Cave *et al.*, 2002). A recent study performed by Omoto (2019), evaluated neonatal deaths in catteries involving Devon Rex and Persian breeders. Excluding stillborn kittens, it is estimated that at least 29.5% (13/44) of kitten deaths could have been due to infection. Immune-mediated disease, poor husbandry and congenital defects are discussed in Chapter 10. Infectious diseases will be discussed in more detail in this chapter.

When a kitten is affected by an infectious cause, dehydration is a major concern because their body composition is 80% water, compared to 60% in adult cats (Little, 2011). This increased water composition, higher proportion of surface area, higher metabolic rate, and lower level of body fat causes kittens to have higher fluid requirements than an adult cat of the same size. Further, a kitten's kidneys are not fully developed at birth, resulting in the excretion of a higher volume of water per unit of body weight than an adult cat. Thus, a kitten can easily become dehydrated if it has diarrhea, vomiting, or reduced fluid/milk intake (Little, 2011). One way to quickly check a kitten's hydration status is to examine its mucous membranes and determine its capillary refill time. If the former appears pale and the latter is delayed, the kitten is at least 10% dehydrated. A dehydrated kitten's urine will be darker in color and have a specific gravity greater than 1.020 (Little, 2011). If a kitten is only slightly dehydrated and does not have any other health issues, it can be treated with warmed subcutaneous fluids or oral milk replacer. However, severe dehydration often requires an intravenous or intraosseous catheter and fluid replacement. In small kittens, an interosseous catheter into the femur can be quickly and easily placed (Fig. 11.1). The kitten's stifle is grasped in one hand (non-dominant) with the operator's thumb resting on the greater trochanter. A 1.0-inch, 22-gauge needle is inserted through the skin just medial to the greater trochanter and advanced along the medial aspect of the greater trochanter to the intertrochanteric fossa. Then, using gentle force, the needle is pushed into the medullary cavity. The boring needle is then removed, and a second 22 G 1-inch needle is inserted through the boring hole and into the bone marrow. Proper positioning of the IO device is confirmed when replacement fluids can be easily flushed into the medullary cavity. Care should be taken to not overhydrate neonatal kittens because they do not have full renal excretory function (Little, 2011).

In addition to kittens that showed signs of infectious disease before death or upon postmortem examination, stillbirths can also be the result of infectious disease. In general, viruses cause feline reproductive loss more often than bacteria or protozoa (Givens and Marley, 2008). In particular, feline panleukopenia virus, feline leukemia virus, feline rhinotracheitis virus, and feline infectious peritonitis virus have been associated with abortion, stillbirth, neonatal death, and fetal mummification (Lefebvre, 2015). Feline immunodeficiency virus can also cause stillbirth (Givens and Marley, 2008). However, without additional testing, it is difficult to determine how many stillbirths are due to infections and how many are due to noninfectious causes.

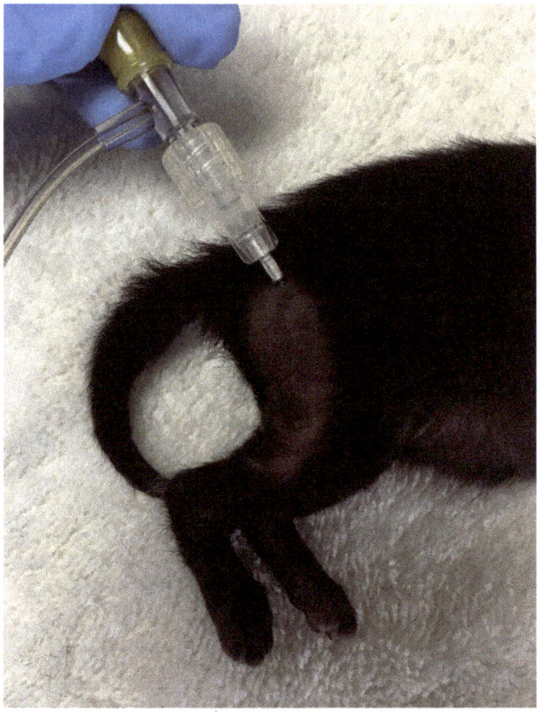

Fig. 11.1. Placement of an interosseous catheter into the femur of the neonatal kitten for fluid therapy. (Image: author's own.)

11.4 Infectious Causes of Kitten Mortality

Cave *et al.* determined in 2002 that out of a total of 274 kitten deaths, infectious disease was the cause of death in over half. Breaking this down further, half of these died from viral infections while the other half died from bacterial infections. Feline herpesvirus and feline calicivirus were determined to have been the main two causes of viral associated death (Cave *et al.*, 2002). Bacterial pathogens isolated from neonates that died included *Escherichia coli*, *Streptococcus*, *Pasteurella*, *Enterobacter*, *Enterococcus*, *Klebsiella*, *Pseudomonas*, *Bordetella*, and *Salmonella* (Mossi-Dieth *et al.*, 1990; Hoskins, 1993). Any of these diseases can cause 'fading kitten syndrome' where the kittens fail to gain weight, cannot maintain body temperature, and 'fade' from an active neonate to death over a short period of time. Infectious causes are more likely to affect more than one kitten in a litter. A careful exam or necropsy should be performed to determine any particular system that may be affected to narrow down the differential list.

11.4.1 Respiratory diseases

The most common types of bacteria isolated from kittens with cases of pneumonia, pleuritis, myocarditis/endocarditis, or meningitis/encephalitis were *Streptococcus* species and *E. coli* (Mossi-Dieth, 1990). Other common causes of upper and lower respiratory tract disease in kittens includes feline herpesvirus-1 (FHV-1), feline calicivirus (FCV), *Bordetella bronchiseptica*, *Mycoplasma* species, and *Chlamydophila* (Little, 2011).

Feline herpes virus is characterized in neonatal kittens as an acute upper respiratory infection. Kittens develop ocular drainage and nasal congestion (Fig. 11.2). They become weak, may have a fever, and display tachypnea or coughing. Kittens may also develop ulceration in their mouths and tongues that make nursing or eating painful (Fig. 11.3). Feline herpes virus can be diagnosed by a swab sample of ocular and/or nasal discharge. When submitted to a laboratory, the swabs are analyzed for presence of the virus by polymerase chain reaction (PCR). Treatment may include broad spectrum antibiotics as secondary bacterial infections are common. Supportive care including fluid therapy, nutritional support, and supplemental warming are also essential. Steam nebulization may assist in clearing the nasal passage and encourage eating. If severe, treatment with famciclovir (90 mg/kg orally every 8 hours for 14 days) may shorten infection or reduce spread to other kittens in the cattery. Additional treatment with oral L-Lysine may also be beneficial for immune support. All kittens in the litter and the queen should be considered for treatment. If the ocular discharge is severe or is causing conjunctivitis neonatorum (accumulation of purulent discharge in the conjunctival sac in kittens that have yet to

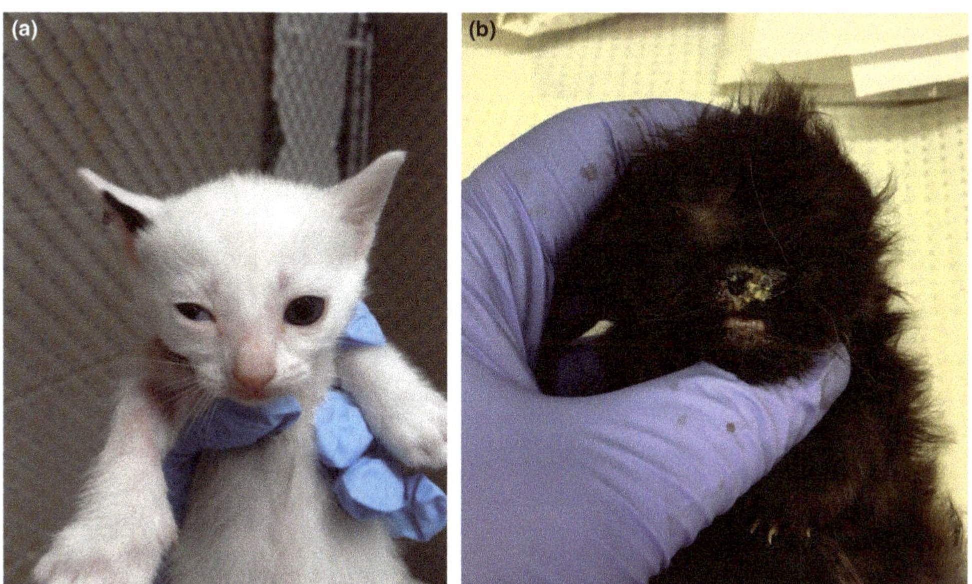

Fig. 11.2 (a) Ocular discharge, prolapsed third eyelid, and blepharospasm in a kitten affected with herpes virus. (Image: author's own.) **(b)** Severe nasal congestion and discharge from a kitten likely infected with herpes virus. (Photo courtesy of Holly Omoto and Dr. Michelle Kutzler, Oregon State University.)

open their eyes), the eyes should be cleaned several times daily with a warm damp gauze or towel. Antibiotic eye ointment may be added to reduce secondary infections. For prevention, strict sanitation and biosecurity are required. The virus does not survive long at room temperature and is easily killed with common disinfectants (Sykes, 2014). Vaccination of the queens against FHV should provide immunity to the kittens, but as maternal antibodies wane, the kittens may be susceptible before their first vaccinations are administered.

Feline calicivius (FCV) is spread through saliva, nasal or ocular discharge, or aerosol. Most kittens develop an upper respiratory infection, but the virus can spread to the lungs causing severe pneumonia. This virus mutates and clinical signs may be dependent on the strain causing the infection. Diagnosis can be made by virus isolation, or, more commonly, reverse transcriptase PCR (RT-PCR). A positive result should accompany clinical signs. False positives after RT-PCR may occur after previous exposure. Treatment includes supportive care, saline nebulization to break up nasal congestion, antibiotics if needed for secondary bacterial infections, and/or nonsteroidal anti-inflammatories in the case of a fever or pain. Vaccinations will help reduce the severity of the disease and queens should be vaccinated prior to pregnancy. Famciclovir or L-Lysine may also be used as discussed with FHV.

Bacterial causes of respiratory disease such as *Chlamydophilia felis*, *Mycoplasma* spp., or *Bordetella bronchiseptica* can be diagnosed with a culture of the nasal secretions and treated with appropriate supportive care and antibiotics. When severe, bacterial or viral infections can lead to pulmonary disease (Fig. 11.4). On necropsy, culture of the cut section of the lungs may aid in the diagnosis. Floating the lung tissue in water will help determine if the lungs are consolidated/congested (sink to the bottom) or aerated (float) (Fig. 11.5).

11.4.2 Gastrointestinal diseases

Infections that cause gastrointestinal (GI) disease include viruses, bacteria, and protozoa. Panleukopenia

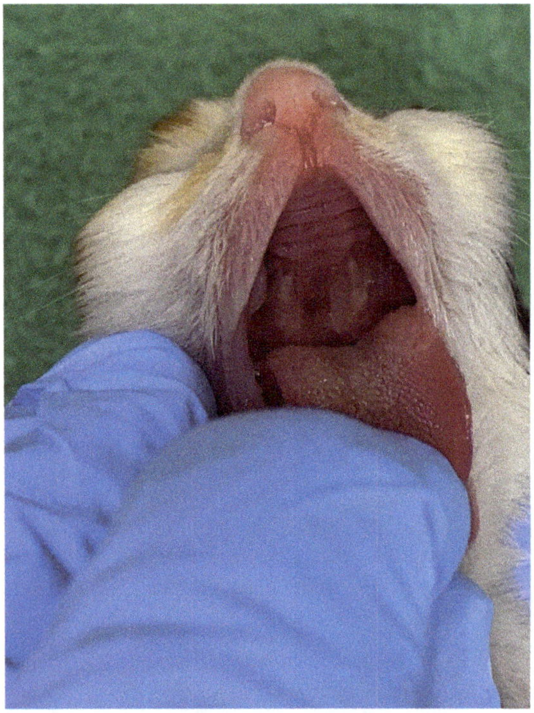

Fig. 11.3. Neonatal kitten with severe ulceration on the caudal aspect of the hard palate and base of the tongue. This kitten was losing weight and required frequent tube feeding to supplement nutrition. (Image: author's own.)

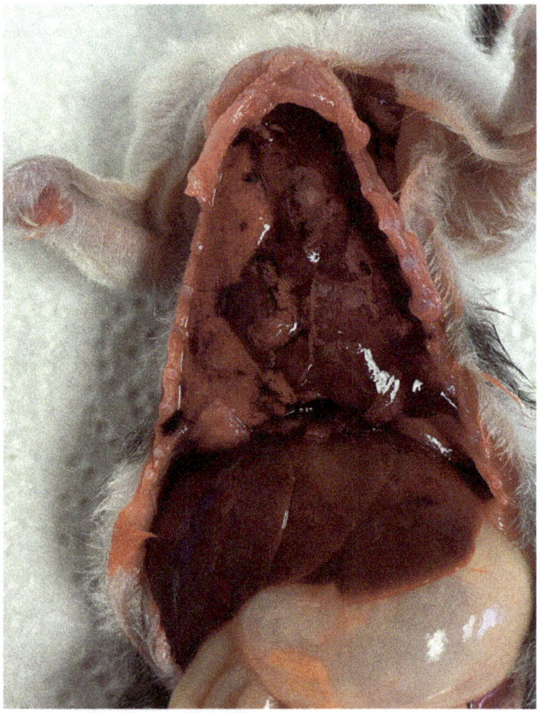

Fig. 11.4. Heart and lungs of a neonatal kitten who died 36 hours after birth. The left lung lobes are diffusely dark red in color indicating severe congestion. (Image: author's own.)

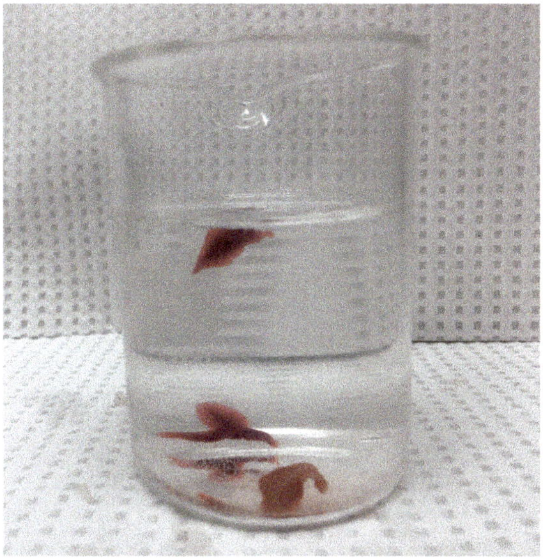

Fig. 11.5. Samples of lung tissue from neonatal kittens that died within the first week of life. The aerated (normal) lung is floating on the top of the water while the consolidated diseased lung has sunk to the bottom. (Photo courtesy of Holly Omoto and Dr. Michelle Kutzler, Oregon State University.)

virus (parvovirus), coliform bacteria, *Tritrichomonas foetus*, *Giardia* spp., *Cytoisopora* spp., and *Cryptosporidium* are common causes of gastrointestinal tract disease in kittens. Gastrointestinal disease can lead to symptoms that include typical GI signs such as diarrhea and vomiting but may also be seen as abdominal distension due to decreased motility in the gastrointestinal tract or ascites (Fig. 11.6).

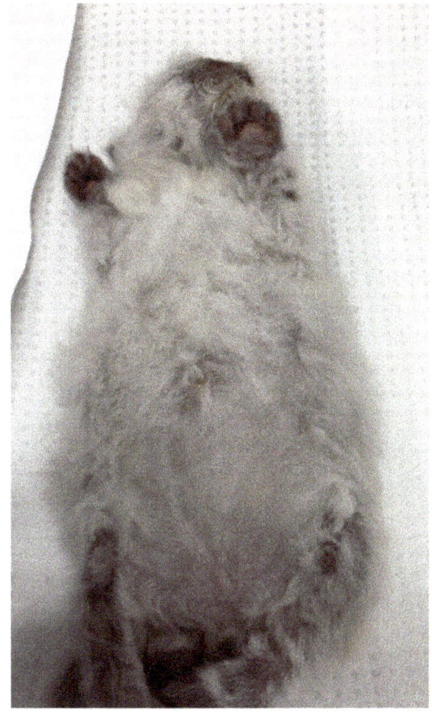

Fig. 11.6. Severe abdominal distension caused by ascites in a kitten (Photo courtesy of Holly Omoto and Dr. Michelle Kutzler, Oregon State University.)

Tritrichomonas foetus has been shown to cause chronic diarrhea in cats, especially young cats. Diarrhea may be transient or may last months to years depending on prompt diagnosis. Transmission is through the fecal-oral route and can easily be passed from one cat to another or from a queen to her kittens. Diagnosis can be confirmed by identifying the organisms in fresh, non-refrigerated feces by a direct smear and observation of the motile trophozoites. However, because this technique requires a large amount of trophozoites in the feces, the sensitivity of this test was less than 5% in one study (Gookin *et al.*, 2003). Diagnosis can be improved by performing serial tests over a few days. Fecal culture can be performed using a commercially available 'In Pouch® TF' system (Biomed Diagnostics, White City, OR). Feces (0.1 g) are placed into the pouch containing specialized media and allowed to incubate at 37°C for up to 6 days. The pouch can be analyzed under a microscope for trophozoites starting at day 2 or 3 and continuing until day 6 if needed. Diamonds media enriched with nutrients and antibiotics can be used as an alternative to the In Pouch® TF system (Gookin *et al.*, 2004). A PCR can be performed on the feces. Gookin *et al.* found almost 95% (34/35 animals) were correctly diagnosed using PCR. Most labs require up to one gram of fresh feces, free of cat litter (some components of the litter may inhibit the PCR test) sent refrigerated. Samples may remain in the refrigerator for several days before shipping and remain stable.

Treatment with ronidazole (30 mg/kg orally once daily for 14 days) has been shown to be effective against *T. foetus*. Retesting 2 weeks after the last dose of antibiotic should be performed to confirm treatment success. Treatment with metronidazole was not effective for treating *T. foetus* in the cat (Gookin *et al.*, 2006).

Giardia spp. causes diarrhea that is often foul smelling, light in color, and contains increased mucus. Infection is more common in kittens and immunocompromised cats. Giardia is transmitted by exposure to the cyst stage. Giardia cysts can remain in the environment for 2–3 months in ideal conditions. Survival of the cysts decreases as temperature increases. Neonatal loss is usually due to dehydration caused by diarrhea and is more common in very young cats. Diagnosis is made by a direct fecal smear and the identification of the cysts or trophozoites. Alternatively, a fecal float using a zinc sulfate flotation solution can also be used to isolate cysts. Because cats shed *giardia* cysts intermittently, serial tests may need to be performed for diagnosis. Treatment with metronidazole (25 mg/kg orally BID for 5 days) will eliminate the trophozoite stage but may not eliminate all cysts leading to recurrence and the need for retreatment. Combination treatment with fenbendazole may improve therapy in cats with refractory diarrhea (Dubey, 1993).

Coccidiosis, typically either *Cystoisospora felis* or *Cystoisospora rivolta*, is a common cause of diarrhea in cats. Infection is fecal-oral. Most cats will be exposed to coccidia at some point in their lifetime. Clinical signs associated with infection tend to appear during times of stress such as the neonatal period, weaning, or in immunocompromised animals. Clinical signs include gastrointestinal signs such as vomiting, diarrhea (often severe), and abdominal pain, but can also be seen as neurologic or respiratory disease depending on the location of the organism (Dubey, 1993). Because the organisms can sporulate in about 6 hours, infection can be rapid and severe in catteries that do not maintain strict sanitation. Diagnosis is made by identifying the organisms in the feces using a fecal float (sugar flotation). The coccidia cysts are small so careful observation should be made so they are not missed. Treatment with sulfadimethoxine has been approved for the treatment of coccidia in cats. Because it is coccidiostatic, treatment should last 5–21 days. The longer the treatment, the more likely that there will not be any viable coccidia remaining after treatment. Trimethoprim sulfonamide is also used (15–30 mg/kg orally for 6 days) but tends to have palatability issues in cats. Furazolidone (8–20 mg/kg once or twice daily for 5 days) has also shown efficacy. Ponazuril has been tested as a treatment in cats. Doses of 20–50 mg/kg orally every 24 hours for 3 days is recommended. However, if the initial oocyst count was high, this dose did not eliminate all oocysts. If oocysts are still detectable, retreatment is recommended (Litster *et al.*, 2014). Prevention is the best way to minimize disease. Litter boxes should be cleaned daily and disinfected at least weekly. Because the oocysts can be transmitted in raw meat, cats that are fed a raw diet or are allowed to hunt are more likely to become infected and shed oocysts, causing problems for younger kittens. Strict sanitation is the best prevention and will reduce further environmental contamination from cats that are shedding the organism.

Feline panleukopenia, caused by feline parvovirus (FPV), infects rapidly dividing cells such as the crypt cells in the small intestine. The infected cells are killed, causing a blunting of the villi leading to malabsorption and diarrhea. The disease is more severe in neonates and younger kittens and may lead to a mortality rate of 90% (Truyen *et al.*, 2009). Signs are often an acute onset of vomiting, diarrhea, and lack of nursing leading to severe dehydration. Fading kitten syndrome is also observed where the kittens die within 24 hours and show only lethargy and anorexia (Addie *et al.*, 1998). Co-infection with other viral agents (such as coronavirus) or bacteria will increase the severity of clinical disease (Truyen *et al.*, 2009). If the queen is infected while pregnant, still births, embryonic absorption, fetal mummification, or fading kitten syndrome can be observed. Alternatively, kittens may be born alive with cerebellar hypoplasia leading to a characteristic neurologic disease (ataxia, hypermetria, and wide based stance) that becomes evident as kittens begin to move around at about 2 weeks of age. Treatment is aggressive supportive care including thermoregulation, nutritional support, and fluid replacement. Confirmation can be made by PCR testing or virus isolation of feces or blood. Clinically, there is a latex agglutination or immunochromatographic test to detect antibodies in feces (Addie *et al.*, 1998). The virus may remain in the environment for months and is resistant to many regular disinfectants. Prevention is by vaccination of all cats within a breeding colony with a modified live vaccine prior to breeding. The disease is more prevalent in shelter or rescue animals but can also occur in pedigree cats (Addie *et al.*, 1998).

11.4.3 Systemic disease

Overall systemic disease in kittens can lead to mortality with minimal clinical signs. Feline leukemia virus, feline immunodeficiency virus, and bacterial septicemia are common causes (Little, 2011) Feline coronavirus

(FCoV) can cause mild symptomatic infection in kittens, but is also associated with a more virulent strain, feline infectious peritonitis. These diseases lead to systemic disease and can be fatal in young kittens. Bacterial septicemia (neonatal sepsis) is also a cause of systemic disease leading to a high mortality rate in neonates. Passive immunity is obtained through nursing colostrum within the first 24 hours of life. If this does not occur, the kittens are at risk of becoming systemically ill. Septicemia occurs when the bacterial load overwhelms the kitten's immune system. Predisposing factors include co-infection with a virus, inadequate nutrition, inadequate thermoregulation, and immunosuppression. Affected kittens often cry, are weak or restless, unable to maintain body temperature, and overall fail to thrive. Diagnosis is made based on history and clinical signs. Confirmation is made by culture of the primary infection (joint, umbilicus, blood, etc.). Treatment is aggressive supportive care and appropriate antibiotics based on culture and sensitivity. Because kittens succumb to infection rapidly, antimicrobial therapy with amoxicillin-clavulanate can be initiated prior to receiving the results. In the neonate, drug dosages should be reduced (possibly 30–50%) or frequency modified based on the neonate's unique body composition and drug distribution (Hoskins, 1993). Oral absorption of antibiotics may be altered in cases of septicemia. Therefore, initial administration of antibiotics via intravenous or interosseous route is recommended (Hoskins, 1993). Prevention should include confirmation that the kittens nurse well within the first 24 hours of birth. The queening area should be clean and sanitary to minimize environmental contamination.

Prevention of infectious neonatal disease is more successful than diagnosis and treatment once disease occurs. Imposition of strict biosecurity is vital by keeping pregnant and lactating queens and their kittens in a separate location from other animals and maintaining a clean environment during the queening and neonatal period. Also, ensure that queens are adequately vaccinated before breeding. Careful examination of sick neonates and submission of any kittens that die to a diagnostic lab for full analysis is essential in obtaining a diagnosis and therefore a plan of treatment and prevention.

11.5 References

Addie, D. D., Toth, S., Thompson, H., Greenwood, N., and Jarrett, J. O. (1998) Detection of feline parvovirus in dying pedigree kittens. *Veterinary Record* 142(14), 353–356. doi: 10.1136/vr.142.14.353

Bücheler, J. (1999) Fading kitten syndrome and neonatal isoerythrolysis. *Veterinary Clinics of North America: Small Animal Practice* 29(4), 853–870.

Casal, M. L., Jezyk, P. F., and Giger, U. (1996) Transfer of colostral antibodies from queens to their kittens. *American Journal of Veterinary Research* 57(11), 1653–1658.

Cave, T. A., Thompson, H., Reid, S. W. J., Hodgson, D. R., and Addie D. D. (2002) Kitten mortality in the United Kingdom: a retrospective analysis of 274 histopathological examinations (1986 to 2000). *Veterinary Record* 151, 497–501. doi: 10.1136/vr.151.17.497

Dolan, E. D., Dolan, E., Tran, H. R., and Slater, M. R. (2020) Pre-mortem risk factors for mortality in kittens less than 8 weeks old at a dedicated kitten nursery. *Journal of Feline Medicine and Surgery.* doi: 10.1177/1098612X20974960

Dubey, J. P. (1993) Intestinal protozoa infections. *Veterinary Clinics of North America: Small Animal Practice* 23(1), 37–55. doi: 10.1016/s0195-5616(93)50003-7

Fournier, A., Masson, M., Corbière, F., Mila, H., Mariani, M., *et al.* (2017) Epidemiological analysis of reproductive performances and kitten mortality rates in 5,303 purebred queens of 45 different breeds and 28,065 kittens in France. *Reproduction in Domestic Animals* 52(2), 153–157. doi: 10.1111/rda.12844

Givens, D. M. and Marley, M. S. D. (2008) Infectious causes of embryonic and fetal mortality. *Theriogenology* 70(3), 270–285. doi: 10.1016/j.theriogenology.2008.04.018

Gookin, J. L., Foster, D. M., Poore, M. F., Stebbins, M. E., and Levy, M. G. (2003) Use of a commercially available culture system for diagnosis of *Tritrichomonas foetus* infection in cats. *Journal of the American Veterinary Medical Association* 222(10), 1376–1379. doi: 10.2460/javma.2003.222.1376

Gookin, J. L., Stebbins, M. E., Hunt, E., Burlone, K., Fulton, M., *et al.* (2004) Prevalence of and risk factors for feline *Tritrichomonas foetus* and *Giardia* infection. *Journal of Clinical* 42(6), 2707–2710. doi: 10.1128/JCM.42.6.2707-2710.2004

Gookin, J. L., Copple, C. N., Papich, M. G., Poore, M. F., Stauffer, S. H., *et al.* (2006) Efficacy of Ronidazole for treatment of feline *Tritrichomonas foetus* infection. *Journal of Veterinary Internal Medicine* 20(3), 536–543. doi: 10.1892/0891-6640(2006)20[536:eorfto]2.0.co;2

Holst, B. S. and Frössling, J. (2009) The Swedish breeding cat: population description, infectious diseases and reproductive performance evaluated by a questionnaire. *Journal of Feline Medicine and Surgery* 11, 793–802. doi: 10.1016/j.jfms.2009.01.008

Hoskins, J. D. (1993) Feline neonatal sepsis. *Veterinary Clinics of North America: Small Animal Practice* 23(1), 91–100. doi: 10.1016/s0195-5616(93)50006-2

Lawler, D. F. and Monti, K. L. (1984) Morbidity and mortality in neonatal kittens. *American Journal of Veterinary Research* 45(7), 1455–1459.

Lefebvre, R. C. (2015) Fetal mummification in the major domestic species: current perspectives on causes and management. *Veterinary Medicine: Research and Reports* 6, 233–244. doi: 10.2147/VMRR.S59520

Litster, A. L., Nichols, J., Hall, K., and Camp, J. (2014) Use of ponazuril paste to treat coccidiosis in shelter-housed cats and dogs. *Veterinary Parasitology* 202(3–4), 319–325. doi: 10.1016/j.vetpar.2014.03.003

Little S. (2011) Feline pediatrics: how to treat the small and the sick. *Compendium: Continuing Education for Veterinarians.* (33)9, E3.

Mossi-Dieth, V., Hauser, B., Corboz, L., Lutz, H., and Pospischil, A. (1990) Todes und erkrankungsursachen bei katzenwelpen. *Schweizer Archiv Tierheilkunde* 132, 587–594. doi: 10.5169/seals-593729

Omoto, H. (2019) Gross causes of neonatal mortality in Devon Rex and Persian kittens. BS Honors College Thesis. Oregon State University, Oregon, United States.

Sparkes, A. H., Rogers, K., Henley, W. E., Gunn-Moore, D. A., May, J. M., *et al.* (2006) A questionnaire-based study of gestation, parturition and neonatal mortality in pedigree breeding cats in the UK. *Journal of Feline Medicine and Surgery* 8, 145–157. doi: 10.1016/j.jfms.2005.10.003

Sykes, J. E. (2014) Pediatric feline upper respiratory disease. *Veterinary Clinics of North America: Small Animal Practice* 44(2), 331–342. doi: 10.1016/j.cvsm.2013.10.005

Truyen U., Addie D., Belák S., Boucraut-Baralon C., Egberink H., *et al.* (2009) Feline panleukopenia. ABCD guidelines on prevention and management. *Journal of Feline Medicine and Surgery* 11(7), 538–546. doi: 10.1016/j.jfms.2009.05.002

12 Termination of Pregnancy

SANDRA GOERICKE-PESCH

Reproductive Unit – Clinic for Small Animals, University of Veterinary Medicine Hannover, Foundation, Hannover, Germany

12.1 Introduction

Feline reproduction is quite efficient, leading to cat overpopulation which can result in severe animal welfare issues, public health risks, and environmental hazards. An ideal contraceptive for cats with private owners would be temporary, reversible contraceptive; whereas an ideal contraceptive for free-roaming cats would be a single treatment that induces life-long sterility in males and females. Prior to performing any method of pregnancy termination, it is important to first confirm the pregnancy status as well as estimate the gestational age (see Chapter 6). This chapter will focus on the surgical and medical methods for terminating pregnancy in queens. Figure 12.1 provides a decision tree for the veterinarian how to proceed in case of (suspected/observed) mismating in the queen. It summarizes all possibilities given in the text below.

12.2 Surgical Termination of Pregnancy

Surgical termination of pregnancy can be performed at any time during gestation. However, in late gestation, kittens may be viable and require euthanasia after removal from the uterus. Alternatively, kittens can be euthanized through the uterine wall without removal. It is important to perform ovariohysterectomy instead of only an ovariectomy as the placenta contributes to the progesterone support of pregnancy. Performing an ovariectomy in a pregnant cat (after day 45) may allow for pregnancy maintenance and delivery of a normal litter (Scott, 1970; Tsutsui *et al.*, 2009). In queens intended for breeding, surgical sterilization for pregnancy termination is not an option. Ethics should be considered, especially in case of late surgical termination.

12.3 Medical Termination of Pregnancy

Knowledge of the different stages and endocrinology of feline pregnancy is necessary to make appropriate medical decisions when and how to terminate pregnancy. Treatment administered before day 13 is to prevent implantation, whereas treatment after day 13 will induce abortion. As in other species, progesterone is necessary for pregnancy maintenance. In cats, both the corpora lutea and the placenta secrete progesterone, with placental progesterone reaching maximal concentrations 6–8 weeks after mating (Tsutsui and Stabenfeldt, 1993). Prolactin from the anterior pituitary gland is luteotrophic and essential for corpora lutea maintenance in the latter half of pregnancy (Tsutsui and Stabenfeldt, 1993). Placenta-derived relaxin may also have a luteotropic effect, as increasing concentrations occur during implantation with a plateau reached at days 30–35 (gestational day 35) (Addiego *et al.*, 1987) until 10–15 days before parturition (Stewart and Stabenfeldt, 1985), and gradually decline to undetectable concentrations 24 hours before parturition (Stewart and Stabenfeldt, 1985; Tsutsui and Stabenfeldt, 1993).

Options for medical termination of pregnancy act by: (i) withdrawal of progesterone either by induction of luteolysis and/or by withdrawal of luteotropic factors; and/or (ii) progesterone receptor antagonism. Single drug and drug combination options are summarized in Tables 12.1 and 12.2, respectively. It is important to mention that an ultrasound examination should be performed at the end of any pregnancy termination protocol to confirm treatment success. In addition, owners should be informed that queens will often return to estrus within 4–8 days after termination so that additional unwanted matings can be avoided. Concomitant

DOI: 10.1079/9781789247107.0012

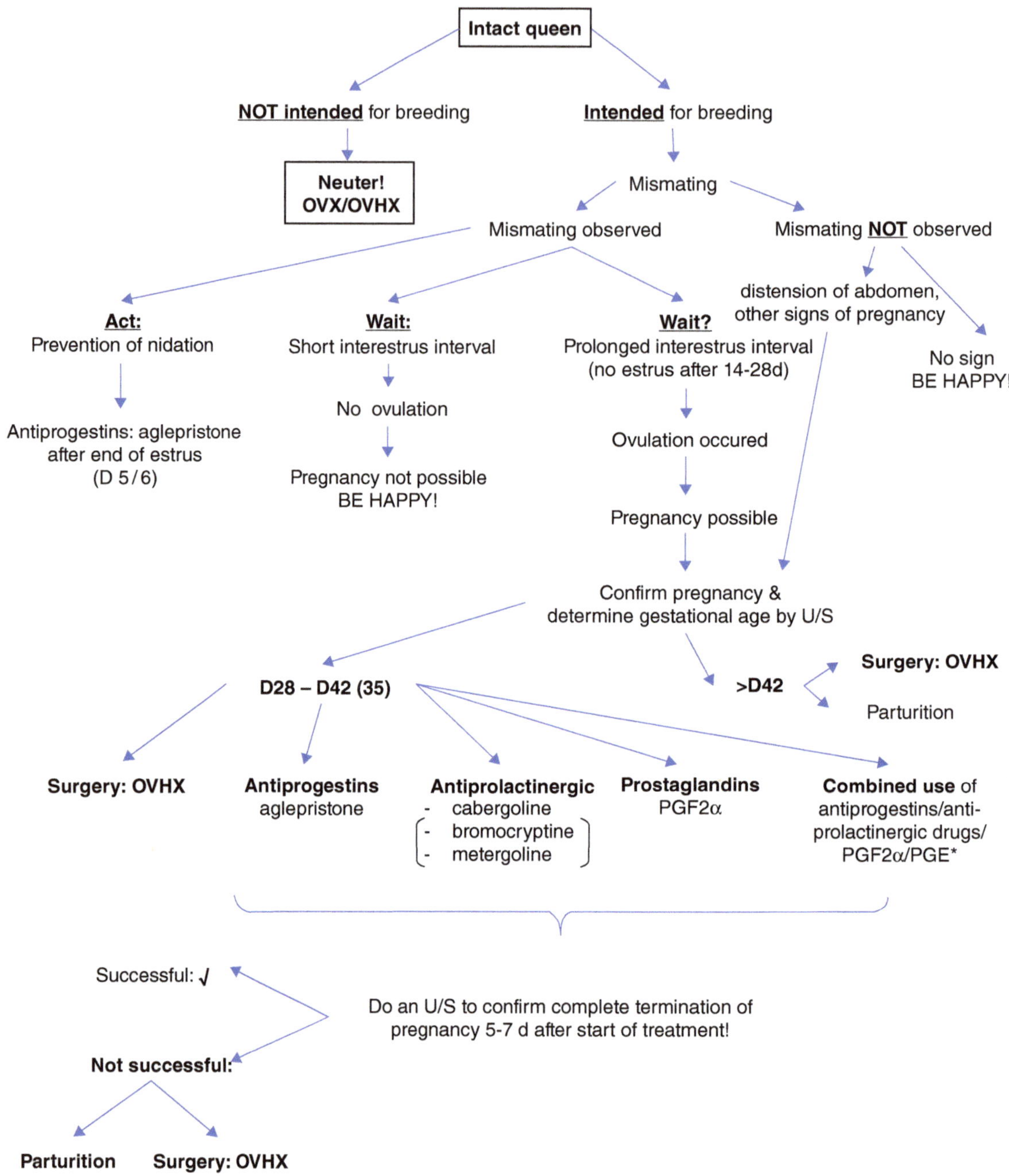

Fig. 12.1. Flow chart – how to proceed with an intact, possibly mismated queen. (Image: author's own.)

use of antibiotics might be considered in case of late termination of pregnancy. The use of estrogens will not be covered here due to the risk of side effects, such as pyometra, etc., and the fact that significantly better drugs are available. Furthermore, estrogens are only effective shortly after mating.

Table 12.1. Single drug medical options for pregnancy termination in queens. (Author's own table.)

Drug	Dosage	Route	Duration	Time of pregnancy to treat
Aglepristone	10–15 mg/kg	SC	Administer twice 24 hours apart (if abortion is incomplete: treat again in 6 days)	D5–D45[a]
Cabergoline	5–15 µg/kg	PO[b]	Once daily for 5–7 days	D28–D42[a]
Dinoprost	20–50 µg/kg	SC/IM	Every 12–24 hours for 5–10 days	D28–42[a]
Cloprostenol	1–5 µg/kg	SC/IM	Every 24 hours for 5–10 days	D28–42[a]

D, day; PO, oral; SC, subcutaneous; IM, intramuscular administration.
[a]Not recommended for use later in pregnancy.
[b]Can give with food.

Table 12.2. Combined drug medical options for pregnancy termination in queens. (Author's own table.)

First drug (dosage, route, duration)	Second drug (dosage, route, duration)
Cabergoline (5 µg/kg, PO, once daily for 5–7 days)	Dinoprost (20–50 µg/kg, SC, twice daily)
Cabergoline (5 µg/kg, PO, once daily for 5–7 days)	Cloprostenol (1 µg/kg, SC/IM, daily or every other day)
Aglepristone (10 mg/kg, SC, twice 24 hours apart beginning at 30–40 days of pregnancy[a])	Misoprostol (200 µg/cat, PO, every 12 hours until abortion starts)

PO, oral; SC, subcutaneous; IM, intramuscular administration.
[a]Not recommended for use later in pregnancy.

12.3.1 Options that act by withdrawal of progesterone

Prostaglandins

Prostaglandin (PG) F2α (dinoprost) has direct luteolytic properties, but also induces smooth muscle contractions. Inducing uterine contractions is beneficial for expulsion of uterine contents. On the other hand, the effect on the smooth muscle is not specific for the reproductive tract and can produce dose-dependent side effects. Dosages of 0.1–2 mg/cat of dinoprost result in vocalization, panting, restlessness, grooming, tenesmus, salivation, diarrhea, kneading, mydriasis, emesis, urination, and lordosis. Side effects start about 30 seconds after PGF2α injection and last up to 60 minutes (Nachreiner and Marple, 1974; Davidson *et al.*, 1992; Verstegen *et al.*, 1993). Even though cats are reported not to be as sensitive as dogs, there is a risk of death with overdosage (median lethal dose: 5.0 mg/kg; Wildt *et al.*, 1979) as described for the dog (Sokolowski and Geng, 1977). One or two subcutaneous (SQ) injections of PGF2α (0.5–1 mg/kg) after day 40 of gestation have been reported to be successful for induction of abortion in one (Nachreiner and Marple, 1974), but not in another study (Wycoff and Ganjam, 1979). Davidson *et al.* (1992) described 0.1–0.25 mg/kg of body weight, SQ, every 12 to 24 hours for 3 or 5 days for successful treatment of open cervix pyometra. Ninety-five percent (20/21) of queens resumed normal estrous cycles and 81% (17/20) delivered normal litter(s) after treatment. These data indicate that treatment is also safe and suitable for pregnancy termination. Dinoprost dosages of 20–50 µg/kg subcutaneously every 12 hours over 5–10 days until complete abortion has been used in clinical practice within minimal side effects (Jöchle, 2016). In general, starting with a lower dose and increasing it slowly to the maximum dose will reduce the likelihood of side effects as has been described for the bitch (Verstegen *et al.*, 2008). Cloprostenol, a PGF2α analog, was described for open cervix pyometra and pregnancy termination at 5 µg/kg (García Mitacek *et al.*, 2014; Jöchle, 2016), but is also effective for pregnancy termination at the dose of 1 µg/kg (author's clinical experience). Feline corpora lutea are refractory to luteolytic substances until day 28 after breeding, which is why these substances are only suitable for use in pregnancy termination after this time. Furthermore, compromised respiratory function in cats is a contraindication for prostaglandin use.

Prostaglandin E (misoprostol) induces uterine contractility and cervical dilation. Oral administration of misoprostol at 400 µg/cat every 12 hours induced abortion in 57% of queens at 30–40 days of gestation, but there were significant side effects (e.g. vomiting) (Ay *et al.*, 2019). It is noteworthy that oral administration of misoprostol at 200 µg/cat every 12 hours did not terminate pregnancy. Based upon the poor efficacy and risk of side effects, oral misoprostol alone cannot be recommended for termination of pregnancy in cats. Misoprostol has been used topically to cause cervical dilation to assist with pregnancy termination in the dog. One study used topical misoprostol at a dose of 400 μg for dogs less than 20kg every other day in combination therapy with cabergoline and a prostaglandin. Cervical dilation occurred within 3 days with misoprostol compared to 5 days without (Cetin *et al.*, 2010). A second study used a lower dose of topical misoprostol in combination with aglepristone. Dogs weighing less than 20 kg received 200 μg of misoprostol daily. The use of misoprostol significantly decreased the time to complete abortion (Agaolu *et al.*, 2014). Clinically, the tablets can be crushed and mixed in sterile saline or sterile lube to a volume of 1–2 mL and inserted into the cranial vagina using an artificial insemination pipette. There are no reports of the use of cervical topical misoprostol in cats, but in selected cases, this treatment may show promise.

It is important to note that the use of any prostaglandins in cats is off label.

Cabergoline

Cabergoline is a dopamine agonist acting like a prolactin antagonist, which withdraws the luteotropic support of prolactin and results in luteolysis. Oral administration of cabergoline between days 28 and 42 after breeding causes a drop in progesterone concentrations within 3–4 days after the start of treatment (unlike 24 hours as seen with high dosages of PGF2α), which induces abortion within 4–6 days after the start of treatment (Verstegen *et al.* 1993). Oral cabergoline administration (5–15 μg/kg) once daily over 5–7 days is safe and effective for pregnancy termination (Jöchle and Jöchle, 1993). At this stage of gestation, external evidence of pregnancy loss is minimal with only light-colored vaginal discharge present for 24–36 hours. If cabergoline is administered after day 42 of gestation, pregnancy may not be terminated because placental progesterone production may be sufficient to maintain the pregnancy. However, cabergoline will prevent colostrum production and lactation as well as normal maternal behavior, resulting in diminished kitten wellbeing or death. Although cabergoline is labeled in cats for suppression of lactation, treatment of eclampsia, and mastitis with concomitant lactation in Europe, it is used extra-label for pregnancy termination.

A combined drug protocol has been established to improve the efficacy of pregnancy termination using cabergoline (5 μg/kg) once daily orally for 5–7 days and PGF2α (Erünal-Maral *et al.*, 2004; Onclin and Verstegen, 1997). Either dinoprost (20–50 μg/kg, once daily, SQ) or cloprostenol (1 μg/kg, every other day, SQ) can be used. The combined drug protocol also has fewer reported side effects due to dose reduction in both cabergoline and PGF2α.

Bromocryptine and metergoline

Similarly to cabergoline, bromocryptine and the serotoninergic antagonist metergoline inhibit prolactin secretion. In the dog, side effects such as nausea and vomiting are more common with bromocryptine compared to cabergoline, making the use of the latter preferable, if available. Although successful use for pregnancy termination in the dog has been described, no corresponding literature provides a dosage and/or confirms efficacy in the cat.

12.3.2 Progesterone receptor antagonism

Aglepristone

Aglepristone (Alizin®, Virbac) binds to the progesterone receptor with nine times higher affinity than progesterone (Alizin product characteristics; reviewed by Gogny and Fiéni, 2016; Goericke-Pesch, 2017). After receptor binding, aglepristone prevents the cellular signaling that normally occurs when progesterone binds to the receptor. The 'effects' of progesterone on the target tissues are blocked, allowing for an increase in uterine contractility and cervical dilation. Aglepristone is currently the most efficient and safest option to prevent nidation and terminate pregnancy in cats. No serious side effects have been reported in queens and aglepristone treatment does not negatively affect subsequent fertility (Georgiev *et al.*, 2010; Goericke-Pesch *et al.*, 2010). However, aglepristone is not available in the US at this time.

Aglepristone is labeled for canine pregnancy termination in Europe but is used off label in queens. Administration of aglepristone (10 mg/kg, SQ) on days 5 and 6 after mating resulted in 100% efficacy in pregnancy prevention (Goericke-Pesch *et al.*, 2010). Administration of aglepristone (10 mg/kg, SQ, two injections 24 hours apart) on days 25–26 after mating (Georgiev and Wehrend, 2006) or 33.3 ± 4.2 after mating (Fiéni *et al.*, 2006) resulted in 87–88.5% efficacy for pregnancy termination. Administration of aglepristone (10 mg/kg, SQ) on days 45 and 46 after mating resulted in 67% efficacy for pregnancy termination (Georgiev *et al.*, 2010). These results show that earlier treatment is preferred due to higher efficacy rates. Furthermore, in case of induction of abortion, an ultrasound examination of the uterus should be performed 6–7 days after the first aglepristone injection to ensure that abortion is complete. In cases of incomplete abortion another injection of aglepristone should be given and the ultrasound examination should be repeated 4–7 days later to confirm complete abortion. In case of vital fetuses still being present, other options including surgery or delivery have to be considered. Owners should be informed about the significantly shortened interestrus interval to avoid further mismating. Even though published studies used the canine dosage of aglepristone (10 mg/kg, SQ, two injections 24 hours apart), the manufacturer recommends the use of 15 mg aglepristone/kg, SQ twice 24 hours apart for higher efficacy.

A combined drug protocol has been established to improve the efficacy of pregnancy termination using aglepristone (10 mg/kg, SQ, two injections 24 hours apart) with misoprostol (200 µg/cat, PO every 12 hours until abortion starts). This combined protocol resulted in 100% efficacy (n = 7) for pregnancy termination and was superior to use of each individual drug alone (Ay *et al.*, 2019).

12.4 References

Addiego, L. A., Tsutsui, T., Stewart, D. R., and Stabenfeldt, G. H. (1987) Determination of the source of immunoreactive relaxin in the cat. *Biology of Reproduction* 37, 1165–1169. doi: 10.1095/biolreprod37.5.1165

Agaoglu, A. R., Aslan, S., Emre, B., Korkmaz, O., Ozdemir Salci, E. S., *et al.* (2014) Clinical evaluation of different applications of misoprostol and aglepristone for induction of abortion in bitches. *Theriogenology* 81(7), 947–951. doi: 10.1016/j.theriogenology.2014.01.017

Ay, S. S., Aslan, S., Önyay, F., Kaya, D., Koldas, E., *et al.* (2019) Effect of oral misoprostol, alone or in combination with aglepristone, on mid-term pregnancy termination in cats. *Journal of Feline Medicine and Surgery* 21, 714–722. doi: 10.1177/1098612X18797139

Cetin, Y., Macun, H. C., Beceriklisoy, H. B., Schäfer-Somi, S., and Aslan, S. (2010) Intravaginal application of misoprostol improves pregnancy termination with cabergoline and alfaprostol in dogs. *Berliner und Münchener Tierärztliche Wochenschrift* 123(5–6), 236–242.

Davidson, A. P., Feldman, E. C., and Nelson, R. W. (1992) Treatment of pyometra in cats, using prostaglandin F2α: 21 cases (1982–1990). *Journal of the American Medical Association* 200, 825–828.

Erünal-Maral, N., Aslan, S., Findik, M., Yüksel, N., Handler, J., *et al.* (2004) Induction of abortion in queens by administration of cabergolin (Galastop™) solely or in combination with the $PGF_{2\alpha}$ analogue Alfaprostol (Gabbrosim™). *Theriogenology* 61, 1471–1475. doi: 10.1016/j.theriogenology.2003.08.014

Fiéni, F., Martal, J., Marnet, P. G., Siliart, B., and Guittot, F. (2006) Clinical, biological and hormonal study of mid-pregnancy termination in cats with aglepristone. *Theriogenology* 66, 1721–1728. doi: 10.1016/j.theriogenology.2006.02.026

García Mitacek, M. C., Stornelli, M. C., Tittarelli, C. M., Nuñez Favre, R., de la Sota, R. L., *et al.* (2014) Cloprostenol treatment of feline open-cervix pyometra. *Journal of Feline Medicine and Surgery* 16, 177–179. doi: 10.1177/1098612X13498248

Georgiev, P. and Wehrend, A. (2006) Mid-gestation pregnancy termination by the progesterone antagonist aglepristone in queens. *Theriogenology* 65, 1401–1406. doi: 10.1016/j.theriogenology.2005.08.011

Georgiev, P., Bostedt, H., Goericke-Pesch, S., Dimitrov, M., Petkov, P., *et al.* (2010) Induction of abortion with aglepristone in cats on day 45 and 46 after mating. *Reproduction in Domestic Animals,* 45, e161–167. doi: 10.1111/j.1439-0531.2009.01540.x

Goericke-Pesch, S. (2017) Antiprogestins in Small Animal Reproduction – more than induction of abortion in dogs. *Turkiye Klinikleri Journal Veterinary Science Obstetrics and Gynecology-Special Topics* 3, 24–31.

Goericke-Pesch, S., Georgiev, P., and Wehrend, A. (2010) Prevention of pregnancy in cats using aglepristone on days 5 and 6 after mating. *Theriogenology.* 74, 304–310. doi: 10.1016/j.theriogenology.2010.02.014.

Gogny, A., and Fiéni, F. (2016) Aglepristone: A review on its clinical use in animals. *Theriogenology* 85, 555–566. doi: 10.1016/j.theriogenology.2015.10.010

Jöchle, W. (2016) Nidationsverhütung und Graviditätsabbruch. In: Günzel-Apel, A., Bostedt, H. *Reproduktionsmedizin und Neonatologie von Hund und Katze.* Schattauer, Stuttgart, Germany, pp. 498–501.

Jöchle, W. and Jöchle, M. (1993) Reproduction in a feral cat population and its control with a prolactin inhibitor, cabergoline. *Journal of Reproduction and Fertility* Supplement 47, 419–424.

Nachreiner, R. F. and Marple, D. N. (1974) Termination of pregnancy in cats with prostaglandin F2α. *Prostaglandins* 7, 303–308. doi: 10.1016/s0090-6980(74)80085-7

Onclin, K. and Verstegen, J. (1997) Termination of pregnancy in cats using a combination of cabergoline, a new dopamine agonist, and a synthetic $PGF_{2\alpha}$, cloprostenol. *Journal of Reproduction and Fertility* Supplement 51, 259–263.

Scott, P. P. (1970) Reproduction and breeding techniques for laboratory animals. In: Hafez, E. S. E. (ed.), *Cats*. Lea & Febiger, Philadelphia, Pennsylvania.

Sokolowski, J. H. and Geng, S. (1977) Effect of prostaglandin F2alpha-THAM in the bitch. *Journal of the American Veterinary Medical Association* 170, 536–553.

Stewart, D. R. and Stabenfeldt, G. H. (1985) Relaxin activity in the pregnant cat. *Biology of Reproduction* 32, 848–854. doi: 10.1095/biolreprod32.4.848

Tsutsui, T. and Stabenfeldt, G. H. (1993) Biology of ovarian cycles, pregnancy and pseudopregnancy in the domestic cat. *Journal of Reproduction and Fertility* Supplement 47, 29–35.

Tsutsui, T., Suzuki, Y., Toyonaga, M., Oba, H., Mizutani, T., *et al.* (2009) The role of the ovary for the maintenance of pregnancy in cats. *Reproduction in Domestic Animals* 2, 120–124. doi: 10.1111/j.1439-0531.2009.01452.x

Verstegen, J. P., Onclin, K., Silva, L. D., and Donnay, I. (1993) Abortion induction in the cat using prostaglandin F2 alpha and a new anti-prolactinic agent, cabergoline. *Journal of Reproduction and Fertility* Supplement 47, 411–417.

Verstegen, J., Dhaliwal, G., and Verstegen-Onclin, K. (2008). Mucometra, cystic endometrial hyperplasia, and pyometra in the bitch: advances in treatment and assessment of future reproductive success. *Theriogenology* 70, 364–374. doi: 10.1016/j.theriogenology.2008.04.036

Wildt, D. E., Panko, W. B., and Seager, S. W. (1979) Effect of prostaglandin F2a on endocrine ovarian function in the domestic cat. *Prostaglandins* 18, 883–892.

Wycoff, J. T., and Ganjam, V. K. (1979) Successful termination of pregnancy in cats by the administration of a combination of adrenocorticotrophic hormone (ACTH) and prostaglandin F2a-tham salt. *Federation Proceedings* 38, 1189.

13 Disorders of the Ovary

AIME K. JOHNSON

Auburn University College of Veterinary Medicine, Department of Clinical Sciences, Auburn, Alabama, USA

13.1 Introduction

The normal anatomy of the ovary is discussed in Chapter 1. Disorders of the ovary are more likely as the queen ages. Ovarian changes may be benign and do not interfere with fertility of the queen, but some cause hormonal changes that may cause concern for the queen's overall health and decrease prognosis for future fertility. One study assessed the records of 106 female cats that presented for routine ovariohysterectomy (OHE). The age of cats undergoing OHE ranged from 4 months to 9 years (average age was about 2 years). Abnormalities of the reproductive tract were detected in 27.4% of cats and included ovarian or paraovarian cysts, uterine pathology (CEH), and endometritis. Of the cats in the age range of 3–5 years, pathologic abnormalities were found in 50%. The percentage increased to 83% when the cats were older than 5 years (Binder *et al.*, 2020).

13.2 Congenital Abnormalities of the Ovary

Sex phenotype is characterized by the appearance of the internal and external genitalia, sexual behavior, and secondary characteristics. Sex determination of the gonads is driven by the sex chromosomes present. The normal female is 38,XX with a total of 38 chromosomes and two copies of the X chromosome, one from each parent. In the normal male who has the genotype XY, the sex determining region of the Y chromosome (the *SRY* gene) drives the development of the testicles by activating other male pathway genes. The *SRY* gene also influences other sex determination genes such as *SOX9 (SRY-box containing gene 9)* and anti-Müllerian hormone influence. In the female, *Wnt4* is upregulated in the presence of two X chromosomes. R-spondins (such as *RSPO1*) act by upregulating the WNT4 pathway which then activates the β-catenin pathway. In the cytoplasm of the early gonadal cells, β-catenin and SOX9 inactivate each other. When the developing embryo reaches a critical point in sexual differentiation, the differentiation pathway is determined by the protein that is higher within the cells. For example, if the chromosomes present are XX, β-catenin is produced in more abundance, it diffuses into the nucleus of the cells and promotes transcription of genes that develop female characteristics, therefore initiating female/ovarian development (Chassot *et al.*, 2008).

Disorders among the female genotype include ovarian dysgenesis (unilateral or bilateral), hermaphroditism, pseudohermaphroditism, supernumerary or accessory ovary, or ovarian aplasia. Ovarian dysgenesis is a common congenital abnormality in the feline and is defined as a lack of development of the ovaries. Other terms that are used are ovarian hypoplasia and streak gonads. Such conditions often result from various chromosomal issues including X monosomy (also referred to as XO or Turner syndrome in the human literature) or trisomy (XXX). In each of these conditions, the ovaries are small, inactive, and underdeveloped. The external genitalia are female and the individuals are sterile. One report of a queen that presented for infertility and primary anestrus had a small, underdeveloped uterus and inactive ovaries. On histopathology, the ovaries showed hypertrophied interstitial cells and fibroblastic stroma. There was no evidence of follicles or corpus lutea on either ovary. The external genitalia of this cat were female. Karyotype revealed 37,XO (Johnston *et al.*, 1983). Other reports of X monosomy have been reported in the cat and have been associated with other conditions such as spina bifida or coarctation of the aorta (Johnston *et al.*, 2001).

 Feline Reproduction (eds. A.K. Johnson and M.A. Kutzler)
DOI: 10.1079/9781789247107.0013

Chimerism and mosaicism, when involving the sex chromosomes, can result in disorders of sexual development. Chimerism is created by a mixing of genetically different tissue, typically due to the fusion of two early embryos. Mosaic animals comprise two genetically different types of cells in a single embryo. The difference between the two is that in a chimera, embryos (usually 2) fuse to create the different cell types while in a mosaic animal, the different cell lines are due to a mutation within a single embryo. Both result in an animal that displays different chromosome numbers in different tissues/cells lines. Thomsen *et al.* reported two unrelated cats that presented for routine ovariohysterectomy at a shelter. Both were pregnant at the time of presentation. Both cats displayed ovarian dysplasia in a single ovary while the contralateral ovary was functioning normally. Karyotype of the lymphocytes in each cat were found to be 37,XO and 39,XXX in the first, and 38,XX and 37,XO in the second. Karyotyping of several of the fetuses showed normal chromosome pattern of 38,XX or 38,XY thereby showing that a mosaic, if only affecting a single ovary, can still result in normal fertility (Thomsen *et al.*, 1987).

Hermaphroditism has been reported in the cat but is much less common than reports involving the dog. One case report of a true hermaphrodite was reported by Schlafer *et al.* in 2011. The phenotypically male cat presented for a bilateral cryptorchid neuter. During surgery, a poorly developed uterus was found with the gonads located where the ovaries would be in a normal female. Histopathology showed a true ovotestis with both female and male duct systems. A karyotype was performed and showed a normal male (38,XY) (Schlafer *et al.*, 2011). There is no known report of a cat that appears female externally but contains both ovarian and testicular tissue. The few reports available of true hermaphroditism are in cats that are phenotypically male. Pseudohermaphrodites are more common than true hermaphrodites. These occur when the phenotypic sex and gonadal sex are different and are classified as either male or female pseudohermaphrodites. Male pseudohermaphrodites have a normal male chromosomal complement of 38,XY but have female-appearing genitalia, while female pseudohermaphrodites have the normal female chromosomes of 38,XX but have male external genitalia. In each of these cases, external development may be a mixture of male and female genitalia. For example, a female pseudohermaphrodite may have an exaggerated and enlarged clitoris, appearing penile-like, but not looking like a 'normal' penis. To differentiate these animals from a true sex reversal case, histology of the gonads and chromosome pattern should be performed. The gonads and chromosomes will agree in pseudohermaphrodite animals while the external genitalia disagree (38,XX and ovaries present, externally appear as male), whereas in sex reversal the chromosomes will not be the same as the gonads (38,XY, testicles or ovotestes present, external genitalia is female). Causes may be genetic or external in origin. For example, female pseudohermaphrodites may occur when the dam is treated with exogenous progestins during the critical window when the external genitalia are forming.

XX sex reversal, where the chromosomes are 38,XX and the gonads are either testes or ovotestes, has been reported in dogs (such as the Cocker Spaniel) but not in the cat. Testicular feminization has been reported in the cat where the chromosomes are 38,XY but the external genitalia is female. In one report, an inherited defect of the cytosolic androgen receptor failed to allow external masculinization to develop. Externally, the cat appeared female. Externally, the chromosomes showed a normal male at 38,XY. Internally, only testicular tissue was found in the gonad. Following a detailed pedigree analysis, this defect appears to be an X-linked disorder, which is the cause of the condition in other species as well (Meyers-Wallen *et al.*, 1989).

Diagnosis of most disorders of sexual development can be confirmed by histopathology of the gonadal tissue and karyotyping. Because many disorders are only found during routine spay or neuter, many owners may decline submission of tissues and karyotyping since their animal is now officially sterile. However, it is important to diagnose and describe these disorders when they occur to determine the frequency in which they do occur and to determine if there is a heritable component. The latter will allow evaluation of the parents, siblings, or any offspring of the affected animal and allow recommendations for future breeding animals.

13.3 Ovarian Remnant Syndrome

Ovarian remnant syndrome (ORS) is a condition that is caused by remaining functional ovarian tissue usually left behind following an ovariohysterectomy (OHE). This happens more commonly in the queen when compared to the bitch because the feline ovary is not encapsulated within a bursa. Rarely, an accessory ovary or tissue nodules may be found as the cause (McEntee, 1990). The ovarian remnant continues to function normally, building follicles and releasing estrogen. The affected queen will continue to display estrus behavior despite a past surgical history of OHE. Signs include lordosis, vocalization, and may accept breeding from a male. The time from OHE to clinical signs varies but may be as early as a few days to weeks or as long as several years, one cat was diagnosed 9 years after OHE) depending on the location and blood supply of the remaining tissue. The average time to clinical signs is 3–4 months (Wallace, 1991).

Ovarian remnant syndrome can be diagnosed by observation of the affected cat when showing signs of estrus. A sample for vaginal cytology can be collected and will be consistent with the presence of estrogen (greater than 70% cornification). Once estrogen is confirmed, the queen can be induced to ovulate with either 500 IU hCG or 25 μg GnRH intramuscularly. This will cause any follicles to luteinize and produce progesterone. A progesterone test should be performed about 1–2 weeks after ovulation induction. If progesterone is high (greater than 2 ng/mL), ovarian tissue is present. Anti-Müllerian hormone (AMH) has been described as an alternative or supplemental diagnostic indicator for the presence of ovarian tissue in several species, including the cat. Unlike progesterone, this hormone is species-specific and each testing method available should be validated in the desired species. In dogs, one study was 100% specific and 90% sensitive in detecting ovarian tissue with a single test (Themmen *et al.*, 2016). Yilmaz *et al.* (2015) showed that AMH was significantly higher in intact bitches than spayed. Anti-Müllerian hormone, as with other hormones, can vary slightly depending on the stage of the cycle and will decrease when luteinizing hormone (LH) is elevated (as with an LH surge) (Nagashima *et al.*, 2016). Combining AMH with progesterone or retesting the AMH several days later may assist in obtaining a correct diagnosis. There also may be a benefit to testing for inhibin-A. This hormone is elevated in intact animals but low or undetectable in spayed animals. Inhibin-A may provide an additional test for confirmation. Diagnosis of ORS is best confirmed by performing multiple tests and receiving multiple positives because no single test is perfect all the time.

Differential diagnostics should be performed to rule out any other sources of estrogen such as diet, adrenal neoplasia, or accidental exposure to human hormone creams. A good history including duration of clinical signs and if the signs are cyclical or constant can help differentiate these from ORS. However, Meler *et al.* reported a case of cyclic behavior in a 15-year-old spayed female that was diagnosed with an adrenocortical carcinoma. The cat showed estrus behavior, but tests were inconclusive for ORS. Hormonal testing showed increased concentrations of estrogen, progesterone, and 17α-hydroxyprogesterone and ultrasound revealed an enlarged adrenal gland (Meler *et al.*, 2011).

Once ovarian tissue has been confirmed, surgery is the treatment of choice. Surgery should be performed 2–3 weeks after induction of ovulation to allow the surgeon to more easily identify the ovarian tissue. The tissue will contain corpora lutea that appear as pale-yellow clusters within the tissue. The ovarian tissue is usually located at the ovarian pedicle, keeping in mind that it may be bilateral. Any tissue removed should be submitted for histopathology to confirm that the ovarian tissue has been removed. Sometimes, the ovarian tissue may have been cut or dropped into the abdomen at the time of the OHE. This tissue can re-vascularize within the omentum and function as an ovarian remnant (Fig. 13.1). During surgery, the entire abdomen should be searched to find all potential ovarian tissue. Ovarian remnant syndrome is curative once the ovarian tissue is removed.

13.4 Ovarian Cysts

Ovarian cysts can be a frequent occurrence in the queen and incidence increases with age. Ovarian cysts typically arise from atretic or mature follicles that are larger than preovulatory follicles and fail to ovulate. Their structure is the same as a normal follicle and includes a layer of thecal and granulosal cells. Many are hormonally functional, producing high concentrations of estrogens. Because of this, a common clinical sign is persistent estrus, but failing to ovulate and become pregnant. Queens with this condition often present for infertility. If hormonally active, the history often includes continued observed estrus behavior, but never diestrus and rarely interestrus. Alternatively, the queen will show irregular cyclicity. The presence of follicular cysts is best confirmed by transabdominal ultrasonography (Fig. 13.2). The ovary can be visualized with the cat restrained in lateral recumbency. An area of hair over the caudal lateral abdomen is clipped. The kidney is visualized, and the ovary is found near the caudal pole of that kidney. Normal preovulatory follicles measure 1–2 mm (Wildt and Seager, 1980). Any cystic structure over 5 mm in diameter is likely an ovarian cyst. This author has observed ovarian cysts as large as 1–2 cm.

Treatment options include attempts to induce luteinization of the cyst(s) by administration of either 500 IU hCG or 25 μg GnRH intramuscularly. Success of treatment can be evaluated by a subsequent rise in serum progesterone, a decrease of cornified epithelial cells on a vaginal cytology, and ultrasound. All diagnostics can be performed as soon as 2–3 weeks after treatment. Surgical resection has also been reported with a return to fertility (Johnston *et al.*, 2001). Clinically, this author aspirated a 2 cm ovarian cyst via laparotomy from a 2-year-old queen that presented for infertility. A uterine biopsy was also obtained at the time of surgery. This queen was bred several months later and became pregnant.

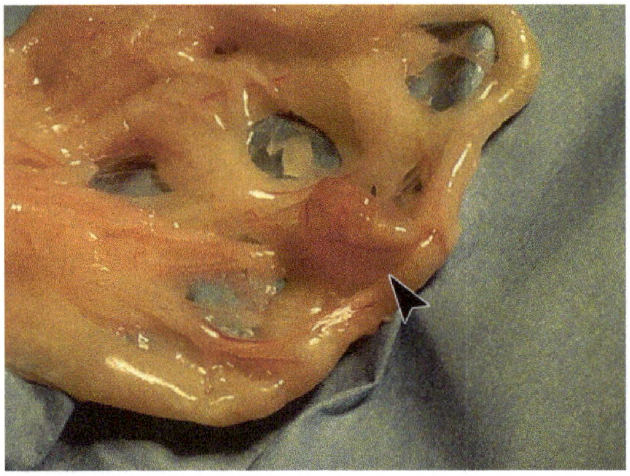

Fig. 13.1. An ovarian remnant located within the omentum (black arrow). This queen presented for continued estrus signs. This queen was in estrus at the time of surgery. The ovarian tissue had re-vascularized. (Image: author's own.)

13.5 Periovarian Cysts

Cysts that arise outside or directly adjacent to the ovary may also be diagnosed via transabdominal ultrasound. The most common of these periovarian cysts originate from the rete ovarii, a collection of blind tubules or cords within the medulla of the ovary. The rete ovarii is analogous to the rete testes in the male. Cysts in this structure tend to be thin walled and may be as large as 2.5 cm in diameter. Cystic rete ovarii are lined with either one or two layers of cuboidal epithelium or ciliated columnar epithelium. These cysts do not appear functional but should be differentiated from follicular cysts as they will not respond to hormonal treatment. Diagnosis can be made based on clinical history of the queen's behavior and histological appearance of the cyst lining (Gelberg *et al.*, 1984).

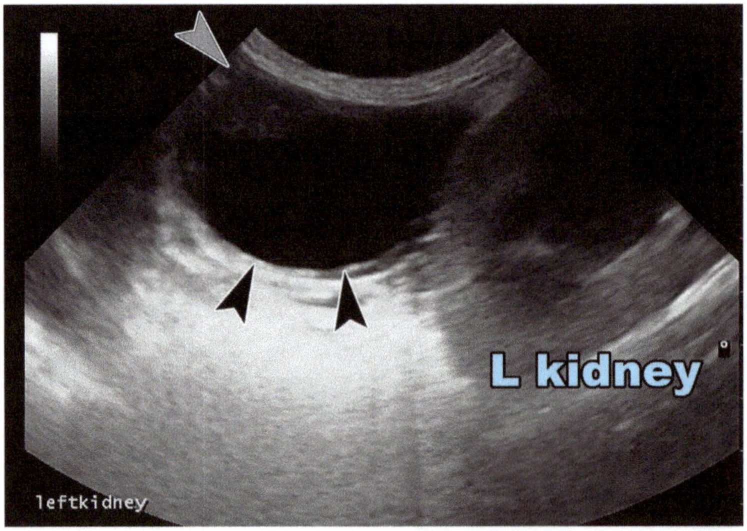

Fig. 13.2. Ultrasound image of a feline ovarian cyst. The ovary is located off the caudal pole of the kidney. The cyst (black arrowhead) is seen as a hypoechoic fluid-filled structure within the ovary (gray arrow). (Image: author's own.)

Cysts that occur in remnants of the mesonephric tubules or tissues beside the ovary are benign but may be confused as a follicular cyst due to their proximity to the ovary. Fluid accumulation within the Wolffian (mesonephric) ducts or the Müllerian (paramesonephric) ducts can be differentiated partially by location. Cysts located near the uterus or caudal ovary or inside the fimbria next to the ovary tend to be caudal or cranial portions of the mesonephric ducts, respectively. Paramesonephric duct remnants are found on the serosal surface of the fimbria near the oviducts. Histology of the cyst structure can allow confirmation of these structures (McEntee, 1990). Other than causing a potential physical blockage of the fimbria or oviducts during ovulation, these cysts are benign.

13.6 Ovarian Neoplasia

Primary neoplasia can arise from any cell present in the affected organ. Therefore, to create a differential list for ovarian neoplasia, one must remember what cells are located in the ovary. Ovarian cell types can be placed into three broad categories: epithelial, stromal, and germinal. The incidence of reported ovarian neoplasia in the cat is low, with only a handful of publications and case reports. This low incidence may be due to the fact that most cats are spayed at a young age. Ovarian neoplasia can be diagnosed by abdominal palpation, ultrasound, or radiography. If an ovarian neoplasia is detected, staging (chest and abdominal radiographs, abdominal ultrasound, complete blood count, and serum chemistry) may be indicated to determine the presence of metastases. Vaginal cytology or hormone assays may also be indicated to assess for functionality of the tumor.

13.6.1 Ovarian epithelial neoplasia

Tumors arise from the ovarian surface tissue and epithelial tissue within the ovary such as the rete ovarii. Cystadenomas and adenomas are rare in cats but have been reported. In a study evaluating primary ovarian neoplasms from 22 cats, only one queen (10 years old) was diagnosed with a cystadenoma. The tumor was bilateral and nodular/cystic in appearance. The cystic areas were lined with low cuboidal or pseudostratified columnar cells containing cilia (Gelberg and McEntee, 1985). Adenocarcinomas are equally rare. A study evaluating ten cats with ovarian tumors showed a single 5-year-old cat with an ovarian adenocarcinoma with spindle cell transformation. The cat presented with ascites, hair loss and an abdominal mass. On further evaluation, metastases were located throughout the abdomen and lungs (Norris *et al.*, 1969).

13.6.2 Ovarian stroma and sex cord neoplasia

Stromal tumors are the most common ovarian tumor in the cat with 14/22 cats diagnosed with stromal cell tumors (Gelberg and McEntee, 1985).

Granulosa cell tumor (GCT)

The GCT is the most diagnosed primary ovarian neoplasia in the cat. This tumor arises from ovarian sex cords and can be malignant in about one-third of cases. This tumor is usually a functional tumor and may produce estrogen, progesterone, or both. Affected cats often present with prolonged estrus, irregular cyclicity, infertility, palpable abdominal mass, alopecia, ascites, or a combination of these. Gross appearance of the ovary can vary but is usually lobulated (Fig. 13.3). Metastases can be found in the uterus (Fig. 13.4a), reginal lymph nodes, liver, kidney, spleen, or lungs (Fig. 13.4b). Histologically, many contain a rosette-type cellular arrangement called Call-Exner bodies (Fig. 13.5). These structures have a pale or eosinophilic center and are surrounded by epithelial cells (Heaps *et al.*, 2017). Many feline granulosa cell tumors also involve thecal cells, but the neoplasia is referred to by the most prominent cell type. Diagnosis is confirmed by histopathology of the affected ovary at the time of

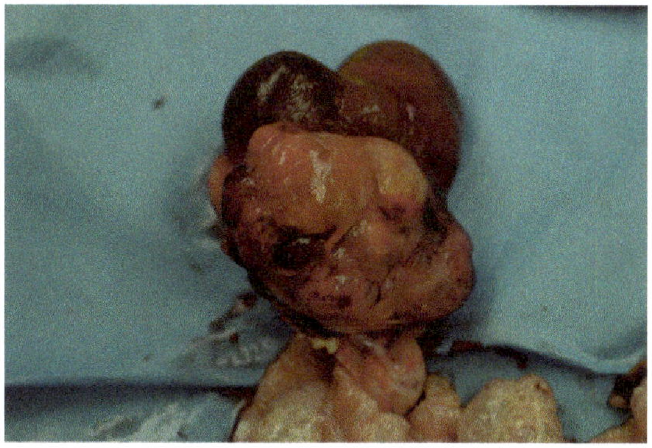

Fig. 13.3. A granulosa cell ovarian tumor in a 14-year-old queen. The queen presented for weight loss and abdominal distension. (Image: author's own.)

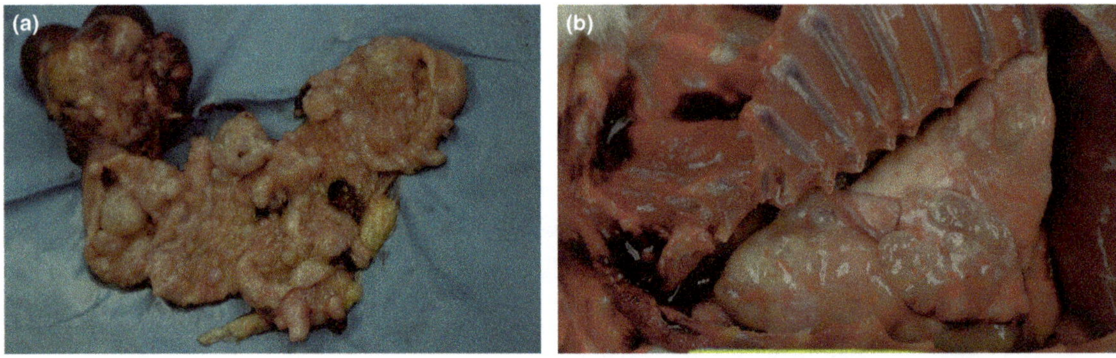

Fig. 13.4 **(a)** The same queen as in Figure 13.3 showing metastases to the uterus. **(b)** On necropsy, the neoplasia was also found throughout the abdomen, with additional metastases to the intestines, liver, chest wall, and lungs. (Images: author's own.)

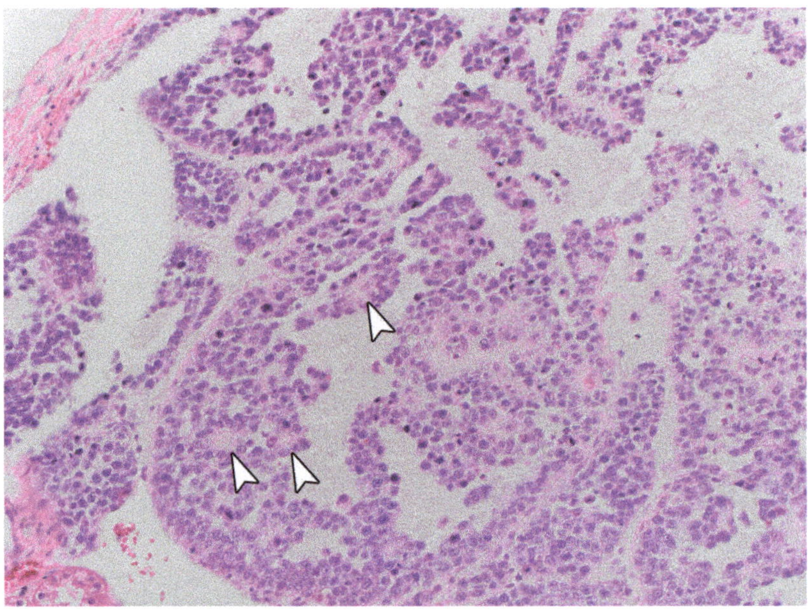

Fig. 13.5. Call-Exner bodies (arrowheads) in a GCT metastasis to the kidney. (Image: author's own.)

removal. One report tested anti-Müllerian hormone before and after removal of a GCT in a 15-year-old cat. Prior to removal, the AMH was elevated even above normal ranges for intact females (5.7 ng/mL vs 1.7 ng/mL in normal intact queens). The AMH decreased to baseline after ovariohysterectomy. This report suggested that AMH may be useful in diagnosing GCT in the cat (Heaps *et al.*, 2017).

Interstitial cell tumor

Interstitial cell tumors have been reported in the queen. The tumors have been described as solid and yellow to brown in color. Histologically, the cytoplasm is vacuolated with a single round nucleus. Out of 22 cats, 5 were diagnosed with interstitial cell tumors. There was no mention of metastasis or paraneoplastic disease. (Gelberg and McEntee, 1985).

13.6.3 Germ cell tumors

Teratoma

Teratomas are tumors that are derived from ectodermal, endodermal, and mesodermal cell types.

Teratomas often include cystic areas lined with hair, bone, muscle, connective tissue, teeth, cartilage, fat, sweat glands, or nervous tissue. Teratomas are also called dermoid cysts. Most teratomas are found in young animals and are rarely malignant. Gelberg and McEntee reported 1 teratoma out of 22 cats (Gelberg and McEntee, 1985). Other reports of teratomas in cats include a 5-month-old cat with abdominal distension and a 10 × 11 cm ovarian teratoma (Basaraba *et al.*, 1998). One case report involved a 5-year-old queen that presented with abdominal distension (Machida *et al.*, 2017). A unilateral immature ovarian teratoma was found on exploratory laparotomy. The tumor contained smooth muscle, neuroectodermal tissue, cartilage, fat, and mesenchymal cells. Estrogen was elevated in the queen's blood and in the neoplastic fluid. This teratoma had metastasized within the abdomen and the cat died about 6 weeks after surgery (Machida *et al.*, 2017).

Dysgerminoma

Dysgerminomas in the female are similar to seminomas in the male. Out of 22 reported cats with ovarian neoplasia, 6 were diagnosed with a dysgerminoma. Two of these were bilateral, a third involved an ovotestis, and two of the six had metastasized (Gelberg and McEntee, 1985). Grossly, the tumors are white to gray in color and firm (Andrews *et al.*, 1974). Histologically, dysgerminomas comprise groups of large round cells separated by cords of connective tissue. Cases of dysgerminoma have been shown to be locally infiltrative and one case involving the ovary and uterine horn was metastatic (Lamm *et al.*, 2020)

13.6.4 Summary

Following diagnosis of an ovarian neoplasia, surgical removal is indicated. All enlarged ovaries should be submitted for histopathology to determine if it is neoplastic, which type, and the metastatic potential. Staging of the cat, including complete blood work, abdominal ultrasound, and chest radiographs, may be indicated if metastasis is suspected. If the tumor is benign, surgical removal is curative. If future fertility is desired, the affected ovary can be removed, allowing the contralateral ovary to resume or continue cyclicity.

13.7 References

Andrews, E. J., Stookey, J. L., Helland, D. R., and Slaughter, L. J. (1974) A histopathological study of canine and feline dysgerminomas. *Canadian Journal of Comparative Medicine* 38(1) 85–89.

Basaraba, R. J., Kraft, S. L., Andrews, G. A., Leipold, H. W., and Small, D. (1998) An ovarian teratoma in a cat. *Veterinary Pathology* 35(2), 141–144. doi: 10.1177/030098589803500208

Binder, C., Reifinger, M., Aurich, J., and Aurich, C. (2020) Histopathological findings in the uteri and ovaries of clinically healthy cats presented for routine spaying. *Journal of Feline Medicine and Surgery* 23(8), 770–776. doi: 10.1177/1098612X20975376

Chassot, A. A., Gregoire, E. P., Magliano, M., Lavery, R., and Chaboissier, M. C. (2008) Genetics of ovarian differentiation: Rspo1, a major player. *Sexual Development* 2, 219–227. doi: 10.1159/000152038

Gelberg, H. B. and McEntee, K. (1985) Feline ovarian neoplasms. *Veterinary Pathology* 22(6), 572–576. doi: 10.1177/030098588502200610

Gelberg, H. B., McEntee, K., and Heath, E. H. (1984) Feline cystic rete ovarii. *Veterinary Pathology* 21(3), 304–307. doi: 10.1177/030098588402100307

Heaps, L. A., Scudder, C. J., Lipscomb, V. J., Steinbach, S. M., Priestnall, S. L., *et al.* (2017) Serum anti-Müllerian hormone concentrations before and after treatment of an ovarian granulosa cell tumour in a cat. *Journal of Feline Medicine and Surgery: Open Reports* 3(2). doi: 10.1177/2055116917722701

Johnston, S. D., Buoen, L. C., Madi, J. E., Weber, A. F., and Smith, F. O. (1983) X-Chromosome monosomy (37, XO) in a Burmese cat with gonadal dysgenesis. *Journal of the American Veterinary Medical Association* 182, 986–989

Johnston, S. D., Root Kustritz, M. V., and Olson, P. N. S. (2001) Disorders of the Ovary. In: Johnston, S. D., Root Kustritz, M. V., and Olson, P. N. S. (eds) *Canine and Feline Theriogenology*. Saunders, Philadelphia, Pennsylvania, pp.453–462.

Lamm, C. G., Foster, R. A., and Swick, A. (2020) Pathology in Practice: Ovarian and uterine dysgerminoma. *Journal of the American Veterinary Medical Association* 257(8), 817–819. doi: 10.2460/javma.257.8.817

Machida, Y., Michishita, M., Wada, M., Hori, T., Kawakami, E., *et al.* (2017) Malignant oestrogen-producing teratoma in a cat. *Journal of Comparative Pathology* 156(2–3), 178–182. doi: 10.1016/j.jcpa.2016.11.273

McEntee, K. (1990) Cysts in and around the ovary. In: McEntee, K. (ed.) *Reproductive Pathology of Domestic Mammals*. Academic Press, San Diego, California, pp. 52–68. doi: 10.1016/B978-0-12-483375-3.50010-X

Meler, E. N., Scott-Moncrieff, J. C., Peter, A. T., Bennett, S., Ramos-Vara, J. *et al.* (2011) Cyclic estrous-like behavior in a spayed cat associated with excessive sex-hormone production by an adrenocortical carcinoma. *Journal of Feline Medicine and Surgery* 13(6), 473–478. doi: 10.1016/j.jfms.2011.02.002

Meyers-Wallen, V. N., Wilson, J. D., Griffin, J. E., Fisher, S., Moorhead, P. H., *et al.* (1989) Testicular feminization in a cat. *Journal of the American Veterinary Medical Association* 195(5), 631–634.

Nagashima, J. B., Hansen, B. S., Songsasen, N., Travis, A. J., and Place, N. J. (2016) Anti-Müllerian hormone in the domestic dog during the anestrus to oestrous transition. *Reproduction in Domestic Animals* 51, 158–164.

Norris, H. J., Garner, F. M., and Taylor, H. B. (1969) Pathology of feline ovarian neoplasms. *The Journal of Pathology* 97, 138–143. doi: 10.1002/path.1710970118

Schlafer, D. H., Valentine, B., Fahnestock, G., Froenicke, L., Grahn, R. A., *et al.* (2011) A case of SRY-positive 38,XY true hermaphroditism (XY sex reversal) in a cat. *Veterinary Pathology* 48(4), 817–822. doi: 10.1177/0300985810382093

Themmen, A. P. N., Kalra, B., Visser, J. A., Kumar, A., Savjani, G., *et al.* (2016) The use of anti-Müllerian hormone as diagnostic for gonadectomy status in dogs. *Theriogenology* 86(6), 1467–1474. doi: 10.1016/j.theriogenology.2016.05.004

Thomsen, P. D., Byskov, A. G., and Basse, E. (1987) Fertility in two cats with X-chromosome mosaicism and unilateral ovarian dysgenesis. *Journal of Reproduction and Fertility* 80, 43–47. doi: 10.1530/jrf.0.0800043

Wallace, M. S. (1991) The ovarian remnant syndrome in the bitch and queen. *Veterinary Clinics of North America Small Animal Practice* 21, 501–507. doi: 10.1016/s0195-5616(91)50056-5

Wildt, D. and Seager, S. (1980) Laparoscopic determination of ovarian and uterine morphology during the reproductive cycle. In: Morrow, D. (ed.). *Current Therapy in Theriogenology*, 2nd edn. W.B. Saunders Co., Philadelphia, Pennsylvania, pp. 828–832.

Yilmaz, Ö. T., Toydemir, T. S. F., Kirsan, I., Ucmak, Z. G., and Karacam, E. C. (2015) Anti-Müllerian hormone as a diagnostic tool for ovarian remnant syndrome in bitches. *Veterinary Research Communications* 39(3), 159–162. doi: 10.1007/s11259-015-9639-0

14 Disorders of the Uterus

Carla Barstow

Highland Pet Hospital, Lakeland, Florida, USA

14.1 Development of the Uterus

The uterus develops from the paramesonephric ducts (mesoderm), along with the oviducts, cervix, and cranial vagina. The caudal vagina and vestibule develop from ectoderm. This occurs during the first and second trimesters of pregnancy (Senger, 2012). In contrast, the ovary develops from the gonadal ridge. This embryologic distinction between ovarian tissue and tubular reproductive tissues may explain why ovaries are typically present with uterine abnormalities (McIntyre *et al.*, 2010).

14.1.1 Abnormal uterine development

Prevalence of congenital uterine abnormalities in cats has been estimated to be 0.09% (Brookshire *et al.*, 2017). The most commonly noted uterine abnormalities are uterus unicornis, segmental aplasia of one uterine horn, and uterine horn hypoplasia. Congenital developmental abnormalities are mainly due to malformation of the paramesonephric ducts (Jones *et al.*, 1997). These congenital defects can be associated with hermaphroditic conditions or with ipsilateral renal agenesis because of the close developmental association of the urinary and genital systems (Johnston *et al.*, 2001). Ipsilateral renal agenesis was present in 29.4% of cats with uterine anomalies (McIntyre *et al.*, 2010; Brookshire *et al.*, 2017). Uterus unicornis is characterized by complete agenesis of one uterine horn (Fig. 14.1). Normal ovaries are commonly reported on the side of the agenesis (McIntyre *et al.*, 2010). Segmental aplasia is characterized by missing portions of the genital tract. This can include the cervix, uterus, and/or the cranial vagina. This results in isolation of the cranial segments of the uterus from the more distal segments (Jones *et al.*, 1997), usually separated by a thin piece of tissue where the uterus should have been. The proximal section is usually dilated by the normal uterine secretions that are unable to be expelled (McIntyre *et al.*, 2010).

Abnormal uterine development is uncommon. Unless it is bilateral, fertility is not necessarily impaired. It is commonly found by exploratory laparotomy or an incidental finding during ovariohysterectomy (Johnston *et al.*, 2001). Identification of uterine developmental anomalies should trigger evaluation of both kidneys because ipsilateral renal agenesis is common and, since both ovaries are likely to be present, it is imperative that they are both removed (McIntyre *et al.*, 2010).

14.2 Endometrial Polyps

Polyps may be single or multiple and occur anywhere in the uterus with their growth projecting into the uterine lumen (Johnston *et al.*, 2001). Some have a pedicle; however, others have a broad base (Gelberg and McEntee, 1984). Evidence suggests that endometrial polyps arise from focal areas of cystic endometrial hyperplasia and are seen in middle age to older cats (Gelberg and McEntree, 1984). Polyps are usually small and often go unnoticed, unless their growth compromises the uterine lumen (Schlafer and Gifford 2008) (Fig. 14.2).

14.3 Hydrometra/Mucometra

The collection of non-inflammatory, sterile watery to viscous fluid within the uterus is hydrometra/mucometra. In most conditions, the accumulation of fluid is the result of a blockage to outflow. Obstruction at the cervix will cause the uterine body and both horns to distend. Endometrial polyps can cause a local obstruction, causing distention proximal to the site. Segmental aplasia, cystic endometrial hyperplasia, and uterine neoplasia are other potential causes of hydrometra/mucometra.

Cats are not usually clinically ill but may show signs of abdominal distention in more severe cases. Ovariohysterectomy is the treatment of choice.

 Feline Reproduction (eds. A.K. Johnson and M.A. Kutzler)
DOI: 10.1079/9781789247107.0014

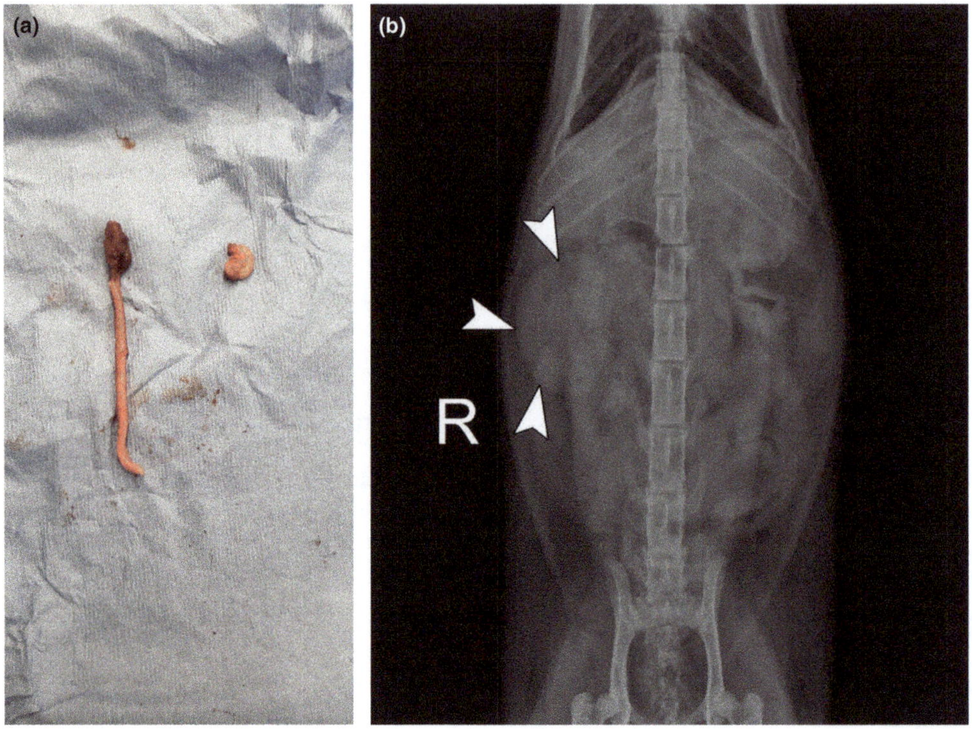

Fig. 14.1. **(a)** Uterus unicornis in a cat that presented for ovariohysterectomy. Both ovaries were present, but only one uterus horn was found. **(b)** Radiograph of the same cat with uterus unicornis. The right kidney is present (arrow heads), but the left kidney is absent. (Images: author's own.)

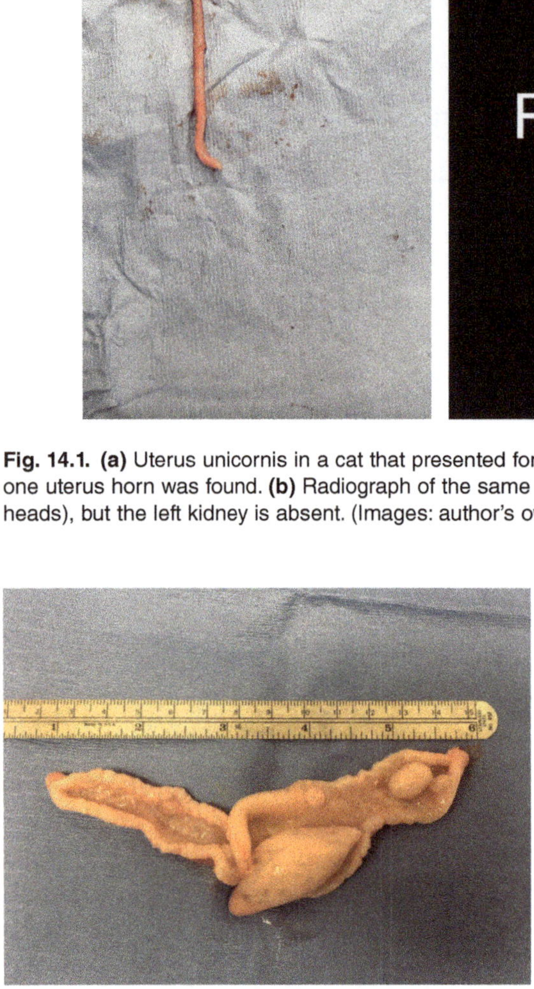

Fig. 14.2. A uterus removed from a subfertile queen that was diagnosed with a uterine mass by ultrasound. Several endometrial polyps are visible protruding into the uterine lumen. On histopathology, the masses were confirmed to be cystic endometrial hyperplasia. (Image courtesy of Dr Aime Johnson, also located in Visual Guide to Animal Reproduction (VISGAR).)

14.4 Cystic Endometrial Hyperplasia-Pyometra Complex

Cystic endometrial hyperplasia-pyometra complex is a disease characterized by hyperplasia of the endometrium with cystic dilatation of the endometrial glands and inflammation of the uterus with or without purulent material in the uterine lumen (Agudelo, 2005). Pyometra occurs in 2.2% of intact cats by age 13 (Hagman *et al.*, 2014). It is the most important reproductive disorder in the queen.

The incidence of cystic endometrial hyperplasia (CEH) is higher in colony queens, whereas no uterine changes were evident in feral cats (Perez *et al.*, 1999). In dogs, it has been discussed that pregnancy has a protective effect against development of CEH/pyometra and the number of nulliparous bitches with pyometra is approximately tenfold greater than in multiparous bitches (Dow, 1958). Nulliparous queens would be more likely to develop the disease; however, there is no correlation between development of the disease, the age of the first parturition, and number of litters delivered (Agudelo, 2005).

14.4.1 Pathophysiology

Repeated exposure of the endometrium to high concentrations of estrogen during estrus, followed by high concentrations of progesterone during the luteal phase, leads to the development of CEH. This predisposes the uterus to ascending secondary bacterial infection and development of pyometra. Progesterone makes the uterine environment suitable for fetal development by promoting gland growth and mucus secretion, closure of the cervix, decreasing muscular activity, and suppressing leukocyte function in the uterus (Hollinshead and Krekeler, 2016). Changes in the uterine microenvironment and decreased contractibility would favor the ascent of normal bacterial flora from the vagina through the open cervix during estrus (Barsanti, 1998). The changes to the endometrium create the perfect conditions for bacterial colonization to occur. *Escherichia coli* is the most frequently isolated microorganism from feline pyometra (Johnston *et al.*, 2001; Agudelo, 2005). Other agents like *Streptococcus* spp., *Staphylococcus* spp., *Klebsiella* spp., *Pseudomonas* spp., *Proteus* spp., *Moraxella* spp., and *Pasteurella* spp. have also been reported (Johnson, 1994).

More recently, it has been discussed as to whether pyometra and CEH are actually two separate disease processes (Hollinshead *et al.*, 2016). Hyperplastic changes have been induced by experimental manipulation of the uterine lumen of bitches. The dog develops endometrial proliferation following minor mechanical irritation (Nomura, 1995). Similar lesions are not reported for the cat (Schlafer and Gifford, 2008). However, it is possible that the presence of CEH in pyometra could merely be the result of a uterine reaction to the bacterial infection (Hollinshead *et al.*, 2016).

Cats are induced ovulators; however, repeated spontaneous ovulation in cats may increase the risk of developing pyometra (Keskin *et al.*, 2009). One study suggested that spontaneous, non-mating induced ovulation occurs in approximately one-third of all queens (Binder *et al.*, 2019). Higher body weight in queens may lead to greater frequency of spontaneous ovulations, as a degree of fatness is pivotal in regulating the cyclic ovarian functions in many species (Binder *et al.*, 2019).

Administration of contraceptive drugs may also increase the risk of pyometra. The use of exogenous steroid hormones (megestrol acetate or medroxyprogesterone acetate) has been shown to induce pyometra in both bitches and queens (Hollinshead *et al.*, 2016).

A CEH classification has been established according to the clinical and histopathological criteria (Table 14.1) (Dow, 1958).

Ovarian remnant syndrome can lead to the development of a stump pyometra, as the remnant ovarian tissue can produce progesterone, coupled with incomplete removal of the uterus below the bifurcation, leading to CEH and pyometra (Johnston *et al.*, 2001).

14.4.2 Signalment, history and physical examination

Cystic endometrial hyperplasia is a major cause of reduced fertility and low litter size and should be evaluated in every subfertile queen. Cystic endometrial hyperplasia was seen in 80% of queens aged 4–5 years old that presented for infertility in one breeding colony.

Pyometra typically occurs within 4 weeks after an estrus cycle and ovulation in middle age to older cats. CEH was more often diagnosed with increasing age of the queens (Perez *et al.*, 1999; Binder *et al.*, 2019). Pyometra was also more commonly diagnosed with

Table 14.1. Cystic endometrial hyperplasia (CEH) classification according to Dow (1958).

Types of CEH	Descriptions of the characteristics
Type I	CEH without inflammatory process, no clinical signs
Type II	CEH with acute endometritis. In most cases have corpora lutea White blood count increases Signs can vary depending on the severity and distention of the uterus, but in general the cats are sick
Type III	Subacute endometritis with mononuclear infiltration of the endometrium and cystic changes of the endometrial glands The clinical signs are more pronounced than in the preceding types
Type IV	Chronic endometritis with endometrial atrophy The severity of clinical signs depends on the amount of abdominal distention and damage to other organs

increasing age (Hagman *et al.*, 2014), indicating that CEH is related to uterine pathologies in queens. However, pyometra has also been diagnosed in queens as young as 1–2 years old without a breeding history. These queens typically do not have pathologic uterine changes and respond well to medical management. Studies of uterine lesions with clinical signs may result in underestimating the actual proportion of queens affected by CEH because of the lack of overt symptoms in mild cases (Binder *et al.*, 2019). Mild cases may present with a slight vaginal discharge and can be associated with implantation failure and subsequent smaller litters or infertility (Johnston *et al.*, 2001).

There appears to be a breed predisposition, with Sphynx's being overrepresented. Other breeds noted to have a higher incidence include Siberian cat, Ocicat, Korat, Siamese, Ragdoll, Maine Coon, and Bengal (Hagman *et al.*, 2014).

14.4.3 Clinical signs

Cats affected only with CEH most often present with reduced litter size or infertility. Cats with an open pyometra may have mucopurulent to hemorrhagic vaginal discharge (Fig. 14.3). Cats can be fastidious groomers, so vulvar discharge may not be noted (Hollinshead and Krekeler, 2016). Discharge can be observed around the vulva or in the bedding when the cat is sitting. Abdominal distension may or may not be noted (Johnson, 1994), but is more likely with a closed cervix. Non-specific clinical signs such as anorexia, fever, vomiting, lethargy, and weight loss can be observed. Polyuria and polydipsia do not occur as often as in dogs. Because of the non-specific clinical signs, pyometra should be ruled out in any ill, intact queen (Hollinshead and Krekeler, 2016). Queens tend to be less systemically ill than their canine counterpart.

14.4.4 Diagnosis

Diagnosis of CEH is best made via ultrasound. On ultrasound, the uterus has a thickened appearance with prominent endometrial folds (Fig. 14.4a). As severity increases, cysts within the endometrium can be visualized (figure 14.4b,c).

Diagnosis of pyometra is made based on history, including stage of cycle and clinical signs. Hematology can show non-regenerative normocytic normochromic anemia and increased white blood counts characterized by neutrophilia with a left shift (Johnson,

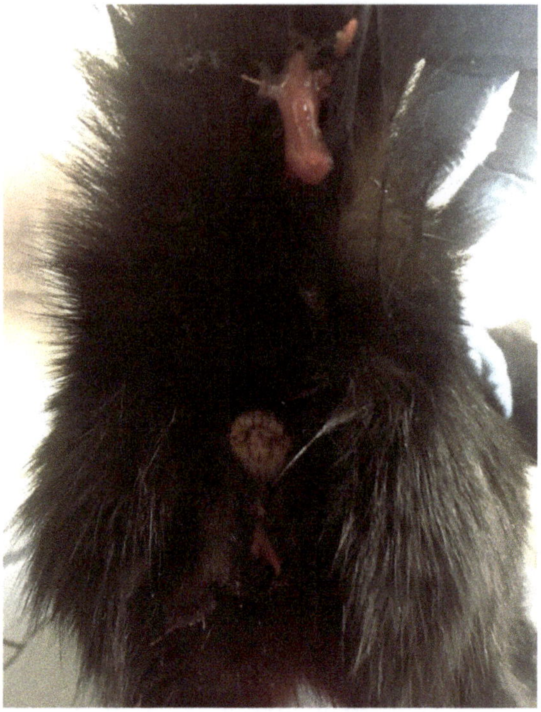

Fig. 14.3. Vaginal discharge in a queen with an open pyometra. (Image courtesy of Dr Aime Johnson, also located in Visual Guide to Animal Reproduction (VISGAR).)

1994). A serum chemistry panel can be normal or show azotemia, similar to dogs. Queens have significantly less evidence of renal damage associated with pyometra than bitches. Hypoglycemia may be noted in cases of sepsis.

A vaginal cytology will have excess amounts of white blood cells and red blood cells. Bacterial culture of vulvar discharge may be helpful in confirming a diagnosis, but normal vaginal flora may also be isolated. However, sensitivity testing is important for making therapeutic decisions as some bacterial strains can be resistant to commonly-used antibiotics (Hollinshead and Krekeler, 2016). Blood progesterone concentrations are usually increased (>5 ng/mL) because of corpora lutea activity, though this is not seen in all cases.

Ultrasound is used to confirm the diagnosis of pyometra as it allows differentiation between a fluid-filled uterus and early pregnancy. The fluid ranges from hypoechoic to hyperechoic; and hyperechoic flecks scattered throughout the fluid may be noted (Fig. 14.5). In the queen, the uterus fills in a segmental pattern similar to a pregnancy rather than a generalized

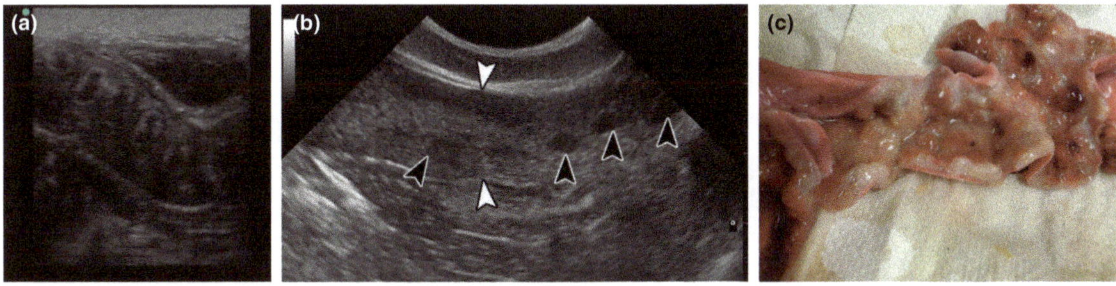

Fig. 14.4. **(a)** Ultrasound image of a 5-year-old queen that presented for infertility. The ultrasound showed moderate CEH with prominent endometrial folds (light and dark striping throughout the uterus). **(b)** Ultrasonographic image of a queen with CEH. The uterus is marked with white arrows. The endometrium is thickened, and multiple small cysts are visualized with in the lumen (black arrows). **(c)** Cut section of uterus following surgical treatment of a pyometra. Cystic endometrium is noted throughout the endometrial surface. (Images courtesy of Dr Aime Johnson, also located in Visual Guide to Animal Reproduction (VISGAR).)

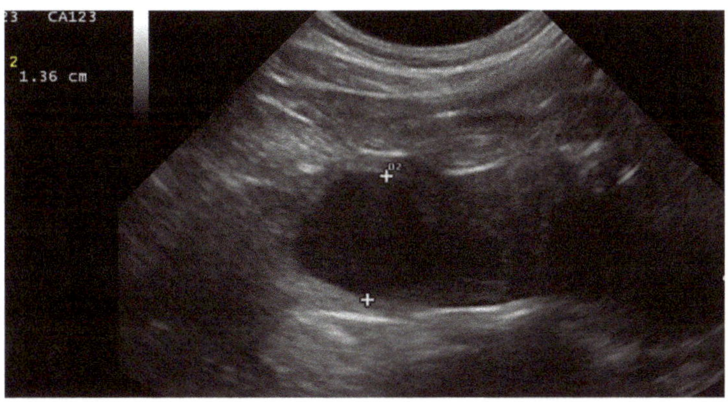

Fig. 14.5. Ultrasound image of the uterus of a queen with pyometra. The loop of distended uterus measured 1.36 cm. Two other distended loops can be seen to the right of the largest loop. (Image courtesy of Dr Aime Johnson, also located in Visual Guide to Animal Reproduction (VISGAR).)

fluid-filled space (Fig. 14.6). It is imperative that pregnancy is ruled out, as medical therapy will cause abortion. There have even been reports of pyometra in one uterine horn and a pregnancy in the other horn (Hollinshead and Krekeler, 2016). Radiographs can be used to identify an enlarged fluid-filled uterus but is not specific for pyometra. It is important to ensure that the queen is not pregnant, as a pyometra and early pregnancy can look similar radiographically.

14.4.5 Treatment

No matter which route is used, broad-spectrum antibiotics should be initiated, while awaiting culture results. Initial options can include ampicillin sodium (11 mg/kg IV every 12 hours), clavulanate + amoxicillin (62.5 mg/cat orally every 12 hours), orbifloxacin (7.5 mg/kg orally every 24 hours), or cephalexin (30 mg/kg orally every 12 hours). If the queen is systemically ill, intravenous fluids (lactated Ringers or Normsol R at 50 mL/kg/day) should be provided to correct any underlying azotemia and maintain hydration/tissue perfusion.

The decision to try medical or surgical therapy is based on the physical status and breeding capacity of the queen. A surgical approach should be considered if a critical or unstable situation exists due to septicemia or shock (Agudelo, 2005), but the patient should be stabilized first. Medical therapy can be offered for queens with minimal systemic compromise, the potential for future fertility, and high reproduction value.

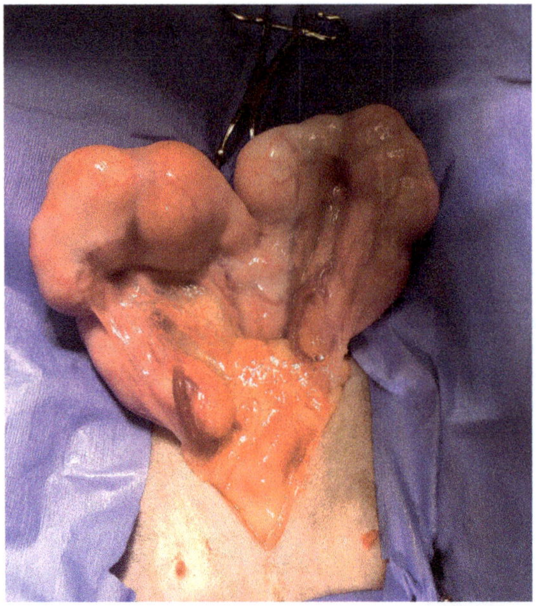

Fig. 14.6. A queen with pyometra at surgery. The fluid-filled uterus is not uniformly filled, rather segmental as is typical in the cat. (Image courtesy of Dr Aime Johnson, also located in Visual Guide to Animal Reproduction (VISGAR).)

Surgical therapy

In queens that are no longer needed reproductively, ovariohysterectomy is considered the treatment of choice, as it is curative. However, surgery is not without risks. Sepsis is the most common cause of death rather than surgical techniques or anesthetic protocols (Agudelo, 2005). The uterine tissue can be friable, so care should be taken when handling the uterus to avoid abdominal contamination. Ensure that the cervix is completely removed. It has been demonstrated in dogs that the inability to decrease azotemia prior to surgery has been associated with higher mortality (Johnson, 1994).

Medical therapy

PROSTAGLANDIN F_{2A} Prostaglandin $F_{2\alpha}$ ($PGF_{2\alpha}$) is an ecbolic agent that is also luteolytic. It causes smooth muscle contraction within the uterus to help expel the uterine contents and decreases progesterone levels via its luteolytic effects on the corpora lutea. $PGF_{2\alpha}$ administration is contraindicated in queens with closed cervix pyometra as it can predispose them to uterine rupture. The resultant reduction in progesterone concentration promotes cervical relaxation and a reduction in uterine secretions. There are two forms of $PGF_{2\alpha}$: natural (dinoprost) or synthetic derivatives (cloprostenol). Cloprostenol has been associated with fewer side effects and requires fewer injections due to its longer half-life. However, natural $PGF_{2\alpha}$ induces greater myometrial contractions and therefore faster evacuation of purulent material from the uterus compared with synthetic $PGF_{2\alpha}$ (Hollinshead and Krekeler, 2016).

Prior to initiating treatment with $PGF_{2\alpha}$, a baseline serum progesterone should be evaluated. $PGF_{2\alpha}$ should be used cautiously as there can be dose-dependent side effects. Side effects include vocalization, panting, restlessness, hypersalivation, urination, defecation, tenesmus, diarrhea, emesis, mydriasis, grooming, lordosis, and kneading (Johnson, 1994; Davidson, 1995; Barsanti, 1998). These effects usually occur within 15 minutes after administration but should resolve after 1 hour. Signs decrease in severity and intensity after subsequent injections (Johnson, 1994; Davidson, 1995). Older treatment protocols with $PGF_{2\alpha}$ range from 0.1–0.25 mg/kg under the skin once to twice daily. It has been observed that the response to higher doses (0.25 mg/kg BID; Johnston *et al.*, 2001) has no benefit over a lower dose of 0.1 mg/kg once daily for 5 to 7 days (Johnson, 1994; Davidson, 1995).

A low dose protocol has been used with good success and side effects are rarely encountered (Hollinshead and Krekeler, 2016). Queens can be administered 10–15 μg/kg dinoprost subcutaneously (SQ) every 6 hours for the first day. The dose can then be increased to 25 μg/kg SQ every 6 hours for day 2 (and day 3 if tolerance to $PGF_{2\alpha}$ is low). The dose should be increased to 50 μg/kg SQ every 8 hours for the next 3–5 days or until vulvar discharge is no longer observed, no fluid is detected in the uterus on ultrasound examination, and systemic progesterone is baseline.

In the case of closed cervix pyometra, a low starting dose of natural $PGF_{2\alpha}$ with incremental increases can be administered to minimize the ecbolic effect of the drug and to reduce the risk of uterine rupture. Once luteolysis has occurred and the cervix opens, the dose can be increased depending on the individual's tolerance of the PGF. Doses greater than 50 μg/kg should not be required (Hollinshead and Krekeler, 2016).

It is important to note that the corpora lutea in the queen are more resistant to the luteolytic effects of $PGF_{2\alpha}$ than that of the bitch. Furthermore, if treatment is started soon after ovulation, the corpora lutea can be refractory to the effects of $PGF_{2\alpha}$ (Johnston *et al.*, 2001; Hollinshead and Krekeler, 2016). Treatment with $PGF_{2\alpha}$ may be prolonged and must continue until the serum progesterone is baseline.

DOPAMINE AGONISTS Dopamine agonists can be used for the treatment of pyometra in the queen either alone or in combination with $PGF_{2\alpha}$ or a progesterone receptor antagonist. The use of a dopamine agonist in combination with $PGF_{2\alpha}$ potentiates the luteolytic effect, causing more rapid luteolysis and leading to cervical opening within 24–48 hours (Hollinshead and Krekeler, 2016).

Cabergoline is the most commonly used dopamine agonist because it is associated with few or no side effects. The recommended dose of cabergoline is 5 µg/kg orally every 24 hours for the duration of treatment (Hollinshead and Krekeler, 2016).

Bromocriptine, a partial agonist of the dopamine receptor, could be used in place of cabergoline. However, it may cause gastrointestinal side effects, such as nausea and vomiting; sedation or hypotension. Bromocriptine has a short half-life, therefore needs to be dosed more frequently. The recommended dose of bromocriptine is 10–30 µg/kg orally every 12 hours.

PROGESTERONE RECEPTOR ANTAGONISTS Progesterone receptor antagonists, such as aglepristone, are synthetic steroids that competitively bind to progesterone receptors with a greater affinity than natural progesterone. This results in a decrease in progesterone activity and induces luteolysis (Galac *et al.*, 2000). Aglepristone has minimal side effects and is a good choice for the treatment of closed cervix pyometra as it results in cervical opening with minimal uterine contractions. In cases of a closed cervix pyometra, aglepristone treatment should be started 2 days prior to $PGF_{2\alpha}$ treatment, as it can reduce the risk of uterine rupture by slowly opening the cervix without the stimulation of strong uterine contractions (Hollinshead and Krekeler, 2016). Contraindications for use are queens with poor liver and/or kidney function. The recommended dosage of aglepristone in the queen is 15 mg/kg SQ, given twice, 24 hours apart, and then a single injection on day 8. A higher dose rate is recommended for queens compared with bitches due to reduced bioavailability in the queen (Hollinshead and Krekeler, 2016). Aglepristone is not commercially available in the US.

Monitoring response to treatment

Clinical improvement is usually seen within 2 days of initiation of medical therapy. Resolution of clinical signs should occur within 7 to 10 days. Antimicrobial therapy should be continued for at least 14 days after resolution of discharge and evacuation of all fluid from the uterine lumen as determined by ultrasound. Ultrasound examination is an important monitoring tool. A decrease in uterine size by 50% should be seen within the first 4 days after initiation of therapy, and usually occurs within the first 2 days. Daily ultrasound examinations are recommended to assess the response to therapy until the uterus is evacuated. When the uterine dimensions have returned to normal, and there is no fluid present in the uterus, and the progesterone is baseline (less than 1 ng/mL), luteolytic treatment can be discontinued. The volume of vulvar discharge should increase as the uterus empties. Treatment must continue until vulvar discharge stops and the uterus returns to its normal size. Progesterone concentrations should be monitored weekly to determine when luteolysis has occurred (indicated by serum progesterone <1 ng/mL). This is particularly valuable if $PGF_{2\alpha}$ alone is used to treat the pyometra or in refractory cases to help determine whether complete luteolysis has occurred.

14.4.6 Outcomes

The overall fatality rate for pyometra is 5.6% (Hagman *et al.*, 2014). In queens with open cervix pyometra, the prognosis for recovery and future pregnancy is excellent if the underlying uterine pathology is not severe. The queen is more likely to have a successful outcome if significant response to treatment is seen within the first 4–5 days. The overall prognosis for future fertility declines the longer treatment is necessary. Most of the treated queens (95%) return to normal estrous cyclicity and successful mating resulting in pregnancy (nearly 85%) (Johnson, 1994; Johnston *et al.*, 2001). Queens should be bred on the next estrous cycle following treatment of pyometra (Hollingshead and Krekeler, 2016) or within a month of when treatment is stopped. Using a proven, fertile tom is essential, as a pregnant queen is less likely to have a reoccurrence of pyometra. Queens no longer intended for breeding should undergo ovariohysterectomy.

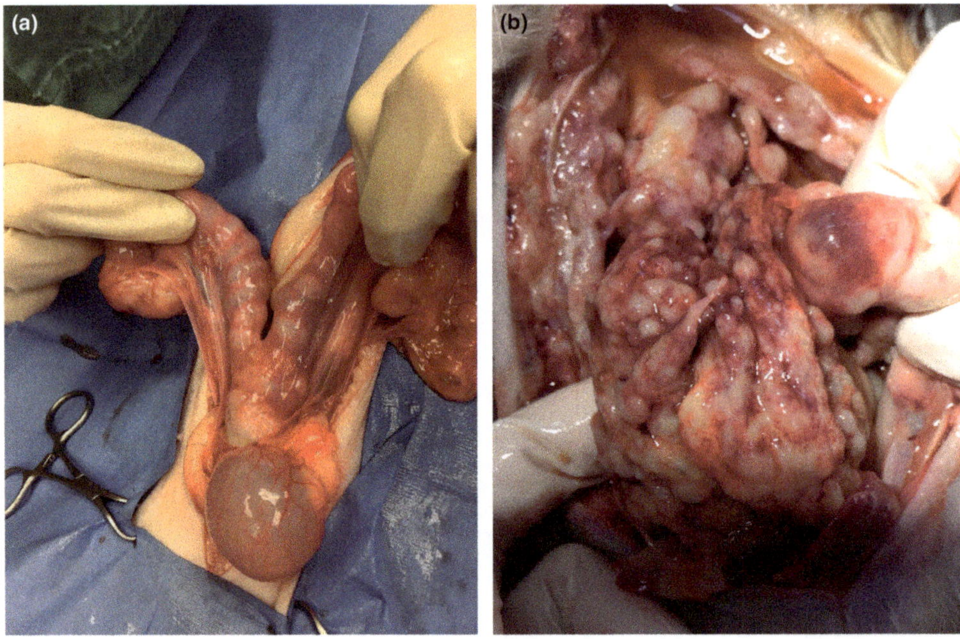

Fig. 14.7. **(a)** An 11-year-old queen presented for bloody vaginal discharge and suspected pyometra. During surgery, the uterus contained multiple masses confirmed to be fibrosarcoma via histopathology. **(b)** The same cat as above at necropsy showing the degree of metastasis within the abdomen. (Photos courtesy of Dr Jessica Cohen, Banfield Legacy Veterinary Hospital, Frisco, Texas.)

14.5 Neoplasia

Uterine neoplasia occurs infrequently in the queen, at a rate of 0.29% of all feline tumors (Miller *et al.*, 2003). This is likely due to the fact that the majority of cats in the US are ovariohysterectomized, essentially eliminating the risk of uterine neoplasia.

The majority of tumors developing in the feline uterus are adenocarcinomas. Other uterine neoplasias are leiomyomas, leiomyosarcoma, lymphoma, and other carcinomas (Johnston *et al.*, 2001; Miller *et al.*, 2003) (Fig. 14.7). Malignant mesenchymal tumors occur rarely in the reproductive tract of cats (MacLachlan and Kennedy, 2002). However, an endometrial stromal sarcoma has been reported (Sato *et al.*, 2007). While it seems logical for these tumors to be noted in intact animals, there is a report of an adenocarcinomas developing in the uterine stump of an ovariohysterectomized cat (Miller *et al.*, 2003).

Middle age to older cats are typically affected (median age of 9 years) and no breed predilection has been noted. Clinical signs are usually not evident until a uterine tumor reaches a large size. In intact queens, it may present as alterations in the estrus cycle (infertility), vaginal discharge, secondary pyometra, or may be an incidental finding. Uterine tumors can be diagnosed via abdominal palpation, radiograph, abdominal ultrasound, exploratory laparotomy and confirmed with histopathology.

Complete ovariohysterectomy is the treatment of choice. Feline uterine adenocarcinomas have well-documented metastatic potential (Miller *et al.*, 2003); therefore, the prognosis must be considered guarded. However, the prognosis for benign tumors, such as leiomyomas, is considered good following surgical removal. Fertility may be maintained with a partial ovariohysterectomy if the mass is located in only one horn.

14.6 References

Agudelo C. F. (2005) Cystic endometrial hyperplasia-pyometra complex in cats. *A review. The Veterinary Quarterly* 27(4), 173–182. doi: 10.1080/01652176.2002.9695198

Barsanti J. (1998) Genitourinary infections. In: Green, C. (ed.) *Infectious Disease of the Dog and Cat,* 2nd edn.

W.B. Saunders Company, Philadelphia, Pennsylvania, pp. 643–644.

Binder, C., Aurich, C., Reifinger, M., and Aurich, J. (2019) Spontaneous ovulation in cats—Uterine findings and correlations with animal weight and age. *Animal Reproduction Science* 209, 106167. doi: 10.1016/j.anireprosci.2019.106167

Brookshire, W., Shivley, J., Woodruff, K., and Cooley, J. (2017) Uterus unicornis and pregnancy in two feline littermates. *Journal of Feline Medicine and Surgery Open Reports* 3(2), 205511691774361. doi: 10.1177/2055116917743614

Davidson, A. (1995) Medical treatment of pyometra with prostaglandin F2α in the bitch and queen. In: Bonagura, J. and Kirk, R. (eds) *Current Veterinary Therapy, XII*. W.B. Saunders, Philadelphia, Pennsylvania, pp.1163–1165.

Dow C. (1958) The cystic hyperplasia-pyometra complex in the bitch. *Veterinary Record* 70, 1102–1110.

Galac, S., Kooistra, H. S., Butinar, J., Bevers, M. M., Dieleman, S. J., *et al.* (2000) Termination of mid-gestation pregnancy in bitches with aglepristone, a progesterone receptor antagonist. *Theriogenology* 53(4), 941–950. doi: 10.1016/S0093-691X(00)00241-7

Gelberg, H. and McEntee, K. (1984) Hyperplastic endometrial polyps in the dog and cat. *Veterinary Pathology* 21(6), 570–573. doi:10.1177/030098588402100604

Hagman, R., Ström Holst, B., Möller, L., and Egenvall, A. (2014) Incidence of pyometra in Swedish insured cats. *Theriogenology* 82(1), 114–120. doi: 10.1016/j.theriogenology.2014.03.007

Hollinshead, F. and Krekeler, N. (2016) Pyometra in the queen. *Journal of Feline Medicine and Surgery* 18(1), 21–33. doi: 10.1177/1098612X15623114

Johnson, C. (1994) Female reproduction and disorders of the female reproductive tract. In: Sherding, R. (ed.) *The Cat: Diseases and Clinical Management*, vol. 2, 2nd edn. Churchill Livingstone, New York, pp.1855–1876.

Johnston, S., Kustritz, M., and Olson, P. (2001) *Canine and Feline Theriogenology*. W.B. Saunders, Philadelphia, Pennsylvania, pp.463–471.

Jones, T., Hunt, R., and King, N. (1997) Genital system. In: *Veterinary Pathology*, 6th edn. Lippincott, Williams & Wilkins, Baltimore, Maryland, pp. 1149–1222.

Keskin, A., Yilmazbas, G., Yilmaz, R., Ozyigit, M., and Gumen, A. (2009) Pathological abnormalities after long-term administration of medroxyprogesterone acetate in a queen. *Journal of Feline Medicine and Surgery* 11(6), 518–521. doi: 10.1016/j.jfms.2008.10.006

MacLachlan, N. and Kennedy, P. (2002) Tumors of the genital systems. In: D. J. Meuten (ed.) *Tumors in Domestic Animals*, 4th edn. Iowa State Press, Ames, Iowa, pp. 547–573.

McIntyre, R., Levy, J., Roberts, J., and Reep, R. (2010) Developmental uterine anomalies in cats and dogs undergoing elective ovariohysterectomy. *Journal of the American Veterinary Medical Association* 237(5), 542–546. doi: 10.2460/javma.237.5.542

Miller, M., Ramos-Vara, J., Dickerson, M., Johnson, G., Pace, L., *et al.* (2003) Uterine neoplasia in 13 cats. *Journal of Veterinary Diagnostic Investigation* 15(6), 515–522. doi: 10.1177/104063870301500602

Nomura, K. (1995) Histological evaluation of the canine decidual reactions induced by intraluminal injection of olive oil. *The Journal of Veterinary Medical Science* 57(1), 71–74. doi: 10.1292/jvms.57.71

Perez, J., Conley, A., Dieter, J., Sanz-Ortega, J., and Lasley, B. (1999) Studies on the origin of ovarian interstitial tissue and the incidence of endometrial hyperplasia in domestic and feral cats. *General and Comparative Endocrinology* 116(1), 10–20. doi: 10.1006/gcen.1999.7331

Sato, T., Maeda, H., Suzuki, A., Shibuya, H., Sakata, A., *et al.* (2007) Endometrial stromal sarcoma with smooth muscle and glandular differentiation of the feline uterus. *Veterinary Pathology* 44(3), 379–382. doi: 10.1354/vp.44-3-379

Schlafer, D. and Gifford, A. (2008) Cystic endometrial hyperplasia, pseudo-placentational endometrial hyperplasia, and other cystic conditions of the canine and feline uterus. *Theriogenology* 70(3), 349–358. doi: 10.1016/j.theriogenology.2008.04.041

Senger, P. (2012) Embryogenesis of the pituitary gland and the male or female reproductive system. In: *Pathways to Pregnancy and Parturition*, 3rd edn. Current Conceptions, Washington, pp. 80–99.

15 Disorders of the Caudal Reproductive Tract

Aime K. Johnson

Auburn University College of Veterinary Medicine, Department of Clinical Sciences, Auburn, Alabama, USA

15.1 Congenital Abnormalities

Congenital abnormalities are most often diagnosed in young females and are usually due to an error in embryonic formation of affected structures. Segmental aplasia of the vagina, vestibule, or vulvar opening are often diagnosed following signs of fluid accumulation cranial to the structure. These cats may present for failure to allow intromission by the tom, chronic licking or grooming of the vulvar area, or infertility following attempted mating. Diagnosis can be made by abdominal ultrasonography to evaluate for fluid accumulation within the tubular tract or vaginoscopy under general anesthesia to allow visualization of the caudal vagina. Surgical correction of segmental aplasia, hypoplasia, and stenosis depends on the severity of the lesion. However, if breeding is desired, the queen may be at a higher risk of dystocia and may require a c-section to avoid the strictured area.

15.2 Vaginitis

The feline vagina is inhabited by a mixed flora of aerobic, non-pathogenic, and facultative pathogenic bacteria. The normal bacterial flora within the queen's vagina has been described following cultures taken during routine ovariohysterectomy (Ström Holst *et al.*, 2003). Aerobic bacteria were isolated in 77% of samples with *Escherichia coli*, *Streptococcus canis*, and *Staphlococcus* spp. being isolated most commonly. Factors that may influence the vaginal flora of the queen include age, stage of the reproductive cycle, external environment (sanitation conditions), and breed. As queens age, the bacterial flora changes such that prepubertal cats show a more diverse population of bacteria than postpubertal queens. Queens in estrus show a more diverse population of bacteria than queens not in estrus. The act of breeding does not appear to greatly affect the vaginal flora in queens.

Although rare in cats, vaginitis may occur. Queens often present clinically with perivulvar irritation, vaginal discharge, excessive licking or grooming, and signs of irritation such as pollakiuria. Other causes of vaginal discharge, such as vaginal foreign body, vaginal neoplasia, pyometra, uterine stump pyometra, or urinary tract infection, should be investigated and eliminated before a diagnosis of primary vaginitis can be made. Diagnostics should include a vaginal cytology to evaluate the presence of inflammatory cells (Fig. 15.1) and a vaginal culture to evaluate what bacteria are present, as well as ultrasound of the uterus or uterine stump and urinalysis with culture (obtained by cystocentesis) to rule out other causes of vaginal discharge.

Treatment consists of targeted antibiotics based on the culture results. Rinsing (douching) the vaginal vault with saline or dilute (5%) betadine solution using a flexible catheter (red rubber or tomcat) may also be beneficial in removing purulent debris. This is typically performed under heavy sedation and a single treatment may be sufficient. If the lavage is performed too frequently, the process may cause additional vaginal irritation and make the condition worse. Recommendations from this author are to perform only as needed, but no more than once daily, and no more than 3–5 days in a row. Probiotics may also be beneficial in restoring normal vaginal flora. Vulvar pyoderma should be treated topically as needed with antibiotics and/or corticosteroids to reduce inflammation. One case of severe vaginitis in a 16-month-old female resulted in adhesion of the vulvar labia, which

DOI: 10.1079/9781789247107.0015

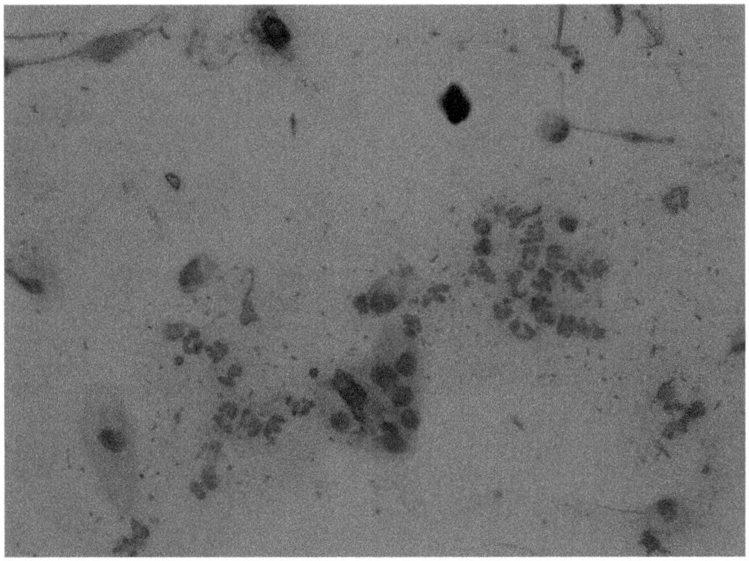

Fig. 15.1. A vaginal cytology from a cat with severe inflammation of the caudal reproductive tract. Note the vaginal cells surrounded by neutrophils. (Image: author's own.)

was corrected surgically and the cat recovered uneventfully (Plavec and Pavlin, 2013).

15.3 Vaginal Prolapse

Vaginal prolapse is rare in the queen when compared to the dog. This condition is caused by excessive vaginal thickening in estrus or late pregnancy when estrogens are high. In one report, a Maine Coon queen presented with a grade III vaginal prolapse 54 days after the first mating (McKelvey *et al.*, 2015). The prolapse was reduced manually and sutured in place. An elective C-section was performed with an ovariohysterectomy due to concerns about future prolapses. The queen recovered uneventfully. If the prolapsed tissue is necrotic or excessively damaged, surgical removal is necessary.

15.4 Neoplasia

Neoplasia of the caudal reproductive tract is uncommon in queens. Clinical signs of vaginal neoplasia include: (i) purulent or serosanguineous vaginal discharge if the neoplasia is causing irritation or is necrotic; (ii) mass effect including protrusion of tissue from the vulva or swelling in the perineum; and (iii) stranguria, pollakiuria, or constipation if the mass is applying pressure to the urethra or colon.

Vaginal leiomyoma is not as common in the cat as it is in the bitch, but has been reported (Wolke, 1963). These tumors are typically benign and can be removed surgically for a good prognosis. An episiotomy is often necessary to allow access to the mass. A vulvar leiomyosarcoma was reported in an 8-year-old intact queen (Firat *et al.*, 2007) and several cases of vulvar adenocarcinoma (apical gland adenocarcinoma) have been reported (Welsh *et al.*, 2010).

Treatment of neoplasia is directed at staging the tumor with blood work, chest and abdominal radiographs, and ultrasound followed by surgical excision. Depending on the tumor type, additional treatments such as chemotherapy or localized radiation treatment may reduce reoccurrence and improve quality of life. With benign neoplasia, the prognosis is good following surgical excision. With vulvar adenocarcinoma, the median reported survival time was 9.2 months (range: 2–18 months) with euthanasia following local recurrence after surgical excision or complications due to metastases (Welsh *et al.*, 2010).

15.5 References

Firat, I., Haktanir-Yatkin, D., Sontas, B. H., and Ekici, H. (2007) Vulvar leiomyosarcoma in a cat. *Journal of Feline Medicine and Surgery* 9, 435–438. doi: 10.1016/j.jfms.2007.04.002

Mckelvey, K. A., Beachler, T. M., Ferris, K. K., Diaw, M., Vasgaard, J. M., *et al.* (2015) Vaginal prolapse in a pregnant Maine coon cat: a case report. *Journal of Small Animal Practice* 56, 473–475. doi: 10.1111/jsap.12310

Plavec, T. and Pavlin, D. (2013) Surgical correction of labial fusion with vaginoplasty in a cat. *Journal of Feline Medicine and Surgery* 15, 520–523. doi: 10.1177/1098612X12470653

Ström Holst, B., Bergström, A., Lagerstedt, A. S., Karlstam, E., Englund, L., *et al.* (2003) Characterization of the bacterial population of the genital tract of adult cats. *American Journal of Veterinary Research* 64, 963–968. doi: 10.2460/ajvr.2003.64.963

Welsh, J. B., Best, S. J., Yager, J. A., and Foster, R. A. (2010) A report of 7 cases of feline vulval adenocarcinoma. *Canadian Veterinary Journal* 51, 764–766.

Wolke, R. E. (1963) Vaginal leiomyoma as a cause of chronic constipation in the cat. *Journal of the American Vet Medical Association* 143. 1103–1105.

16 Disorders of the Mammary Glands

Diane Delmain

Auburn University College of Veterinary Medicine, Department of Clinical Sciences, Auburn, Alabama, USA

16.1 Anatomy

Queens have four pairs of mammary glands that are bilaterally symmetrical from the cranial ventral thorax to the caudal ventral abdominal region. These pairs are usually numbered from 1 to 4, cranial to caudal, but are sometimes referred to as the axillary, thoracic, abdominal, and inguinal mammary glands. Supernumerary glands occasionally occur. In non-lactating females and male cats, the mammary glands are mostly composed of stroma and fat. Secretory epithelial tissue develops and expands during pregnancy and during lactation. Lactating mammaries comprise glandular lobular tissue drained by a series of ducts to a teat sinus, then to the teat opening. The teat is composed of smooth muscle which has three layers in the cat: two longitudinal and one circular. Stellate myoepithelial cells surround the glandular tissue and ducts contract in response to oxytocin or stretching (Silver, 1966).

Blood supply to the mammary glands is provided by the perforating branches of the thoracic arteries, cutaneous branches of the intercostal arteries, the lateral thoracic arteries, the superficial epigastric arteries, the caudal intercostal arteries, and the cutaneous branches of the deep circumflex iliac artery. Blood is drained by the axillary veins, branches of the internal thoracic veins within the pectoral muscles, the cranial superficial epigastric veins, penetrating intercostal veins, and the caudal superficial epigastric veins. Small veins may penetrate the chest wall or cross the midline, serving as a potential route for metastasis of mammary neoplasia (Silver, 1966).

Lymphatic drainage of the two cranial pairs of glands is toward the axillary lymph nodes, and the fourth glands drain toward the superficial inguinal lymph nodes. The third glands may drain to either the axillary or superficial inguinal lymph nodes. Drainage of the third and fourth glands to the median iliac lymph node may occur rarely (Papadopoulou *et al.*, 2009).

16.2 Mammary Neoplasia

Mammary tumors are fairly common in cats, accounting for approximately 17% percent of all neoplasms in this species (Zappulli *et al.*, 2015). Most mammary tumors are aggressive carcinomas which metastasize readily. The overall prognosis is poor, with most affected cats dying within 12 months of diagnosis. Early detection and treatment may result in longer survival.

Mammary tumors are more likely to occur in older female cats but may also rarely occur in males. The average age at onset is between 10–12 years (Zappulli *et al.*, 2015). The Siamese breed has a highest incidence, and disease may occur at a younger age in these cats. While the etiology is not fully understood, reproductive status is linked to incidence. Intact queens are significantly more likely to develop disease. Age at the time of hysterectomy is also linked to disease incidence, with earlier ovariohysterectomy (OHE) significantly reducing occurrence. In one study, cats undergoing OHE prior to 6 months of age had a 91% reduction in occurrence relative to intact cats, while OHE prior to a year showed an 86% reduction (Overley *et al.*, 2005). The role of estrogen and progesterone in development of feline mammary carcinomas is unclear, as the majority of these neoplasms are negative for receptors for these hormones (Zappulli *et al.*, 2015). Progesterone-induced, cyclical growth hormone stimulation and release by mammary glandular tissue is surmised to be related to carcinogenesis in dogs, and this may also be the case in cats (Sorenmo *et al.*, 2020). Exogenous progestin administration may also lead to development

 Feline Reproduction (eds. A.K. Johnson and M.A. Kutzler)
DOI: 10.1079/9781789247107.0016

of mammary neoplasia. However, further research is needed in cats to elucidate the etiology and hormone interaction of mammary neoplasia.

While epidemiological studies vary, feline mammary masses are more likely to be malignant than benign, with as many as 90% being malignant (Hayes *et al.*, 1981). Benign tumors in cats include simple adenoma, ductal adenoma, fibroadenoma, and intraductal papillary adenoma (duct papilloma) (Sorenmo *et al.*, 2020). Carcinomas are the most common mammary malignancy and nomenclature is variable. These tumors may be referred to as adenocarcinomas or carcinomas and may be ductal, complex, tubular, papillary, or solid. For purposes of this chapter, feline malignant mammary tumors will be referred to as mammary gland carcinomas (MGC). Nodules may occur in any gland, but the caudal four glands are most commonly affected (Fig. 16.1). Masses may affect a single gland or be multifocal at diagnosis. Clipping the hair on the ventrum and positioning the cat in dorsal recumbency for examination may aid in palpation and diagnosis of smaller nodules. Ulceration and inflammation of larger masses is common (Fig. 16.2).

MGC tend to be aggressive and locally invasive of vasculature and lymphatics. Masses in the cranial four glands tend to metastasize to the axillary lymph nodes, while masses in the caudal four glands metastasize to the inguinal glands. However, anatomic variability of connections between glands and lymphatics is possible with some crossover of metastasis. Metastasis to the lungs and pleura is common and many cats will present initially for respiratory distress. Metastasis may also involve the thoracic or abdominal lymph nodes, liver, and, rarely, bone. Queens with more disseminated disease carry a worse prognosis.

MGC in cats share many characteristics with mammary carcinomas in humans. Therefore, prognostic markers and targeted therapies commonly used in human medicine may have clinical relevance in cats in the future. Many markers are used to direct targeted therapy in humans. This is an area of great interest in cats and may lead to better future treatment options in cats. The data related to estrogen and progesterone receptors as prognostic indicators is controversial, probably due to differing methodologies in studies. The majority of feline MGC are estrogen receptor negative and these tumors may carry a worse prognosis (Zappulli *et al.*, 2015). Human epidermal growth factor

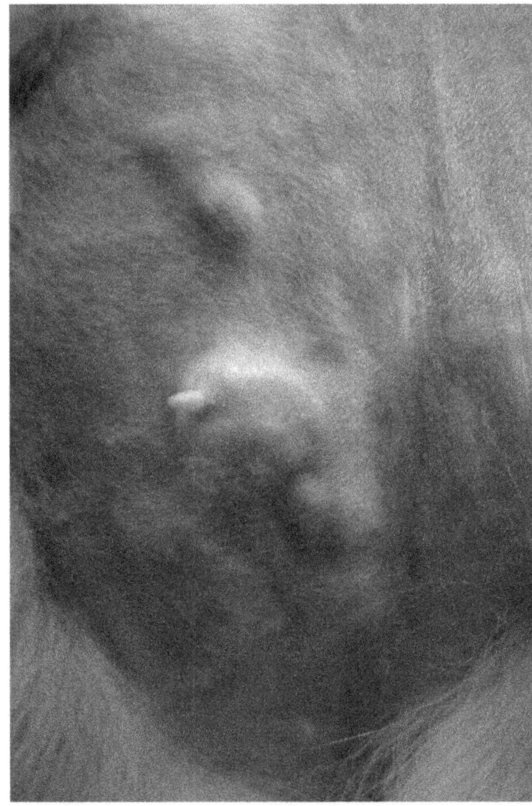

Fig. 16.1. Multifocal mammary gland carcinoma. The right caudal mammary gland has several nodules surrounding the nipple. Nodules extend cranially to the next mammary gland which was also affected. The cranial nodules are noticeable only after shaving the hair. (Photo courtesy of Dr Aime Johnson, also located in Visual Guide of Animal Reproduction (VISGAR).)

(HER-2) is a protein that promotes the growth of cancer cells and is caused by a gene mutation in humans. In women, HER-2-positive breast cancers tend to be more aggressive and less sensitive to hormone therapy. The role of HER-2 in feline mammary neoplasia is unclear, but in one study, HER-2-positive cats had shorter overall survival (Zappulli *et al.*, 2015). Ki-67, a nuclear protein and proliferation marker frequently used to aid staging in human patients, has been investigated in cats and may be useful in predicting whether disease is disseminated (Soares *et al.*, 2016). Cytotoxic T-lymphocyte-associated antigen (CTLA-4) plays an important role in breast cancer progression in women and appears to be increased in feline MGC. This may be useful for developing targeted

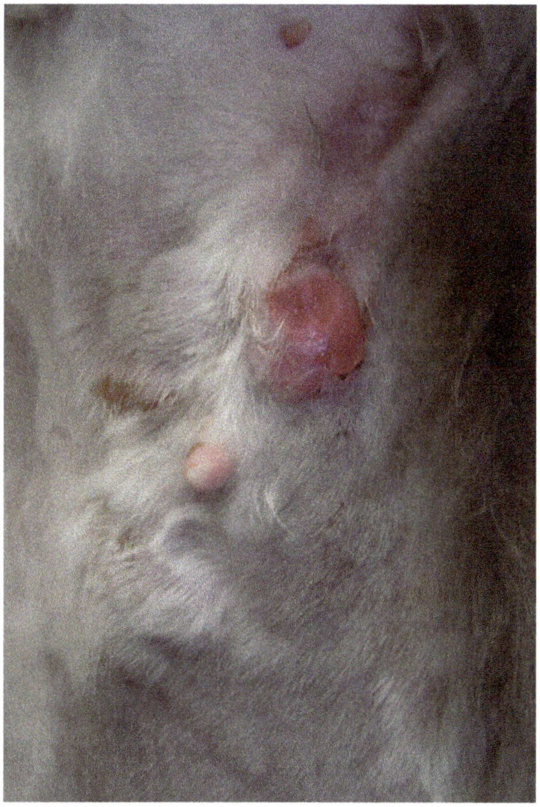

Fig. 16.2. Ulcerated mammary gland carcinoma. (Photo courtesy of Dr Aime Johnson, also located in Visual Guide of Animal Reproduction (VISGAR).)

therapies for cats (Urbano *et al.*, 2020). Cyclooxygenase-2 (COX-2) expression has been reported in feline MGC, and may be associated with a poorer prognosis (Millanta *et al.*, 2006).

Inflammatory mammary carcinoma (IMC) is a particularly aggressive form of MGC. In described cases, IMC developed postoperatively and was characterized by extreme local pain, firmness, severe edema, erythema, absence of mammary nodules, and extremity involvement. Histology revealed malignant mammary papillary adenocarcinomas, severe inflammation, and dermal tumor embolization of lymphatic vessels. Two of the three cats in the report showed rejection of surgical suture. All cats were rapidly euthanized, and the two that were necropsied showed metastasis to the lungs and regional lymph nodes. All tumors had a high Ki-67 index and were positive for estrogen, progesterone and androgen receptors (Pérez-Alenza *et al.*, 2004).

16.2.1 Diagnosis and staging

Any mass involving the ventral area in a cat warrants careful evaluation, as most mammary masses are malignant and disseminate rapidly. Careful physical examination and fine needle aspirate cytology should be performed to evaluate and rule out other cutaneous or subcutaneous growths. Cytology may not be diagnostic for MGC as it is difficult to differentiate epithelial tumors in this manner, and histopathology would be required for diagnosis. The cat should be evaluated for the number of masses, ulceration, and enlargement of regional lymph nodes. Fine needle aspiration and cytology should be performed on palpable regional lymph nodes to screen for metastasis.

A complete blood count (CBC), chemistry panel, thyroid, feline leukemia and immunodeficiency virus testing, and urinalysis should be performed to screen for concurrent conditions or systems affected by metastases. Three-view thoracic radiographs (right and left lateral and ventrodorsal views) are important to evaluate for pulmonary, mediastinal or pleural lesions. Lung lesions may appear as fluffy or nodular interstitial densities (Fig. 16.3) or miliary pleural densities. Pleural effusion may be evident. A CT or MRI, if available, will detect smaller metastatic lesions and may better identify the extent of the disease. Abdominal radiography, ultrasound, and fine needle aspiration of the regional abdominal lymph nodes may further elucidate the extent of disease.

The most reliable predictors of survival time are related to tumor size and presence of metastasis at the time of diagnosis. While it is intuitive that cats with greater tumor burden should expect shorter disease-free intervals and survival times, studies have varied in measurement methodology. A tumor diameter of 3 cm has been shown to be significant (Viste *et al.*, 2002). Cats with MGC greater than 3 cm in diameter had a poor prognosis with mean survival period of 5 months and median survival periods of 4–12 months. Survival periods in cats with tumors less than 3 cm had a mean survival of 21 months, but the median ranged from 3–54 months, making prediction of prognosis more difficult with smaller tumors. Other significant factors for progression included tumor ulceration, lymph node metastasis at the time of surgery, and tumors in the caudal (inguinal) gland (Viste *et al.*, 2002).

Several systems have been proposed for grading and staging MGC and were based upon those

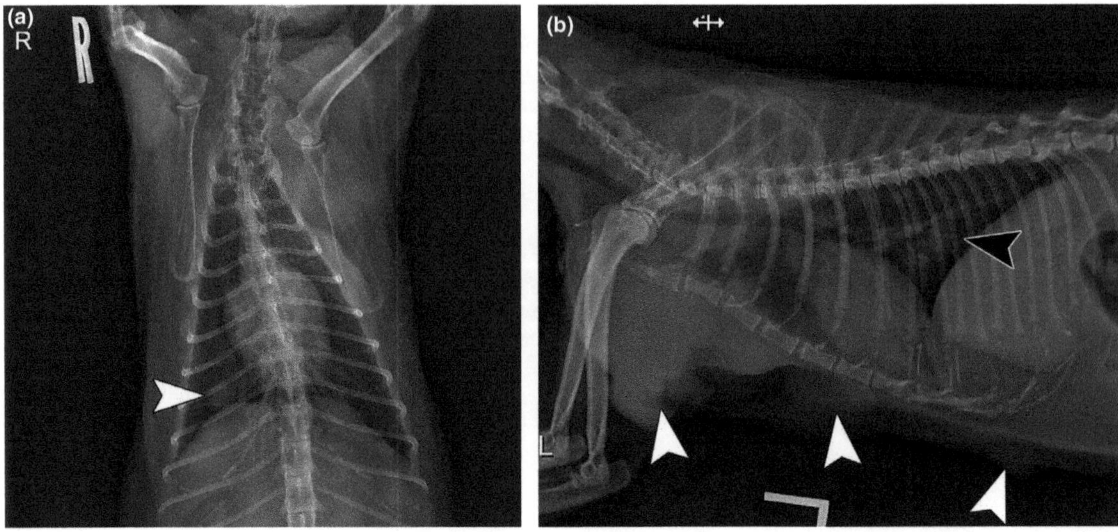

Fig. 16.3. (a) Metastatic mammary gland carcinoma. A large nodule is present in the right caudo-dorsal lung field (arrow). **(b)** Metastatic mammary gland carcinoma left lateral view. The pulmonary nodule is apparent in the caudal lung (black arrow). Mammary masses are present in the regions of the first, second and third glands, with the largest in the region of the first glands (white arrows). (Images: author's own.)

used for humans. The modified World Health Organization staging system ranges from I to IV, depending upon tumor size, regional lymph node involvement and distant metastasis. Stage I includes tumors <1 cm diameter without metastasis. Stage II includes tumors from 1–3 cm in diameter, with or without involvement of regional lymph nodes and no distant metastasis. Stage III includes any tumor >3 cm in diameter and any inflammatory carcinomas without distant metastasis, regardless of regional lymph node involvement. Any tumor with distant metastasis is considered to be stage IV. This system is of use in guiding clinical decisions regarding chemotherapy, as it is typically recommended for cats with stage III and IV disease (Ito *et al.*, 1996).

Recently, Mills, *et al.* (2015) proposed a novel grading system based upon lymphovascular invasion, nuclear form, and mitotic count, which showed significant correlation with overall survival. Using these criteria, low-grade carcinomas are categorized as grade I, with a median survival time of 31 months and 82% survival at 18 months. Grade II or intermediate carcinomas had a 14-month median survival time, with 37% survival at 18 months. Grade III or high-grade carcinomas had a worse prognosis, with 8-month median survival and only 18% surviving to 18 months (Mills *et al.*, 2015).

16.2.2 Treatment

Surgery is the mainstay of treatment for MGC. Based upon presentation, physical examination and staging diagnostics, the clinician must decide whether to perform an incisional biopsy for diagnosis prior to mastectomy or proceed to mastectomy and perform histopathology en bloc. Since feline mammary masses are highly likely to be malignant and metastasize quickly, clinicians often choose to perform immediate mastectomy. Full-chain mastectomy has been the recommended approach, even if only one gland is affected, due to the possibility of connections between glands and lymphatics. Removal of regional lymph nodes should also be performed, if possible. A recent large multicenter study showed that cats receiving bilateral radical mastectomies had significantly longer progression-free and survival times compared to cats that underwent unilateral mastectomy. Progression-free time was defined as time from mastectomy to local recurrence, regional or distant metastasis, or tumor-related death. Median progression-free and survival times were 542 and 1,140 days, respectively, for cats undergoing bilateral mastectomy versus 289 and 473 days, respectively, for those undergoing unilateral mastectomy. Cats with unilateral mastectomy were more likely to develop metastasis. However, unilateral mastectomy had less surgical complications, while simultaneous bilateral mastectomy had the highest complication rate, likely due to the large amount of tissue removed. For this reason, staged bilateral mastectomies several weeks apart, are recommended to maximize survival and minimize surgical complications (Gemignani *et al.*, 2018). Wide surgical margins should be taken, and all tissue submitted for histopathology. There is no evidence that concurrent OHE at the time of mastectomy is beneficial, and this procedure has the possibility of disseminating malignancy to the abdomen. Some clinicians recommend concurrent OHE to lessen hormonal influence on any remaining mammary tissue. The OHE should be performed first, the abdomen closed, and then the mastectomy to follow.

16.2.3 Chemotherapy

While early detection and an aggressive surgical approach can improve quality of life and survival times, cats with disseminated disease and larger tumors are not as effectively treated with surgery alone. Since MGC metastasizes rapidly, the possibility for undetectable, microscopic, disseminated disease is possible, even if all diagnostics are 'clear' of evidence. For that reason, chemotherapy may be considered for all cats with MGC, but effective client communication is essential in making this decision. In general, tumors less than 3 cm without evidence of lymph node involvement, may be treated with surgery alone. Higher histological grading, lymphovascular involvement, or size of greater than 3 cm warrants consideration for chemotherapy (Sorenmo *et al.*, 2020). Chemotherapy regimens are usually doxorubicin based but may include a large variety of additional chemotherapeutic agents or other medications. In a large retrospective study, chemotherapy after unilateral or bilateral radical mastectomy was associated with a significant decrease in risk of death related to MGC. Since many MGC express COX-2 receptors, it has been theorized that adding a COX-2 inhibitor may improve treatment outcome. However, this did not improve the overall survival or disease-free interval in one study (Borrego *et al.*, 2009). The lack of prospective, randomized studies of MGC in cats hampers clinical decision making in this area, and consultation with a veterinary oncologist is recommended.

16.3 Mammary Hyperplasia

16.3.1 Signalment, history and physical examination

Mammary hyperplasia (MH), also known as fibroadenomatous mammary hyperplasia or mammary hypertrophy, is a benign condition characterized by profound, rapid, diffuse enlargement of the mammary glands (Fig. 16.4). Dramatic mammary enlargement may occur within several weeks. This condition most commonly occurs in young intact cyclic (diestrus) or pregnant queens under the influence of progesterone but may occur in cats of either sex after administration of exogenous progesterone or analogs. Affected glands exhibit rapid diffuse enlargement, but in some cases, nodules are palpable mimicking the appearance of neoplasia. Secondary mastitis may occur with necrosis and ulceration (Johnston *et al.*, 2001; Choy, 2012).

16.3.2 Pathogenesis

Endogenous progesterone and exogenous progestogens play an important role in pathogenesis of mammary hyperplasia. Mammary hyperplasia is theorized to be caused by an exaggerated response to progestin compounds. In one study, progesterone receptors were found in the mammary tissue of most cats with mammary hyperplasia, while estrogen receptors were only found 50% of the time

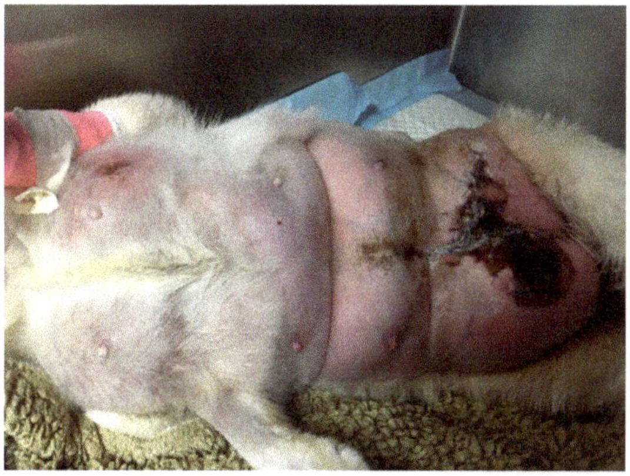

Fig. 16.4. Mammary hypoplasia in a 1-year-old queen. The caudal mammary glands contained areas of necrosis which required additional treatments and pain management. (Photo courtesy of Dr Aime Johnson, also located in Visual Guide of Animal Reproduction (VISGAR).)

(De Las Mulas *et al.*, 2000). Increased progesterone concentrations with false pregnancy after an induced ovulation may also result in MH (Burton, 2007; Ferrer and Miller, 2007). Administration of exogenous progestins, especially megastrol acetate or methyprogesterone acetate, has been shown to induce MH in cats of either sex (Hayden *et al.*, 1989; MacDougall, 2003; Loretti *et al.*, 2005). This typically resolves with cessation of these medications. Pathogenesis may also involve growth hormone, prolactin and insulin-like growth factor (Loretti *et al.*, 2005)

16.3.3 Diagnosis

Tentative diagnosis of MH can typically be made by history, signalment, and characteristic findings on physical examination. Fine needle aspiration and cytology of the glands may reveal mammary epithelial or glandular cells but should not show evidence of neoplasia. Inflammation may be present if mastitis or ulceration occurs secondary to the MH. Biopsy should be considered with great care, as healing of surgical incisions may be prolonged in these patients. Mammary hyperplasia is characterized histologically by benign, unencapsulated fibroglandular proliferation without evidence of inflammation or neoplasia. Testing for endogenous progesterone should be performed but may not be definitive as concentrations may be normal by the time of diagnosis. In one study, only one third of affected cats with MH had increased progesterone levels (Norsworthy and Romeo, 2018).

16.3.4 Treatment

Mammary hyperplasia may resolve spontaneously with naturally-occurring luteolysis in pregnant or cyclic queens. These cats may be painful, and appropriate analgesic measures should be used. Ovariohysterectomy of intact cats is usually curative, with lesions resolving within weeks to months. A flank incision should be used if the OHE is performed while the mammary tissue is enlarged (Fig. 16.5). Cessation of exogenous progestins in iatrogenic cases usually results in resolution within several weeks, although cats receiving a sustained release product may take much longer.

Medical therapy may be considered in cats with MH intended for breeding, or when removing the source of progesterone does not result in resolution.

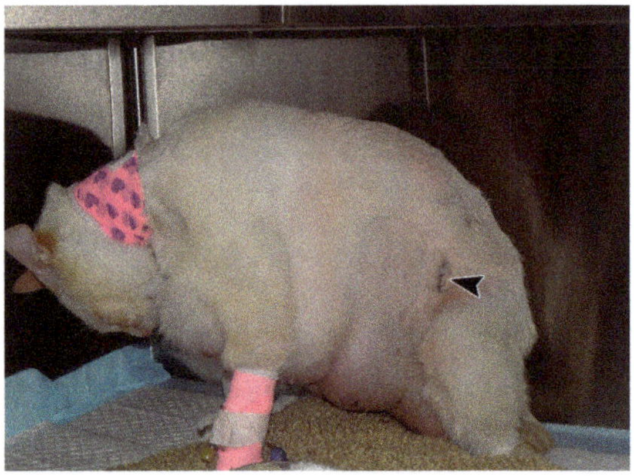

Fig. 16.5. Image shows the location of a flank incision for OHE in a cat with mammary hyperplasia. A ventral midline incision was not possible due to the gland enlargement and inflammation. (Photo courtesy of Dr Aime Johnson.)

There is no labeled product for treatment of MH in cats, and client communication regarding use and potential side effects is vital.

Treatment with the progesterone receptor blocker aglépristone has been reported. Subcutaneous injections were administered on 1 (7 cats, 20 mg/kg) or 2 consecutive days (15 cats, 10 mg/kg/d) once. All but one cat responded with a complete and lasting remission of signs within 1–4 weeks of treatment. Two cats had short-term skin irritation at the site of the aglépristone injection. Two pregnant cats with MH aborted after treatment with aglépristone and subsequently developed endometritis (Görlinger *et al.*, 2002). Aglépristone is not currently available in the US.

Treatment with a prolactin inhibitor such as a dopamine agonist (cabergoline at 5 mcg/kg every 24 hours or bromocriptine mesylate at 0.25 mg per cat once by mouth), or testosterone (50–150 mg/cat intramuscular or subcutaneously every 30 days) has also been recommended, but there are no reports of the safety or efficacy of these products in MH (Schmidt, 2018). Bromocriptine may cause nausea, anorexia, or vomiting, and is thought to be hallucinogenic in cats at high doses. Concurrent administration of maropitant may alleviate gastrointestinal side effects (Gonzalez-Lima *et al.*, 1984). Maropitant is labeled for subcutaneous or intravenous administration at 1 mg/kg for up to 5 consecutive days. It is also widely used in an extra-label manner at 1 mg/kg every 24 hours by mouth.

Mastectomy may be considered as a treatment of last resort in cases of MH with necrosis or severe infection. Complications may be encountered due to the large amount of tissue to be removed and the vascularity of the affected glands, and closure will be difficult. Surgical drainage of abscessed glands and debridement of necrotic areas was successful in a queen with mastitis secondary to MH (Burstyn, 2010).

16.3.5 Prognosis

The prognosis for MH is generally good, with most cats having complete resolution once the source of progesterone is removed.

16.4 Mastitis

Mastitis is an infection of the mammary gland or glands and occurs in postpartum queens. Typical presentation is 1–3 weeks after queening when milk production is maximal but may also occur after weaning when mammary glands become distended. Mastitis occurs uncommonly in queens compared to other species but can be diagnosed secondary to trauma to the teats and surrounding skin, milk retention, lack of sanitation, or ascending infections. Symptoms include fever, anorexia, or tachycardia. Affected glands are typically swollen, warm to the touch, discolored or painful, and milk may be discolored (Fig. 16.6). Kittens of affected queens may fail to gain weight, be weak, or cry excessively (O'Brien, 2014). In severe cases, abscessation or gangrene may occur. If gangrene or necrosis occurs, surgical debridement is indicated, and healing allowed to occur by second intention. In these cases, the kittens should be removed and bottle fed. Antibiotic therapy is indicated for these queens (Wilson, 2013) (Fig. 16.7).

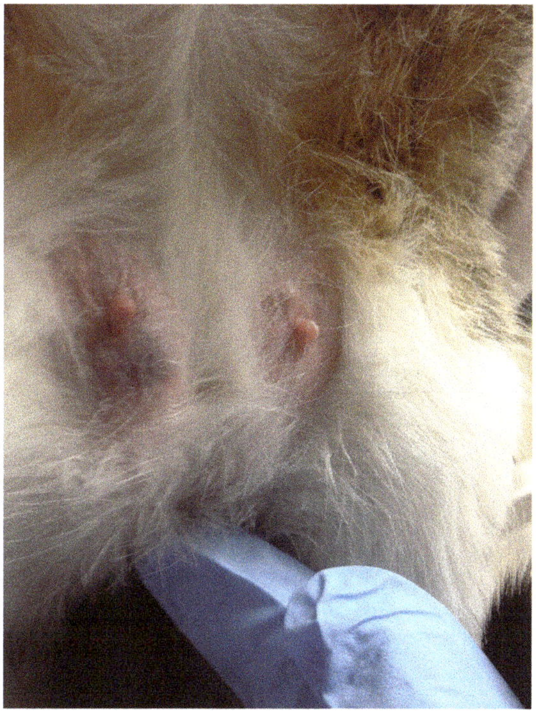

Fig. 16.6. The caudal right gland is affected in this postpartum queen. Note the discoloration of the mammary gland. On palpation, the gland was firm, warm, and painful on palpation. The milk extruded from the gland was discolored. This queen was placed on antibiotics and the gland was treated topically with warm compresses. The kittens remained with the queen and the mastitis resolved without incident. (Photo courtesy of Dr Aime Johnson, also located in VISGAR.)

16.4.1 Diagnosis

Diagnosis of mastitis is based upon history and clinical signs and confirmed with cytology and bacterial (aerobic) culture. The most common causative organisms are *Escherichia coli*, *Staphylococcus* spp., and *Streptococcus* spp. All are opportunistic bacteria, and infections are predisposed by trauma to the mammary area, unsanitary conditions, or poor condition of the queen. Culture and sensitivity testing of milk or draining material should be performed as soon as possible and prior to the administration of antibiotics. *Escherichia coli* is normally part of the intestinal flora, and reproductive infections may be caused by strains containing virulence genes producing endotoxins. Virulent strains of *E. coli* may pose a zoonotic risk. *Staphylococcus* spp. and *Streptococcus* spp. are part of the skin microflora and are thought to cause mastitis through ascending infection. *Staphylococcus felis* is the major species in cats, but *Staphylococcus pseudointermedius* is occasionally isolated. Cytology of impression smears of mammary discharge may be helpful in making a tentative diagnosis. *Staphylococcus* spp. will appear as gram positive cocci in 'bunches of grapes,' while *Streptococcus* spp. occurs in pairs or chains. Beta-hemolytic *Streptococcus* spp. have also sporadically been isolated from queens with mastitis. More than one gland may be affected and the queen is often systemically

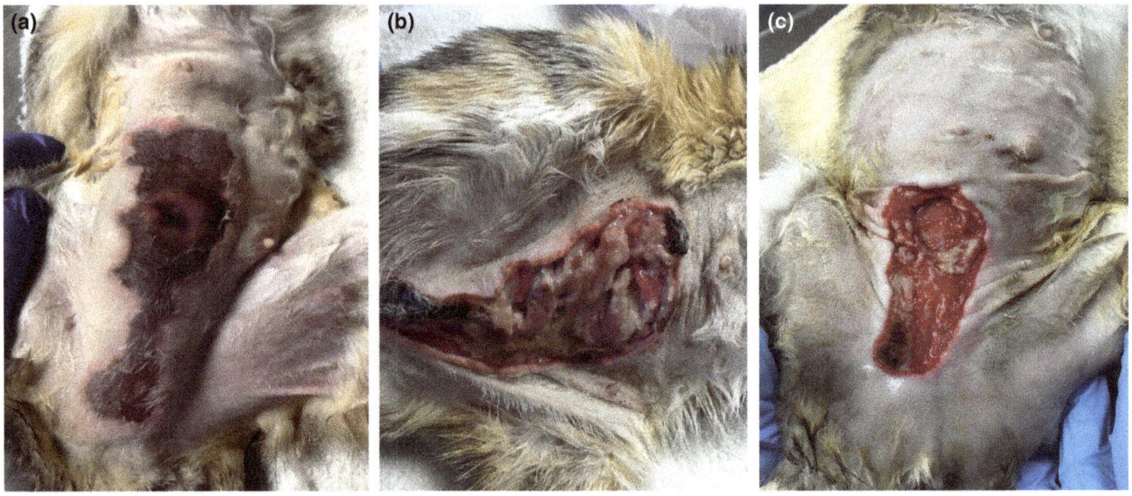

Fig. 16.7. **(a)** A cat with gangrenous mastitis in the caudal right mammary gland. The surrounding tissues are also affected and are devitalized. The kittens were removed from this queen and cross fostered to another female. The queen was systemically ill and was no longer producing milk in any of the glands. This queen was treated with intravenous fluids, intravenous antibiotics, and anti-inflammatories. The gland was treated directly with warm compresses and bandaging. **(b)** The same queen 3 days later. The tissue has sloughed leaving an open wound. The degree of necrotic tissue required surgical debridement and bandaging to keep this area clean. **(c)** Ten days later after several consecutive surgical debridement episodes with bandaging. The necrotic tissue has been removed and a bed of granulation tissue is now apparent. This wound was allowed to heal by second intention. If the wound does not heal completely, primary wound closure can be performed to provide complete healing. (Photos courtesy of Dr Aime Johnson, also located in VISGAR.)

ill (Graham and Taylor, 2012). Screening for Feline leukemia and immunodeficiency viruses, CBC, and serum chemistry should be performed to rule out predisposing or concurrent conditions and determine the extent of systemic illness. Radiology or ultrasound imaging should be performed if the clinician suspects concurrent reproductive problems, such as a retained fetus or metritis.

16.4.2 Treatment

Correction of predisposing conditions is vital. Providing a clean, safe environment and ensuring good nutrition for the queen and her kittens is of utmost importance. Supportive care including intravenous or subcutaneous fluids should be provided to maintain hydration, especially with the increased fluid demand with milk production. When possible, hospitalization should be avoided, unless the queen is systemically ill, as this may cause excess stress and interfere with her nutritional intake and willingness to care for the kittens. Warm compresses of affected glands two to four times daily is helpful to provide relief and draw out infection.

Analgesia should be provided; however, none are licensed for use in nursing queens. Informed consent should be obtained from the client prior to using any. Opioids may pass into the milk at low levels but are unlikely to cause risk to neonates. While several non-steroidal anti-inflammatory drugs (NSAIDs) are labeled for short-term use in cats, these will also pass into the milk at low levels. NSAIDs are relatively contraindicated in human neonates, but there is no literature concerning their use in nursing queens (Meyer, 2007). Short-term use (1–3 doses total) has been used anecdotally in clinical cases without detrimental effects on the kittens and can provide effective analgesia.

Antibiotics safe for nursing neonates should be administered prior to receiving culture results. If culture and sensitivity necessitate the use of an antibiotic potentially unsafe for neonates, removal of kittens and either supplemental feeding or cross fostering would be required. Amoxicillin/clavulanic acid or cephalexins are good empirical antibiotic choices pending culture and sensitivity. Clindamycin achieves good levels in milk, but may cause gastroenteritis in nursing kittens (O'Brien, 2014).

16.4.3 Kitten management

Escherichia coli and beta-hemolytic *Streptococcus* spp. are a major cause of neonatal death. Kittens are usually infected through vaginal discharge but can contract pathogenic bacteria through mastitic milk. Fatal septicemia may develop. *Streptococcus canis* septicemia may be problematic in catteries, resulting in neonatal death. Litters of young queens are more likely to be affected, as they tend to have higher bacteria loads in the vagina. Kittens may need to be removed from the queen and hand-reared if they are unable or unwilling to nurse.

Mastitis is common in nursing women, with approximately a 10% incidence in the US. As in cats, teat trauma and milk retention are among the predisposing causes. Treatment involves changing breastfeeding techniques to minimize trauma, emptying of the breasts, and antibiotics if needed (Spencer, 2008). The effectiveness of antibiotics versus other therapies has been questioned, and more research is needed in this area (Jahanfar *et al.*, 2013). Treatment with *Lactobacilli* probiotics was superior to antibiotic treatment in one study of women with mastitis (Arroyo *et al.*, 2010). The use of probiotics in queens with mastitis warrants investigation and consideration.

16.5 References

Arroyo, R., Martín, V., Maldonado, A., Jiménez, E., Fernández, L., *et al.* (2010) Treatment of infectious mastitis during lactation: antibiotics versus oral administration of *Lactobacilli* isolated from breast milk. *Clinical Infectious Diseases* 50, 1551-1558. doi: 10.1086/652763

Borrego, J. F., Cartagena J. C., and Engel, J. (2009) Treatment of feline mammary tumours using chemotherapy, surgery and a COX-2 inhibitor drug (meloxicam): a retrospective study of 23 cases (2002-2007). *Veterinary and Comparative Oncology* 7, 213–221. doi: 10.1111/j.1476-5829.2009.00194.x

Burstyn, U. (2010) Management of mastitis and abscessation of mammary glands secondary to fibroadenomatous hyperplasia in a primiparturient cat. *Journal of The American Veterinary Medical Association* 236, 326–329. doi: 10.2460/javma.236.3.326

Burton, J. (2007) Mammary gland hyperplasia – cat. In: Smith, T., *et al.* (eds) *The 5-Minute Veterinary Consult: Canine and Feline.* Lippincott Williams & Wilkins, Hoboken, New Jersey, pp. 865–866.

Choy, K. (2012) Mammary hyperplasia. In: Little, S. (ed.) *The Cat: Clinical Medicine and Management.* Elsevier, St. Louis, Missouri, pp. 1203–1204.

De Las Mulas, J. M., Millán, Y., Bautista, M. J., Pérez, J. and Carrasco, L. (2000) Oestrogen and progesterone receptors in feline fibroadenomatous change: an immunohistochemical study. *Research in Veterinary Science* 68, 15–21. doi: 10.1053/rvsc.1999.0327

Ferrer, M. and Miller, L. (2007) Mammary gland hyperplasia – cat. In: Smith, T., *et al.* (eds) *The 5-Minute Veterinary Consult: Canine and Feline.* Lippincott Williams & Wilkins, Hoboken, New Jersey, pp. 864.

Gemignani, F., Mayhew, P. D., Giuffrida, M. A., Palaigos, J., Runge, J. J., *et al.* (2018) Association of surgical approach with complication rate, progression-free survival time, and disease-specific survival time in cats with mammary adenocarcinoma: 107 cases (1991–2014). *Journal of the American Veterinary Medical Association,* 252, 1393–1402. doi: 10.2460/javma.252.11.1393

Gonzalez-Lima, F., Stiehl, W. L., and Medina, R. (1984) Long-lasting behavioral effects of bromocriptine in cats. *European Journal of Pharmacology* 102, 279–287. doi: 10.1016/0014-2999(84)90259-0

Görlinger, S., Kooistra, H. S., van den Broek, A., and Okkens, A. C. (2002) Treatment of fibroadenomatous hyperplasia in cats with aglépristone. *Journal of Veterinary Internal Medicine* 16, 710–713. doi: 10.1892/0891-6640(2002)016<0710:tofhic>2.3.co;2

Graham, E. M. and Taylor, D. J. (2012) Bacterial reproductive pathogens of cats and dogs. *Veterinary Clinics of North America – Small Animal Practice* 42, 561–582. doi: 10.1016/j.cvsm.2012.01.013

Hayden, D. W., Barnes, D. M., and Johnson, K. H. (1989) Morphologic changes in the mammary gland of megestrol acetate-treated and untreated cats: a retrospective study. *Veterinary Pathology* 26, 104–113. doi: 10.1177/030098588902600202

Hayes Jr, H. M., Milne, K. L., and Mandell, C. P. (1981) Epidemiological features of feline mammary carcinoma. *Veterinary Record* 108, 476–479. doi: 10.1136/vr.108.22.476

Ito, T., Kadosawa, T., Mochizuki, M., Matsunaga, S., Nishimura, R., and Sasaki, N. (1996) Prognosis of malignant mammary tumor in 53 cats. *Journal of Veterinary Medical Science* 58, 723–726. doi: 10.1292/jvms.58.723

Jahanfar, S., Ng, C. J., and Teng, C. L. (2013) Antibiotics for mastitis in breastfeeding women. *Cochrane Database of Systemic Reviews* 28, CD005458. doi: 10.1002/14651858.CD005458.pub3

Johnston, S. D., Root Kustritz, M. V., and Olson, P. S. (2001) Disorders of the Mammary Glands of the Queen. In: Johnston, S. D., Root Kustritz, M. V., and Olson, P. S. (eds) *Canine and Feline Theriogenology,* W.B. Saunders, Philadelphia, Pennsylvania, pp. 474–485.

Loretti, A. P., Ilha, M. R., Ordás, J., and De Las Mulas, J. M. (2005) Clinical, pathological and immunohistochemical study of feline mammary fibroepithelial hyperplasia following a single injection of depot medroxyprogesterone acetate. *Journal of Feline Medicine and Surgery* 7, 43–52. doi: 10.1016/j.jfms.2004.05.002

MacDougall, L. D. (2003) Mammary fibroadenomatous hyperplasia in a young cat attributed to treatment with megestrol acetate. *The Canadian Veterinary Journal* 44, 227–229.

Meyer, R. (2007) Paediatric patients. In: Seymour, C. and Duke-Novakovski, T. (eds) *BSAVA Manual of Canine and Feline Anaesthesia and Analgesia*, British Small Animal Veterinary Association., Quedgeley, Gloucester, UK, pp. 265–273.

Millanta, F., Citi, S., Santa, D.D., Porciani, M., and Poli, A. (2006) COX-2 expression in canine and feline invasive mammary carcinomas: correlation with clinicopathological features and prognostic molecular markers. *Breast Cancer Research and Treatment* 98, 115–120. doi: 10.1007/s10549-005-9138-z

Mills, S. W., Musil, K. M., Davies, J. L., Hendrick, S., Duncan, C., *et al.* (2015) Prognostic value of histologic grading for feline mammary carcinoma: a retrospective survival analysis. *Veterinary Pathology* 52, 238–249. doi: 10.1177/0300985814543198

Norsworthy, G. D. and Romeo, A. (2018) Mammary hyperplasia In: Norsworthy, G. D. and Restine, L. M. (eds) *The Feline Patient*. Wiley-Blackwell, Hoboken, New Jersey, pp. 385–386.

O'Brien, M. (2014) Reproductive Emergencies. In: McMichael, M. (ed.) *Handbook of Canine and Feline Emergency Protocols*, Wiley Blackwell, West Sussex, UK, pp. 198–199.

Overley, B., Shofer, F. S., Goldschmidt, M. H., Sherer, D., and Sorenmo, K. U. (2005) Association between ovarihysterectomy and feline mammary carcinoma. *Journal of Veterinary Internal Medicine,* 19, 560–563. doi: 10.1111/j.1939-1676.2005.tb02727.x

Papadopoulou, P. L., Patsikas, M. N., Charitanti, A., Kazakos, G. M., Papazoglou, L. G., *et al.* (2009) The lymph drainage pattern of the mammary glands in the cat: a lymphographic and computerized tomography lymphographic study. *Anatomia Histologia Embryologia* 38, 292–299. doi: 10.1111/j.1439-0264.2009.00942.x

Pérez-Alenza, M. D., Jiménez, A., Nieto, A. I., and Peña, L. (2004) First description of feline inflammatory mammary carcinoma: clinicopathological and immunohistochemical characteristics of three cases. *Breast Cancer Research* 6, R300–R307. doi: 10.1186/bcr790

Schmidt, B. (2018) Mammary neoplasia. In: Norsworthy, G. D. and Restine, L. M. (eds) *The Feline Patient*. Wiley-Blackwell, Hoboken, New Jersey, pp. 385–386.

Silver, I. A. (1966) The anatomy of the mammary gland of the dog and cat. *Journal of Small Animal Practice* 7,689–696. doi: 10.1111/j.1748-5827.1966.tb04394.x

Soares, M., Ribeiro, R., Carvalho, S., Peleteiro, M., Correia, J., *et al.* (2016) Ki-67 as a prognostic factor in feline mammary carcinoma: what is the optimal cutoff value? *Veterinary Pathology* 53, 37–43. doi: 10.1177/0300985815588606

Sorenmo, K., Worley, D., and Zappulli, V. (2020) Tumors of the mammary gland. In: Vail, D. M., Thamm, D., and Liptak, J. (eds) *Withrow and MacEwen's Small Animal Clinical Oncology*. Elsevier, St. Louis, Missouri, pp. 615–620.

Spencer, J. P. (2008) Management of mastitis in breastfeeding women. *American Family Physician* 78, 727–731.

Urbano, A. C., Nascimento, C., Soares, M., Correia, J., and Ferreira, F. (2020) Clinical Relevance of the serum CTLA-4 in Cats with Mammary Carcinoma. *Scientific Report* 10, 3822. doi: 10.1038/s41598-020-60860-3

Viste, J. R., Myers, S. L., Singh, B., and Simko, E. (2002) Feline mammary adenocarcinoma: tumor size as a prognostic indicator. *The Canadian Veterinary Journal* 43, 33–37.

Wilson, C. R. (2013) Feline gangrenous mastitis. *The Canadian Veterinary Journal* 54, 292–294.

Zappulli, V., Rasotto, R., Caliari, D., Mainenti, M., Peña, L., *et al.* (2015) Prognostic evaluation of feline mammary carcinomas: a review of the literature. *Veterinary Pathology* 52, 46–60. doi: 10.1177/0300985814528221

17 Reproductive Anatomy and Puberty in the Tom

MICHELLE ANNE KUTZLER

Department of Animal and Rangeland Sciences, Oregon State University, Corvallis, Oregon, USA

17.1 Embryology

17.1.1 External genitalia

The external genitalia of the male feline embryo originate from the urogenital tubercle which forms at the level of the embryonic cloacal membrane around day 25 of gestation (Noden and de la Hunta, 1985). At a crown–rump length of 2.2 cm (around day 25 of gestation), seminiferous tubules develop within the testes (Knospe, 2002; Inomata *et al*., 2009). When male feline fetuses have a crown–rump length of 3.2 cm (around day 28 of gestation), the anogenital raphe appears and the caudal portion of the genital swellings fuse to form the scrotum (Knospe, 2002; Inomata *et al*., 2009). The hormone dihydrotestosterone induces formation of the prepuce from a circular plate of ectoderm at the distal tip of the penis that thickens and invaginates (Noden and de la Hunta, 1985).

17.1.2 Internal tubular tract

The Wolffian duct develops just beneath the surface of the mesonephros when the male feline embryo has a crown–rump length of 1.2 cm (around day 19 of gestation) (Knospe, 2002; Inomata *et al*., 2009). The Wolffian duct begins to develop into the epididymal duct at a fetal crown–rump length of 7 cm (around day 48 of gestation), which is an androgen-dependent process (Knospe, 2002; Inomata *et al*., 2009).

17.2 Puberty

In male mammals, puberty is the time when a male can mate with a female to result in a pregnancy. In tomcats, puberty is reported to occur at 8–10 months (range 6–15 months) (Roberts, 1986) and coincides with several physiological and anatomical events (Tiptanavattana *et al*., 2015). It is important to mention that the attainment of puberty does not signify full reproductive capacity. In addition, some breeds of cats (e.g. Maine Coon, Persian, Chartreux) may not be able to sire a litter until closer to 2 years of age (Malandain *et al*., 2006).

Testosterone produced by the testes causes separation of the penis from the prepuce, which begins at 1 month of age and is completed by 6 months of age in tomcats. From 4–7 months of age, the mean plasma testosterone concentrations are ≤0.8 ng/mL (Tsutsui *et al*., 2004). However, using fecal testosterone measurements, puberty occurred at 14.3 ± 0.3 weeks with a corresponding fecal testosterone of 61.4 ± 7.9 ng/g (Faya *et al*., 2013). Plasma testosterone concentrations peak around 10 months of age (2.64 ± 0.68 ng/mL) and then plateau at 2 years of age (1.52 ± 0.37 ng/mL) (Tsutsui *et al*., 2004). It is important to note that plasma testosterone concentrations in the normal tomcat can fluctuate greatly throughout the day (from 0.25–2.50 ng/mL), depending on the individual, with no definite pattern (Tsutsui *et al*., 1990). The percentage of cats with sperm present in the testicular seminiferous tubule lumen increases over time from 0% (at 2–2.5 months old), 17% (at 3–4 months old), 67% (at 5–6 at months old), and 100% (at 12–24 months old). Some toms had sperm present in the vas deferens by 4 months old (Fig. 17.1) (Bohrer *et al*., 2015). Accessory sex gland secretions begin at 5 months of age.

17.3 Prepuce and Penis

17.3.1 Prepuce

At birth, the prepuce of the tom consists of a short fold surrounding the caudally directed preputial

 Feline Reproduction (eds. A.K. Johnson and M.A. Kutzler)
DOI: 10.1079/9781789247107.0017

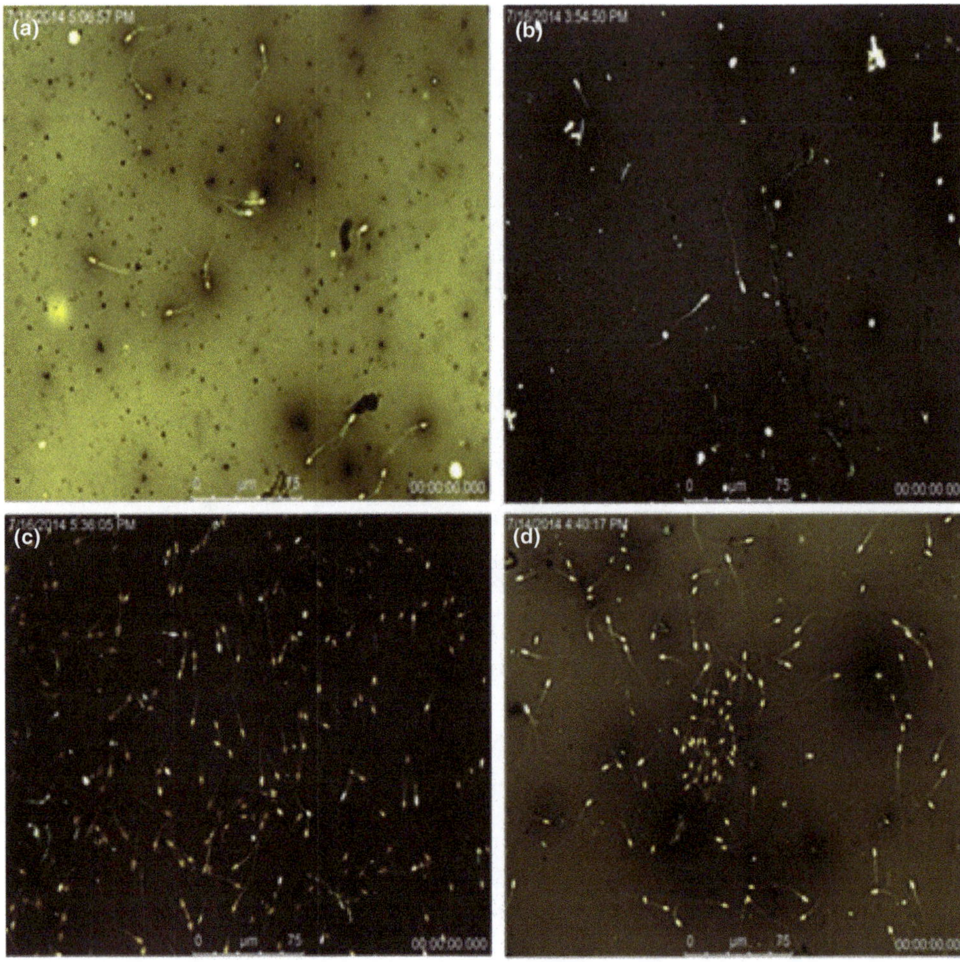

Fig. 17.1. Vas deferens secretions in: **(a)** 2-month-old; **(b)** 4-month-old; **(c)** 6-month-old; and **(d)** 12-month-old tom. (Images: author's own.)

orifice (Roberts, 1986) (Fig. 17.2). The balanopreputial fold connects the preputial and penile mucosa until it separates at puberty due to the influence of androgens (Romagnoli and Schlafer, 2006) (Fig. 17.3). In the sexually mature tom, the prepuce is attached to the proximal end of the shaft of the penis.

17.3.2 Penis

The cat penis is short, and the urethral opening is located dorsally (Schummer *et al.*, 1979). In the non-erect state, the penis is directed caudally (toward the tail) and downward. Erection causes the penis to point forward. Erection is achieved by engorgement of two penile erectile bodies: corpus spongiosum penis and corpus cavernosum penis (Fig. 17.4). Engorgement results from a combination of arterial vasodilatation, venous occlusion or constriction, and pumping of blood into erectile tissue by striated penile muscles (Hart, 1974). Vascular drainage from the corpus spongiosum penis is from the penile bulb for the proximal part and from the glans for the distal part (Amiri *et al.*, 2014). Vascular drainage for the corpus cavernosum penis is only from the crura proximally (Amiri *et al.*, 2014).

Os penis

The feline penis can contain a bone (os penis), but it is rarely present in young toms. Unlike in dogs,

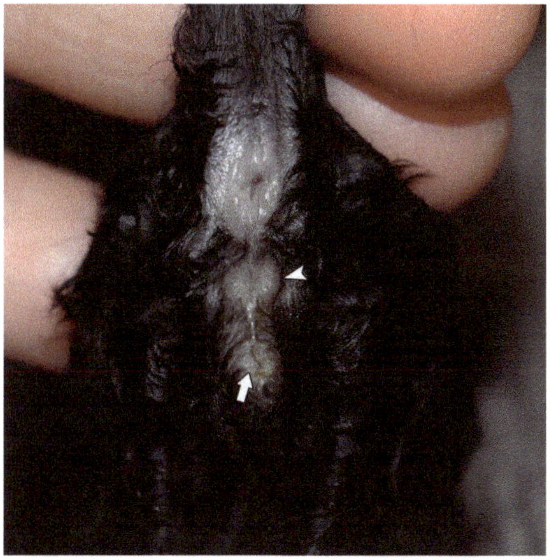

Fig. 17.2. At birth, the prepuce of the tom consists of a short fold surrounding the caudally directed preputial orifice (arrow). The testes may be fully descended in the scrotum (arrowhead) at birth or descend within the first week after birth. (Used with permission from Tina Chittick.)

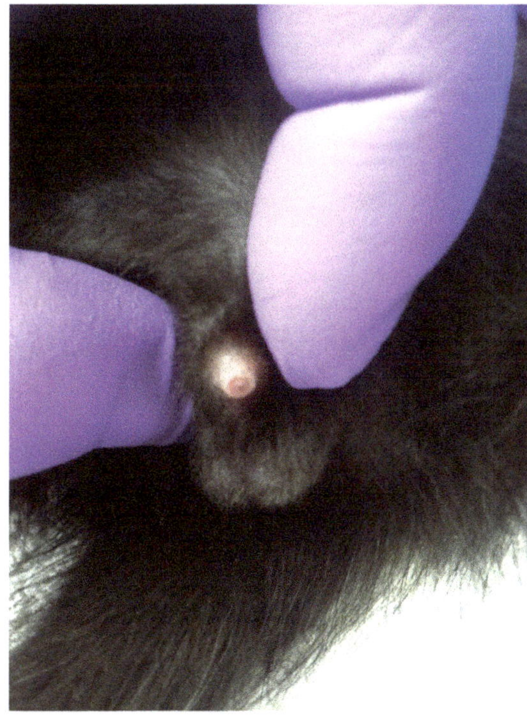

Fig. 17.3. Everted preputial mucosa connected to the penile mucosa at the balanopreputial fold in the pre-pubertal tomcat. The balanopreputial fold separates at puberty due to the influence of androgens. (Image: author's own.)

the development of the feline os penis is an age-related change that results from ossification of the distal end of the septum between the penile corpus cavernosum (Jackson, 1902). When present, the os penis is 3–5 mm long (Schummer *et al.*, 1979). The os penis can be visualized on standard radiographs of the pelvis (Fig. 17.5).

Penile spines

By 9–13 weeks of age, there is sufficient testosterone to initiate the eruption of conical papillae (spines) encircling the glans of the penis in intact toms (Ives *et al.*, 1975). Penile spines increase in size as androgen levels rise (Aronson and Cooper, 1967) and reach their full size when the tom is 8 months old (Ives *et al.*, 1975). The spines are larger proximally on the penis compared to distally (closer to the glans) and measure from 0.7–0.1 mm in diameter at the base of the spine (Aronson and Cooper, 1967). At sexual maturity, there are 100–200 keratinized penile spines present (Shille and Stabenfeldt, 1980; Roberts, 1986) (Fig. 17.6). Growth or regression of the penile spines is strongly correlated with the presence of

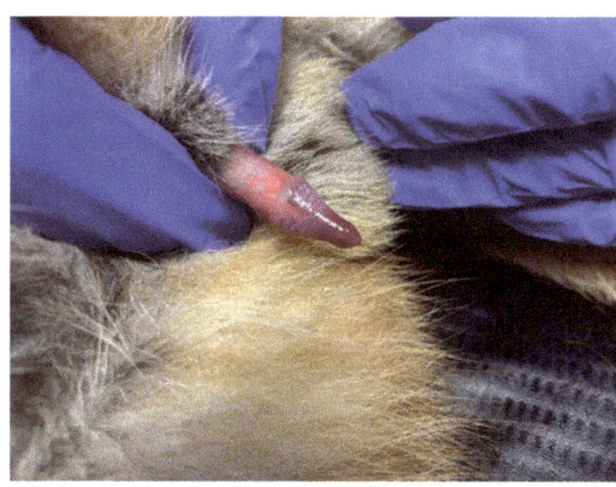

Fig. 17.4. An erect penis on a caracal during an electroejaculation session. Note the full extension of the penis out of the sheath with erect glans penis. (Image courtesy of Dr Aime Johnson.)

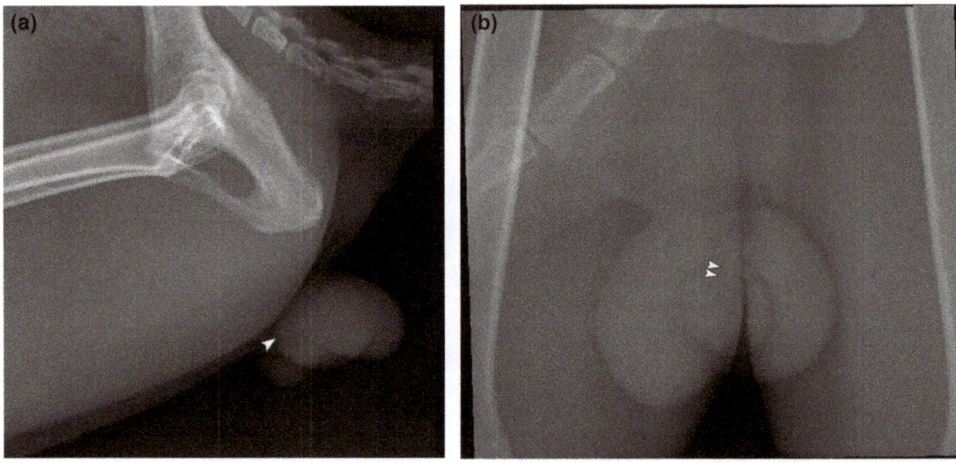

Fig. 17.5. (a). Lateral radiograph of a 6-year-old intact male feline pelvis. The os penis is faintly visualized below the testicles/scrotum and within the prepuce (arrow). **(b)** A ventrodorsal radiograph of the pelvis of an intact 6-year-old tom. The os penis can be seen near midline (arrows). (Image courtesy of Dr Aime Johnson.)

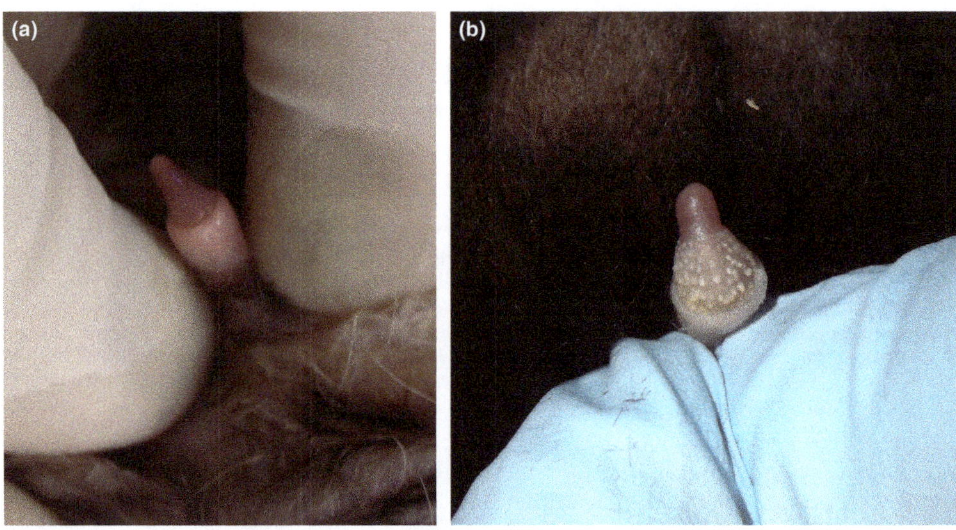

Fig. 17.6. The glans penis from: **(a)** a 2-month-old; and **(b)** adult tomcat have been exteriorized. Note the presence of 100–200 keratinized spines on the mature tomcat. (Images: author's own.)

circulating androgens. The penile spines regress quickly following castration and can redevelop if a castrated tom is treated with androgens (McEntee, 1990). Although the exact function of penile spines is not clearly understood, it is commonly believed that the spines are used to induce ovulation in the female during mating (Goodrowe *et al.*, 1989).

17.4 Scrotum and Testes

17.4.1 Scrotum

The tom scrotum is in the perineum ventral to the anus and proximal to the prepuce. Except for hairless breeds, the feline scrotum is normally covered with dense hair (Schummer *et al.*, 1979) (Fig. 17.8).

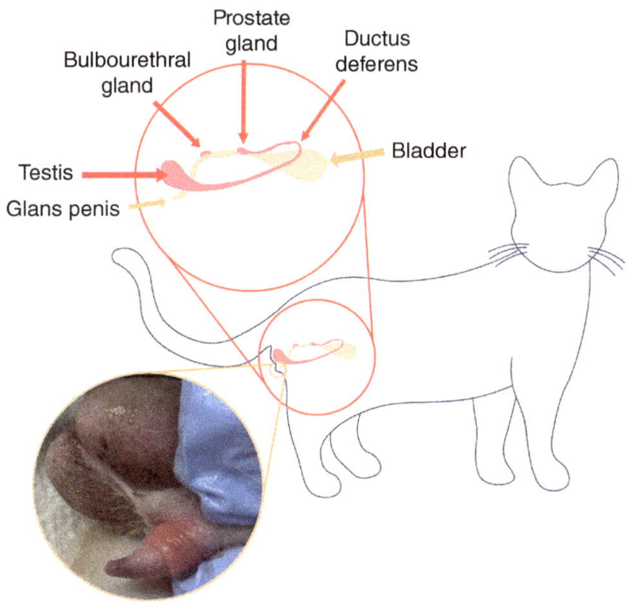

Fig. 17.7. Diagram of the male reproductive tract (created by Dr Jamie Douglas, used with permission from Johnson, *Journal of Feline Medicine and Surgery*, 2022).

17.4.2 Testes and epididymides

The testes may be fully descended at birth (Scott and Scott, 1957) or descend within the first week after birth. The feline testis contains a strand-like central mediastinum that extends through the cranial three-fourths of the testis (Wrobel and Gürtler, 2001). The intratesticular rete is inside the mediastinum. The rete penetrates the tunica albuginea at the cranial end of the testis and continues as an extensive extratesticular rete that covers the testis in a cap-like manner (Wrobel and Gürtler, 2001). Thirteen to eighteen efferent ductules leave the extratesticular rete and empty into the head of the epididymis (McEntee, 1990). The long axes of the testes are nearly vertical with the free border of the testis and tail of the epididymis located dorsocaudally (Schummer *et al.*, 1979). In the cat, the epididymis is uniform in size throughout its entire length (McEntee, 1990).

The feline testes are surrounded by a dense connective tissue layer that is rich in collagen fibers called the tunica albuginea (Diagone *et al.*, 2011). The feline tunica albuginea thickens with age, such that tomcats aged over 8 years have a thicker tunica albuginea compared to other male mammals (Elcock and Schoning, 1984; Diagone *et al.*, 2011).

The feline spermatic cord is relatively long due to the distance between the superficial inguinal ring and the scrotum (Schummer *et al.*, 1979). The vascular cone of the spermatic cord is formed by the convoluted testicular artery and the venous pampiniform plexus, which together are embedded in a fatty body that contacts the cranial end of the testis (Wrobel and Gürtler, 2001). Basal values of blood flow through the feline spermatic cord range from 20–64 mL/100 g/min (Chiocchio *et al.*, 1999). The ductus deferens, originating from the tail of the epididymis at the caudal end of the testis, runs separate from the spermatic cord (Wrobel and Gurtler, 2001) (Fig. 17.7). The cat possesses a broad mesodeferens that runs between the ductus deferens and the testicular epididymal margin (Wrobel and Gürtler, 2001). The cremaster muscle is poorly developed in tomcats (Schummer *et al.*, 1979).

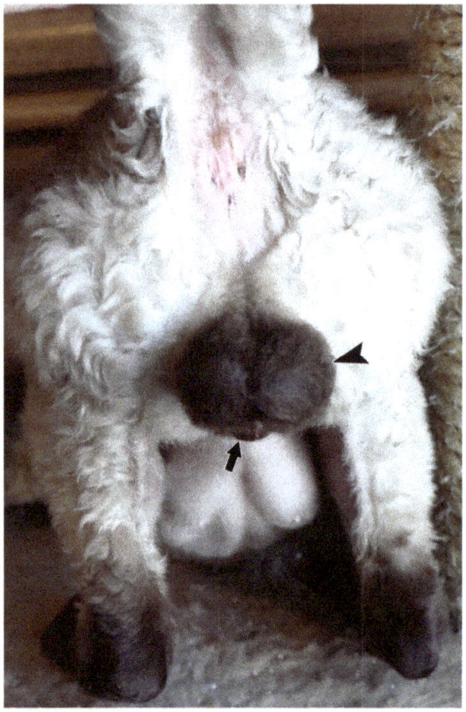

Fig. 17.8. The tom scrotum (arrowhead) is in the perineum ventral to the anus and proximal to the prepuce (arrow). Note the dense hair covering the scrotum. (Image: Tina Chittick.)

The feline testes can be easily imaged ultrasonographically within the scrotum. The normal testis is uniform in texture with echogenicity similar to the spleen (Davidson and Baker, 2009) (Fig. 17.9). The mediastinum testis is a thin, centrally located, very hyperechoic line (Davidson and Baker, 2009). The epididymis (head, body, tail) is less echogenic than the testis (Davidson and Baker, 2009). The ductus deferens is difficult to visualize (Davidson and Baker, 2009). The spermatic cord is adjacent to the head of the epididymis and has obvious, tortuous, small diameter veins (Davidson and Baker, 2009). Doppler ultrasonography can also be performed on feline testes. Doppler examination of the testicular artery shows monophasic-patterned waves with low vascular resistance (0.53–0.54) (Brito *et al.*, 2015). The values for the vascular indices of right and left testicular artery do not differ significantly (Brito *et al.*, 2015). For peak systolic velocity and end diastolic velocity, the values are 6.23–6.73 cm/s and 2.77–2.80 cm/s, respectively (Brito *et al.*, 2015).

Each mature feline testis measures 1.2–2 cm in length and 0.7–1.5 cm in width (Roberts, 1986) (Fig. 17.10). Testicular measurements are most accurately taken using ultrasound and measuring the width, length, and height of each testicle. These measurements allow estimation of the volume of testicular tissue present. Images should be obtained

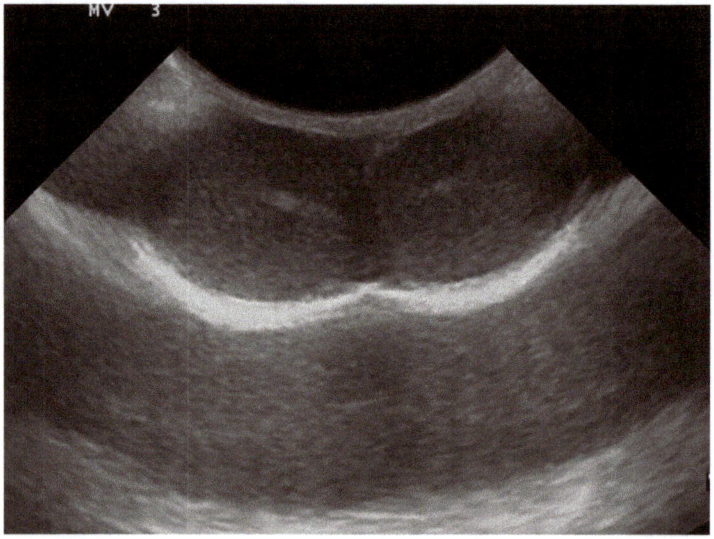

Fig. 17.9. Ultrasonographic image of normal feline testes. The mediastinum can be visualized as a hyperechoic structure in the center of each testis. (Image courtesy of Dr Aime Johnson.)

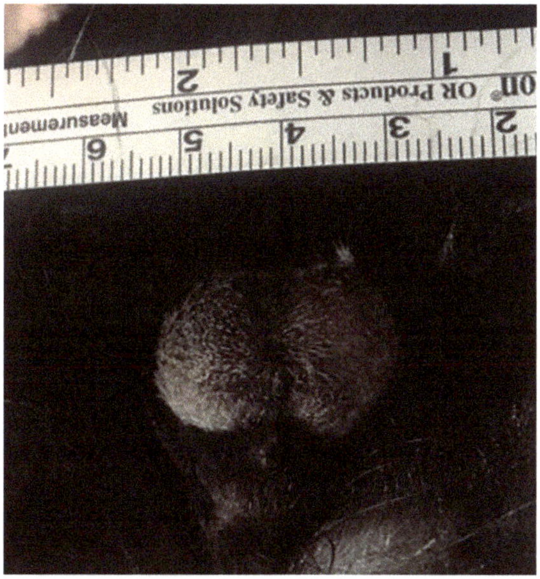

Fig. 17.10. The mature feline testis measures 1.2–2 cm in length and 0.7–1.5 cm in width. (Image courtesy of Dr Aime Johnson.)

in a heavily sedated or anesthetized tom to reduce error. Each testicle should be isolated individually by gently pushing one testicle cranially to prevent interference with the measurement of the other testicle. The testicle to be measured is then stabilized by gently grasping the base of the scrotum and trapping the testicle within the scrotum with the index finger and the thumb positioned between the testicle and the body. The testicle should be wet thoroughly with alcohol (or ultrasound gel) to allow sufficient contact between the skin and the probe. The ultrasound probe is then placed on the scrotal skin to measure the testicle underneath. The probe is placed at a 90° angle to the desired measurement (length, width, or height), taking care not to rotate or measure the testicle obliquely (Fig. 17.11). Care must also be taken not to apply pressure with the probe to the testicle as it will falsely decrease the measurement due to the compression. Once the operator is certain that the probe is oriented correctly and no compression of the testicle is present, the image can be frozen and measured from one tunica albuginea, across the testicular parenchyma, to the other tunica albuginea. The same measurement should be obtained two to four separate times (remove probe, replace, and remeasure). By obtaining more than one measurement, error is decreased. The measurements obtained from each attempt are averaged to provide a single value (length, width, and height of each testicle). Testicular volume of each testicle can be calculated using the formula for an ellipse ($TV=4/3\pi \times L/2 \times W/2 \times H/2$). The equation can be simplified to $TV=0.2533 \times L \times W \times H$. These measurements are best used to monitor testicular volume (and changes) over time in an individual tom rather than evaluating the amount of testicular tissue present and comparing it to all cats (as is commonly done in bulls).

The size of the feline testes varies depending on age and time of year. However, there is no correlation between testis size and body weight (Tsutsui *et al.*, 1990, 2004). At birth, the combined weight of the testes is 20 mg and increases to 100 mg in the first 2 months after birth (Scott and Scott, 1957). At sexual maturity, the individual weight of the feline testis is 1.2–2.0 g, with no significant difference between the left and right testes (Scott and Scott, 1957). Testicular weights are higher during the long day reproductive season (1.46 ± 0.06 g) compared to the short day non-reproductive season (1.29 ± 0.05 g) (Blottner and Jewgenow, 2007).

The testes secrete reproductive hormones (i.e. testosterone) and produce sperm. Within the testes, there are two morphologically and functionally different compartments: the interstitial tissue (for androgen production) and the seminiferous tubules (for sperm production). The interstitial tissue contains clusters of Leydig cells, which occupy approximately 50% of the interstitial space (Franca and Godinho, 2003). In the cat, Leydig cells occur not only in intertubular locations, but also as intratunical and mediastinal Leydig cells (Wrobel and Gürtler, 2001). Androgenic activity is detectable in feline Leydig cells at birth, which then decreases to negligible amounts until around 4 months of age when androgenic activity resumes (Sánchez *et al.*, 1993a). The production of testosterone is positively correlated with photoperiod in tom cats (Joffre, 1977; Kirkpatrick, 1985; Blottner and Jewgenow, 2007). However, testicular histology studies reveal the presence of sperm in the seminiferous tubules during all four seasons of the year.

In the testes, the seminiferous tubules contain Sertoli cells and germ cells. The Sertoli cells support the development of the germ cells from

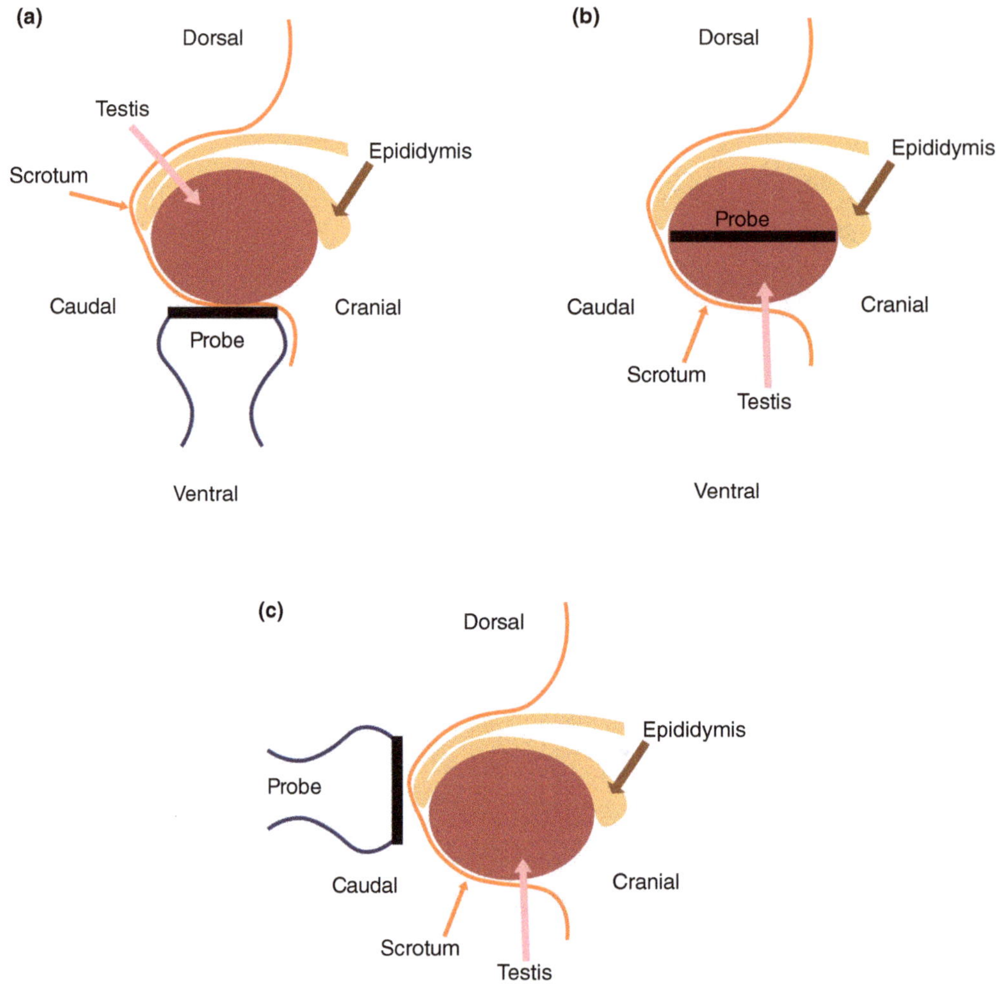

Fig. 17.11. Diagram of placement of the ultrasound probe on the testicle for measurement of: **(a)** testicular height; **(b)** testicular width; and **(c)** testicular length. These measurements can be combined to determine total testicular volume for each testicle and used to follow changes over time in a single cat. (Created by Dr Jamie Douglas, used with permission from Johnson, *Journal of Feline Medicine and Surgery*, 2022.)

spermatogonia to spermatocytes. In mature toms, the daily sperm production per testis is 15.8 ± 2.5 million, for an average total daily output of 30 million sperm (Franca and Godinho, 2003; Tsutsui *et al.*, 2012). The daily sperm production is significantly correlated with the total number of germ cells and the number of round spermatids per seminiferous tubule cross section at stage 1 of the cycle (Franca and Godinho, 2003). Approximately 200 million sperm are stored in the epididymis and ejected during frequent ejaculations (Tsutsui *et al.*, 2012). Tomcats can perform multiple consecutive copulations to induce ovulation in queens, but about 75% of the sperm stored in the epididymis are released in the first two ejaculations (Tsutsui *et al.*, 2012). Because the minimum number of spermatozoa necessary to achieve conception in cats through intravaginal insemination is 80 million (Tanaka *et al.*, 2000), the spermatozoa stored in the epididymis are sufficient to fertilize at least two female cats (Tsutsui *et al.*, 2012).

Seminiferous tubule diameter size is correlated with sexual maturity. In the adult tom, the mean seminiferous tubular diameter is 223 μm and the mean seminiferous tubular epithelium height is 81 μm (Franca and Godinho, 2003). The seminiferous tubular diameter (mean ± standard deviation) increases steadily from 2–2.5 months old (88.10 ± 10.88 μm), 3-4 months old (109.8 ± 8.89 μm), and 5-6 months old (142.2 ± 16.89 μm) to 12-24 months old (237.90 ± 52.45 μm) (Fig. 17.12). At birth, the seminiferous tubules consist of a monolayer of Sertoli cells with few spermatogonia and no tubular lumen present (Sánchez *et al.*, 1993b; Siemieniuch and Wocławek-Potocka, 2007). It is important to mention that there are approximately 23 meters of seminiferous tubules per gram of testis, which is higher than what is observed in other species (Franca and Godinho, 2003).

Spermatogenesis

Spermatogenesis is a complex yet highly organized process within the seminiferous tubule by which spermatozoa are produced from primordial germ cells (spermatogonia) via mitosis and meiosis (Franca and Godinho, 2003). Spermatogenesis is increased at the onset of the breeding season with enhanced mitosis of spermatogonia and increased meiotic transformation (Blottner and Jewgenow, 2007).

Sperm cells mature from spermatogonia in the outer epithelium of the seminiferous tubule and progress in maturation stage through the epithelium until they reach the lumen, where mature sperm may be observed. The arrangement and location of sperm in different times of development within the seminiferous tubule is arranged in 'stages' (Courot *et al.*, 1970; Berndtson, 1977). In

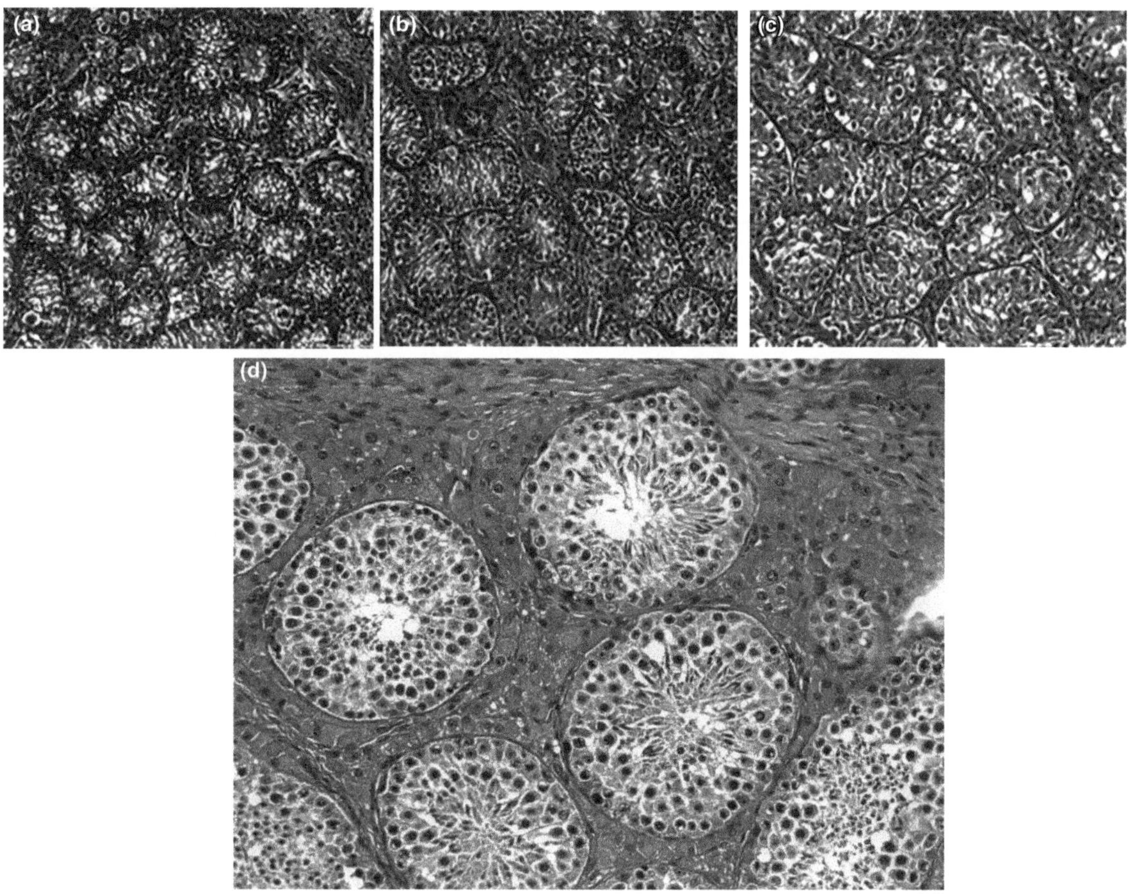

Fig. 17.12. Representative seminiferous tubule cross-sections from: **(a)** a 2-month-old tom; **(b)** a 4-month-old tom; **(c)** a 6-month-old tom; and **(d)** a 12-month-old tom. (Images: author's own.)

cats, there are eight stages of the spermatogenic cycle. The percentage of time these stages are observed varies. Stage 1 is the most frequent and stage 7 is the least frequent (Fig. 17.13). The length of the spermatogenic cycle in cats is 10 to 11 days, which is similar of other mammals.

Spermatogenesis is regulated by follicle-stimulating hormone. Follicle-stimulating hormone also stimulates Sertoli cells to produce androgen-binding protein, which binds to intratesticular testosterone to increase its concentration within the seminiferous tubule (Diagone *et al.*, 2011).

Sperm morphology

Specific morphological characteristics of the sperm can dictate whether it can fertilize an egg. The percentage of morphologically normal and abnormal sperm in the ejaculate can determined by examining 200 sperm using phase-contrast microscopy or by routine light microscopy following staining with eosin-nigrosin stain (Johnston *et al.*, 2001). There are many different sperm morphological abnormalities to consider in semen analysis. Various parts of the sperm are integral for the transportation of the spermatozoa to the egg (e.g. tail) and the fusion with the zona pellucida (e.g. acrosome), the first step in the process of fertilization. Some of the most common morphologic abnormalities of feline sperm include macroencephaly, microencephaly, double head, double tail, proximally coiled tail, bent mid-piece, proximal and distal retained cytoplasmic droplet, detached head, and bent tail (Howard *et al.*, 1990).

An acceptable overall normal percentage of spermatozoa morphology has been debated. Toms with less than 40% morphologically normal spermatozoa (teratospermic) have lower zona pellucida penetration rates than did toms with greater than 60% normal spermatozoa (Howard *et al.*, 1993). However, according to Wildt *et al.* (1999), it is not unusual to find fertile tomcats with more than 60% abnormally shaped sperm. It is important to note that the median percentage of morphologically normal spermatozoa in a population of random domestic cats during the reproductive season was 56.1% (Axner and Linde Forsberg, 2007).

The mean percentage of morphologically normal spermatozoa is significantly higher during the reproductive season (long days) than during the non-reproductive season (short day) (Blottner and Jewgenow, 2007). The mean percentages of proximal droplets, distal droplets, detached heads, acrosomal abnormalities, and sperm tail abnormalities

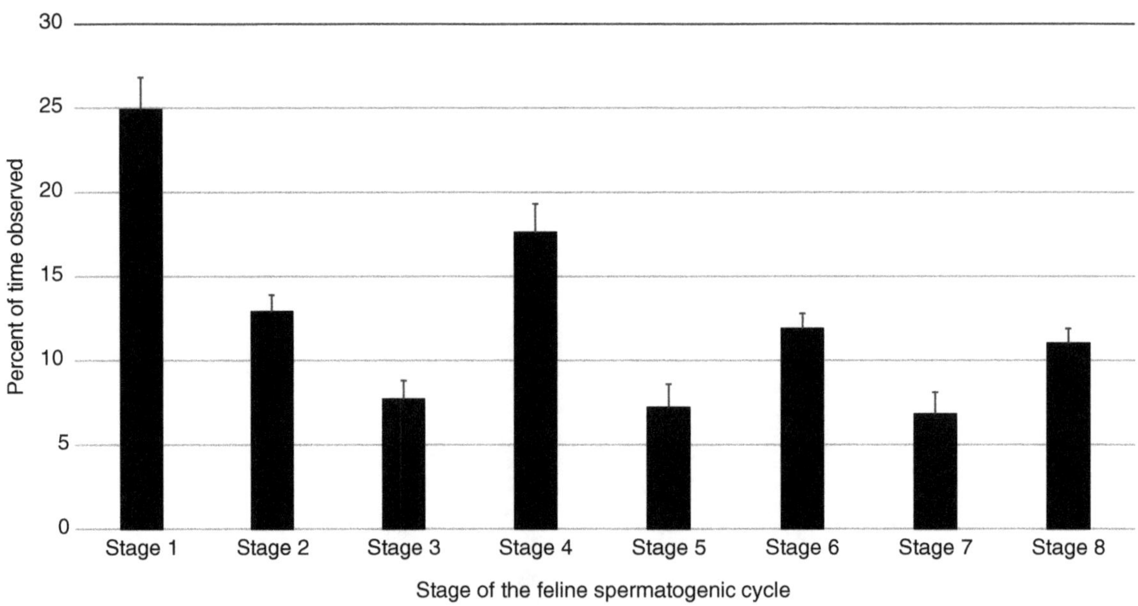

Fig. 17.13. Percent of time each stage of the spermatogenic cycle was observed. The length of the feline spermatogenic cycle in cats is 10–11 days. (Data modified from Franca and Godinho (2003).)

have been found to be higher during the non-reproductive season. Acrosomal abnormalities seem to be particularly affected by seasonality (Axner and Linde Forsberg, 2007).

Age can also influence sperm morphology in toms. It was observed histologically that tomcats older than 4 years old with normal-appearing testes exhibit spermatogonia irregularity (Diagone *et al.*, 2011).

Semen collection for sperm analysis is discussed in Chapter 18. Spermatozoa can also be collected following removal of the testicle by squeezing or slicing the tail of the epididymis. This technique is frequently used for research with the advantage to obtain tissues after routine orchiectomy. However, epididymal samples generally demonstrate greater proportions of abnormal spermatozoa (36%) than do ejaculated cells (26%).

17.5 Accessory Glands

17.5.1 Prostate

The feline prostate is 10–12 mm long and 5–6 mm in diameter and can increase slightly with age (Mialot, 1988). The feline prostate has two lateral lobes that are divided by a longitudinal median groove as well as divided into cranial and caudal (disseminate) lobes by a wide connective septum. Ultrasonographically, the feline prostate is a dense tissue that has a ultrasonographically homogenous, medium to fine echotexture (Zambelli and Levy, 2010). The feline prostate is close to the pelvic brim and covers the urethra dorsally and laterally, but not ventrally (Hewitt, 1998) (Fig. 17.7). The disseminate part of the prostate consists of small lobules that extend into the urethralis muscle (Aitken and Aughey, 1964).

The feline prostate is a compound tubular gland with tubules of varying diameter lined by a secretory epithelium (Aughey, 1973). The composition of feline prostatic fluid includes a secretory protein, glycogen, acid phosphatase, 5-nucleotidase, and zinc (Aughey, 1970).

17.5.2 Bulbourethral glands

The feline bulbourethral glands are two pea-shaped glands about 5 mm in diameter that lie dorsolateral to each penile bulb at the level of the ischial symphysis (Sikorski, 1978; McEntee, 1990; Zambelli and Levy, 2010) (Fig. 17.7). The ultrasonographic appearance of the feline bulbourethral glands is similar in echotexture to that of the prostate (Zambelli and Levy, 2010). The feline bulbourethral gland parenchyma consists of spacious, sinus-like intraglandular ducts and short, narrow, mostly unbranched tubular endpieces (Wrobel, 1969). The feline bulbourethral gland has a very thin, incomplete fibrous capsule, such that some of the peripheral tubules are situated directly between fibers of the surrounding bulboglandularis muscle (Wrobel, 1969; Schummer *et al.*, 1979; McEntee, 1990).

The feline bulbourethral gland parenchyma is rich in β-D-glucuronidase, β-D-galactosidase, aldolase, α-glycerophosphate dehydrogenase, lactate dehydrogenase, alcohol dehydrogenase, NAD-dependent isocitrate dehydrogenase, succinate dehydrogenase, and cytochrome oxidase (Wrobel, 1969). The composition of feline bulbourethral gland fluid is mainly sulfated mucopolysaccharides (i.e. mucin) (Herron, 1989; McEntee, 1990; Johnston *et al.*, 2001).

17.5.3 Urethra

The feline male urethra is 8.5–10.5 cm long and divided into the pelvic urethra and the penile urethra (Fletcher, 1996). The prostate is present in the middle of the pelvic urethra, such that the pelvic urethra can be divided into pre-prostatic, prostatic, and post-prostatic urethra (Fletcher, 1996). The internal urethral sphincter occupies the bladder neck and pre-prostatic urethra (Fletcher, 1996). The pre-prostatic urethra is cylindrical, 0.9–2.0 mm in diameter, and 3–5 cm long (Wang *et al.*, 1999). The urethral crest in the dorsal wall of the pre-prostatic urethra leads to the colliculus seminalis of the prostatic urethra (Fletcher, 1996). The colliculus seminalis is a submucosal thickening with multiple openings for the prostatic ducts as well as openings for the paired ductus deferens openings into the prostatic urethral lumen (Fletcher, 1996). The prostatic urethra travels ventral to the prostate, and 4.5–5.0 mm in diameter and 1.5–1.9 cm long (Wang *et al.*, 1999).

The bulbourethral gland ducts empty into the post-prostatic urethra at the level of the ischial arch (Fletcher, 1996). The bulbourethral glands are situated dorsolateral to the post-prostatic urethra. Occasionally disseminated bulbourethral glandular tissue can be found around the urethral wall (Johnston *et al.*, 2001). The post-prostatic urethra is 1.9–2.6 mm in diameter and 1.2–1.8 cm long (Wang *et al.*, 1999). The striated urethralis muscle encircles the post-prostatic urethra to form the external urethral sphincter before blending with bulboglandularis and bulbospongiosus muscles to cover the bulbourethral glands and the bulb of the penis, respectively (Martin *et al.*, 1974; Cullen *et al.*, 1983; Wang *et al.*, 1999). The penile urethra runs along the dorsal aspect of the penis and is surrounded by the corpus cavernosus (Wang *et al.*, 1999).

17.6 References

Aitken, R. N. C. and Aughey, E. (1964) A histochemical study of the accessory genital glands of the male cat. *Research in Veterinary Science* 5, 268–273. doi: 10.1016/S0034-5288(18)34791-X

Amiri, A. A., Gilanpour, H., and Veshkini, A. (2014) Contrast radiographic study of venous drainage of the corpus cavernosum and the corpus spongiosum of the cat penis. *Italian Journal of Anatomy and Embryology* 119(3), 193–200.

Aronson, L. R and Cooper, M. L. (1967) Penile spines of the domestic cat: their endocrine-behavior relations. *The Anatomical Record* 157, 71–78.

Aughey, E. (1970) Zinc in the cat prostate. *Journal of Reproduction and Fertility* 22, 65–68.

Aughey, E. (1973) The ultrastructure of the prostate gland in the cat. *Journal of Reproduction and Fertility* 33, 351–352.

Axner, E. and Linde Forsberg, C. (2007) Sperm morphology in the domestic cat, and its relation with fertility: a retrospective study. *Reproduction in Domestic Animal* 42, 282–291. doi: 10.1111/j.1439-0531.2007.00780.x

Berndtson, W. E. (1977) Methods for quantifying mammalian spermatogenesis: a review. *Journal of Animal Science* 44, 818–833. doi: 10.2527/jas1977.445818x

Blottner, W. and Jewgenow, K. (2007) Moderate seasonality in testis function of domestic cat. *Reproduction in Domestic Animals* 42, 536–540. doi: 10.1111/j.1439-0531.2006.00817.x

Bohrer, E., Mihalyo, A., and Kutzler, M. A. (2015) Histologic and morphometric evaluation of testes of feral tom kittens and cats. *Clinical Theriogenology* 7(3), 312.

Brito, M. B. S, Feliciano, M., Coutinho, L. N., Uscategui, R. R., Simões, A., *et al.* (2015) Doppler and contrast-enhanced ultrasonography of testicles in adult domestic felines. *Reproduction in Domestic Animals* 50(5), 730–734.

Chiocchio, S. R., Suburo, A. M., Vladucic, E., Zhu, B. C., Charreau, E., *et al.* (1999) Differential effects of superior and inferior spermatic nerves on testosterone secretion and spermatic blood flow in cats. *Endocrinology* 140(3), 1036–1043. doi: 10.1210/endo.140.3.6569

Courot, M., Hochereau-de Reviers, M. T., and Ortavant R. (1970) Spermatogenesis. In: Johnson, A. D., Gomes, W. R., and Vandemark, N. L. (eds) *The Testis*. Academic Press, New York City, New York, pp.339–432.

Cullen, W. C., Fletcher, T. F., and Bradley, W. E. (1983) Morphometry of the male feline pelvic urethra. *Journal of Urology* 129, 186–189. doi: 10.1016/s0022-5347(17)51979-5

Davidson, A. P. and Baker, T. W. (2009) Reproductive ultrasound of the dog and tom. *Topics in Companion Animal Medicine* 24(2), 64–70. doi: 10.1053/j.tcam.2008.11.003

Diagone, K. V., Feliciano, M. A. R., Pacheco, M. R., and Vicente, W. R. R. (2011) Histology and morphometry of the testes of adult domestic cats (*Felis catus*). *Journal of Feline Medicine and Surgery* 14(2), 124–130. doi: 10.1177/1098612X11431531

Elcock, L. H. and Schoning, P. (1984) Age-related changes in the cat testis and epididymis. *American Journal of Veterinary Research* 45(11), 2380–2384.

Faya, M., Carranza, A., Miotti, R., Ponchón, T., Furlan, P., *et al.* (2013) Fecal estradiol-17β and testosterone in prepubertal domestic cats. *Theriogenology* 80(6), 584–586. doi: 10.1016/j.theriogenology.2013.05.026

Fletcher, T. F. (1996) Applied anatomy and physiology of the feline lower urinary tract. *Veterinary Clinics of North America: Small Animal Practice* 26(2), 181–196. doi: 10.1016/S0195-5616(96)50201-9

Franca, L. R. and Godinho, C. L. (2003) Testis morphometry, seminiferous epithelium cycle length, and daily sperm production in domestic cats (*Felis catus*). *Biology of Reproduction* 68, 1554–1561. doi: 10.1095/biolreprod.102.010652

Goodrowe, K. L., Howard, J. G., Schmidt, P. M., and Wildt, D. E. (1989) Reproductive biology of the domestic cat with special reference to endocrinology, sperm function, and in-vitro fertilization. *Journal of Reproduction and Fertility Supplement* 39, 73–90.

Hart, B. L. (1974) Physiology of sexual function. *Veterinary Clinics of North America* 4(3), 557–571. doi: 10.1016/s0091-0279(74)50059-0

Herron, M. A. (1989) Feline physiology of reproduction. In: Burke, T. J. (ed.) *Small Animal Reproduction and Infertility: A Clinical Approach to Diagnosis and Treatment*. Lea & Febiger. Philadelphia, Pennsylvania, pp 13–23.

Hewitt, D. (1998) Physiology and endocrinology of the male. In: Simpson, G. M., England, G. C. W., and Harvey, M. (eds) *Manual of Small Animal Reproduction and Neonatology*. British Small Animal Veterinary Association, Cheltenham, UK, pp. 61–69.

Howard, J. G., Brown, J. L., Bush, M., and Wildt, D. E. (1990) Teratospermic and normospermic domestic cats: ejaculate traits, pituitary-gonadal hormones, and improvement of spermatozoal motility and morphology after swim-up processing. *Journal of Andrology* 11, 204–215.

Howard, J. G., Donoghue, A. M., Johnston, L. A., and Wildt, D. E. (1993) Zona pellucida filtration of structurally abnormal spermatozoa and reduced fertilization in teratospermic cats. *Biology of Reproduction* 49, 131–139. doi: 10.1095/biolreprod49.1.131

Inomata, T., Ninomiya, H., Sakita, K., Kashiwazaki, N., Ito, J., *et al.* (2009) Developmental changes of Müllerian and Wolffian ducts in domestic cat fetuses. *Experimental Animals* 58(1), 41–45. doi: 10.1538/expanim.58.41

Ives, P. J., McArthur, N. H., and Sis, F. R. (1975) Scanning electron microscopy of the penile spines of the domestic cat. *Southwestern Veterinarian* 28, 58–59.

Jackson, C. M. (1902) On the structure of the corpus cavernosa in the domestic cat. *American Journal of Anatomy* 2, 73–80.

Joffre, M. (1977) Relationships between testicular blood flow, testosterone secretion and spermatogenic activity in young and adult red foxes (*Vulpes vulpes*). *Journal of Reproduction and Fertility* 51, 35–40. doi: 10.1530/jrf.0.0510035

Johnston, S. D., Root-Kustritz, M. V., and Olson, P. N. S. (2001) Sexual differentiation and normal anatomy of the tom cat. In: Johnston, S. D., Root-Kustritz, M. V., and Olson, P. N. S. (eds) *Canine and Feline Theriogenology*. Elsevier Health Sciences, St. Louis, Missouri, pp. 497–507.

Kirkpatrick, J. (1985) Seasonal testosterone levels, testosterone clearance, and testicular weights in male domestic cats. *Canadian Journal of Zoology* 63, 1285–1287.

Knospe, C. (2002) Periods and stages of the prenatal development of the domestic cat. *Anatomia, Histologia, Embryologia* 31(1), 37–51. doi: 10.1046/j.1439-0264.2002.00360.x

Malandain, E., Little, S., Casseleux, G., Shelton, L., Pibot, P., *et al.* (2006) Reproduction from oestrus to kittening. In: Malandain, E., Little, S., Casseleux, G., Shelton, L., Pibot, P., *et al.* (eds) *Practical Guide to Cat Breeding*. Aniwa SAS, Lyon, France, pp. 63–79.

Martin, W. D., Fletcher, T. F., and Bradley, W. E. (1974) Perineal musculature in the cat. *Anatomical Record* 180, 3–13. doi: 10.1002/ar.1091800103

McEntee, K. (1990) Penis and prepuce. In: McEntee, K. (ed.) *Reproductive Pathology of Domestic Mammals*. Academic Press, Inc., San Diego, California, pp. 359–383.

Mialot, J. P. (1988) *Patologia da reprodução dos carnivoros domésticos*. A Hora Veterinária, Porto Alegra, Brazil.

Noden, D. N. and de la Hunta, A. (1985) Derivatives of intermediate mesoderm: reproductive organs. In: Noden, D. N. and de la Hunta, A. (eds) *The Embryology of Domestic Animals*. Williams & Wilkins, Baltimore, Maryland, pp. 330.

Roberts, S. J. (1986) *Veterinary Obstetrics and Genital Diseases (Theriogenology)*, 3rd edn. Roberts, S. J. published by the author, Woodstock, Vermont.

Romagnoli, S. and Schlafer, D. H. (2006) Disorders of sexual differentiation in puppies and kittens: a diagnostic and clinical approach. *Veterinary Clinics of North America, Small Animal Practice* 36(3), 573–606. doi: 10.1016/j.cvsm.2005.12.007

Sánchez, B., Pizarro, M., García, P., and Flores, J. M. (1993a) Histological study of Leydig cells in the cat from birth to sexual maturity. *Journal of Reproduction and Fertility Supplement* 47, 349–353.

Sánchez, B., Pizarro, M., García, P., and Flores, J. M. (1993b) Postnatal development of seminiferous tubules in the cat. *Journal of Reproduction and Fertility Supplement* 47, 343–348.

Schummer, A., Nickel, R., and Sack, W. A. (1979) In: Nickel, A., Schummer, A., Seiferle, E. (eds) *The Viscera of the Domestic Mammals*, 2nd ed. Springer Verlag, Berlin, pp. 304–389.

Scott, M. G. and Scott, P. P. (1957) Some factors affecting the maturation of the reproductive organs of the cat. *Proceedings of the Societal Study Fertility* 9, 72–89.

Shille, V. M. and Stabenfeldt, G. H. (1980) Current concepts in reproduction of the dog and cat. *Advances in Veterinary Science and Comparative Medicine* 24, 211–243.

Siemieniuch, M. J. and Wocławek-Potocka, I. (2007) Morphological features of the seminiferous epithelium in cat (*Felis catus*, L. 1758) testes. *Journal of Reproduction and Development* 53(5), 1125–1130. doi: 10.1262/jrd.19053

Sikorski, A. (1978) Comparative anatomy of the bulbourethral glands. (Preliminary report). *Folia Morphologica (Warsz)* 37(2), 151–156.

Tanaka, A., Takagi, Y., Nakagawa, K., Fujimoto, Y., Hori, T., *et al.* (2000) Artificial intravaginal insemination using fresh semen in cats. *Journal of Veterinary Medical Science* 62, 1163–1167. doi: 10.1292/jvms.62.1163

Tiptanavattana, N., Radtanakatikanon, A., Hyttel, P., Holm, H., Buranapraditkun, S., *et al.* (2015) Determination phase at transition of gonocytes to spermatogonial stem cells improves establishment efficiency of spermatogonial stem cells in domestic cats. *Journal of Reproduction and Development* 61(6), 581–588. doi: 10.1262/jrd.2015-094

Tsutsui, T., Murao, I., Kawakami, E., Ogasa, A., and Stabenfeldt, G. H. (1990) Androgen concentration in the blood and spermatogenic function of tom cats during the breeding season. *Japanese Journal of Veterinary Science* 52(4), 801–806.

Tsutsui, T., Kuwabara, S., Kuwabara, K., Kugota, Y., Kinjo, T., *et al.* (2004) Development of spermatogenic function in the sex maturation process in male cats. *Journal of Veterinary Medical Science* 66(9), 1125–1127. doi: 10.1292/jvms.66.1125

Tsutsui, T., Oba, H., Fujimoto, S., and Toyonaga, M. (2012) Spermatogenic function in cats. *Reproduction in Domestic Animals* 47(6), 247–249. doi: 10.1111/rda.12074

Wang, B., Bhadra, N., and Grill, W. M. (1999) Functional anatomy of the male feline urethra: morphological and physiological correlations. *Journal of Urology* 161(2), 654–659. doi: 10.1016/S0022-5347(01)61989-X

Wildt, D. E., Brown, J. L., and Swanson, W. F. (1999) Cats. In: Knobil, E. and Neill, J. (eds) *Encyclopedia of Reproduction*, vol. 1. Academic Press, New York, pp. 497–510.

Wrobel, K. H. (1969) Morphologische Untersuchungen an der Glandula bulbourethralis der Katze [Morphological studies on the bulbourethral gland of the cat]. *Zeitschrift fur Zellforschung und Mikroskopische Anatomie* 101(4), 607–620.

Wrobel, K. H. and Gürtler, A. (2001) The nerve distribution in the testis of the cat. *Annals of Anatomy* 183(4), 297–308. doi: 10.1016/S0940-9602(01)80167-9

Zambelli, D. and Levy, X. (2010) Clinical approaches to the infertile male. In: England, G. and von Heimendahl, A. (eds) *BSAVA Manual of Canine and Feline Reproduction and Neonatology*. BSAVA, Gloucester, UK, pp. 70–79.

18 Semen Collection and Evaluation

Daniele Zambelli[1] and Marco Cunto[1]

[1]Animal Reproduction Unit, Department of Veterinary Medical Sciences, Alma Mater Studiorum, University of Bologna, Bologna, Italy

18.1 Introduction

Practitioners are more frequently asked to collect cat semen for artificial insemination or diagnostic purpose, especially when fertility must be investigated. The technique of artificial insemination has improved from the first report by Sojka *et al.* (1970). In the last decades, much research has been performed concerning the number of spermatozoa to be used and the anatomical site of insemination to obtain the best results (Tsutsui *et al.*, 2000a,b). Important steps have also been made with the development of the endoscopic intrauterine insemination technique (Zambelli *et al.*, 2015a,b). Many advantages to using artificial insemination (AI) with fresh or preserved spermatozoa include the control of disease (e.g. respiratory infections) and bypass of psychological or physical breeding problems. Another important source of interest in cat reproduction derives from its use as a model in the study of endangered wild felids or for human diseases.

Ejaculates collected should have good quality in relation to the final use, with minimal stress for the animal during collection. Sperm may be collected in practice using different methods. Artificial vagina and electroejaculation were first described in the seventies (Scott, 1970; Sojka *et al.*, 1970; Platz *et al.*, 1976, 1978; Platz and Seager, 1978; Johnstone, 1984; Pineda *et al.*, 1984; Dooley and Pineda, 1986; Dooley *et al.*, 1991; Howard *et al.*, 1990). More recently, urethral catheterization after pharmacological induction has been described as a new and simple method for collection (Zambelli *et al.*, 2006, 2008; Filliers *et al.*, 2010; Cunto *et al.*, 2015, 2018, 2019; Prochowska *et al.*, 2015; Romagnoli *et al.*, 2016, 2020; Jelinkova *et al.*, 2018). Researchers frequently obtain large amounts of epididymal sperm for studies by slicing or squeezing the tail of the epididymis following castration (Bowen, 1977; Hay and Goodrowe, 1993; Yu and Leibo, 2002). Both for practice and research purposes, sperm should be evaluated immediately after collection and before its use. The first limitation in sperm evaluation is the low ejaculate volume, so only a small amount can be sacrificed for this reason. Sperm is usually evaluated for macroscopic and microscopic parameters, volume, color, concentration, percentage of total and progressive sperm motility, and morphology. For particular needs, other parameters may be evaluated including pH, seminal plasma chemistries (Zambelli *et al.*, 2010), or ejaculate culture.

18.2 Sperm Collection

18.2.1 Artificial vagina (AV)

Sojka *et al.* (1970) reported the first paper about sperm collection with AV and the technique to construct the device. This technique is used in catteries or in research colonies where the animals are properly trained and frequently collected for AI, sperm preservation, or other purposes. However, for a single collection that is frequently requested in practice in an untrained cat, this is usually a fruitless method. The advantages to using an AV are the low cost of the equipment, no restraint needed for the cat, a single technician can perform the collection, and multiple collections can be made in a single week. The training necessary for the use of an AV is possible in many cats and can be completed after 2 weeks of gentle handling during exposure to estrus queen (Sojka *et al.*, 1970). The need for training and a teaser queen is the most common disadvantage of this method. A simple AV has been described by Sojka using a plastic tube (such as an

 Feline Reproduction (eds. A.K. Johnson and M.A. Kutzler)
DOI: 10.1079/9781789247107.0018

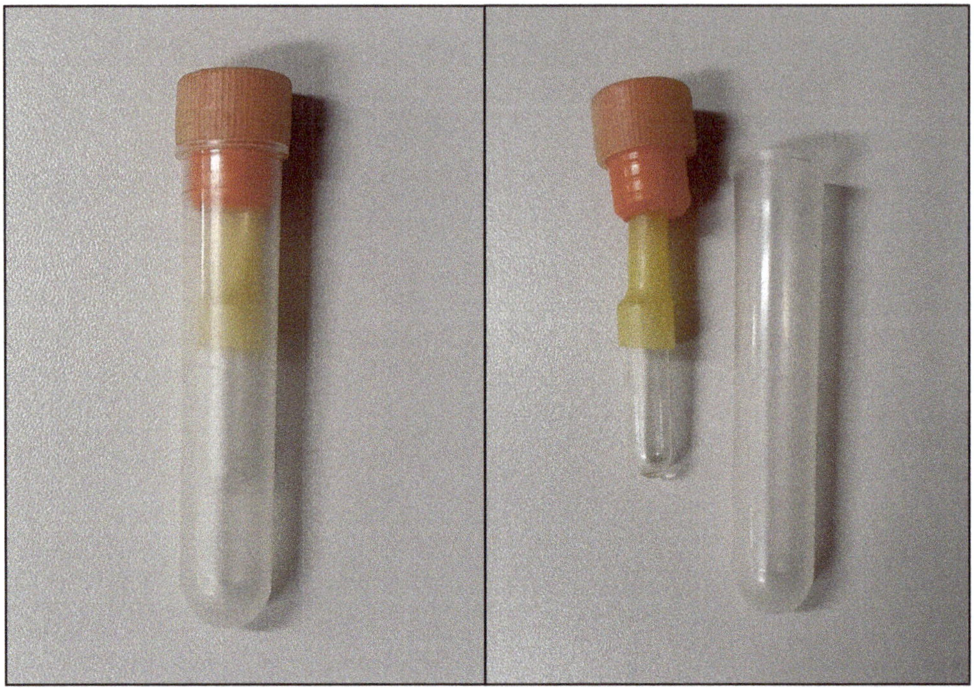

Fig. 18.1. A simple AV constructed using a plastic tube (such as an Eppendorf) and a rubber bulb from a Pasteur pipette. (Image: author's own.)

Eppendorf) and a rubber bulb from a Pasteur pipette (Sojka *et al.*, 1970) (Fig. 18.1). Another model can be made using a 5-mL plastic tube (external part), Penrose drainage and a small glass tube. The 5-mL tube is filled with water (40°C) to maintain the sperm temperature and reduce the thermal shock (Zambelli *et al.*, 2006). Before the collection, it is necessary to permit the male to have a normal approach to the female to get maximal sexual arousal. When he mounts the queen, the operator's gloved hand slips the AV over the erected penis. After a few coital movements, the cat will ejaculate. If the cat is well trained, it is possible to collect the semen without an estrus female by simply allowing the male to mount the operator's protected arm (to avoid the male bite during collection). A second ejaculate can be collected as soon as 10 minutes later; however, the frequency of collection may influence the sperm quality. It has been reported that three collections per week does not change the sperm volume and concentration, but daily collection caused a rapid drop in these two parameters starting on the fourth day (Sojka *et al.*, 1970).

18.2.2 Electroejaculation (EE)

Transrectal electrostimulation is used in many wild species in which training to an AV is not possible. Additionally, it has been used in some zootechnical species and in humans with spinal cord injuries. First reports of use are in 1936 and 1948, respectively, for collection of ejaculates in sheep (Gunn, 1936) and humans (Horne *et al.*, 1948). The first report of its use in the cat species was in 1970 by Scott. The ejaculate collected with EE typically has a sufficient volume to be more easily manipulated. Electroejaculation may be used in all males that can be safely anesthetized (Sojka, 1986) and when collection with an AV is not possible with untrained or aggressive males or in the absence of a teaser queen. The procedure has been shown to be safe and does not induce histological or colonoscopic lesions in the rectum (Furthner *et al.*, 2018). All these advantages lead many clinicians to consider EE as the best elective method. Disadvantages include the necessity to anesthetize the patient, the skills to perform the procedure, and the investment in the equipment. Different anesthesiologic protocols and drugs have been proposed in the literature, but ketamine is the most commonly used drug alone (20 mg/kg IM) or preferably in association with medetomidine (5 mg/kg IM and 80 μg/kg IM, respectively). Other drugs associated in anesthetic protocols with ketamine include xylazine, diazepam, phenothiazine derivatives (e.g. acepromazine maleate), use of inhalation anesthetics (e.g. isoflurane or sevoflurane), or propofol have also been reported (Johnston *et al.*, 1988; Howard, 1992; Axnér and Linde-Forsberg., 2002; Chatdarong *et al.*, 2006; Zambelli *et al.*, 2007). The effect of medetomidine on the quality of electroejaculated sperm has been reported in a comparative study with ketamine (Zambelli *et al.*, 2007). The addition of medetomidine produced an ejaculate with higher number of sperm than after ketamine administration alone and provided good pharmacological restriction and adequate analgesia. In the same study, a high concentration of spermatozoa in urethra was observed after medetomidine administration; this important aspect has opened the doors to the introduction of a new method to collect seminal material: urethral catheterization after pharmacological induction (Zambelli *et al.*, 2006).

Medetomidine does not influence the percentage of sperm retrograde flow in the urinary bladder, a normal process during ejaculation in the cats (Dooley *et al.*, 1991). If medetomidine is not available, studies show that dexmedetomidine, at half dose of medetomidine, induces sedative, analgesic, and cardiorespiratory and body temperature effects comparable with those of medetomidine (Ansah *et al.*, 1998). An anesthetic protocol that includes 30–40 μg/kg of dexmedetomidine combined with 3–5 mg/kg ketamine IM is used by some US practitioners for semen collection by EE when medetomidine is not available (Johnson, 2018), but data about this topic has never been published. In our experience, use of inhalation anesthetics is associated with an increase of urine contamination during collection with EE. Effects of voltage, number of collections, and presence of sperm retrograde flow on seminal characteristics have been reported (Pineda and Dooley 1984; Pineda *et al.*, 1984; Dooley *et al.*, 1991). Volume and total number of sperm collected with EE are variable within and between cats. Voltage of stimulation and number of electrical stimuli appear to influence the number of sperm, but not the volume of ejaculate. It has been reported that stimulation between 0 and 1 V is the minimum threshold for release of accessory gland secretion. Voltages higher than 2 V but lower than 8 V (because of an increased risk of urine contamination) is the threshold for the maximal number of sperm in the ejaculate (Pineda and Dooley, 1984; Pineda *et al.*, 1984). Sperm motility and viability did not change in relation with voltage of stimulation, week of collection (in repeated collections), or method of sperm collection (EE versus AV) (Dooley and Pineda, 1986). For sperm collection with EE, an electro-ejaculator connected with a rectal probe (1 cm in diameter and 12 cm in length) is required, equipped with three longitudinal stainless-steel electrodes (Fig. 18.2). After inducing anesthesia, it is necessary to verify the absence of feces in the rectum which could be interposed between the mucosa and the electrodes. The glans portion of the penis should be cleaned using gauze moistened with saline. The lubricated probe, with electrodes oriented ventrally, is gently introduced into the rectum for 7–8 cm, then pushed ventrally on the urinary neck bladder to ensure a good contact with rectal mucosae and the pelvic plexus located dorsally to membranous urethra, between prostate and bulbourethral gland. The prepuce is retracted, the glans penis is exposed and introduced into a sterile Eppendorf tube before the start of the electrical protocol. Different electrical protocols have been reported in literature, but the one proposed by Howard *et al.* (1990) is the most used in the practice. It consists of a total of 80 stimuli divided into three sets (30, 30, and 20, respectively) with 2–3 minutes of rest between sets. In particular, the first set consists of ten stimuli at 2 V, ten at 3 V and ten at 4 V. The second set consists of ten stimuli at 3 V, ten at 4 V and ten at 5 V. The third set consists of ten stimuli at 4 V and ten at 5 V.

It is recommended to change tubes between each set of stimuli, because higher voltage can induce urine contamination, resulting in the loss of the entire sample. During the electrical stimulation, the male responds with a rigid and symmetric extension of both hind

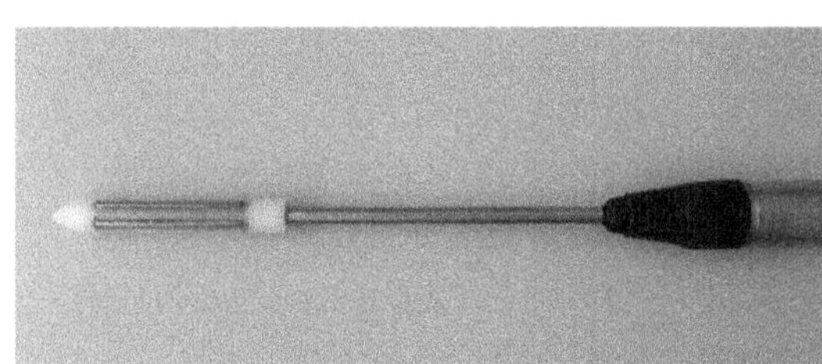

Fig. 18.2. The electroejaculation probe used by authors (Minitube®) has two electrodes, a diameter of 1.27 cm and a length of 6.35 cm. (Image: author's own.)

limbs. Assessing this extension is very important. Absent, weak, or asymmetrical movement of the hind limbs means that the contact between electrodes and rectal mucosae is not good and could be due to a wrong position of the rectal probe or in the interposition of fecal material.

18.2.3 Urethral catheterization after pharmacological induction (Ur.Ca.P.I.)

A new sperm collection technique described in the last decades (Zambelli *et al.*, 2006) allows clinicians the ability to overcome some of the most important disadvantages encountered with collection by AV and EE. Medetomidine or other alpha-2-adrenergic agonist administration in the cat may have similar effects also reported in other species. In the rat, the contraction of the vas deferens and the consequent release of sperm cells into the urethra without inducing ejaculation after alpha-2-adrenergic agonist administration has been reported (MacDonald and McGrath, 1980). In the stallion, administration of these medications can induce ejaculation (McDonnell and Odian, 1994) characterized by a low volume and extremely high sperm concentration ideal for freezing (Turner *et al.*, 1995). Ur.Ca.P.I. does not require any specific equipment (artificial vagina or electroejaculator) or training necessary for collection with AV and can be performed in any country without restrictions. In practice, this technique allows collection, evaluation, and use of sperm with reduced cost, additional equipment, and extensive training. Spermatozoa collected with Ur.Ca.P.I. can be cryopreserved (Zambelli *et al.*, 2008), used for *in vitro* fertilization (Zambelli *et al.*, 2008) or artificial fertilization (Zambelli *et al.*, 2015a,b). A peculiarity of this technique is to provide ejaculates with a small volume and very high concentration of spermatozoa (Zambelli *et al.*, 2006). This can be considered an advantage for artificial fertilization and *in vitro* procedures but requires very careful handling to avoid damage to the spermatozoa. Ur.Ca.P.I. allows retrieval of sperm that have the same or better quality than those obtained by epididymal slicing and which may be successfully cryopreserved. The quality of frozen-thawed sperm obtained with Ur.Ca.P.I. did not differ from that of cryopreserved epididymal spermatozoa.

A disadvantage of this technique, as for electroejaculation, is the need for heavy sedation before the collection. The dosage used for the collection is within the limits tested and reported by the manufacturer of the drug, and, in our experience, has never induced any type of animal health problem. Despite this, many anesthetists are reluctant to use the high dosage required and therefore do not recommend the method. The effects of high doses of medetomidine (0.13 mg/kg) used on healthy cats have been extensively studied. Although changes in systolic and diastolic heart function and systolic blood pressure were observed, they were not clinically relevant or dangerous for healthy cats. These changes are also observed using lower doses, therefore they must be considered intrinsic to the action of the molecule and not dose dependent. The dose of medetomidine used was well tolerated by all subjects (Romagnoli *et al.*, 2016).

The breeding subjects are also chosen based on their good physical conditions. In any case, as it is always advisable to do in case of anesthesia, it is advisable to perform a cardiological examination and exclude the use of subjects with cardiovascular diseases. The use of dexmedetomidine as an alternative to medetomidine for sperm collection is now reported due to the discontinuation of medetomidine. Cunto *et al.* (2019) reported two different dosages of both sedatives. High dosages of medetomidine (120 μg/kg) and dexmedetomidine (60 μg/kg) and low dosages of the two drugs (50 μg/kg and 25 μg/kg, respectively) were compared. It has been observed that at high dosages, both drugs allow the collection of sperm. It is noteworthy that slight movement of the caudal limbs during catheterization was observed in some animals receiving dexmedetomidine. The results with low dosages were both unsatisfactory for both sperm collection and sedation level. Use of low doses of dexmedetomidine (25 μg/kg) combined with ketamine (10 mg/kg) has been reported for Ur.Ca.P.I. in a study in which only three cats were enrolled, with results similar to those obtained using high dose of medetomidine (Swanson *et al.*, 2017). Three different sperm collection protocols were tested after medetomidine administration (130 μg/kg IM): immediately upon reaching the pharmacological effect of the drug, three times every 5 minutes after the pharmacological effect was reached, and 20 minutes after the pharmacological effect was reached. The results suggest that a single catheterization immediately after the onset of the pharmacological effect leads to good quality sperm without clinically detectable damage to the urethra (Cunto *et al.*, 2015). Although no clinical problems have been found, collection with three successive catheterizations could more easily induce urethral damage. For collection by Ur.Ca.P.I., an open-ended tomcat urinary catheter is used (Fig. 18.3). Catheterization is performed when level 5 of sedation is obtained (about 10–15 minutes after injection, depending on animal individual response to drug) using a numeric rating scale described by Carter *et al.* (2013), where zero stands for no sedation and five stands for lying in lateral recumbency and unresponsive.

The penis is exposed and the catheter is introduced gently and slowly into the urethra to a total depth of 9 cm in the domestic cat, pulling back the prepuce. This ensures that the tip of the catheter does not reach the bladder and collect urine. When the catheter has been fully introduced, it is removed immediately. Catheterization allows collection by capillarity action and sperm already present in the urethra after pharmacological effect enters the catheter rapidly. There is a risk of urine contamination if the catheter remains in the urethra for a prolonged period of time (several minutes). The sperm collected into the catheter by capillarity is flushed into an Eppendorf tube with an insulin syringe. Because of the simple collection procedure, the possibility of multiple collection from the same male and the ability to obtain high-quality sperm samples makes Ur.Ca.P.I. a good method of collection for sperm banking. Unsuccessful semen collection (no spermatozoa in the catheter or visible urine contamination) is possible in 1.7–8% (Zambelli *et al.*, 2008; Prochowska *et al.*, 2016).

18.3 Sperm Evaluation

This is a tool that represents the cornerstone of the diagnostic process for the evaluation of male fertility. It permits the ability to establish the quality of spermatozoa including morphology, total number,

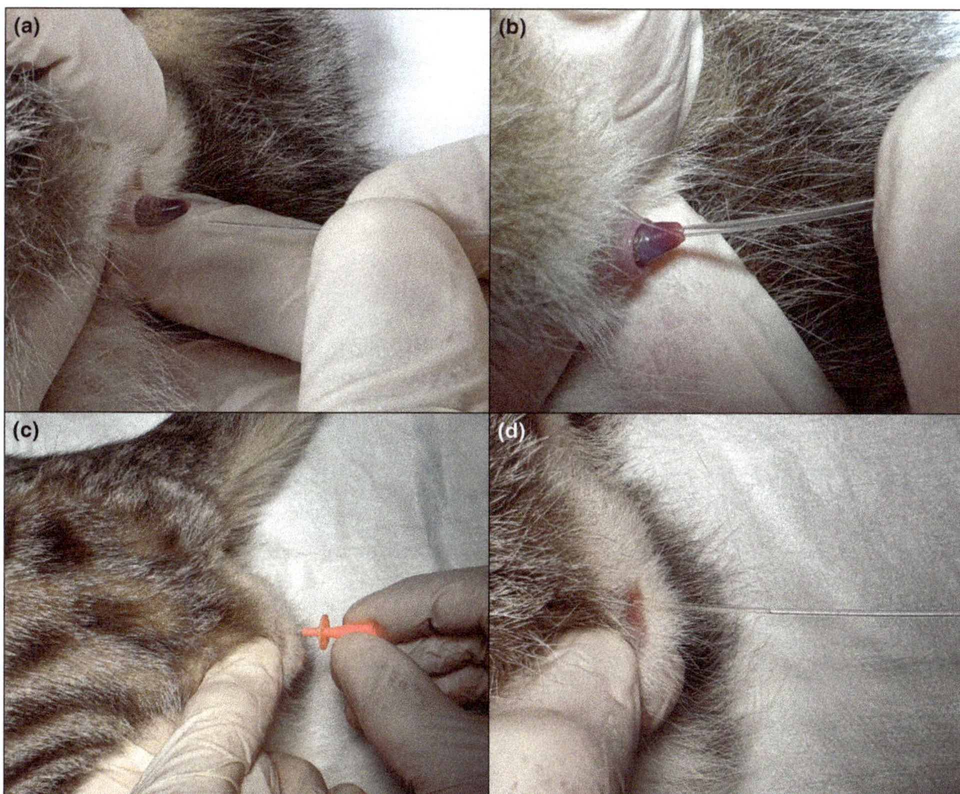

Fig. 18.3. Ur.Ca.P.I. semen collection. **(a)** An open-ended tomcat urinary catheter is used. **(b)** The penis is exposed and the catheter is introduced into the urethra to a total depth of 9 cm, pulling back the prepuce **(c)**. **(d)** When the catheter has been fully introduced, it is removed immediately. (Images: author's own.)

motility, and other parameters. However, even if sperm quality is excellent, fertility cannot be guaranteed since many of the functional characteristics that contribute to fertility are still not well known today (Rodríguez-Martínez, 2003). Sperm quality can also be affected by external factors such as method of collection, environmental conditions, or handling techniques. Sperm must be handled carefully to avoid causing damage to the sperm. The low volume of the feline ejaculate is the biggest limitation to a full evaluation because of difficulty maintaining constant environmental parameters (temperature, protection form light, etc.). Moreover, when sperm is needed for fertilization or preservation, the low volume may not allow the clinician enough material for a complete examination. The clinician can improve skills with manipulation and evaluation of small volumes of ejaculate by practicing using sperm obtained through epididymal squeezing or slicing after routine cat orchiectomies.

Depending on low volume and high concentration of sperm collected, dilution of a little sample could be necessary in order to permit a correct evaluation and to dispose of an adequate amount of material without use of an excessive part of ejaculate. Tris-glucose-citrate and TALP have been reported for this purpose (Zambelli *et al.*, 2008; Buranaamnuay, 2013).

A basic spermiogram should include the evaluation of macroscopic parameters such as appearance and volume, and microscopic parameters such as motility, morphology, and viability. Additional tests may include the evaluation of pH, osmolarity, sperm culture, membrane integrity, acrosomal integrity, and seminal chemistry.

Macroscopic parameters

Semen should appear homogeneous and creamy white. Samples that appear with traces of blood (appear pink), inflammation, or urine (sample smells of urine) should alert the clinician to fully examine the animal. Volume of the ejaculate can be assessed with a variable volume calibrated pipette to obtain an accurate volume in microliters.

Microscopic parameters

To allow a larger volume to be available for evaluation, extender may be added after the initial ejaculate volume is obtained. Motility of the sperm can be evaluated subjectively using a phase-contrast microscope at 400× magnification and a prewarmed slide or objectively using a computer-assisted sperm analysis (CASA). Motility is expressed as percent total motility (TMOT), percent progressive motility (PMOT), or sperm motility index that provides an overall estimate of sperm motility characteristics calculated using the formula [% TMOT + (PMOT x 20): 2)] (Howard *et al.*, 1990). Using a phase-contrast microscope (preferably with a warming stage), a small drop of ejaculate (2–3 µL) is placed on a warmed slide with a coverslip. The TMOT is determined by the percentage of sperm moving. Progressive motility is determined by the percentage of total sperm that are moving in a straight line. Development of CASA allows the objective evaluation of sperm motility, giving detailed motion characteristics such as the percentage of motile spermatozoa (TMOT, %); the percentage of spermatozoa with a PMOT, %); average path velocity (VAP, mm/s); straight line velocity (VSL, mm/s); curvilinear velocity (VCL, mm/s); amplitude of lateral head displacement (ALH, mm); beat cross-frequency (Hz); the straightness (STR, %); and the linearity (LIN, %) (Contri *et al.*, 2012; Prochowska *et al.*, 2016).

Morphologic assessment can be performed using a phase-contrast microscope. Sperm fixed with a formole-saline solution (Axnér *et al.*, 1999) can be counted and, if necessary, stored for several months while maintaining the morphology of the spermatozoa and their defects. Sperm staining allows a simpler morphological evaluation even if many techniques can create artifacts that influence the count of anomalies. Different staining methods, such as air-dried stain (Giemsa-Wright) or wet stain (eosin-nigrosin), and conventional light microscopy can also be used to determine the proportions of normal and abnormal spermatozoa (Perez-Marin *et al.*, 2016) (Fig. 18.4). Fast green FCF-rose Bengal staining allows good differentiation of the sperm structures and induces a low number of artifacts (Zambelli *et al.*, 1993). For each sample, at least 100–200 sperm should be counted at 1000× magnification (oil). For a complete evaluation, morphologic abnormalities of heads, acrosomes, midpieces, and sperm tails should be considered. In literature, different methods to count the sperm anomalies have been reported. Sperm are divided into normal and abnormal, and the last ones classified on the basis of their anomaly: proximal droplet, head abnormalities, acrosome abnormalities, midpiece defects, distal droplet, bent tail, detached head, and coiled tail. If a sperm has more than one abnormality,

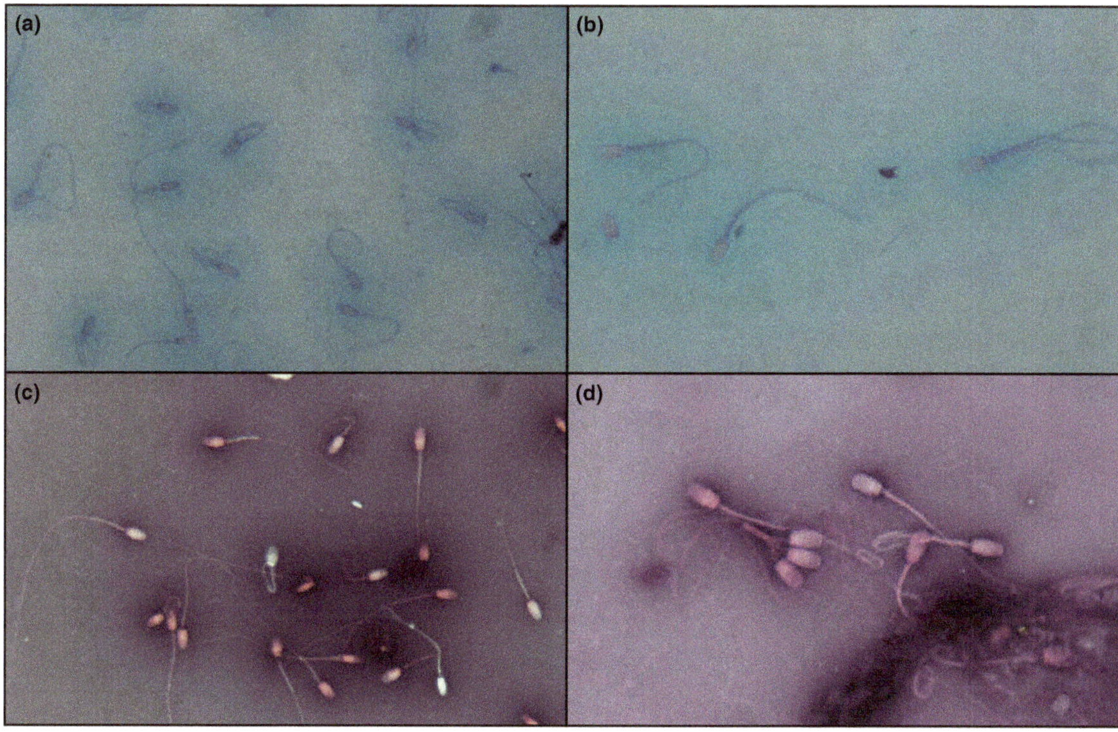

Fig. 18.4. Two spermatozoa staining methods: **(a)** and **(b)** fast green FCF – rose Bengal stain is suggested for a good sperm structure differentiation and sperm abnormalities evaluation. **(c)** and **(d)** Eosin-nigrosin stain is used for viability evaluation (live sperm are white, dead sperm are pink) and for normal and abnormal spermatozoa determination. (Images: author's own.)

some researchers consider only the most important defect while other clinicians count all the anomalies in a single sperm so the total percentage may be higher than 100 while the total cells counted are a consistent 100 cells.

In the literature, two useful indices to evaluate sperm defects are reported: the Teratozoospermia Index (TZI) (Menkveld and Kruger, 1996) and the Sperm Deformity Index (SDI) (Aziz *et al.*, 1996). The TZI is an indication of how many defects, including head abnormality, neck/midpiece abnormality, tail abnormality, or the presence of a cytoplasmic droplet, are present simultaneously per abnormal sperm. The total number of abnormalities recorded are added together and divided by the total number of abnormal sperm. TZI can range from 1 to 4 and this means that one spermatozoon can contain a single defect, or a combination of two, three, or all four defects simultaneously. The SDI is defined as the average number of defects per sperm evaluated. In human medicine, it has been reported that SDI is a more reliable predictor of the outcome of *in vitro* fertilization (higher sensitivity, specificity, positive predictive value, and negative predictive value) than the percentage of normal sperm morphology (Aziz *et al.*, 1996). The SDI is calculated by dividing the total number of anomalies counted from the total sperm count (normal plus abnormal) randomly selected and evaluated for this count. Acrosome integrity is one of the determinant factors of the success of fertilization. Only acrosome-intact spermatozoa are able to penetrate the zona pellucida and fuse with oocyte plasma membrane. It can be determined after staining with pisum sativum agglutinin conjugated with fluorescein isothiocyanate (FITC) and evaluated under a fluorescence microscopy (Filliers *et al.*, 2010). In the practice sperm viability and morphology can be assessed with eosin-nigrosin stain (Zambelli *et al.*, 1993). Sperm concentration (expressed in million sperm per mL) is determined after diluting an aliquot of the sample in formol–saline with a ratio based on concentration of sperm collected and counting the spermatozoa in a hemocytometer chamber or a Bürker counting chamber with a final density of 6–7 spermatozoa/field, under a phase-contrast microscope. Once total volume and concentration are determined, the total number of spermatozoa obtained can be calculated (volume x concentration).

Mean values of osmolality and pH of seminal plasma, prostatic and bulbourethral fluid, and prostatic fluid were reported to be 323, 327, and 331 mOsm/L (osmolality) and 6.6, 6.7, and 7.8 (pH), respectively (Johnston *et al.*, 1988). The biochemical characterization of seminal plasma is poorly reported in the literature due to the difficulty of performing these analyses on very small volumes of ejaculate. Johnston *et al.* (1988) evaluated the characteristics of seminal plasma, prostate, and bulbourethral gland sample. They reported that the secretion of the bulbourethral glands is preponderant, the pH of the prostatic secretion is alkaline, and that alkaline phosphatase in the ejaculate originates from the testis and/or epididymis. The characteristics of sperm can vary in relation to the collection method used. The ejaculate collected with an AV is certainly similar to what is deposited in the vagina during natural mating. On the contrary, EE, by causing greater stimulation of the accessory glands, induces a higher volume of ejaculate than that collected with AV. Finally, Ur.Ca.P.I. provides sperm with reduced volume due to minimal accessary gland contribution. Table 18.1 shows the mean values of the sperm collected with AV, EE and Ur.Ca.P.I. If further diagnostics are desired, a sample of the sperm can be submitted to a specialized laboratory for transmission electron microscope analysis or fluorescence microscope using different fluorescent probes; in particular isothiocyanate conjugated peanut agglutinin (FITC-PNA) and fluorophores EthD-1 and SYBR-14 probes can be used respectively for acrosomal status and plasma membrane integrity evaluation (Axnér *et al.*, 2004).

18.4 Sperm Dosage and Site for Artificial Insemination

Using fresh sperm, intravaginal insemination doses with 20 × 10^6, 40 × 10^6, and 80 × 10^6 spermatozoa have been reported to obtain conception rates of 6.6, 33.3, and 77.8%, respectively (Tanaka *et al.*, 2000a). The higher insemination dose was comparable to the number of sperm collected with two consecutive ejaculations (Tanaka *et al.*, 2000b) and could be justified considering cats copulate several times during estrus, probably to ensure high sperm dosage (Tanaka *et al.*, 2000a). Tsutsui *et al.* (2000a) reported a conception rate of 80.0% by surgical insemination of 8 × 10^6 fresh sperm into one uterine horn. The ratio of ten times the number of sperms needed for high fertilization rates for intravaginal (80 × 10^6) versus intrauterine (8 × 10^6) insemination is the same reported for the dog (Tsutsui *et al.*, 1988, 1989).

Conception after artificial intrauterine insemination using 2.4–19.2 × 10^6 fresh sperm was also reported (Howard *et al.*, 1992). In particular, for transcervical uterine insemination, a dose of 200 μL of fresh or frozen-thawed semen containing 10 × 10^6 or 30 × 10^6 motile sperm, respectively, was compared and a conception rate of 100% was obtained in queens where transcervical catheterization was possible (Zambelli and Cunto, 2005). Successful uterine endoscopic transcervical insemination has been reported in three queens using 8.1–53.3 × 10^6 of fresh spermatozoa collected by Ur.Ca.P.I. In the last case, each queen was inseminated twice and conception rate was 100% (Zambelli *et al.*, 2015a,b).

Table 18.1. Characteristics of cat semen collected by artificial vagina (AV), electroejaculation (EE), and urethral catheterization after pharmacological induction (Ur.Ca.P.I.). Values in table represent ranges of means reported by several authors. Superscript numbers indicate references: 1 = Sojka *et al.* (1970); 2 = Dooley and Pineda (1986); 3 = Platz and Seager (1978); 4 = Platz *et al.* (1978); 5 = Jelinkova *et al.* (2018); 6 = Howard *et al.* (1990); 7 = Zambelli and Cunto (2006); 8= Zambelli *et al.* (2006); 9 = Prochowska *et al.* (2015); 10 = Cunto *et al.* (2015).

Technique	Motility (%) Progressively motile sperm	Motility (%) Total motility	Forward progressive motility (1–5)	Volume (μl)	Concentration (10^6 × mL)	Total number of spermatozoa (10^6)
AV	58–82 [1,2,3]			34–60 [1,2,3]	57–60.97 [1,2,3]	
EE	60–84.4 [2,4,5,6]	78.1–91.11 [8,9]	4.5–5 [1,2,4]	67.1–260 [2,4,5,6,8]	28–542.9 [2,4,5,6,8]	19.11–33.6 [5,7,8]
Ur.Ca.P.I.	34.1–46.06 [5,9]	63.0–78.1 [8,9,10]	4.2–4.7 [9,10]	10.5–21.06 [5,8,9,10]	412.6–3257.8 [5,8,9,10]	5.36–47.7 [5,8,9,10]

Table 18.2. Characteristics of cat semen used for vaginal or intrauterine artificial insemination and relative conception rates in queens inseminated with fresh or frozen-thawed semen.

Semen	Total number of spermatozoa (10^6)	Volume (μl)	Site of insemination	Conception rate (%)	Author
Fresh	5	100	Intravaginal	42.9	Sojka *et al.* (1970)
Fresh	80	50–100	Intravaginal	77.8	Tanaka *et al.* (2000a)
Frozen	50–100	100	Intravaginal	10.6	Platz *et al.* (1978)
Fresh	4.2–7.5	200	Bilateral intrauterine (surgical)	34.4	Howard *et al.* (1992)
Fresh	8	30	Unilateral intrauterine (surgical)	80	Tsutsui *et al.* (2000a)
Fresh	50	30	Unilateral intrauterine (surgical)	57.1	Tsutsui *et al.* (2000b)
Fresh	10	200	Intrauterine (transcervical)	100[a]	Zambelli and Cunto (2005)
Frozen	30	200	Intrauterine (transcervical)	100[a]	Zambelli *et al.* (2005)
Fresh	8.1–53.3	18–32	Intrauterine (endoscopic transcervical)	100	Zambelli *et al.* (2015a,b)

[a]Conception rate in queens where transcervical insemination was possible.

Numerous reports subsequently reported varying conception rates with different doses of fresh or frozen semen (Platz *et al.*, 1978; Howard *et al.*, 1992; Tsutsui *et al.*, 2000a,b) (Table 18.2).

18.5 References

Ansah, O. B., Raekallio, M., and Vainio, O. (1998) Comparison of three doses of dexmedetomidine with medetomidine in cats following intramuscular administration. *Journal of Veterinary Pharmacology and Therapeutics* 21, 380–387. doi: 10.1046/j.1365-2885.1998.00155.x

Axnér, E. and Linde-Forsberg, C. (2002) Semen collection and assessment, and artificial insemination in the cat. In: Concannon, P. W., England, G., Verstegen, J., and Linde-Forsberg, C. (eds) *Recent Advances in Small Animal Reproduction*. International Veterinary Information Service, Ithaca, New York.

Axnér, E., Linde-Forsberg, C., and Einarsson, S. (1999) Morphology and motility of spermatozoa from different regions if the epididymal duct in the domestic cat. *Theriogenology* 52, 767–778. doi: 10.1016/S0093-691X(99)00170-3

Axnér, E., Hermansson, U., and Linde-Forsberg, C. (2004) The effect of Equex STM paste and sperm morphology on post-thaw survival of cat epididymal spermatozoa. *Animal Reproduction Science* 84, 179-191. doi: 10.1016/j.anireprosci.2003.11.003

Aziz, N., Buchan, I., Taylor, C., Kingsland, C. R., and Lewis-Jones, I. (1996) The sperm deformity index: a reliable predictor of the outcome of oocyte fertilization in vitro. *Fertility and Sterility* 66, 1000–1008. doi: 10.1016/S0015-0282(16)58697-X

Bowen, R.A. (1977) Fertilization in vitro of feline ova by spermatozoa from ductus deferens. *Biology of Reproduction* 17, 144–147. doi: 10.1095/biolreprod17.1.144

Buranaamnuay, K. (2013) Sperm-TALP: An alternative extender for retrieving and diluting epididymal sperm in the domestic cat. *Reproduction in Domestic Animals* 48, 912–917. doi: 10.1111/rda.12185

Carter, J. E., Lewis, C., and Beths T. (2013) Onset and quality of sedation after intramuscular administration of dexmedetomidine and hydromorphone in various muscle groups in dogs. *Journal of the American Veterinary Medical Association* 243, 1569–1572. doi: 10.2460/javma.243.11.1569

Chatdarong, K., Ponglowhapan, S., Manee-in, S., and Pongphet, K. (2006) The use of propofol for electroejaculation in domestic cats. *Theriogenology* 66, 1615–1617. doi: 10.1016/j.theriogenology.2006.01.006

Contri. A, Zambelli, D., Faustini, M., Cunto, M., Gloria, A., *et al.* (2012) Artificial neural networks for the definition of kinetic subpopulations in electroejaculated and epididymal spermatozoa in the domestic cat. *Reproduction* 144, 339–347. doi: 10.1530/REP-12-0125

Cunto, M., Küster, D. G., Bini, C., Pietra, M., and Zambelli, D. (2015) Influence of different protocols of urethral catheterization after pharmacological induction (Ur.Ca.P.I.) on semen quality in the domestic cat. *Reproduction in Domestic Animals* 50, 999–1002. doi: 10.1111/rda.12626

Cunto, M., Mariani, E., Ballotta, G., Anicito Guido, E., and Zambelli, D. (2018) Influence of two anesthesiological protocols on quality of cat semen collected by urethral catheterization after pharmacological induction (Ur.Ca.P.I.). In: *Proceedings of the 21st European Veterinary Society for Small Animal Reproduction (EVSSAR) Congress*. Venice, Italy, pp. 103.

Cunto, M., Anicito Guido, E., Ballotta, G., and Zambelli, D. (2019) Effect of medetomidine and dexmedetomidine administration at different dosages on cat semen quality using urethral catheterization after pharmacological induction (Ur.Ca.P.I.). *Reproduction in Domestic Animals* 54, 96–97.

Dooley, M. P. and Pineda, M. H. (1986) Effect of method of collection on seminal characteristics of the domestic cat. *American Journal of Veterinary Research* 47, 286–292.

Dooley, M. P., Pineda, M. H., Hopper, J. G., and Hsu, W. H. (1991) Retrograde flow of spermatozoa into urinary bladder of cat during electroejaculation, collection of semen with an artificial vagina, and mating. *American Journal of Veterinary Research* 52, 687–691.

Filliers, M., Rijsselaere, T., Bossaert, P., Zambelli, D., Anastasi, P., *et al.* (2010) In vitro evaluation of fresh sperm quality in tomcats: a comparison of two collection techniques. *Theriogenology* 74(1), 31–39. doi: 10.1016/j.theriogenology.2009.12.016

Furthner, E., Cordonnier, N., Le Dudal, M., Fontbonne, A., and Freiche, V. (2018) Is electroejaculation a safe procedure in cats? An endoscopic and histological prospective blinded study. *Theriogenology* 119, 69–75. doi: 10.1016/j.theriogenology.2018.06.013

Gunn, R. M. C. (1936) Fertility in sheep: Artificial production of seminal ejaculation and the characters of the spermatozoa contained therein. In: *Bulletin for Council Scientific Industrial Research*. Melbourne: Government Printer, Melbourne, Australia, pp 1–116.

Hay, M. and Goodrowe, K. (1993) Comparative cryopreservation and capacitation of spermatozoa from epididymis and vasa deferentia of domestic cat. *Journal of Reproduction and Fertility* 47, 297–305.

Horne, H. W., Paull, D. P., and Munro, D. (1948) Fertility studies in the human male with traumatic injuries of the spinal cord and cauda equina. *Journal of Medicine* 239, 959–961. doi: 10.1056/NEJM194812162392504

Howard, J. G. (1992) Feline semen analysis and artificial insemination. In: Kirk, R. W. and Bonagura, J. D. (eds) *Kirk's Current Veterinary Therapy XI: Small Animal Practice.* W.B. Saunders, Philadelphia, Pennsylvania, pp. 929–938.

Howard, J. G., Brown, J. L., Bush, M., and Wildt, D. E. (1990) Teratospermic and normospermic domestic cats: ejaculate traits, pituitary-gonadal hormones, and improvement of spermatozoa motility and morphology after swim up processing. *Journal of Andrology* 11, 204–215. doi: 10.1002/j.1939-4640.1990.tb03229.x

Howard, J. G., Barone, M. A., Donoghue, A. M., and Wildt, D. E. (1992) The effect of pre-ovulatory anaesthesia on ovulation in laparoscopically inseminated domestic cat. *Journal of Reproduction and Fertility* 96, 175–186. doi: 10.1530/jrf.0.0960175

Jelinkova, K., Vitasek, R., Novotny, R., and Bartoskova, A. (2018) A comparison of quality parameters of fresh feline ejaculates collected by three different collection techniques. *Reproduction in Domestic Animals* 53, 1068–1074. doi: 10.1111/rda.13205

Johnson, A. K. (2018) Assisted reproduction in the male cat. *Veterinary Clinics of North America: Small Animal Practice* 48, 511–521. doi: 10.1016/j.cvsm.2018.02.001

Johnston, S. D., Osborne, C. A., Lipowitz, A. J. (1988) Characterization of seminal plasma, prostatic fluid and bulbourethral gland secretions in the domestic cat. In: *Proceedings of the 11th International Congress Animal Reproduction and Artificial Insemination*, vol IV, pp. 560.

Johnstone, I. P. (1984) Electroejaculation in domestic cat. *Australian Veterinary Journal* 61, 155–158. doi: 10.1111/j.1751-0813.1984.tb07220.x

MacDonald, A. and McGrath, J. C. (1980) The distribution of adrenoreceptors and other drug receptors between the two ends of the rat vas deferens as revealed by selective agonists and antagonists. *British Journal of Pharmacology* 71, 445–458. doi: 10.1111/j.1476-5381.1980.tb10957.x

McDonnell, S. M. and Odian, M. J. (1994) Imipramine and xylazine-induced ex copula ejaculation in stallions. *Theriogenology* 41, 1005–1010. doi: 10.1016/S0093-691X(05)80023-8

Menkveld, R. and Kruger, F. T. (1996) Basic semen analysis. In: Acosta, A.A. and Kruger, T.F. (eds), *Human Spermatozoa in Assisted Reproduction*. Parthenon Publishing, Carnforth, UK, pp. 53–71.

Perez-Marin, C. C., Jimenez, E., and Aguera, E. (2016) Choice of staining technique affects the morphological assessment of epididymal feline sperm. *Veterinarni Medicina* 61, 560–566.

Pineda, M. H. and Dooley, M. P. (1984) Effect of voltage and order of voltage application on seminal characteristics of electroejaculates of the domestic cat. *American Journal of Veterinary Research* 45, 1520–1525.

Pineda, M. H., Dooley, M. P., and Martin, P. A. (1984) Long term study on the effects of electroejaculation on seminal characteristics of the domestic cat. *American Journal of Veterinary Research* 45, 1038–4010.

Platz, C. C. and Seager, S. W. J. (1978) Semen collection by electroejaculation in the domestic cat. *Journal of the American Veterinary Medical Association* 173, 1353–1355.

Platz, C. C., Fallis, T., Demorest, N., and Seager, S. W. J. (1976) Semen collection, freezing and insemination in the domestic cat. In: *Proceedings of the 8th International Congress on Animal Reproduction and Artificial Insemination*, vol. IV, pp. 1053–1056.

Platz, C. C., Wildt, D. E., and Seager S. W. J. (1978) Pregnancy in the domestic cat after artificial insemination with previously frozen spermatozoa. *Journal of Reproduction and Fertilitiy* 52, 279–282. doi: 10.1530/jrf.0.0520279

Prochowska, S., Niżański, W., Ochota, M., and Partyka, A. (2015) Characteristics of urethral and epididymal semen collected from domestic cats – A retrospective study of 214 cases. *Theriogenology* 84, 1565–1571. doi: 10.1016/j.theriogenology.2015.08.005

Prochowska, S., Nizanski, W., and Partyka, A. (2016) Comparative analysis of in vitro characteristics of fresh and frozen-thawed urethral and epididymal spermatozoa from cats (*Felis domesticus*). *Theriogenology* 86, 2063–2072. doi: 10.1016/j.theriogenology.2016.07.002

Rodríguez-Martínez, H. (2003) Laboratory semen assessment and prediction of fertility: still utopia?

Reproduction in Domestic Animals 38, 312–318. doi: 10.1046/j.1439-0531.2003.00436.x

Romagnoli, N., Zambelli, D., Cunto, M., Lambertini, C., Ventrella, D., *et al.* (2016) Non-invasive evaluation of the haemodynamic effects of high-dose medetomidine in healthy cats for semen collection. *Journal of Feline Medicine and Surgery* 18, 337–343. doi: 10.1177/1098612X15583345

Romagnoli, N., Lambertini, C., Zambelli, D., Cunto, M., *et al.* (2020) Plasma concentration rise after the intramuscular administration of high dose medetomidine (0.13 mg/kg) for semen collection in cats. *Veterinary Sciences* 7, 17. doi: 10.3390/vetsci7010017

Scott, P. (1970) Cats. In: Hafez, E. S. E. (ed.). *Reproduction and Breeding Techniques for Laboratory Animals*. Lea and Febiger, Philadelphia, Pennsylvania, p. 205.

Sojka, N. J. (1986) Management of artificial breeding in cats. In: Morrow, D. A., (ed.) *Current Therapy in Theriogenology: Diagnosis, Treatment and Prevention of Reproductive Diseases in Large and Small Animals*, 2nd edn. W.B. Saunders, Philadelphia, Pennsylvania, pp. 805–808.

Sojka, N. J., Jennings, L. L., and Hamner, C. E. (1970) Artificial insemination in the cat (*Felis catus* L.). *Laboratory Animal Care* 20, 198–204.

Swanson, W. F., Bateman, H. L., and Vansandt, L. M. (2017) Urethral catheterization and sperm vitrification for simplified semen banking in felids. *Reproduction in Domestic Animals* 52, 255–260. doi: 10.1111/rda.12863

Tanaka, A., Takagi, Y., Nakagawa, K., Fujimoto, Y., Hori, T., *et al.* (2000a) Artificial intravaginal insemination using fresh semen in cats. *Journal of Veterinary Medical Science* 62, 1163–1167. doi: 10.1292/jvms.62.1163

Tanaka, A., Kuwabara, S., Takagi, Y., Nakagawa, K., Fujimoto, Y., *et al.* (2000b) Effect of ejaculation intervals on semen quality in cats. *Journal of Veterinary Medical Science* 62, 1157–1161. doi: 10.1292/jvms.62.1157

Tsutsui, T., Tezuka, T., Shimizu, T., Murao, I., Kawakami, E., *et al.* (1988) Artificial insemination with fresh semen in beagle bitches. *The Japanese Journal of Veterinary Science* 50, 193–198. doi: 10.1292/jvms1939.50.193

Tsutsui, T., Shimizu, T., Ohara, N., Shiba, Y., Hironaka, T., *et al.* (1989) Relationship between the number of sperms and the rate of implantation in bitches inseminated into unilateral uterine horn. *The Japanese Journal of Veterinary Science* 51, 257–263. doi: 10.1292/jvms1939.51.257

Tsutsui, T., Tanaka, A., Takagi, Y., Nakagawa, K., Fujimoto, Y., *et al.* (2000a) Unilateral intrauterine horn insemination of fresh semen in cats. *Journal of Veterinary Medical Science* 62, 1241–1245. doi: 10.1292/jvms.62.1241

Tsutsui, T., Tanaka, A., Takagi, Y., Nakagawa, K., Fujimoto, Y., *et al.* (2000b) Unilateral intrauterine horn insemination of frozen semen in cats. *Journal of Veterinary Medical Science* 62, 1247–1251. doi: 10.1292/jvms.62.1247

Turner, R. M., McDonnell, S. M., and Hawkins, J. F. (1995) Use of pharmacologically induced ejaculation to obtain semen from a stallion with a fractured radius. *Journal of the American Veterinary Medical Association* 206, 1906–1908.

Yu, I. and Leibo, S. P. (2002) Recovery of motile, membrane intact spermatozoa from canine epididymis stored for 8 days at 4 degrees C. *Theriogenology* 57, 1179–90. doi: 10.1016/s0093-691x(01)00711-7

Zambelli, D. and Cunto, M. (2005) Transcervical artificial insemination in the cat. *Theriogenology* 64, 698–705. doi: 10.1016/j.theriogenology.2005.05.020

Zambelli, D. and Cunto, M. (2006) Semen collection in cats: Techniques and analysis. *Theriogenology* 66, 159–165. doi: 10.1016/j.theriogenology.2006.01.054

Zambelli, D., Bergonzoni, M. L., De Fanti, C., and Carluccio, A. (1993) Techniques for cat, dog and rabbit spermatozoa morphologic evaluation *Proceedings of XLVII S.I.S. Vet* (Italian Society of Veterinary Sciences). *Congress Riccione*, pp. 279–283.

Zambelli, D., Prati, F., Merlo, B., and Cunto, M. (2006) Collection of semen by urethral catheterization after pharmacologically induced spermatozoa releasing in the domestic cat. In: *Proceedings of 5th Biannual Congress*, European Veterinary Society for Small Animal Reproduction (EVSSAR), Budapest, p. 300.

Zambelli, D., Cunto, M., Prati, F., and Merlo, B. (2007) Effects of ketamine or medetomidine administration on quality of electroejaculated sperm and on sperm flow in the domestic cat. *Theriogenology* 68, 796–803. doi: 10.1016/j.theriogenology.2007.06.008

Zambelli, D., Prati, F., Cunto, M., Iacono, E., and Merlo, B. (2008) Quality and in vitro fertilizing ability of cryopreserved cat spermatozoa obtained by urethral catheterization after medetomidine administration. *Theriogenology* 69, 485–490. doi: 10.1016/j.theriogenology.2007.10.019

Zambelli, D., Raccagni, R., Cunto, M., Andreani, G., and Isani, G. (2010) Sperm evaluation and biochemical characterization of cat seminal plasma collected by electroejaculation and urethral catheterization. *Theriogenology* 74, 1396–1402. doi: 10.1016/j.theriogenology.2010.06.011

Zambelli, D., Bini, C., and Cunto, M. (2015a) Endoscopic transcervical catheterization in the domestic cat. *Reproduction in Domestic Animals* 50, 13–16. doi: 10.1111/rda.12442

Zambelli, D., Bini, C., Küster, D. G., Molari, V., and Cunto, M. (2015b) First deliveries after estrus induction using deslorelin and endoscopic transcervical insemination in the queen. *Theriogenology* 84(5), 773–778. doi: 10.1016/j.theriogenology.2015.05.010

19 Causes of Infertility in the Tom

Cristina Gobello

Director Center of Reproductive Physiology, Veterinary Sciences, National University of La Plata and National Research Council, La Plata, Argentina

19.1 Introduction

With the increasing interest in breeding purebred cats, the requests to investigate cases of reproductive failure have become more frequent. In comparison to female cat infertility, male cat infertility has been less described in the literature. A systematic approach, including a detailed history and physical examination with ancillary tests, can lead to a diagnosis in most cases. Therapy should only be initiated if a definitive diagnosis has been established. Indiscriminate use of 'fertility drugs' is usually ineffective and potentially dangerous. The aim of this chapter is to guide the clinician through the systematic approach used to achieve a definitive diagnosis and determine the appropriate treatment options for cases of infertility in tom cats.

19.2 Signalment and History

The signalment of the affected cat (age, breed, color pattern) should be used for correct interpretation of the presenting complaint. Very young and old male cats may have a reduced fertility. Certain breeds (e.g. Persians) are prone to a higher incidence of reproductive problems (Axnér *et al.*, 1996). The calico (black, white, and orange) or tortoiseshell (black and orange) coat patterns can be associated with an abnormal karyotype (Fig. 19.1; Table 19.1) (Centerwall and Benirschke, 1975).

As discussed in Chapter 4, information pertaining to any change in husbandry (e.g. housing, new animals, medications, diet supplements, vaccinations, exposure to environmental toxins, shows, travel, etc.) should be gathered. In addition, general health history (illness, hyperthermia, or fever) and results from previous laboratory tests should be recorded. The development of infertility in relation to husbandry changes or health disorders should be carefully evaluated. Testicular infertility problems do not typically appear simultaneously with insults but rather after at least one spermatic cycle (approximately 47 days; Franca and Godinho, 2003). Furthermore, these problems may also take more than one cycle to reverse. Conversely, infertility from epididymal insults may be apparent in less than one or two weeks.

A complete reproductive history with special attention to mating frequency, breeding practices, and previous reproductive problems in the tom or any of his relatives is also important to record. Finally, the coefficient of inbreeding (COI) should be calculated using pedigree analyses as this may explain infertility in some cases.

19.3 Physical Examination

A complete physical examination should be performed before focusing on the reproductive tract. Special attention should be given to determine if there is ongoing concurrent disease (e.g. urinary tract infection or dermatological problems suggestive of endocrine diseases).

A careful evaluation of the genital tract should be performed. The scrotal skin should be examined for dermatitis or lesions (e.g. wounds, scars). The testes should be firm and resilient in consistency and smooth in texture. Palpable abnormalities (e.g. hard, soft or lumpy testes) warrant additional investigation. Soft and small testes are correlated with abnormal spermatogenesis and may be indicative of testicular degeneration. Epididymides are difficult to individualize unless they are enlarged due to inflammation or obstructions. The skin of the prepuce should also be normal with a clean orifice. The penis should have a pink mucosa with small, keratinized spicules in mature non-castrated cats. In these cats, the penis should be easily extruded from the prepuce.

DOI: 10.1079/9781789247107.0019

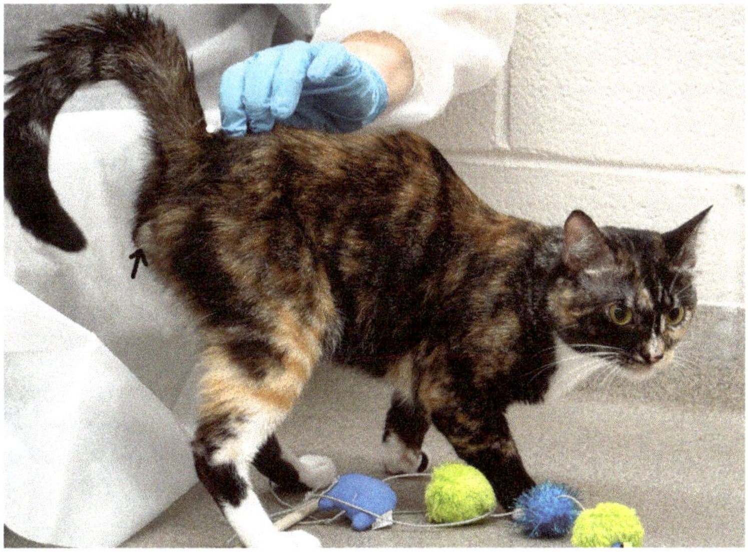

Fig. 19.1. A calico male. The coat color is a combination of orange and black, both carried on the X chromosome. This cat is a male making him genetically XXY (arrow showing the testicles). (Photo courtesy of Dr Aime Johnson.)

Table 19.1. Infertility of the male cat. (Table: author's own.)

Categories	Desired information
Date	
Owner	
Presenting Complaint	
Signalment	Name
	Breed
	Age
	Body weight
	Coat
History	General health
	Reproductive history
Physical examination	General examination
	Reproductive examination: testes, epididymis, prepuce, penis
Ancillary tests	
Diagnosis	
Therapy	

The impossibility to achieve this maneuver indicates sexual immaturity or a persistent frenulum. If possible, the owner should provide an estrus female so that the act of mating can be observed to determine what functional problems may exist.

19.4 Causes of Infertility

Infertility can arise from congenital or acquired causes. If previous litters were never produced by the tom cat, congenital etiologies should be suspected. If infertility appears later in life, then acquired causes are more likely. From a practical point of view, tom cat infertility can be categorized as: (i) poor or lack of libido; (ii) inability to mate; and (iii) failure to produce litters after mating.

19.4.1 Poor or lack of libido

Poor libido can be due to generalized illness or psychological causes. For instance, stress caused by strange surroundings or social changes can cause a temporary decrease in libido (Long, 1979). Dominant queens can also diminish the male sex drive.

9.4.2. Inability to mate

When a tom shows good libido but fails to copulate successfully, then dental, locomotor, and penile problems should be considered. Pelvic or lumbar back pain may prevent intromission. Because the tom bites the back of the queen's neck during coitus, severe gingivitis may prevent female immobilization and penile penetration. On occasion, size differences between the tom and queen can prevent intromission. Penile and preputial problems (e.g. persistent penile frenulum, phimosis, paraphimosis, priapism) are covered in Chapter 22.

19.4.3 Failure to produce litters after mating

Failure to produce litters after mating can be caused by incorrect management, retrograde ejaculation, or primary testicular problems (covered in Chapter 20). Administration of glucocorticoids, ketoconazole, chemotherapeutic agents, or sexual hormones like androgens, progestins, or estrogens can cause infertility in tom cats. In addition, male overuse or insufficient number of matings to induce ovulation can also result in perceived infertility (Johnston *et al.*, 2001b).

Retrograde movement of sperm into the bladder is common in tom cats and has been reported in 14–90% of feline ejaculates (Dooley *et al.*, 1991). Severe retrograde ejaculation can cause infertility due to the decreased number of spermatozoa ejaculated. Genital or urinary tract pain can induce a complete retrograde ejaculation. Oligo or azoospermia from retrograde ejaculation must be distinguished from partial or complete epididymal obstructions resulting from sperm granulomas. Collection of urine and assessment of sperm concentration following centrifugation allows diagnosis.

19.5 Diagnosis and Ancillary Tests

Diagnosis is based upon the results of a thorough medical and breeding history, complete physical examination, and laboratory blood work. There are online computer programs that can calculate the COI automatically. As a general rule, this coefficient should be lower than 10%. The undesirable effects of inbreeding start when the coefficient is higher than 5%, which is just below the value obtained for mating between cousins (Vella *et al.*, 1999). Researchers found that the percentage of normal sperm dropped from 55% to 15% after just one generation of mother–son or father–daughter mating showing the dramatic effect of inbreeding (Pukazhenthi *et al.*, 2006).

Complete blood cell count, serum biochemistry, thyroid hormone panel, and testing for infectious diseases (e.g. FeLV, FIV, FIP) should be included. If abnormal sexual differentiation is suspected, karyotyping of lymphocytes from heparinized whole blood is indicated (Centerwall and Benirschke, 1975).

19.5.1 Semen collection and evaluation

Usually, the first test performed in cases of male fertility, performing a semen evaluation in toms, is difficult because of the challenges related to semen collection. However, performing a semen evaluation is indicated because this test will not only determine if the problem is related to sperm production, but the evaluation may also define the severity of the problem and allow for priorities to be made for additional diagnostic testing. Multiple semen evaluations may be required before determining if the problem is reversible. Methods used for semen collection are described in Chapter 18. To quantify the severity of retrograde ejaculation, sperm can be recovered from the urine via cystocentesis. One report showed the mean percentage of sperm found in the bladder after natural ejaculation was 46.8 ± 31.7% (range 14.6–90.32%) (Dooley *et al.*, 1991). A second study showed the percentage of sperm retrograded in the bladder after electroejaculation ranged from 0–93.7% (mean of 40.9%) (Herron *et al.*, 1986).

Normal values for semen evaluation parameters are discussed in Chapter 18. The normal color of the feline semen is white, and the clarity of sample reflects the concentration of the spermatozoa (with clearer samples having lower sperm concentrations). A yellow semen sample may reflect urinary contamination or the presence of inflammatory cells. Urine contamination in the ejaculate can be diagnosed by evaluating a seminal plasma creatinine. This value would be high, as it is in a urine sample. White blood cells can be identified by performing a routine cytology stain on the ejaculate (diff quick, etc.) that will allow the neutrophils to become apparent.

Progressive sperm motility <25% (*asthenozoospermia*) could be the first sign of infection. However, contamination of equipment with detergent, water, urine, or lubricants, or evaluation of cold-shocked sperm samples can result in low sperm motility. Sperm become motile during epididymal transit so any alteration in the epididymides can reduce sperm motility without altering other semen characteristics. It is important to note that complete lack of motility does not confirm that sperm are dead as ciliary dyskinesis and other hereditable conditions can present with 100% immotile sperm. In these cases, additional testing such as sperm chromatin structure assay to evaluate the DNA fragmentation in the sperm or membrane integrity to evaluate the sperm cell should be performed. Alkaline phosphatase (ALP) can be measured directly from the seminal plasma to confirm epididymal and ductal tubular patency in cases of *oligospermia* or *azoospermia* (Valiente *et al.*, 2014). If the sample originates from the testes or epididymides, the ALP is extremely high. Values over 5,000 U/L typically indicate a testicular/epididymal sample (mean ALP in feline semen 160,000 U/L) (Johnston *et al.*, 1996).

Purebred toms tend to have a high percentage of abnormally-shaped sperm (*teratozoospermia*) within an ejaculate due to lack of genetic variation. Conversely, sperm morphologic abnormalities are infrequently observed in unrelated crossbred cats (unpublished observations). Other than inbreeding, causes of teratozoospermia include inflammation, neoplasia, infectious diseases of the genital tract, and fever which would increase intratesticular temperature. The presence of primary morphologic defects (coiled tail, microcephalic, macrocephalic) is associated with a greater severity of infertility as these abnormalities originate during spermatogenesis (Fig. 19.2). Toms with normal sperm motility, concentration, and morphology should have additional sperm functional testing performed to determine acrosome integrity, sperm chromatin structure assay, and if any ultrastructural morphologic abnormalities exist through electron microscopy.

19.5.2 Other diagnostic tests

In males, serum testosterone is secreted in a pulsatile manner, such that a single determination typically does not reflect the endocrine status of the testes. To test the pituitary–gonadal axis, gonadotropin-releasing hormone (gonadorelin) should be administered at a single dose of 50 µg intramuscularly following collection of a baseline blood sample, and a second blood sample should be collected 1 hour later. Serum testosterone should be significantly higher post-stimulation in comparison to the prestimulation sample (Romagnoli *et al.*, 2017).

Two-dimensional ultrasonography is a noninvasive diagnostic technique that has been widely used in andrology to evaluate size and echogenicity of accessory glands (prostate and bulbourethral glands), testicles, and epididymis. Testicular parenchyma is commonly described as a structure of medium echogenicity and homogeneous echotexture (Nyland and Mattoon, 1995) (Fig. 19.3). Testicular measurements can be taken using a high-frequency ultrasound and measuring the width, length, and height of each testicle. These measurements allow estimation of the volume of testicular tissue present. If necessary, images can be obtained in a sedated tom to reduce error. Each testicle should be isolated individually by gently pushing one testicle cranially to prevent interference with the measurement of the other testicle. The testicle to be measured is then isolated by grasping the base of the scrotum and trapping the testicle within the scrotum with the index finger and the thumb. The index finger and thumb should gently hold the scrotum between the testicle and the body. The testicle should be wet thoroughly with alcohol or ultrasound gel to allow sufficient contact between the skin and the probe. The ultrasound probe is then placed on the scrotal skin to measure the testicle underneath (Fig. 19.4). The testicle should not be obliqued or rotated. The probe is placed at a 90° angle to the desired measurement (length, width, or height) making sure the testicle is not measured obliquely. Too much pressure with the probe should not be applied to the testicle as it will falsely decrease the measurement due to the compression. The width can be obtained by placing the probe on the medial surface (and measuring laterally) of the 'down' testicle and on the lateral surface of the 'up' testicle (with the cat

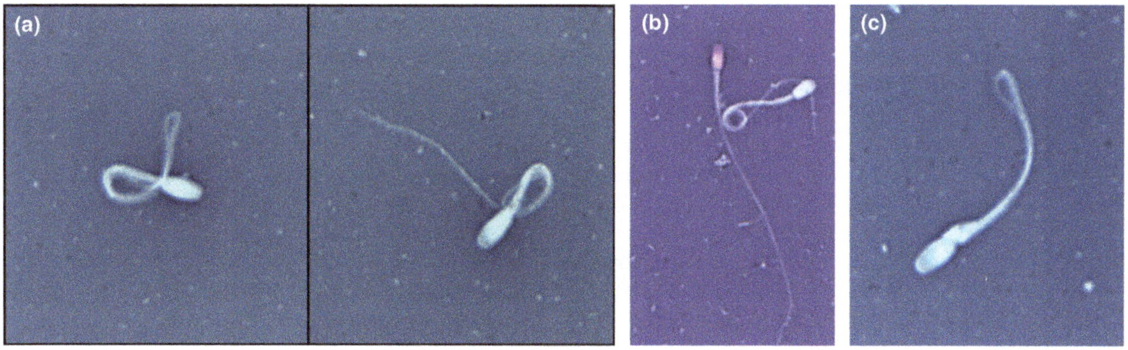

Fig. 19.2. **(a)** Coiled midpiece and tail. **(b)** Abnormal head and abnormal midpiece. **(c)** Abnormal midpiece. (Photos courtesy of Dr Aime Johnson.)

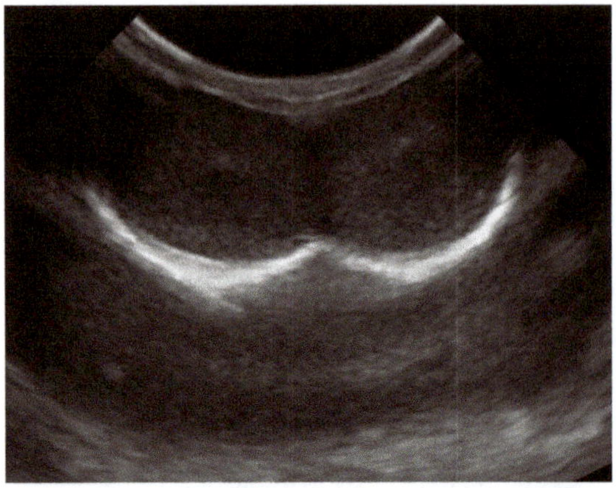

Fig. 19.3. Ultrasound of both testicles in cross section. The tunica albuginea can be seen as the hyperechoic line surrounding the testicles. (Photo courtesy of Dr Aime Johnson.)

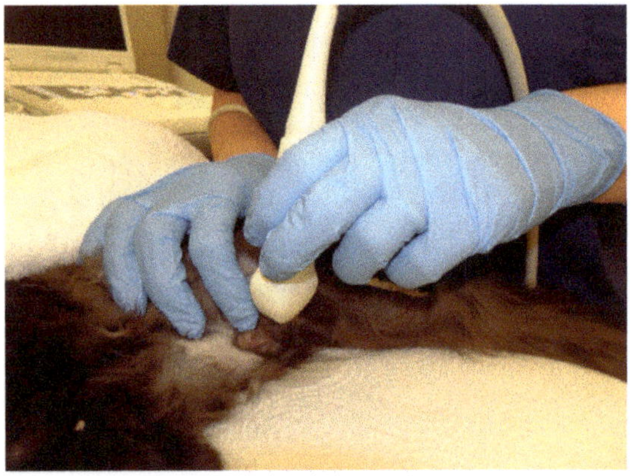

Fig. 19.4. Placement of the probe on the sedated tom's scrotum to measure the width of the testicle. The probe is moved to a different axis for height and length. Tom positioned in right lateral recumbency, head to the left of the photo, tail to the right. Examiner's right index finger is positioned between the testicle and prepuce. (Photo courtesy of Dr Aime Johnson.)

in lateral recumbency). For the height, the probe is placed on the ventral surface of each testicle with the measurements traveling ventral to dorsal. The length is the most difficult to obtain and does require patience and practice. The probe is placed on the caudal surface of the testicle (over the tail of the epididymis) and the testicle is measured cranially. It may be easier to gently grasp the testicle between the thumb and forefinger to align the longitudinal axis of the testicle with the probe. The measurement is taken from the caudal pole to the cranial pole. Once the operator is certain that the probe is oriented correctly and no compression of the testicle is present, the image can be frozen and measured from the one tunica albuginea, across the testicular parenchyma, to the other tunica albuginea (Fig. 19.5). The measurement should be repeated two to four times (remove probe, replace, and remeasure). By obtaining more than one measurement, error is decreased. The measurements obtained from each attempt are averaged to provide a single value (length, width, and height of each testicle). Testicular volume of each testicle can be calculated using the formula for an ellipse ($TV=2/3\pi \times L/2 \times W/2 \times H/2$). The equation can be simplified to $TTV=0.2533 \times L \times W \times H$. These measurements are best used to monitor testicular volume over time in a single tom rather than evaluating the amount of testicular tissue in a single animal. The average daily sperm output for an average weight tom has been estimated at 32 million (Franca and Godinho, 2003).

An abnormal decrease of 34% of the feline germinal epithelium height caused a significant diminution of parenchyma echogenicity (Francisco *et al.*, 2020). A testicular biopsy is indicated in cases of persistent oligo or azoospermia. Adequate testicular biopsies can be obtained using punch technique, but an open wedge biopsy permits better evaluation of tissues (Johnston *et al.*, 2001a). The biopsy should be fixed in Bouin´s, Zenker´s, or modified Davidson's solution because the artifacts produced by formalin make the interpretation of the biopsy less accurate. The biopsy should be examined by a trained pathologist with expertise in reproductive histopathology. Because the procedure must be done aseptically, part of the tissue obtained can also be cultured for microbial agents.

Although fine needle aspiration of the testes is a simple procedure to perform, the diagnostic usefulness of this technique is very limited to diagnosing active spermatogenesis from the finding of mature spermatozoa. On the other hand, a testicular biopsy can be used to determine the adequacy and completeness of spermatogenesis as well as for the presence of neoplastic or inflammatory lesions. In the case of autoimmune orchitis, testicular biopsy will only identify lymphoplasmacytic inflammation if performed early in the course of disease. In many cases of prolonged oligo/azoospermia, the etiologic agent cannot be identified at the time of histological evaluation, but the diagnosis of testicular degeneration can be confirmed. However, testicular histological examination

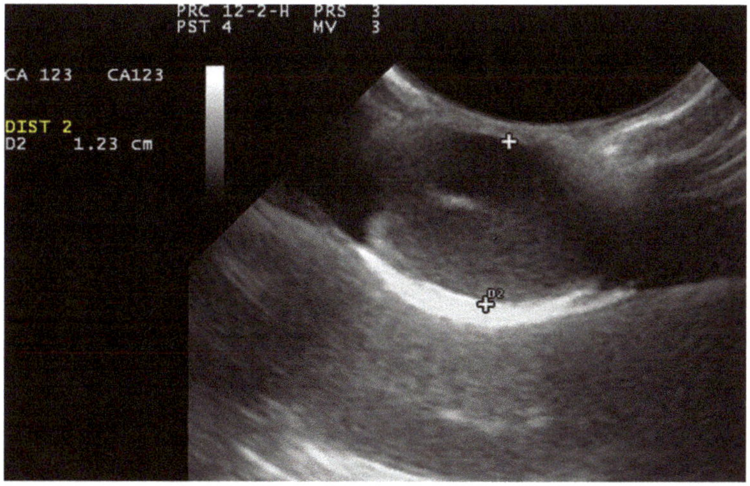

Fig. 19.5. A measurement of the width of the testicle. The testicle is measured from one side of the tunica albuginea to the other. The mediastinum can be visualized as the hyperechoic area in the center of the testicle and indicates the probe is placed across the center of the testicle. (Photo courtesy of Dr Aime Johnson.)

may differentiate between an acquired testicular degeneration and a congenital testicular hypoplasia (Johnston *et al.*, 2001a). Prior to performing a testicular biopsy, the risks of inducing immune intolerance by disruption of the blood–testis barrier and of hemorrhage that may affect thermoregulation of both testes should be discussed with the client.

19.6 Treatment

Treatment should be directed at the primary source of the infertility. In some cases, improving housing, husbandry, sanitation, and breeding management can resolve the problem. In catteries with high inbreeding coefficients, the lineage of inbred toms should be diversified by including outcrossed queens. Competition among males should be avoided. Pheromones could also reduce psychological stress (Beck, 2013). In cases of poor libido, gonadorelin (25 µg IM) should be administered 1 hour prior to mating to naturally boost the testosterone (Johnston *et al.*, 2001b). When retrograde ejaculation is inducing oligo/azoospermia, phenylpropanolamine (1–2 mg/kg orally) can be administered every 8 to 12 hours (Cohn and Cote, 2020). Phenylpropanolamine should be used with caution in animals with hyperthyroid, heart disease, hypertension, glaucoma, or diabetes.

Persistent penile frenula are easily treated by sharply incising with scissors. In cases of phimosis, treatment is not needed for toms not intended for breeding, but neutering should be performed to prevent pain associated with arousal. Paraphimosis is a medical emergency because the exposed penis quickly becomes swollen, dry, and painful. If paraphimosis is found early, treatment consists of treating the inciting cause (such as trimming the entangled hair), cleaning, lubricating, and replacing the exposed penis. If the urethra is damaged, a urinary catheter may be needed temporarily. If the penile damage is severe, amputation of the penis may be necessary.

Acute inflammatory disorders of the genital tract require prompt treatment because inflammation can cause permanent damage. Because of the cat's sensitivity to nonsteroidal anti-inflammatory (NSAIDS) agents, short-term use with an NSAID that is safe for cats should be used. In case of bacterial infections, antibiotics that cross into the reproductive tract such as oxacillin, trimethoprim-sulfonamide, aminoglycoside or enrofloxacin should be initiated until specific antibiotics based on culture and sensitivity are identified. Antibiotics should be administered for 3–4 weeks. In cases of unilateral testicular injury, the severely injured testis should be hemi-orchiectomized as soon as possible to minimize thermal injury of the contralateral testis.

With respect to prognosis following the diagnosis of infertility, the prognosis for return to fertility is guarded if there is no improvement after the first spermatogenic cycle (47 days; Franca and Godinho, 2003) and the prognosis is poor if there is no improvement after two or three spermatogenic cycles (94–141 days).

19.7 References

Axnér, E., Ström, B., Linde-Forsberg, C., Gustavsson, I., Lindblad, K., *et al.* (1996) Reproductive disorders in 10 domestic male cats. *Journal of Small Animal Practice* 37(8), 394–401. doi: 10.1111/j.1748-5827.1996.tb02427.x

Beck, A. (2013) Use of pheromones to reduce stress in sheltered cats. *Journal of Feline Medicine and Surgery* 15(9), 829–830. doi: 10.1177/1098612X13500882

Centerwall, W. R., and Benirschke, K. (1975) An animal model for the XXY Klinefelter's syndrome in man: tortoiseshell and calico male cats. *American Journal of Veterinary Research* 36(9), 1275–1280.

Cohn, L.A. and Cote, E. (2020) Drug compendium. In: Cohn, L. and Cote, E. (eds) *Cote's Clinical Veterinary Advisor Dogs and Cats*. Elsevier, St Louis, Missouri, pp. 1461–1510.

Dooley, M. P., Pineda, M. H., Hopper, J. G., and Hsu, W. H. (1991) Retrograde flow of spermatozoa into the urinary bladder of cats during electroejaculation, collection of semen with an artificial vagina, and mating. *American Journal of Veterinary Research* 52(5), 687–691.

Franca, L. R. and Godinho, C. L. (2003) Testis morphometry, seminiferous epithelium cycle length, and daily sperm production in domestic cats (*Felis catus*). *Biology of Reproduction* 68(5), 1554–1561. doi: 10.1095/biolreprod.102.010652

Francisco, F. D., Lapuente, C., Merlo, M. L., Barbeito, C., and Gobello, C. (2020) Feline testicular ultrasonogram differentiates pre vs. postpubertal and normal vs. disrupted spermatogenesis. *Theriogenology* 157, 503–507. doi: 10.1016/j.theriogenology.2020.08.012

Herron, M. A., Barton, C. L., and Applegate, B. (1986) A modified technique for semen collection by electroejaculation in the domestic cat. *Theriogenology* 26(3), 357–364. doi: 10.1016/0093-691x(86)90155-x

Johnston, S. D., Root, M. V., and Olson, P. N. S. (1996) Ovarian and testicular function in the domestic cat: clinical management of spontaneous reproductive disease. *Animal Reproduction Science* 42, 261–274. doi: 10.1016/0378-4320(96)01485-6

Johnston, S.D., Root Kustritz, M.V., and Olson, P.N. (2001a) Disorders of the feline testes and epididymides. In: Johnston, S. D., Root Kustritz, M. V., and Olson, P. N. (eds) *Canine and Feline Theriogenology*. W.B. Saunders, Philadelphia, Pennsylvania, pp. 525–536.

Johnston, S.D., Root Kustritz, M.V., and Olson, P.N. (2001b) Clinical approach to the complaint of infertility in the male cat. In: Johnston, S. D., Root Kustritz, M. V., and Olson, P. N. (eds) *Canine and Feline Theriogenology*. W.B. Saunders, Philadelphia, Pennsylvania, pp.544–548.

Long, S. E. (1979) Infertility in male animals with special reference to the cat. *Pedigree Digest* 6, 13.

Nyland, T. G. and Mattoon, J. S. (1995) *Veterinary Diagnostic Ultrasound*. W.B. Saunders, Philadelphia, Pennsylvania, p. 357.

Pukazhenthi, B. S., Neubauer, K., Jewgenow, K., Howard, J., and Wildt, D. E. (2006) The impact and potential etiology of teratospermia in the domestic cat and its wild relatives. *Theriogenology* 66(1), 111–121. doi: 10.1016/j.theriogenology.2006.03.020

Romagnoli, S., Baldan, A., Righetti, C., Fontaine, C., Scenna, L., *et al.* (2017). Use of the gonadotropin-releasing hormone (GnRH) stimulation test to monitor gonadal function in intact adult male cats. *Reproduction in Domestic Animals* 52(1), 24–27. doi:10.1111/rda.12771

Valiente, C., de la Sota, P. E., Arauz, S., and Gobello, C. (2014). Ejaculation training, seminal alkaline phosphatase and semen preservation through cooling in a milk-based extender in domestic cats. *Journal of Feline Medicine and Surgery*, 16(4), 312–316. doi:10.1177/1098612X13508192

Vella, C. M., Shelton, L. M., McGonagle, J. J., and Stanglein, T. W. (1999) *Robinson's Genetics for Cat Breeders and Veterinarians*, 4th edn. Elsevier Health Sciences, Oxford.

20 Disorders of the Testicles and Scrotum

Michelle Anne Kutzler

Department of Animal and Rangeland Sciences, Oregon State University, Corvallis, Oregon, USA

20.1 Congenital Disorders

20.1.1 Cryptorchidism

Although the process is probably similar to the dog, much less is known about the descent of the feline testes. Feline testicular migration through the inguinal canal and into the scrotum occurs before birth (Romagnoli and Schlafer, 2006). Cryptorchidism is a disorder of sexual development because the condition results from defective transmigration of one or both testes into the scrotum (Centerwall and Benirschke, 1975; Millis *et al.*, 1992; Yates *et al.*, 2003).

Cryptorchidism is one of the most common congenital defects in cats, along with umbilical hernias, cerebellar hypoplasia and eye and lid defects (Priester *et al.*, 1970). The reported incidence of feline cryptorchidism ranges from 1.3–3.8% (Millis *et al.*, 1992; Richardson and Mullen, 1993; Yates *et al.*, 2003). The testes can be retained inside the abdomen, just beneath the skin in the groin tissue (ectopic) or in the inguinal canal, with the latter location accounting for about 50% of cases of cryptorchidism (Richardson and Mullen, 1993; Steckel, 2011). There is no side predilection (left or right) for the development of feline cryptorchidism (Richardson and Mullen, 1993).

The condition may have a genetic basis and is reported to be more prevalent in pure breed cats (Johnston *et al.*, 2001). Persians are overrepresented in reports on cryptorchidism, with an incidence of 29% in one study (Millis *et al.*, 1992; Richardson and Mullen, 1993). Cryptorchidism can be inherited from either parent (even though females are unaffected). Although sperm production is absent in a cryptorchid testis, the tomcat will still be fertile if there is one descended testis (Fig. 20.1). However, tomcats with bilateral cryptorchidism are typically azoospermic.

Cryptorchidism can also result from a chromosomal anomaly (e.g. XX/XY chimerism) and occur with other reproductive defects (e.g. ambiguous genitalia or absence of portions of the internal reproductive tract) (Meyers-Wallen and Patterson, 1989). In addition, the presence of non-reproductive congenital abnormalities has also been reported with cryptorchidism including patellar luxation, tarsal deformity, supranumerary kidney with ureteral hypoplasia, a shortened or kinked tail, tetralogy of Fallot, microphthalmia, and upper eyelid agenesis (Richardson and Mullen, 1993; Paradise and Clark, 2013).

Although cryptorchidism can be suspected at an earlier age, definitive diagnosis cannot be made until puberty when the inguinal rings close, making scrotal descent of retained testes impossible. Movements of the testes up and down the inguinal canal before puberty is more common in cats than in dogs, which explains why a high percentage of patients diagnosed as cryptorchid kittens have normal scrotal testes by 6 months of age (Henderson, 1951) (Fig. 20.2).

Cryptorchidism should be distinguished from monorchidism or anorchidism, which rarely occur (see Section 20.1.2). The presence of penile spines can be used to differentiate from these conditions since testosterone production is maintained in cryptorchid testes (Richardson and Mullen, 1993) (Fig. 20.3). As a result, tomcat phenotype, behavior (e.g. libido, aggressiveness), and urine odor are also maintained (Diaz, 1947; Mason, 1976; Memon *et al.*, 1992).

If there is any doubt in the retention of testicular tissue, serum testosterone should be measured

DOI: 10.1079/9781789247107.0020

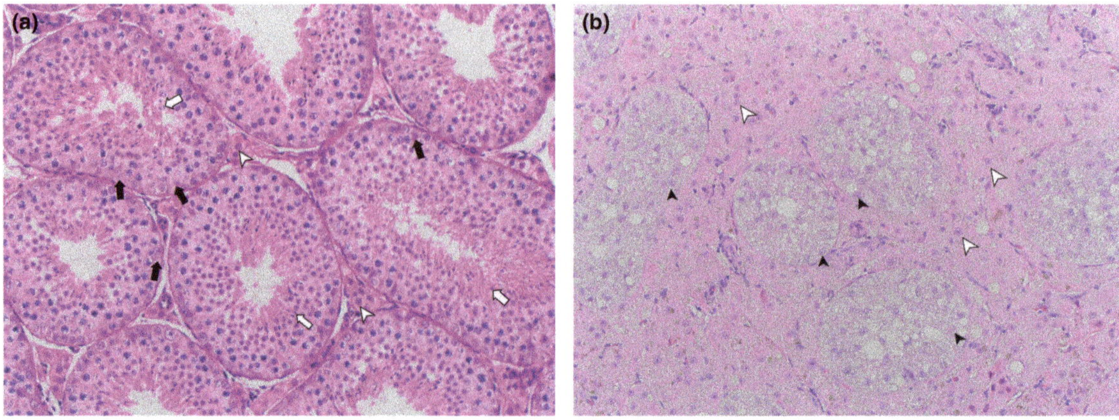

Fig. 20.1. Histologic images from: **(a)** normal testis; and **(b)** a cryptorchid testis (20×). The normal testis (a) has active spermatogenesis within the tubules as evidenced by tubules containing spermatocytes to elongated spermatids (white arrows). Normal germ cells are evident on the basement membrane of the seminiferous tubule (black arrows). The interstitial (Leydig) cells are located outside the tubules (white arrowheads). In the cryptorchid testis (b), there is no evidence of spermatogenesis with the tubules containing only Sertoli cells (black arrowhead) and no germ cells. Outside the tubules, there is a relative increase of interstitial (Leydig) cells (white arrowheads). (Images courtesy of Dr Russell Cattley; Auburn University Pathobiology Department.)

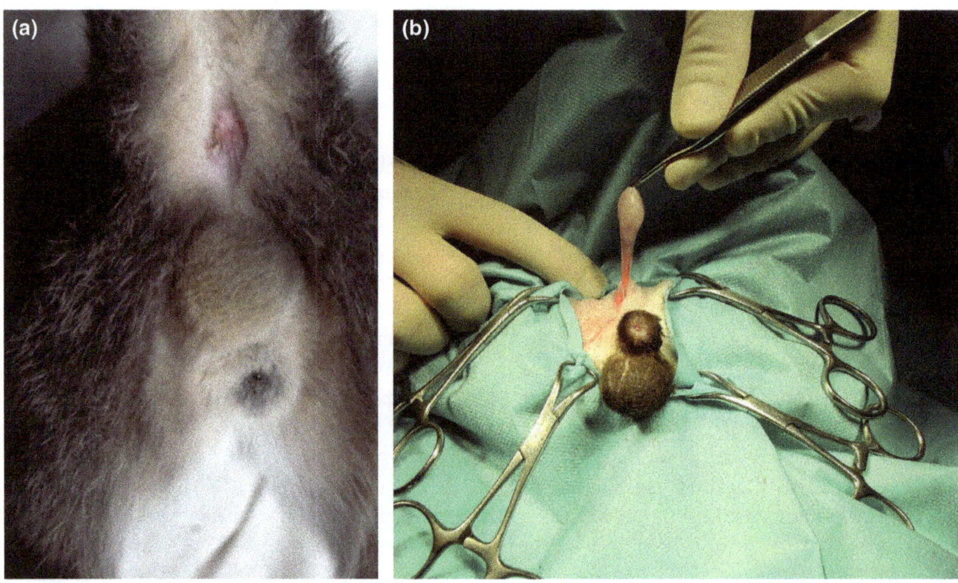

Fig. 20.2. (a). This is a post-pubertal tomcat with a descended left testis and cryptorchid right testis. **(b)** Surgical removal of the cryptorchid right testis. Note the smaller size of the cryptorchid testis (removed surgically) compared to the descended testis (still in scrotum). (Images courtesy of Dr Hasan Sontas.)

before and 2 hours after the intravenous administration of human chorionic gonadotropin (hCG; 500 mg/cat). Baseline testosterone concentration for sexually intact tomcats ranges from 1.0–6.0 ng/mL and is <0.5 ng/mL in castrated tomcats (Reimers, 1989). Following hCG administration, serum testosterone concentrations in intact tomcats will increase by fivefold over baseline but remain unchanged in castrated tomcats (Memon *et al.*, 1992). Transcutaneous ultrasonography is helpful

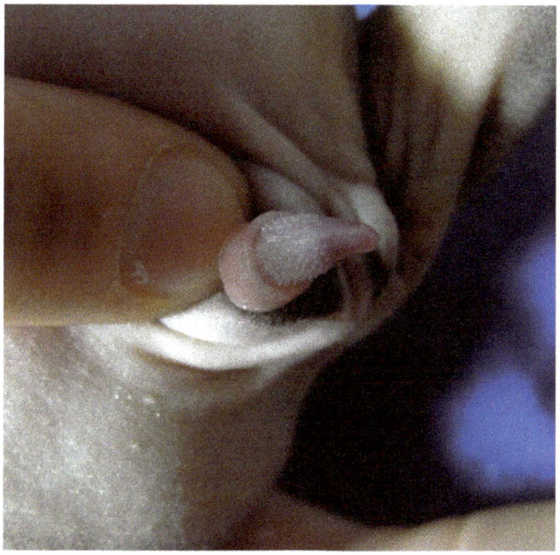

Fig. 20.3. Penile spines present in a tomcat with a history of castration. Based upon the appearance of penile spines, testosterone is still present and this tomcat likely still has at least one testis. (Image: author's own.)

to confirm palpation findings for a cryptorchid testis under the skin in the inguinal region (Fig. 20.4). Transabdominal ultrasonography to locate an abdominally cryptorchid testis is largely unrewarding but can be attempted by scanning between the kidney and the inguinal ring.

There is no medical treatment that has been shown to be effective for inducing or hastening testicular descent in cryptorchid animals. However, as previously stated, the testes may descend spontaneously before 6 months of age. Tomcats with one or two cryptorchid testes should be castrated to prevent against the genetic transmission of this condition as well as neoplastic transformation in the cryptorchid testes.

If a cryptorchid testis is palpable in the inguinal region, a paramedian incision should be made over the testis for removal. However, if the testis cannot be palpated, then a ventral midline incision should be made. Because the testis is most commonly in an inguinal location in cases of feline cryptorchidism, dissection deep to the inguinal fat pad should be made following the ventral midline incision to allow visualization of the external inguinal ring (Millis *et al.*, 1992). Caution must be used to differentiate the external inguinal ring from the femoral triangle (Millis *et al.*, 1992). If the testis is not found in the inguinal region, then the ventral midline incision is extended cranially for an abdominal exploratory. Most abdominal testes are found lying lateral to the bladder with the vas deferens and spermatic vessels, or near the caudal pole of the kidney (Wolff, 1981; Hakala, 1984; Millis *et al.*, 1992; Paradise and Clark, 2013)

20.1.2 Monorchidism and anorchidism

The congenital absence of one (monorchidism) or both (anorchidism or aplasia) of the testes is a rare condition in cats but has been reported (McEntee, 1990a). Three cases of monorchidism have been reported in tomcats (including two cases in a series of 23 cryptorchid cats) (Millis *et al.*, 1992; Backhaus and Krauss, 2019). Two cases of anorchidism/testicular aplasia were reported from a series of 50 cryptorchid cats (Richardson and Mullen, 1993). Confirming the diagnosis of monorchidism and anorchidism requires identification of the blunt end of the spermatic cord(s) and testicular blood vessels during an exploratory search for the missing testis. The epididymis may be found in the location of the missing testis (Backhaus and Krauss, 2019).

20.1.3 Polyorchidism

Polyorchidism is a rare anomaly defined as the presence of more than two histologically proven testes. Two cases of polyorchidism have been reported in tomcats (Milwright and Smith, 1999; Roca-Ferrer *et al.*, 2015). In one case, the tomcat had one testis in the left scrotum and two testes in the right scrotum (Milwright and Smith, 1999). The two right testes had fused epididymides and joined a common ductus deferens. Spermatozoa were present in all three epididymides. In the other case, the tomcat had four cryptorchid testes, one on the left side and three on the right side (Fig. 20.5) (Roca-Ferrer *et al.*, 2015). A presumptive diagnosis can be made by ultrasonography and intra-operative examination but definitive diagnosis requires histological confirmation.

20.1.4 Testicular hypoplasia

Testicular hypoplasia is a condition in which the testis (or testes) is underdeveloped and significantly smaller in size, usually due to a reduced number of germ cells (Roberts, 1986; McEntee, 1990a).

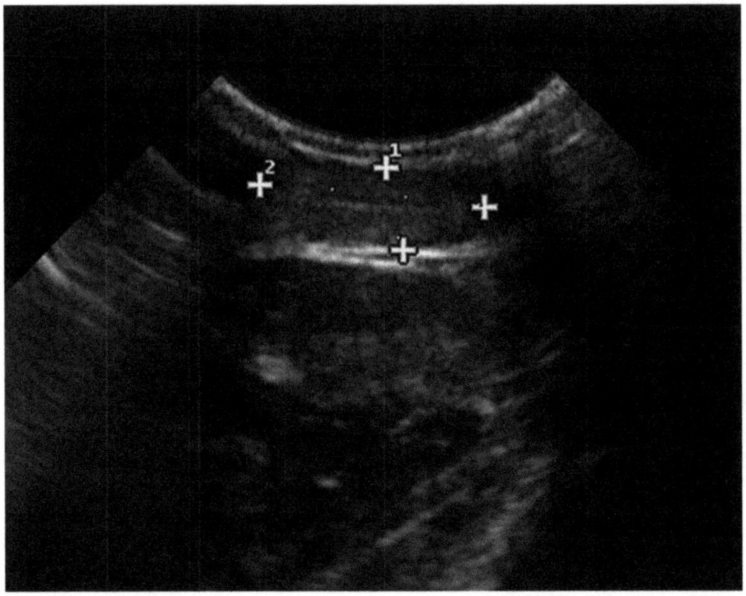

Fig. 20.4. Ultrasonographic image of an inguinal cryptorchid testis measuring 0.57 cm × 1.52 cm. Note the appearance of the hyperechoic mediastinum across the middle of the testis. (Image courtesy of Dr Hasan Sontas.)

Kittens with testicular hypoplasia may be indistinguishable from their normal counterparts until their testes fail to grow with puberty. Tomcats with testicular hypoplasia are phenotypically male with a scrotum containing two very small testes with normal-sized epididymides and have a normal-sized penis and prepuce (Fig. 20.6). Tomcats with testicular hypoplasia often have normal sexual behavior since the Leydig cells within the testes are unaffected. However, they are often azoospermic or oligospermic and fertility is usually compromised. Therefore, the treatment of choice is castration.

Feline Kleinfelter's syndrome (39,XXY) results in bilateral testicular hypoplasia with only Sertoli cells, a few spermatogonia, and no evidence of spermatogenesis present in the seminiferous tubules (Axnér *et al.*, 1996). Over time, degenerative changes within the seminiferous tubule will develop including hyaline sclerosis and tubule atrophy (Bishop, 1972). The presence of more than one X-chromosome is known to be deleterious to spermatogenesis. The trisomic condition can result from meiotic nondisjunction of the sex chromosomes during male or female gametogenesis or by mitotic nondisjunction in the early zygote (Meyers-Wallen and Patterson, 1989). Nondisjunctional events leading to abnormal sex chromosome constitutions occur randomly and are not the result of a heritable defect (Meyers-Wallen and Patterson, 1989).

Tomcats with more than one X-chromosome can present with a calico or tortoiseshell coat color because the genes for orange and black coat color are X-linked alleles (Malandain *et al.*, 2006; Pedersen *et al.*, 2014). For a cat to have both an orange and black coat color, all (or at least part) of the karyotype must have two X chromosomes. The variegated pattern of coat color is produced following the random inactivation of one of the two X chromosomes (Lyon, 1961). In cats, this occurs at the 12-day embryo stage (Austin and Amoroso, 1957). Although the 39,XXY karyotype is the most common condition to result in the calico or tortoiseshell coat color (Fig. 20.7), 38XY/38XX, 38XY/39XXY, and 38XY/38XY have also been reported (Ishihara, 1956; Thuline and Norby, 1961; Malouf *et al.*, 1967; Pyle *et al.*, 1971; Centerwall and Benirschke, 1973, 1975; Long *et al.*, 1981; Moran *et al.*, 1984). Tomcats that are XX/XY, XY/XXY, or XY/XY chimeras typically do not have testicular hypoplasia and are fertile with normal spermatogenesis because they have at least one normal 38XY cell line (Long *et al.*, 1981; Pedersen *et al.*, 2014). Fertile XY/XY mosaics also occur in cats but are rare (Loughman *et al.*, 1970).

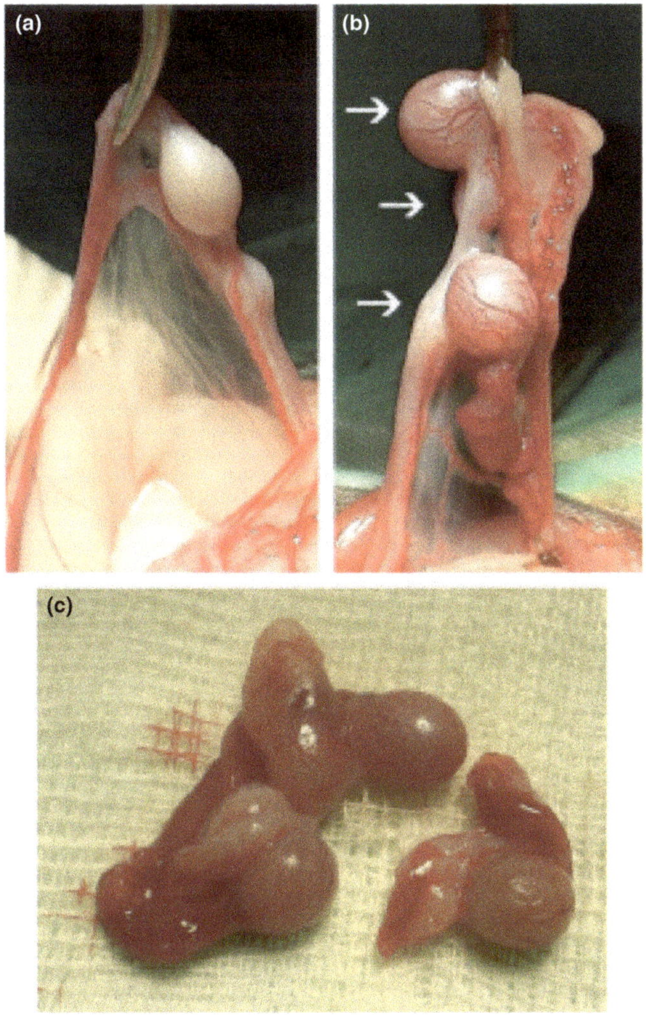

Fig. 20.5. A rare case of polyorchidism in a cat with four intra-abdominal testes. There was one testis on the left side **(a)** and three testes on the right side **(b)** All four testes removed following castration of a cat with polyorchidism **(c)**. (Used with permission from J. Roca-Ferrer *et al.*)

- Chimera: An individual with cell populations of more than one genotype arising from a mixture of different embryos during gestation.
- Mosaic: An individual with cell populations of more than one genotype derived from a mutational event within a single embryo.

20.1.5 Ovotestes

The occurrence of an ovotestis (combination of both ovary and testis) in the cat is extremely rare. In one report, the tomcat presented with a normal penis, prepuce, and unilaterally descended testis, along with an undescended ovotestis with a corresponding normal uterine tube and uterine horn that connected to a prostate (Harman, 1917). In another report, the tomcat presented with bilateral ovotestes and a thin-walled uterus that had resulted in long-lasting urinary incontinence and hematuria, which was corrected by surgical removal of the gonads and uterus (Felts *et al.*, 1982). An ovotestis can occur with XX/XY and XY/XY chimeras. In the normal condition, the XY karyotype gives rise to the development of a testis; whereas the XX karyotype gives rise to the development of an ovary (Meyers-Wallen and Patterson, 1989). Mixture of these two karyotypes to various degrees can produce different varieties of ovotestis or an individual with one ovary and one testicle (true hermaphrodite) (Meyers-Wallen and Patterson, 1989). A true hermaphrodite with an XX/XY karyotype has been reported in a cat (Biggers and McFeeley, 1966).

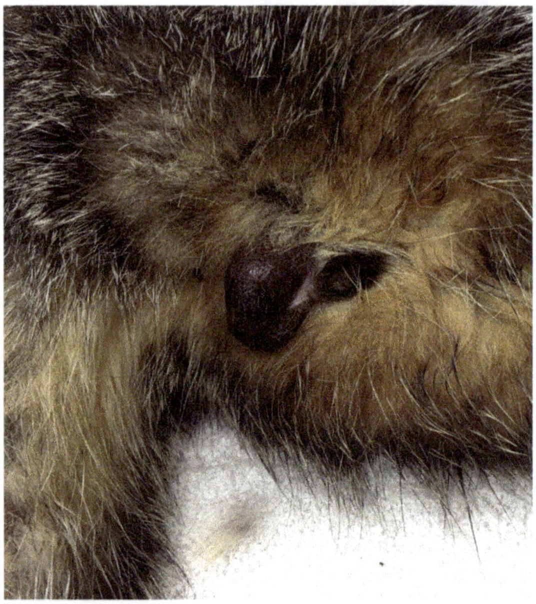

Fig. 20.6. Testicular hypoplasia in an adult tom. The testicles remained small as the tom aged from a kitten to an adult. This tom showed some male characteristics but had reduced/absent libido and never produced a pregnancy. (Image: Dr Aime Johnson.)

20.1.6 Cystic rete testis

Cystic rete testis is a congenital cystic condition of the testis, specifically the rete testis. The rete testis is a series of interconnected channels between the seminiferous tubules and the efferent ducts. The rete testis acts as a one-way valve for the passage of sperm and fluid, opening only when the pressure in the tubule rises above that in the rete and efferent ducts. The rete testis also serves to absorb seminiferous tubule fluid (Haschek *et al.*, 2009). There has been one report of a cystic rete testis in an 8-month-old cat (Gelberg and McEntee, 1983). The tomcat was asymptomatic, and the condition was identified during routine castration. The cystic area occupied approximately half of the right testis and communicated with a smaller cyst in the head of the epididymis, which originated from cystic efferent ductules. Although there were areas of active spermatogenesis within the right testis, there was no sperm present in the right epididymis. The left testis and epididymis were unaffected. In this case, the cystic dilation of the rete testis occurred secondary to blockage of the excurrent ducts caused by the epididymal cyst (Gelberg and McEntee, 1983). Removal of the affected testicle is curative.

20.2 Acquired Disorders of the Testes and Scrotum

20.2.1 Testicular neoplasia

Testicular tumors in cats are uncommon (Zambelli and Levy, 2010). In a review of 395 feline tumors, there were no testicular tumors identified (Brodey,

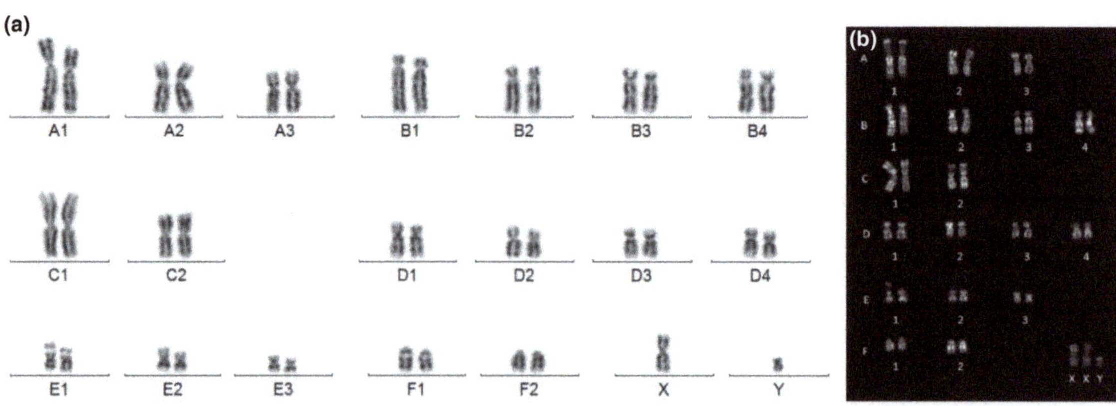

Fig. 20.7. (a) A karyotype of a normal male, 38 XY with a single X and Y chromosome. **(b)** A 39XXY karyotype from a tortoiseshell male cat showing the extra X-chromosome. (Used with permission from A.S. Pedersen.)

1970). Having said this, several Sertoli cell tumors (Meier, 1956; Moulton, 1961; Whitehead, 1967; Cotchin, 1984; Baptista and Silva, 1985; McEntee, 1990b; Silva, 2002; Benazzi *et al.*, 2004) and Leydig cell tumors (Rosen and Carpenter, 1993; Withrow and Reeves, 1996) have been reported in tomcats.

A Sertoli cell tumor is a primary tumor of the sustenacular cells within the testis that support the development of the germ cells as well as secrete estradiol, inhibin, androgen binding protein, and anti-Müllerian hormone. At least two of the five reported feline Sertoli cell tumors in one case series developed in a cryptorchid testis (Benazzi *et al.*, 2004). Estrus behavior for a 6-week duration from a Sertoli cell tumor was reported in a 3-year-old bilaterally cryptorchid tomcat that was resolved by castration (Mason, 1976). In addition, Sertoli cell tumors can be malignant and metastasize to the liver and spleen in tomcats (Meier, 1956).

A Leydig cell tumor is a primary tumor of the interstitial cells within the testis that secrete testosterone. Leydig cell tumors are typically incidental findings at necropsy (McEntee, 1990b). However, there have been six cases of Leydig cell tumors that developed in geriatric castrated tomcats (Rosen and Carpenter, 1993; Doxsee *et al.*, 2006). In each case, clinical signs associated with testosterone production (e.g. large jowls, urine marking) were noted. These neoplasms could have arisen from an embryological testicular remnant, transplantation of testicular parenchymal cells at the time of castration, or an incomplete castration.

Teratomas are complex tumors with recognizable elements of multiple germ layers in various stages of maturation and are thus composed of multiple tissues foreign to the part of the body in which they arise (Miyoshi *et al.*, 2001). A single feline case of a malignant teratoma has been reported in a cryptorchid testis (Miyoshi *et al.*, 2001). The teratoma metastasized to the omentum near the cryptorchid testis and the cat died secondary as a result of metastatic disease about a month after the neoplastic testis was removed (Miyoshi *et al.*, 2001).

Seminomas are primary tumors of the testicular germ cells. A single feline case of a malignant seminoma has been reported in a cryptorchid testis (Carpenter *et al.*, 1987). The seminoma metastasized to the sublumbar lymph nodes and adjacent soft tissues surrounding the cryptorchid testis (Carpenter *et al.*, 1987).

It is important to mention that multiple tumors may be present within the same feline testis. There was one report in a 9-year-old Russian Blue cat with a cryptorchid testis that had a Leydig cell tumor and Sertoli cell tumor in it (Miller *et al.*, 2007). There was another report of a cat with a descended testis containing a Sertoli cell tumor and seminoma (Meier, 1956). Diagnosis is made via ultrasound examination. The mass may appear as a hyperechoic or hypoechoic lesion within or adjacent to the testicular parenchyma. The affected testicle should be removed at the time of diagnosis. Because metastasis has been reported for all tumor types, a minimum data base and tumor staging should be performed to assess the presence of any metastases.

20.2.2 Testicular trauma

Scrotal and testicular trauma can result from blunt force trauma (e.g. vehicular accidents), bite wounds (Fig. 20.8), or penetrating injuries (Fig. 20.9). The peritoneal recess that forms the vaginal tunic surrounding the testes is susceptible to local infection and inflammation (periorchitis) (Foster, 2012). Periorchitis is usually fibrinosuppurative and the scrotum becomes distended and painful. This may be indistinguishable externally from clinical signs of testicular trauma, which also include swelling of the affected testicle or scrotum possibly with a corresponding hind limb lameness.

Diagnosis of scrotal and testicular trauma is made by careful physical examination for the presence of fluid in the scrotum, pain, and discomfort with or without discoloration of the scrotum, or changes in size, shape, or consistency of the scrotal contents. Scrotal swelling and bruising may be seen externally in cases of severe testicular trauma. Severe blunt trauma to the testes may result in local hemorrhage and rupture of the tunica albuginea covering the testes, which could lead to the development of sperm granulomas. Rupture of the tunica albuginea may be difficult to detect by palpation alone because of local swelling. The extent of the testicular damage or involvement of the vaginal tunics may be evident using ultrasonography.

In all cases of scrotal or testicular trauma, systemic antibiotics and anti-inflammatories should be administered. Most scrotal injuries should be treated as open wounds with the goal to minimize inflammation which may result in periorchitis and pressure necrosis with subsequent testicular

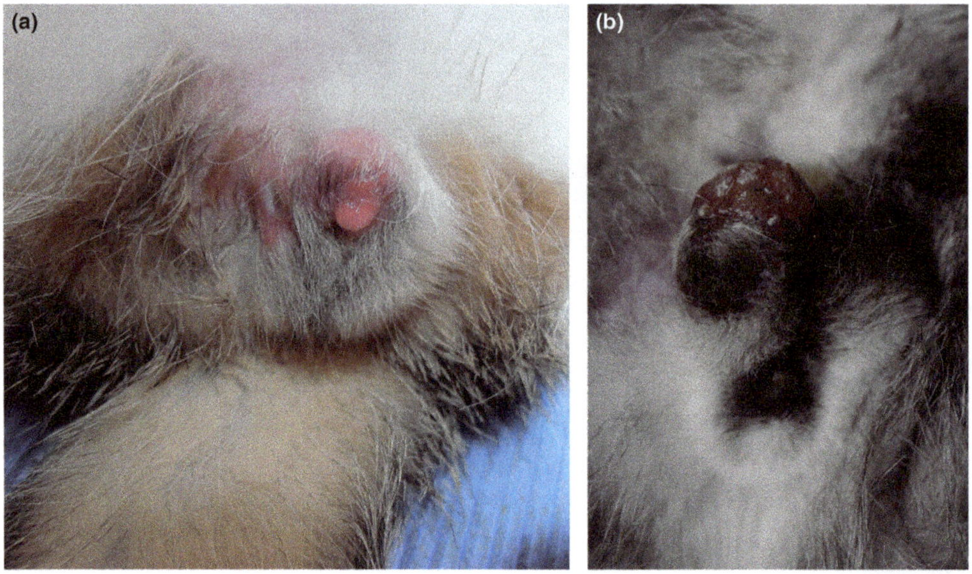

Fig. 20.8. (a) An acute bite injury to the penis and preputium; and **(b)** a chronic bite wound affecting the testicle. (Images courtesy of Dr Hasan Sontas.)

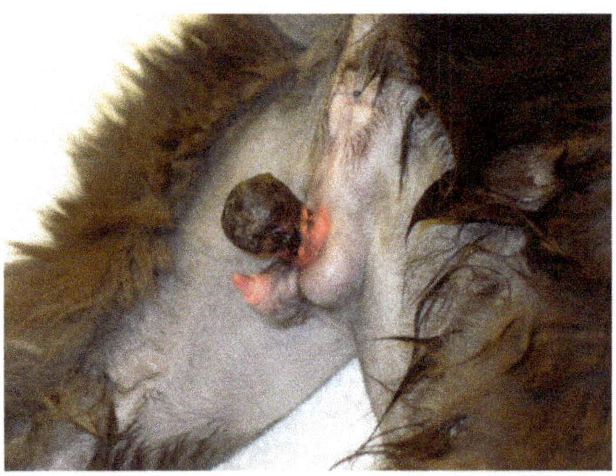

Fig. 20.9. Trauma to the scrotum of an intact adult male. The testicle is exposed and necrotic. (Image courtesy of Dr S.H. Cheong, also, in Library of Reproductive Images (LORI).)

atrophy. Other secondary changes to the testis can occur, including testicular necrosis or infarction (Foster, 2012). Most cases of severe testicular trauma require unilateral or bilateral castration. It is important to note that unlike other species, mature cats do not develop compensatory hypertrophy within 60 days of unilateral castration (Romero *et al.*, 2012).

Testicular torsion

Testicular torsion is rare in tomcats likely due to the anatomy of testicular placement within the scrotum. In the acute presentation, the tomcat is severely painful (Verstegen, 1998; Graves, 2006). There has also been one report of chronic testicular torsion in an asymptomatic prepubertal tomcat (Giuliano, 2013). All cases of testicular torsion involved descended testes. On examination, the scrotum will be enlarged and painful on palpation. Removal of the affected testis is required as testicular degeneration is likely to occur secondary to the inflammation and ischemia. During castration, the testis is usually ischemic and dark in color.

20.2.3 Inflammatory and/or infectious conditions

Inflammation of the testes (orchitis) or epididymis (epididymitis) are rare in cats unless due to trauma (e.g. bite wound) (Davidson, 2016). Lower urinary tract infections with and without crystalluria can also predispose to orchitis and epididymitis. Inflammation of the vaginal tunics surrounding the testes (periorchitis) can occur as a complication of castration when there is a post-surgical infection (Foster, 2012). Periorchitis can also occur secondarily to orchitis or epididymitis but this is very rare in cats (Foster, 2012). Ultrasonographic examination of testes with orchitis will reveal greater echogenicity and occasional irregularly shaped hypoechoic areas within the testicular parenchyma (Foster *et al.*, 1996). Adhesions between the vaginal tunics from periorchitis may be visible ultrasonographically. Treatment for orchitis should be hemicastration if future fertility is desired. Removing the affected testicle will provide the best chance for the unaffected testicle to remain functional. Excessive heat and inflammation from the affected testicle can lead to testicular degeneration in the unaffected testicle (Fig. 20.10).

Feline infectious peritonitis (FIP) can present as a primary orchitis and periorchitis (Fig. 20.11) (Wolfe and Griesemer, 1971; Sigurdardóttir *et al.*, 2001). In some cases of FIP, scrotal or testicular enlargement is the first indication of the infection (Foster, 2012; Sigurdardóttir *et al.*, 2001). Diagnosis of FIP is challenging because there are so many different manifestations of the disease. Differentiating FIP from traumatic/bacterial periorchitis may not be possible, but concurrent lesions of the scrotal skin would increase the likelihood of trauma (Foster, 2012). The histological changes seen in the testis from cats expressing the full clinical signs of FIP include vasculitis, fibrinogen exudation, and infarction (Foster *et al.*, 1996). The overall prognosis for FIP is grave, especially if the infection co-exists with feline leukemia virus (Foster *et al.*, 1996).

20.2.4 Degeneration

Any inflammatory, immune-mediated, nutritional, thermal, endocrine, or metabolic insult may progress to testicular degeneration or atrophy. For example, there have been two reports in young growing tomcats fed solely raw heart that developed epididymal intraepithelial cysts and hyperplasia (Leathern, 1970; Anver and Cohen, 1979). Age-related histological changes of the testes and epididymides have been reported, but unlike in dogs, there are no corresponding ultrasonographic descriptions of these changes in tomcats (Mantziaras, 2020).

Testicular and epididymal tunica adventitia thickness as well as interstitial cell number increase significantly with tomcat age (Elcock and Schoning, 1984). Conversely, spermatogonia A, spermatogonia B, and secondary spermatocyte number

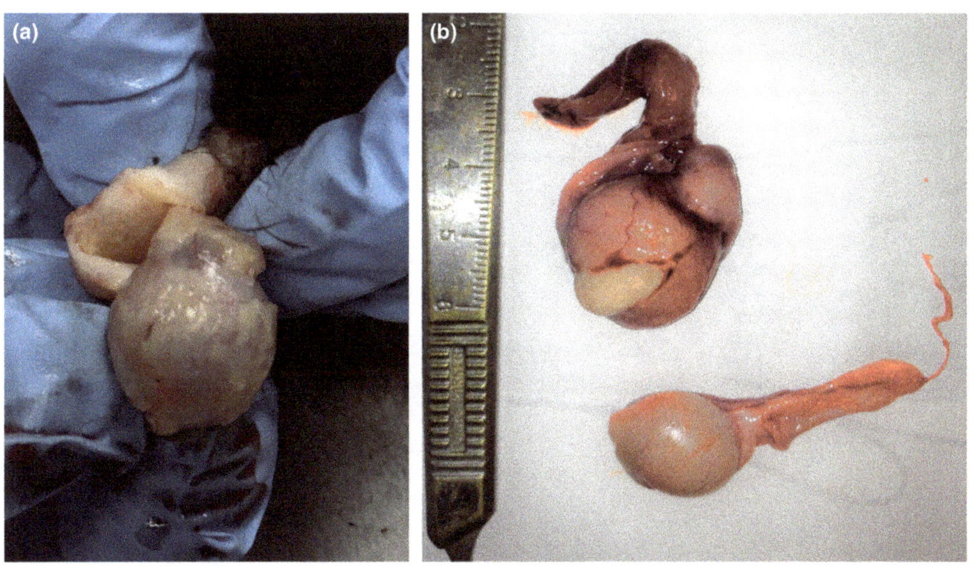

Fig. 20.10. **(a)** Male with unilateral orchitis during an open castration. The external surface of the testicle (tunica albuginea) is covered with fibrin. There were several adhesions between the testicle and the scrotum. **(b)** Same tom following removal of both testicles. The affected testicle is enlarged and is cut open showing severe inflammation and purulent material within the testicle. The spermatic cord is also enlarged and inflamed. The other testicle is slightly smaller than expected. (Images courtesy of Dr Aime Johnson.)

decrease significantly as the tomcat ages (Elcock and Schoning, 1984). The presence of seminiferous tubule degeneration, seminiferous tubular basement membrane thickness, Sertoli cell cytoplasmic vacuolation, proteinaceous tubular luminal debris, interstitial cell lipofuscin, interstitial cell cytoplasmic bodies, and epididymal ductal spermatozoa are all significantly related to age (Elcock and Schoning, 1984).

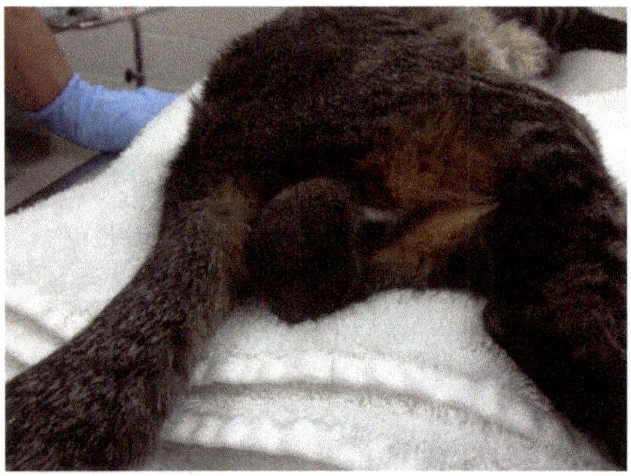

Fig. 20.11. Bilateral orchitis in a tomcat presumably from a systemic infection (e.g. feline infectious peritonitis). Note the large size of both testes. (Image courtesy of Dr Aime Johnson.)

Seminiferous tubular degeneration is most common in young (0.5–1 years old) or old (≥7 years old) tomcats (Elcock and Schoning, 1984). The severity of the degeneration varies from degeneration of mature germinal cells to degeneration of both mature and immature cells, including increased amount of Sertoli cell cytoplasmic vacuolation, varying amounts of spermatocyte vacuolation, karyorrhexis and pyknosis of Sertoli cells, spermatogonia, and spermatocytes, and sloughed germinal cells into the tubular lumen (Elcock and Schoning, 1984). Mononuclear and multinuclear spermatid giant cells observed histologically are early degenerative findings (Elcock and Schoning, 1984). Seminiferous tubular basement membranes are significantly thickened and wavy in older tomcats and interstitial cell lipofuscin is also significantly increased (Elcock and Schoning, 1984). Other histological findings may include the arrest of spermatogenesis.

Epithelial hyperplasia and intraepithelial cysts in the epididymal duct are evident in 70% of cats 0.5–1 years old and 20% of cats ≥ 5 years old (Elcock and Schoning, 1984). Spermatoceles have

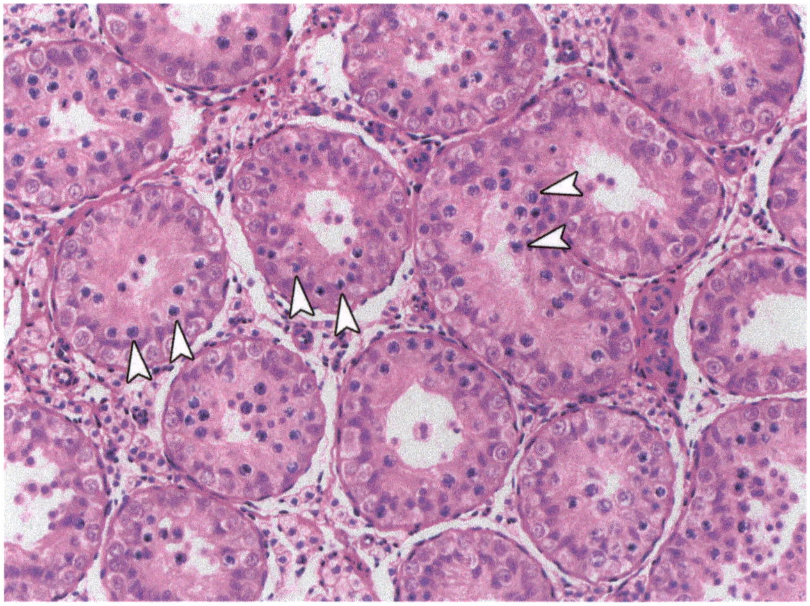

Fig. 20.12. Histological section of a testicle in an azoospermic tom (20×). Within the tubules, there are spermatocytes and early spermatids (arrowheads) but there is complete lack of mature spermatids and overall germ cell depletion. (Image courtesy of Dr Aime Johnson.)

been reported in older tomcats within the testis (n = 2) and head of the epididymal duct (n = 1) (Elcock and Schoning, 1984). Testicular spermatoceles are characterized by dilated tubules with no observable germinal epithelium or Sertoli cells and tightly packed luminal spermatozoa (Elcock and Schoning, 1984). The epididymal spermatocele consisted of a dilated duct with numerous tightly packed spermatozoa and spermatid giant cells (Elcock and Schoning, 1984).

Prognosis for future fertility with testicular degeneration is poor but will depend on the inciting factor. If the underlaying cause is treated, fertility may improve over one spermatogenic cycle (approximately 60 days). Subsequent semen collections and testicular measurements are necessary to fully evaluate the testicles over time. Examining the tom every 30–60 days provides information on any improvement or decline. When a definitive diagnosis is needed, a testicular biopsy should be performed to assess the stages of spermatogenesis within the tubules and if mature sperm are present. If not, prognosis is poor (Fig. 20.12).

20.3 References

Anver, M. R. and Cohen, B. J. (1979) Lesions associated with aging. In: Baker, H. J., Lindsey, J. R., and Weisbroth, S. H. (eds) *The Laboratory Rat*. Academic Press Inc, London, pp 378–396.

Austin, C. R. and Amoroso, E. C. (1957) Sex chromatin in early cat embryos. *Experimental Cell Research* 13(2), 419–421. doi: 10.1016/0014-4827(57)90027-7

Axnér, E., Ström, B., Linde-Forsberg, C., Gustavsson, I., Lindblad, K., *et al.* (1996) Reproductive disorders in 10 domestic male cats. *Journal of Small Animal Practice* 37(8), 394–401. doi: 10.1111/j.1748-5827.1996.tb02427.x

Backhaus, S. and Krauss, M. (2019) Monorchismus bei einem Kater [Monorchism in a tomcat]. *Tierarztl Prax Ausg K Kleintiere Heimtiere* 47(3), 202–208. doi: 10.1055/a-0886-0854

Baptista, R. and Silva, M. C. (1985) Animal tumors-statistical data. *Repos Trabalhos Lab Nac Invest Vet* 17, 95–110.

Benazzi, C., Sarli, G., and Brunetti, B. (2004) Sertoli cell tumour in a cat. *Journal of Veterinary Medicine, A Physiology, Pathology, Clinical Medicine* 51, 124–126. doi: 10.1111/j.1439-0442.2004.00608.x

Biggers, J. D. and McFeeley, R. A. (1966) Intersexuality in domestic animals. *Advanced Reproductive Physiology* 1, 29–60.

Bishop, M. W. H. (1972) Genetically determined abnormalities of the reproductive system. *Journal of Reproduction and Fertility and Supplement* 15, 51–78.

Brodey, R. S. (1970) Canine and feline neoplasia. *Advances in Veterinary Science and Comparative Medicine* 14, 309–354.

Carpenter, J. L., Andrews, L. K., and Holzworth, J. (1987) Tumors and tumor-like lesions. In: Holzworth, J. (ed.) *Diseases of the Cat: Medicine and Surgery*. W.B. Saunders, Philadelphia, Pennsylvania, pp. 517–518.

Centerwall, W. R. and Benirschke, K. (1973) Male tortoiseshell and calico (T-C) cats: Animal models of sex chromosome mosaics, aneuploids, polyploids, and chimerics. *Journal of Heredity* 64, 272–273. doi: 10.1093/oxfordjournals.jhered.a108410

Centerwall, W. R. and Benirschke, K. (1975) An animal model for XXY Klinefelter's syndrome in man: tortoiseshell and calico male cats. *American Journal of Veterinary Research* 36, 1275–1280.

Cotchin, E. (1984) Neoplasia. In: Wilkinson, G. T. (ed.) *Diseases of the Cat and Their Management*. Blackwell, Oxford, pp 366–387.

Davidson, A. P. (2016) Reproductive diseases of the male small animal. In: Aiello, S. E. (ed.) *The Merck Veterinary Manual*, 11th edn. Merck & Co, Inc., Kenilworth, New Jersey, pp. 1400–1402.

Diaz, J. A. (1947) Cryptorchid on a cat. *Veterinary Medicine* 42, 159.

Doxsee, A. L., Yager, J. A., Best, S. J., and Foster, R. A. (2006) Extratesticular interstitial and Sertoli cell tumors in previously neutered dogs and cats: a report of 17 cases. *The Canadian Veterinary Journal* 47(8), 763–766.

Elcock, L. H. and Schoning, P. (1984) Age-related changes in the cat testis and epididymis. *American Journal of Veterinary Research* 45(11), 2380–2384.

Felts, J. F., Randell, M. G., Greene, R. W., and Scott, R. C. (1982) Hermaphroditism in a cat. *Journal of the American Veterinary Medicine Association* 181, 925–926.

Foster, R. A. (2012) Common lesions in the male reproductive tract of cats and dogs. *Veterinary Clinics of North America, Small Animal Practice* 42, 527–545. doi: 10.1016/j.cvsm.2012.01.007

Foster, R. A., Caswell, J. L., and Rinkardt, N. (1996) Chronic fibrinous and necrotic orchitis in a cat. *The Canadian Veterinary Journal* 37(11), 681–682.

Gelberg, H. B. and McEntee, K. (1983) Cystic rete testis in a cat and fox. *Veterinary Pathology* 20, 634–636.

Giuliano, A. (2013) Testicular torsion in a normally descended testicle in a cat. *Journal of Small Animal Practice* 54(3), 164. doi: 10.1111/jsap.12030

Graves, T. K. (2006) Diseases of the testes and scrotum. In: Birchard, S. J. and Sherding, R. G. (eds) *Saunders Manual of Small Animal Practice*, 3rd edn. Elsevier, St. Louis, Missouri, pp. 963.

Hakala, J. E. (1984) Reproductive tract anomalies in 2 male cats. *Modern Veterinary Practice* 65(8), 629.

Harman, M. T. (1917) Another case of gynandromorphism. *Anatomical Record* 13, 425–435.

Haschek, W. M., Rousseaux, C. G., and Wallig, M. A. (2009) Male reproductive system. In: Haschek, W. M., Rousseaux, C. G., and Wallig, M. A. (eds) *Fundamentals of Toxicologic Pathology*, 2nd Edn. Elsevier, St. Louis, Missouri, pp. 553–597.

Henderson, W. (1951) Cryptorchidism in the adult cat. *North American Veterinarian* 32, 634–636.

Ishihara, T. (1956) Cytological studies on tortoiseshell male cats. *Cytologia* 21, 391.

Johnston, S. D., Root-Kustritz, M. V., and Olson, P. N. S. (2001) *Canine and Feline Theriogenology*. Elsevier Health Sciences, St. Louis, Missouri.

Leathern, J. H. (1970) Nutrition. In: Johnson, A. D., Gomes, W. R., and Vandemark, N. L. (eds) *The Testis*. Academic Press Inc, New York, pp 170–197.

Long, S. E., Gruffydd-Jones, T., and David, M. (1981) Male tortoiseshell cats: an examination of testicular histology and chromosome complement. *Research in Veterinary Science* 30, 274–280.

Loughman, W. D., Frye, F. L., and Condon, T. B. (1970) XY/XXY bone marrow mosaicism in three male tricolor cats. *American Journal of Veterinary Research* 31, 307-314.

Lyon, M. F. (1961) Gene action in the X-chromosome of the mouse (*Mus musculus* L.). *Nature* 190, 372–373. doi: 10.1038/190372a0

Malandain, E., Little, S., Casseleux, G., Shelton, L., Pibot, P., *et al.* (2006) *Practical Guide to Cat Breeding*. Aniwa SAS, Lyon, France.

Malouf, N., Bernischke, K., and Hoefnagel, D. (1967) XX/XY chimerism in a tricolored male cat. *Cytogenetics* 6, 228–241.

Mantziaras, G. (2020) Imaging of the male reproductive tract: Not so easy as it looks like. *Theriogenology* 150, 490–497. doi: 10.1016/j.theriogenology.2020.03.009

Mason, K. V. (1976) Oestral behaviour in a bilaterally cryptorchid cat. *Veterinary Record* 99, 296–297. doi: 10.1136/vr.99.15.296

McEntee, K. (1990a) Scrotum and testis: anatomy and congenital anomalies. In: McEntee, K. (ed.) *Reproductive Pathology of Domestic Mammals*. Academic Press, San Diego, California, pp. 224–251.

McEntee, K. (1990b) Scrotum, spermatic cord and testis: proliferative lesions. In: McEntee, K. (ed.) *Reproductive Pathology of Domestic Mammals*. Academic Press, San Diego, California, pp. 276–306.

Meier, H. (1956) Sertoli-cell tumor in the cat: report of two cases. *North American Veterinary* 37, 979–981.

Memon, M. A., Ganjam, V. K., Pavletic, M. M., and Schelling, S. H. (1992) Use of human chorionic gonadotropin stimulation test to detect a retained testis in a cat. *Journal of the American Veterinary Medical Association* 201(10), 1602.

Meyers-Wallen, V. N. and Patterson, D. F. (1989) Sexual differentiation and inherited disorders of sexual development in the dog. *Journal of Reproduction and Fertility Supplement* 39, 57–64.

Miller, M. A., Hartnett, S. E., and Ramos-Vara, J. A. (2007) Interstitial cell tumor and Sertoli cell tumor in the testis of a cat. *Veterinary Patholoīgy* 44(3), 394–397. doi: 10.1354/vp.44-3-394

Millis, D. L., Hauptman, J. G., and Johnson, C. A. (1992) Cryptorchidism and monorchidism in cats: 25 cases (1980–1989). *Journal of the American Veterinary Medical Association* 200, 1128–1130.

Milwright, R. D. and Smith, K. C. (1999) Polyorchidism in a cat. *Veterinary Record* 145(23), 679–680.

Miyoshi, N., Yasuda, N., Kamimura, Y., Shinozaki, M., and Shimizu, T. (2001) Teratoma in a feline unilateral cryptorchid testis. *Veterinary Pathology* 38(6), 729–730. doi: 10.1354/vp.38-6-729

Moran, C., Gillies, C. B., and Nicholas, F. W. (1984) Fertile male tortoiseshell cats. Mosaicism due to gene instability? *Journal of Heredity* 75(5), 397–402. doi: 10.1093/oxfordjournals.jhered.a109964

Moulton, J. E. (1961) *Tumors of Domestic Animals*. University of California Press, Berkeley, California.

Paradise, D. and Clark, D. (2013) Supernumerary kidney with ipsilateral cryptorchidism in a cat. *Journal of the American Animal Hospital Association* 49(5), 338–341. doi: 10.5326/JAAHA-MS-5885

Pedersen, A. S., Berg, L. C., Almstrup, K., and Thomsen, P. D. (2014) A tortoiseshell male cat: chromosome analysis and histologic examination of the testis. *Cytogenetic and Genome Research* 142(2), 107–111.

Priester, W. A., Glass, A. G., and Waggoner, N. S. (1970) Congenital defects in domesticated animals: general considerations. *American Journal of Veterinary Research* 31, 1871–1879.

Pyle, R. L., Patterson, D. F., Hare, W. C. D., Kelly, D. F., and Digiulia, T. (1971) XXY sex chromosome constitution in a Himalayan cat with tortoise-shell points. *Journal of Heredity* 62, 220–222. doi: 10.1093/oxfordjournals.jhered.a108154

Reimers, T. J. (1989) Feline reproductive endocrinology. *Proceedings from the Cornell Feline Specialists Seminar*. Ithaca, New York, USA.

Richardson, E. F. and Mullen, H. (1993) Cryptorchidism in cats. *Compendium on Continuing Education for the Practicing Veterinarian* 15, 1342–1345.

Roberts, S. J. (1986) *Veterinary Obstetrics and Genital Diseases (Theriogenology)*, 3rd edn. Roberts, S. J. (published by the author), Woodstock, Vermont.

Roca-Ferrer, J., Rodríguez, E., Ramírez, G. A., Moragas, C., and Sala, M. (2015) A rare case of polyorchidism in a cat with four intra-abdominal testes. *Reproduction in Domestic Animals* 50(1):172–176. doi: 10.1111/rda.12461

Romagnoli, S. and Schlafer, D. H. (2006) Disorders of sexual differentiation in puppies and kittens: a diagnostic and clinical approach. *Veterinary Clinics of North America, Small Animal Practice* 36(3), 573–606. doi: 10.1016/j.cvsm.2005.12.007

Romero, G. G., Barbeito, C., Fernandez, P., Gimeno, E., and Gobello C. (2012) Unilateral orchidectomy in mature cats is not followed by compensatory hypertrophy. *Reproduction in Domestic Animals* 47(6), 226–228. doi: 10.1111/rda.12024

Rosen, D. K. and Carpenter, J. L. (1993) Functional ectopic interstitial cell tumor in a castrated male cat. *Journal of the American Veterinary Medicine Association* 202, 1865–1866.

Sigurdardóttir, O. G., Kolbjørnsen, O., and Lutz, H. (2001) Orchitis in a cat associated with coronavirus infection. *Journal of Comparative Pathology* 124(2-3), 219–222. doi: 10.1053/jcpa.2000.0443

Silva, J. F. (2002) Sertolinoma maligno em testículo ectópico de gato (*Felis catus*). [Malignant Sertoli cell tumor in an ectopic testis of a cat (*Felis catus*).] *Revista Portuguesa de Ciencias Veterinarias* 97, 87–92.

Steckel, R. R. (2011) Use of an inguinal approach adapted from equine surgery for cryptorchidectomy in dogs and cats: 26 cases (1999–2010). *Journal of the American Veterinary Medical Association* 239, 1098–1103. doi: 10.2460/javma.239.8.1098

Thuline, H. C. and Norby, D. E. (1961) Spontaneous occurrence of chromosome abnormality in cats. *Science* 134, 554–555. doi: 10.1126/science.134.3478.554

Verstegen, J. P. (1998) Condition of the male. In: Simpson, G., England, G., and Harvey, M. (eds) *BSAVA Manual of Small Animal Reproduction and Neonatology*, 1st edn. BSAVA, Gloucester, UK, pp. 81.

Whitehead, J. E. (1967) Neoplasia in the cat. *Veterinary Medicine, Small Animal Clinician* 62(1), 44–45.

Withrow, S. J. and Reeves, N. P. (1996) Tumors of the male reproductive tract. In: Withrow, S. G. and MacEwen, E. G. (eds) *Small Animal Clinical Oncology*, 2nd edn. W.B. Saunders, Philadelphia, Pennsylvania, pp. 373–379.

Wolfe, L. G. and Griesemer, R. A. (1971) Feline infectious peritonitis: review of gross and histopathologic lesions. *Journal of the American Veterinary Medical Association* 158(6), 987–993.

Wolff, A. (1981) Castration, cryptorchidism, and cryptorchidectomy in dogs and cats. *Veterinary Medicine, Small Animal Clinician* 76(12), 1739–1741.

Yates, D., Hayes, G., Heffernan, M., and Beynon, R. (2003) Incidence of cryptorchidism in dogs and cats. *Veterinary Record* 152(16), 502–504. doi: 10.1136/vr.152.16.502

Zambelli, D. and Levy, X. (2010) Clinical approaches to the infertile male. In: England, G. and von Heimendahl, A. (eds) *BSAVA Manual of Canine and Feline Reproduction and Neonatology*. BSAVA, Gloucester, UK, pp. 70–79.

21 Disorders of the Accessory Sex Glands

MICHELLE ANNE KUTZLER

Department of Animal and Rangeland Sciences, Oregon State University, Corvallis, Oregon, USA

21.1 Overview

The accessory glands of the tom are the prostate and bulbourethral gland. Congenital bulbourethral abnormalities have never been reported in cats (Romagnoli and Schlafer, 2006). Congenital prostatic hypoplasia or aplasia is rare in the cat and is usually associated with other developmental anomalies (e.g. pseudohermaphroditism) (Romagnoli and Schlafer, 2006). Acquired diseases of the accessory glands in cats are also rare. Cystitis and urethritis can extend to both the prostate and bulbourethral glands resulting in urethroadenocystitis (Foster, 2012). Bacterial prostatitis, abscessation, paraprostatic cysts, squamous metaplasia of the prostate, and prostatic adenocarcinoma have all been reported in cats, where the latter is the most common (McEntee, 1990; Foster and Ladds, 2007). Prostatic hyperplasia, a common condition in intact male dogs, has not been reported in cats; even those with prostatitis.

In cats, clinical signs alone cannot be used to diagnose prostatic disease or differentiate between prostatic adenocarcinoma and non-neoplastic prostatic disease. Clinical signs most associated with prostatic disease in cats involve symptoms associated with the gastrointestinal tract and lower urinary tract. Vomiting, anorexia, constipation, obstipation, tenesmus, and dyschezia have been reported. Hematuria, dysuria, pollakiuria, bladder atony, and signs of urinary obstruction have also been reported. Pyrexia can occur in cases of prostatic abscessation.

When prostatic enlargement is identified in cats, an aggressive diagnostic approach should be pursued. General laboratory testing (e.g. complete blood count (CBC), serum biochemistry, urinalysis) should be performed. In most cases, the results of the CBC and serum biochemistry will be within normal limits. Occasionally, in cases of bacterial prostatitis and prostatic abscessation, a mature neutrophilia is present. Analysis of a urine sample collected by cystocentesis will likely yield erythrocytes and neutrophils in cases of bacterial prostatitis or prostatic abscessation, but this does not rule out prostatic adenocarcinoma.

A cursory examination of the prostate can be performed by digital rectal palpation. Rectal palpation permits examination of only the dorsal aspect of the prostate. Unlike in dogs where concomitant abdominal palpation allows for improved palpation of the prostate, the feline prostate is positioned more caudal and located between the root of the penis and neck of the bladder (Caney *et al.*, 1998). During palpation per rectum, the prostate should be evaluated for size, symmetry, surface contour, movability, and pain. The normal prostate is bilobed, symmetric, smooth, movable and nonpainful. In contrast to dogs, cats with bacterial prostatitis or prostatic abscessation do not present with a painful prostate on rectal palpation.

Survey abdominal radiographs are unrewarding for assessing the feline prostate. If the prostatic enlargement is causing lower gastrointestinal signs, dorsal deviation of a feces-filled colon may be present. However, intravenous urography, double-contrast cystourethrography, and voiding urethrography have all been used to delineate the extent of urologic involvement with prostatic disease. Intravenous urography is also known as intravenous pyelography or excretory urography. This test is indicated for several conditions including to check for anatomical abnormalities of the kidneys,

DOI: 10.1079/9781789247107.0021

ureters, and bladder. Briefly, an intravenous catheter is placed and survey abdominal radiographs are taken. Then a bolus of non-ionic water-soluble iodinated contrast medium (e.g. lopamidol) is administered (880 mg/kg iodine). Abdominal radiographs are repeated at 10-minute intervals for 1 hour. Compared to negative or positive contrast cystourethrography, double-contrast cystourethrography provides the most information about the bladder wall and bladder contents. Under general anesthesia or deep sedation, a urinary catheter is placed and a small amount of 2% lidocaine is injected into the bladder to reduce straining. Then, positive contrast medium (3 mL/cat of non-ionic water-soluble iodinated, e.g. lopamidol) is injected through the urinary catheter to label intraluminal structures. The cat should be rolled over (e.g. from right to left lateral recumbency) to ensure that the entire bladder mucosa is covered with media. Leaving the cat in left lateral recumbency (to prevent air embolism) and while palpating the bladder to prevent overdistention, the bladder is filled with negative contrast medium (2–3 mL/kg or room air) to outline the bladder wall. The bladder must be palpated during injection and rupture. Abdominal radiographs are then taken. Voiding urethrography is also performed under general anesthesia or deep sedation. An enema should be administered prior to obtaining the initial lateral and ventrodorsal radiographs. Then, a urinary catheter is inserted into the tip of the penis and 2 mL of 2% lidocaine is injected to prevent urethral spasm. The urinary catheter is then passed completely to the bladder and any urine present in the bladder is emptied. The bladder is then filled (5–10 mL) with diluted non-ionic water-soluble iodinated contrast medium (1 part contrast medium to 2 parts sterile saline) and the catheter is removed. Gentle external pressure is then applied to the bladder. Radiographs should be taken when urine is seen flowing from the urethra.

Intravenous urography can be used to diagnose a paraprostatic cyst by filling the bladder with contrast medium, leaving a second fluid-filled structure visible on radiographs without contrast (the paraprostatic cyst) (Newell *et al.*, 1992). In addition, double-contrast cystourethrography or voiding urethrography can reveal irregularity in the prostatic urethra and intraprostatic reflux of contrast medium, which are consistent with prostatic adenocarcinoma (Hawe, 1983; Hubbard *et al.*, 1990). Normal accessory glands in tomcats have been described using computed tomography (CT) but there have been no reports of its use for diagnosis of feline accessory gland disorders (Mantziaras *et al.*, 2019; Mantziaras, 2020) (Fig. 21.1).

Transabdominal ultrasonography is an excellent imaging modality for evaluating the prostate, but the technique is more difficult in cats compared to dogs owing to the mostly intrapelvic location of the feline prostate. The ultrasonographic appearance of a prostate should be uniformly fine-medium texture and moderately hyperechoic, similar to that of the spleen, with a capsule that is echoic and has smooth margins (Fig. 21.2). Changes in echogenicity and/or echotexture can be associated with disease making the prostate more easily visible via ultrasound.

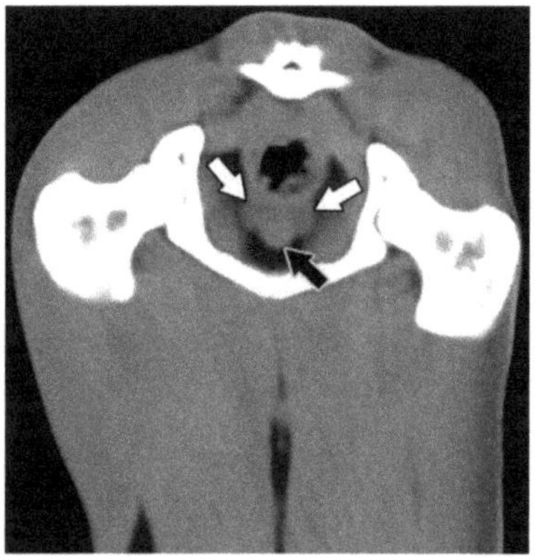

Fig. 21.1. A CT image of a normal adult male cat. Visible is the bilobed prostate (white arrows). The urethra can be seen between the prostate (black arrow). (Image: Dr Rachel Moon.)

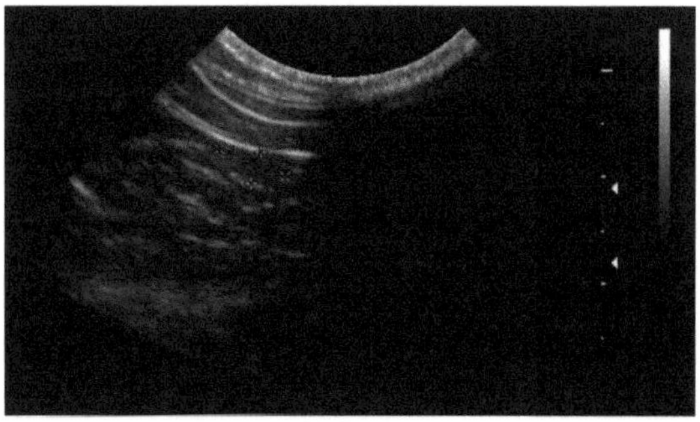

Fig. 21.2. Ultrasound image of a normal feline prostate (marked by cross hairs). (Image courtesy of Dr Judith Hudson.)

Ultrasound-guided fine-needle aspiration of the prostate is performed when lesions are observed, but not all aspirates are diagnostic. In cases of bacterial prostatitis or prostatic abscessation, numerous neutrophils (usually degenerate) and a variable amount of macrophages, lymphocytes, and/or plasma cells are visualized (Roura *et al.*, 2002; Pointer and Murray, 2011). Intracellular and/or extracellular bacteria are often not observed with bacterial prostatitis but are found in prostatic abscessation (Mordecai *et al.*, 2008). With prostatic adenocarcinoma, sheets of epithelioid cells with numerous acini and numerous mitotic figures would be confirmatory (Hubbard *et al.*, 1990). Performing a fine-needle aspiration of the prostate in cases of suspected prostatitis, abscess, or neoplasia has the risk of seeding the needle tract with infection or tumor cells. Histopathology is required in most cases to obtain a definitive diagnosis. Histopathology can be performed on excisional biopsies or following prostatectomy or necropsy. Although there have been few reports, urinary incontinence following excisional biopsies of the feline prostate have not been reported. Results from the histopathology will vary depending upon the etiology. However, it is important to mention again that benign prostatic hyperplasia has not been reported before in cats.

21.2 Bacterial Prostatitis

Bacterial prostatitis is rare but has been reported in adult intact and neutered cats (Roura *et al.*, 2002; Pointer and Murray, 2011). The anatomic and physiologic features of the feline lower urinary tract typically create an adverse environment for bacterial growth (Bartges and Barsanti, 2000). However, urinary tract infections are more common in cats with underlying disease (e.g. hyperthyroidism, chronic renal disease, diabetes mellitus) (Mayer-Roenne *et al.*, 2007). With bacterial prostatitis, the prostate will be enlarged and ultrasonographically will be well defined with echogenic margins and a parenchyma of mixed echogenicity (hyperechoic and hypoechoic) (Fig. 21.3). This diagnosis can be confirmed via cytology and culture of a fine-needle aspirate of the prostate. As observed in dogs, the most common culture findings in cats with prostatitis is a pure growth of *Escherichia coli.*

A long-term course of an antibiotic that features good penetration into prostatic tissue is necessary when treating bacterial prostatitis. However, most

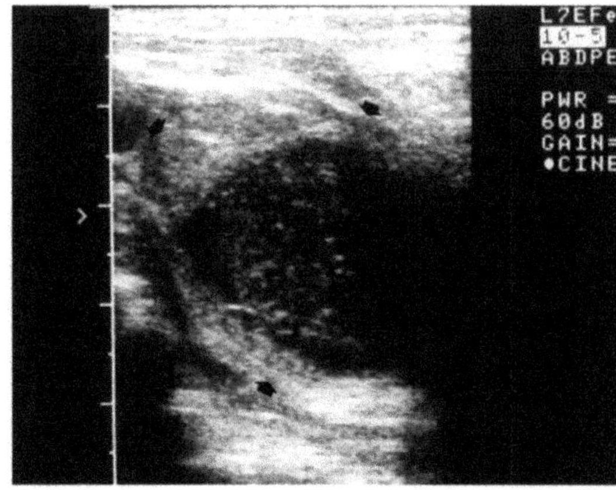

Fig. 21.3. Image of an enlarged prostate with well-defined echogenic margins and a mixed parenchyma typical of prostatitis. (Image used with permission from X. Roura *et al.* (2002).)

antimicrobial agents useful against uropathogenic bacteria diffuse poorly into prostatic tissue due to an intact blood-prostate barrier. For example, amoxicillin with clavulanic acid does NOT penetrate into the prostate. The blood-prostate barrier permits access only to lipophilic drugs and those not highly bound to proteins (Dorfman and Barsanti, 1995). In addition, basic drugs (e.g. trimethoprim-sulfamethoxazole, erythromycin) diffuse easily from the blood (pH 7.4) into the more acidic prostatic environment (pH 6.1–6.5) (Fair and Cordonnier, 1978). Both chloramphenicol and enrofloxacin can readily cross epithelial membranes regardless of their pH (Dorfman *et al.*, 1995). Cases of bacterial prostatitis have been successfully treated in cats using enrofloxacin (5 mg/kg PO q24h for 1 month) (Roura *et al.*, 2002).

21.3 Prostatic Abscessation

Prostatic abscessation is extremely rare in cats and is a possible sequela of bacterial prostatitis. There is a single case report of a prostatic abscess in a 6-year-old castrated domestic shorthair that presented with an acute onset of straining to defecate, lethargy, vomiting, and anorexia (Mordecai *et al.*, 2008). The pathogenesis of prostatic abscessation in cats is not known but is considered the consequence of chronic and severe bacterial prostatitis similar to dogs. Chronic bacterial prostatitis progresses to parenchymal microabscesses which ultimately coalesce into larger abscesses (White and Williams, 1995). Palpation per rectum and survey abdominal radiology were not conclusive. However, abdominal ultrasonography revealed a hypoechoic prostate (2.2 cm) with anechoic foci. Fine-needle aspiration of the prostate was grossly purulent, and the cytology was predominately degenerate neutrophils with rare macrophages and large numbers of intracellular and extracellular pleomorphic bacteria.

Omentalization of a prostatic abscess is often the best course of action for treatment. Omentalization is performed via a ventral midline incision made into the abdomen under general anesthesia. The prostate should be isolated with moistened laparotomy sponges. The prostate is then incised on the ventrolateral aspect of both the left and right prostatic lobes and the contents are removed by suction. A single prostatic cavity that communicates between the left and right lobes is then created by breaking down the abscessed prostatic parenchyma with a Poole suction tip. The prostatic abscess is then omentalized by passing the omentum sequentially through the right lateral incision, through the prostatic cavity ventral to the prostatic urethra, and through the left lateral incision. The omentum is then sutured back onto itself. Following completion of prostatic omentalization, the abdomen should be thoroughly lavaged and a standard closure of the body wall, subcutaneous layer, and skin should be performed.

As in dogs (White and Williams, 1995; Basinger *et al.*, 2003), omentalization is the recommended treatment for prostatic abscesses because success rates are good with minimal postoperative complications (DeHoff *et al.*, 1972; Mordecai *et al.*, 2008). In the prostatic abscess case report, the abscess was drained via a ventral midline laparotomy (Mordecai *et al.*, 2008). The abscessed prostatic parenchyma was broken down in both sides of the prostate and an incision was made between the two sides resulting in a single prostatic cavity (Mordecai *et al.*, 2008). The prostatic abscess was omentalized and the abdomen was thoroughly lavaged (Mordecai *et al.*, 2008). Histopathological evaluation of tissue obtained during the laparotomy confirmed the presence of chronic, suppurative, granulomatous prostatitis with a single isolate of *E. coli* cultured (Mordecai *et al.*, 2008). Following surgery and after-care for the constipation and anorexia, the cat made a full recovery and remained free of symptoms for at least 3 years (Mordecai *et al.*, 2008).

21.4 Urethroadenocystitis

Urethroadenocystitis is a bacterial infection of the prostate, but it differs from bacterial prostatitis. Presenting signs of urethroadenocystitis are similar to those of cystitis (e.g. stranguria, hematuria) (Meier, 1967). Urethroadenocystitis results from a *Pseudomonas aeruginosa* or *P. maltophilia* infection of the prostate and/or bulbourethral glands in cats of any age or sex status (castrated or intact). The causative organism can be aerobically cultured from the urine to make the diagnosis (Meier, 1967). Urethroadenocystitis can complicate the management of feline lower urinary tract disease. However, all reported cases responded to chloramphenicol or oxytetracycline therapy (Meier, 1967). The reported recurrence rate is approximately 50%, with recurrence occurring 6 weeks to 6 months later (Meier, 1967).

21.5 Paraprostatic Cyst

The etiology of paraprostatic cysts is not fully understood, but they are believed to develop from the uterus masculinus, an embryologic remnant of the Müllerian duct (see section on persistent Müllerian duct syndrome in Chapter 22). Histologically, these cysts are lined by one to two layers of transitional epithelium that are continuous with prostatic ductules in several locations. Radiographically, a paraprostatic cyst appears as a large circular density similar to a 'second' bladder. Contrast radiography can be diagnostic because the contrast medium will delineate the bladder and not the paraprostatic cyst (DeHoff *et al.*, 1972; Newell *et al.*, 1992). There have only been two reports of paraprostatic cysts in cats. In both cases, the cyst communicated with the urethra and in one case, the paraprostatic cyst/cystic uterus masculinus became septic (Schulman and Levine, 1989). The latter case resolved successfully following surgical excision. However, the cat in the other case was euthanized for an unrelated problem (Newell *et al.*, 1992).

21.6 Squamous Metaplasia of the Prostate Gland

Squamous metaplasia of the prostatic epithelium has been well described in dogs with estrogen-secreting testicular tumors, but there has only been one published report in cats (Tucker and Smith,

2008). In this report, a 10-year-old male domestic short-haired cat that was presumed to be castrated but was unilaterally cryptorchid presented with chronic intermittent stranguria and pollakiuria. The patient could not be managed by urethral catheterization or perineal urethrostomy and was euthanized. Postmortem examination revealed squamous metaplasia of the prostate and an interstitial cell tumor within the retained testis. Unfortunately, there was no endocrinology performed to support the diagnosis of an estrogen-secreting testicular tumor so the pathogenesis for the prostatic squamous metaplasia in this case is unknown.

21.7 Prostatic Adenocarcinoma

Prostatic adenocarcinoma is rare in cats but is the most reported accessory gland disorder in cats (Hornbuckle and Kleine, 1980; Hawe, 1983; Hubbard *et al.*, 1990; Caney *et al.*, 1998; LeRoy and Lech, 2004; Tursi *et al.*, 2008; Zambelli *et al.*, 2010). All reported cases of prostatic adenocarcinoma have been in neutered cats. Clinical signs of prostatic adenocarcinoma are indistinguishable from non-neoplastic conditions of the feline prostate. Although prostatic reflux of contrast material during double-contrast cystography and voiding urethrography can be highly suggestive of prostatic adenocarcinoma, definitive diagnosis must come from cytology or histopathology. Fine-needle aspirate of a prostatic adenocarcinoma reveals sheets of epithelioid cells with numerous acini and numerous mitotic figures (Hubbard *et al.*, 1990). However, there is risk of seeding the needle tract with tumor cells if a fine-needle aspirate is performed. Thoracic and abdominal radiography should be performed to rule out evidence of metastatic disease prior to treatment. A complete prostatectomy with urethral anastomosis and bilateral pubic osteotomy if necessary has been used to treat prostatic adenocarcinoma in a cat (Hubbard *et al.*, 1990; LeRoy and Lech 2004; Zambelli *et al.*, 2010). However, even with post-prostatectomy chemotherapy with doxorubicin (30 mg/m^2 of body surface) and cyclophosphamide (300 mg/m^2 of body surface) once every 4 weeks for four treatments, this cat became dyschezic 10 months after surgery (Hubbard *et al.*, 1990). Euthanasia was performed and necropsy revealed a 4-cm pelvic mass associated with the urethra in addition to metastases within the lung and pancreas (Hubbard *et al.*, 1990).

21.8 Prognosis

Prognosis for acquired accessory gland diseases in cats is guarded to grave. Cats with non-neoplastic conditions of the prostate can be successfully treated with prolonged antimicrobial therapy that may include surgery (e.g. abscessation, paraprostatic cysts). However, most cats with the prostatic adenocarcinoma die or are euthanized within 3 months of diagnosis (Fan and de Lorimer, 2007).

21.9 References

Bartges, J. W. and Barsanti, J. A. (2000) Bacterial urinary tract infection in cats. In: Bonagura, J. D. (ed.) *Kirk's Current Veterinary Therapy XIII*. W. B. Saunders, Philadelphia, Pennsylvania, pp. 880–882.

Basinger, R. R., Robinette, C. L., and Spaulding, K. A. (2003) Prostate. In: Slatter, D. (ed.) *Textbook of Small Animal Surgery*, 3rd edn. W. B. Saunders, Philadelphia, Pennsylvania, pp. 1542–1557.

Caney, S. M., Holt, P. E., Day, M. J., Rudorf, H., and Gruffydd-Jones, T. J. (1998) Prostatic carcinoma in two cats. *Journal of Small Animal Practice* 39, 140–143. doi: 10.1111/j.1748-5827.1998.tb03619.x

DeHoff, W. D., Greene, R. W., and Greiner, T. P. (1972) Surgical management of abdominal emergencies. *Veterinary Clinics of North America* 2(2), 301–330. doi: 10.1016/s0091-0279(72)50032-1

Dorfman, M. and Barsanti, J. (1995) CVT update: treatment of canine bacterial prostatitis. In: Bonagura, J. D. (ed.) *Kirk's Current Veterinary Therapy*, 12th edn. W. B. Saunders, Philadelphia, Pennsylvania, pp. 1029–1032.

Dorfman, M., Barsanti, J., and Budsberg, S. C. (1995) Enrofloxacin concentrations in dogs with normal prostate and dogs with chronic bacterial prostatitis. *American Journal of Veterinary Research* 56, 386–390.

Fair, W. R. and Cordonnier, J. J. (1978) The pH of prostatic fluid: a reappraisal and therapeutic implications. *Journal of Urology* 120, 695–698. doi: 10.1016/s0022-5347(17)57333-4

Fan, T. E. and de Lorimer, L. (2007) Tumors of the male reproductive system. In: Withrow, S. J. and Vail, D. M. (eds) *Withrow and MacEwen's Small Animal Clinical Oncology*, 4th edn. W. B. Saunders, St. Louis, Missouri, pp. 637–648.

Foster, R. A. (2012) Common lesions in the male reproductive tract of cats and dogs. *Veterinary Clinics of North America Small Animal Practice* 42, 527–545. doi: 10.1016/j.cvsm.2012.01.007

Foster, R. A. and Ladds, P. W. (2007) The male genital system. In: Maxie, G. (ed.). *Jubb, Kennedy & Palmer's Pathology of Domestic Animals*, vol. 3, 5th edn. Saunders, Toronto, Canada, pp. 565–619.

Hawe, R. S. (1983) What is your diagnosis? Prostatic adenocarcinoma. *Journal of the American Veterinary Medical Association* 182, 1257–1258.

Hornbuckle, W. E. and Kleine, L. J. (1980) Medical management of prostatic disease. In: Kirk, R. W. (ed.) *Current Veterinary Therapy VII*. W. B. Saunders, Philadelphia, Pennsylvania, pp. 1146–1150.

Hubbard, B. S., Vulgamott, J. C., and Liska, W. D. (1990) Prostatic adenocarcinoma in a cat. *Journal of the American Veterinary Medical Association* 197(11), 1493–1494.

LeRoy, B. E. and Lech, M. E. (2004) Prostatic carcinoma causing urethral obstruction and obstipation in a cat. *Journal of Feline Medicine and Surgery* 6, 397–400. doi: 10.1016/j.jfms.2004.04.005

Mantziaras, G. (2020) Imaging of the male reproductive tract: not so easy as it looks like. *Theriogenology* 150, 490–497. doi: 10.1016/j.theriogenology.2020.03.009

Mantziaras, G., Choudeloudis, A., Flarakos, M., and Grivas, I. (2019) Computed tomography of the accessory glands in clinically normal intact tomcats. Preliminary results. *Reproduction in Domestic Animals* 54(S2), 108 (abstract).

Mayer-Roenne, B., Goldstein, R. E., and Erb, H. N. (2007) Urinary tract infections in cats with hyperthyroidism, diabetes mellitus and chronic kidney disease. *Journal of Feline Medicine and Surgery* 9(2), 124–132. doi: 10.1016/j.jfms.2006.09.004

McEntee, K. (1990) Bulbourethral, vesicular, and prostate glands. In: *Reproductive Pathology of Domestic Mammals*. Academic Press, San Diego, California, pp. 333–358.

Meier, F. W. (1967) Urethroadenocystitis in the male cat. *Journal of the American Veterinary Medical Association* 151(8), 1059–1071.

Mordecai, A., Liptak, J. M., Hofstede, T., Stalker, M., and Kruth, S. (2008) Prostatic abscess in a neutered cat. *Journal of the American Animal Hospital Association* 44, 90–94. doi: 10.5326/0440090

Newell, S. M., Mahaffey, M. B., Binhazim, A., and Greene, C. E. (1992) Paraprostatic cyst in a cat. *Journal of Small Animal Practice* 33, 399–401. doi: 10.1111/j.1748-5827.1992.tb01186.x

Pointer, E. and Murray, L. (2011) Chronic prostatitis, cystitis, pyelonephritis, and balanoposthitis in a cat. *Journal of the American Animal Hospital Association* 47, 258–261. doi: 10.5326/JAAHA-MS-5627

Romagnoli, S. and Schlafer, D. H. (2006) Disorders of sexual differentiation in puppies and kittens: a diagnostic and clinical approach. *Veterinary Clinics of North America Small Animal Practice* 36(3), 573–606. doi: 10.1016/j.cvsm.2005.12.007

Roura, X., Camps-Palau, M. A., Lloret, A., Garcia, F., and Espada, I. (2002) Bacterial prostatitis in a cat. *Journal of Veterinary Internal Medicine* 16, 593–597. doi: 10.1111/j.1939-1676.2002.tb02393.x

Schulman, J. and Levine, S. H. (1989) Pyometra involving *uterus masculinus* in a cat. *Journal of the American Veterinary Medicine Association* 194, 690–691.

Tucker, A. R. and Smith, J. R. (2008) Prostatic squamous metaplasia in a cat with interstitial cell neoplasia in a retained testis. *Veterinary Pathology* 45(6), 905–909. doi: 10.1354/vp.45-6-905

Tursi, M., Costa, T., Valenza, F., and Aresu, L. (2008) Adenocarcinoma of the disseminated prostate in a cat. *Journal of Feline Medicine and Surgery* 10(6), 600–602. doi: 10.1016/j.jfms.2008.02.008

White, R. A. and Williams, J. M. (1995) Intracapsular prostatic omentalization: a new technique for management of prostatic abscesses in dogs. *Veterinary Surgery* 24, 390–395. doi: 10.1111/j.1532-950x.1995.tb01349.x

Zambelli, D., Cunto, M., Raccagni, R., Merlo, B., Morini, M., *et al.* (2010) Successful surgical treatment of a prostatic biphasic tumour (sarcomatoid carcinoma) in a cat. *Journal of Feline Medicine Surgery* 12, 161–165. doi: 10.1016/j.jfms.2009.07.016

22 Disorders of the Prepuce and Penis

MICHELLE ANNE KUTZLER

Department of Animal and Rangeland Sciences, Oregon State University, Corvallis, Oregon, USA

22.1 Overview

Disorders of the feline prepuce and penis can be congenital or acquired. In some cases (e.g. phimosis), the etiology of the condition could be both congenital and acquired factors. Congenital conditions may arise from chromosomal abnormalities or genetic conditions that affect sexual differentiation. It is important to mention that not all congenital abnormalities are hereditable. Congenital defects of the prepuce and penis are rare in cats. In one report of over 19,646 cats seen at ten North American veterinary colleges, none of the male cats with single or multiple congenital urogenital anomalies had defects of the penis or prepuce (Priester *et al.*, 1970). Acquired disorders of the feline prepuce and penis can be non-neoplastic (e.g. balanoposthitis, phimosis, paraphimosis) or neoplastic.

22.2 Congenital Disorders

22.2.1 Ambiguous genitalia

Although the external genitalia of newborn kittens may appear similar to the untrained eye, there should be no evidence of ambiguity by the time of weaning. Cats with ambiguous genitalia or genitalia that does not 'match' their gonadal sex are referred to as pseudohermaphrodites (Fig. 22.1). Male pseudohermaphrodites have testes (which may be retained) with female-like external and internal genitalia (e.g. vulva and uterus masculinus) (Schulman and Levine, 1989; Romagnoli and Schlafer, 2006). Several abnormal karyotypes have been reported with these conditions in cats including 39,XX7 trisomy, 38,XX/XY chimerism, 37,X/38,XY chimerism, and 38,XX (SRY-positive) (Szczerbal *et al.*, 2015, 2017, 2018). This condition is caused by failure of the embryologic Müllerian duct remnants to regress and/or failure of fetal androgens to masculinize the internal and external genitalia (testicular feminization) (Meyers-Wallen, 1993). Female pseudohermaphrodites have ovaries with male-like genitalia (e.g. prepuce and penis). This masculinization is caused from exposure of female fetuses to exogenous androgens or progestogens transplacentally or excessively high androgens endogenously (as in the case of 11 beta hydroxylase deficiency) (Knighton, 2004).

Male pseudohermaphrodite – persistent Müllerian duct syndrome

Failure of Müllerian ducts to regress occurs because of a mutation in the gene for anti-Müllerian hormone (AMH) receptors (Kutzler, 2011). Cats with persistent Müllerian duct syndrome (PMDS) are genetically male (38, XY) and have a small/rudimentary penis, normal accessory glands, and testes (which are usually cryptorchid). They are pseudohermaphrodites because PMDS cats also have bilateral uterine tubes, a complete uterus with a cervix, and a cranial vagina (Fig. 22.2) (Balogh *et al.*, 2015). Although PMDS has been reported in domestic short hair and domestic long hair cats (Herron and Boehringer, 1975; Kutzler, 2011), it results from an autosomal recessive gene in Persians and Himalayans (Meyers-Wallen and Patterson, 1989a,b; Bredal *et al.*, 1997). Only males homozygous for the recessive gene will be affected. The condition has also been reported in a Bengal cat (Balogh *et al*, 2015). Most male pseudohermaphrodites are presumed to be 'normal' males until they develop a pyometra (ascending infection into the uterus from the prostatic urethra), which can present as persistent dysuria (Osborne *et al.*, 1984; Schulman and Levine, 1989). The dysuria will resolve following hysterectomy. If the male is unilaterally or bilaterally cryptorchid, the testes are found at the ends of

 Feline Reproduction (eds. A.K. Johnson and M.A. Kutzler)
DOI: 10.1079/9781789247107.0022

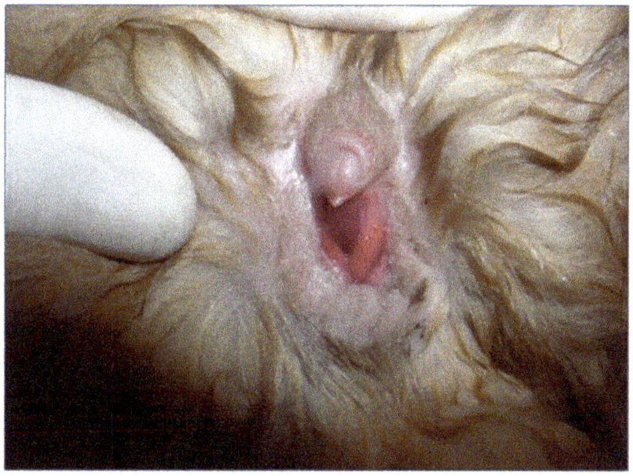

Fig. 22.1. Sexual ambiguity in a cat. There is a vulvar opening with a prominent clitoris or rudimentary penis. (Image courtesy of Dr Alain Fontbonne.)

the uterine horns, where ovaries would typically be located.

Male pseudohermaphrodite – testicular feminization

Failure of normal male genitalia to develop occurs because of a mutation in the gene for androgen receptors (Meyers-Wallen *et al.*, 1989; Kutzler, 2011). Cats with testicular feminization are genetically male (38, XY) and have testes (which are bilaterally cryptorchid), but have a vulva, vestibule, and caudal vagina. Affected males are presumed to be females by their owners until puberty when male secondary sex characteristics develop. Testicular feminization is caused by a recessive X-linked gene. Half (50%) of the male offspring from females carrying this defect will be affected with testicular feminization (Meyers-Wallen, 1993).

Female pseudohermaphrodite – congenital adrenal hyperplasia

Development of male external genitalia (penis, prepuce, scrotum) in genetically female (38, XX) cats with normal uterus and ovaries occurs because of 11-beta hydroxylase deficiency, which results in congenital adrenal hyperplasia (Knighton, 2004). The enzyme deficiency results in an overproduction of testosterone from the adrenal glands, which masculinizes the female embryos. Affected females are presumed to be cryptorchid males by their owners until puberty when estrous behaviors develop (Diegman *et al.*, 1978).

22.2.2 Other congenital abnormalities of the penis and prepuce

Even if the genitalia are not ambiguous, other congenital abnormalities of the feline penis and prepuce have been reported including penile frenulum, penile hypoplasia, hypospadias, and cloacal duplication.

Penile frenulum

During feline embryonic development, the balanopreputial fold circumferentially connects the penis to the prepuce (Fig. 22.3). The dissolution of the balanopreputial fold is an androgen-dependent process. Occasionally, the balanopreputial fold does not completely dissolve, such that a thin membrane of fibrous connective tissue joining the ventral aspect of the penis to the prepuce remains (penile frenulum) (Romagnoli and Schlafer, 2006, Foster, 2011). When the penis is extended or erect, a penile frenulum will cause a ventral or lateral penile deviation (phallocampus), which can prevent intromission (Kutzler, 2011) (Fig. 22.4). The heritability of penile frenulum is unknown in cats, but there is no known pattern of inheritance in the dog (Hutchinson, 1973). Tomcats affected with a persistent frenulum may be asymptomatic or may show discomfort during urination or copulation (erection). Diagnosis is made by visual inspection. Treatment is made by transecting the frenulum with scissors, which can be under a light plane of general anesthesia without risk of hemorrhage. If diagnosed in a prepubertal tomcat, delaying castration in nonbreeding animals until after puberty (>6 months) may result in spontaneous correction.

Penile hypoplasia

Underdevelopment of the penis (penile hypoplasia) is reported in male cats with chromosomal intersex (e.g. male tortoiseshell cats with XXY karyotype) (Malouf *et al.*, 1967; Pyle *et al.*, 1971; Centerwall and Bernischke, 1975). In addition to penile hypoplasia, testicular hypoplasia and persistent Müllerian ducts may be present. Severe cases of penile hypoplasia may have signs of urinary incontinence, dysuria, hematuria, dripping of urine secondary to urine pooling and infection within the prepuce, and phimosis (inability to extend penis beyond preputial

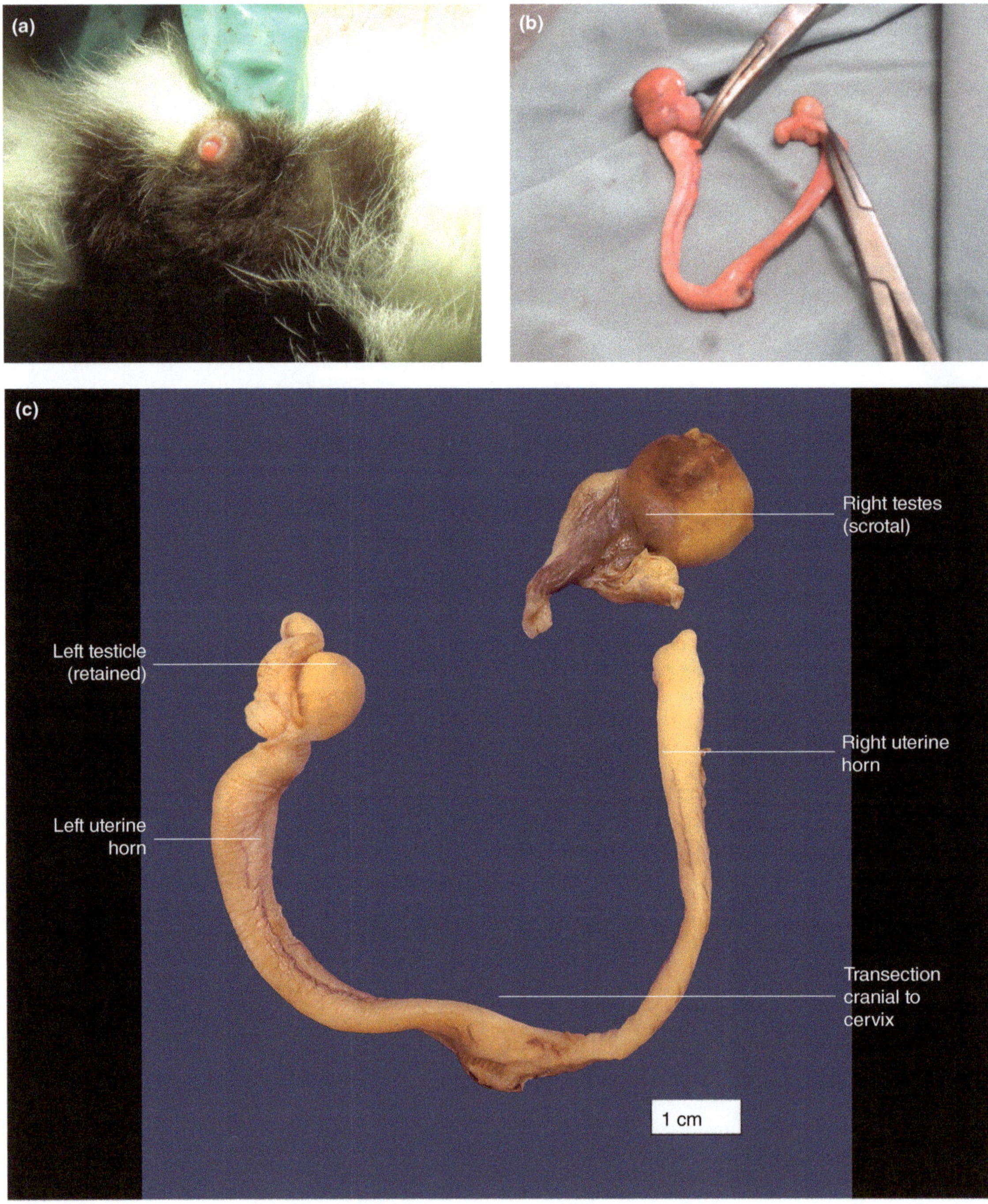

Fig. 22.2. An adult cat presented for surgical sterilization through a trap/neuter/return clinic. **(a)** External genitalia consisted of a small external penis and one testicle in the scrotum. The second testicle was located in the abdomen. (**b**) Abdominal exploration revealed a structure that appeared to be uterus, with the left horn extending cranially ending in a gonad just distal to the left kidney. The right horn looped caudal out through the inguinal canal, ending in a larger gonad in the scrotum. **(c)** Confirmed to be persistent Müllerian duct syndrome. (Images courtesy of Heather M. Hillier. Image (c) is included in Library of Reproductive Images (LORI).)

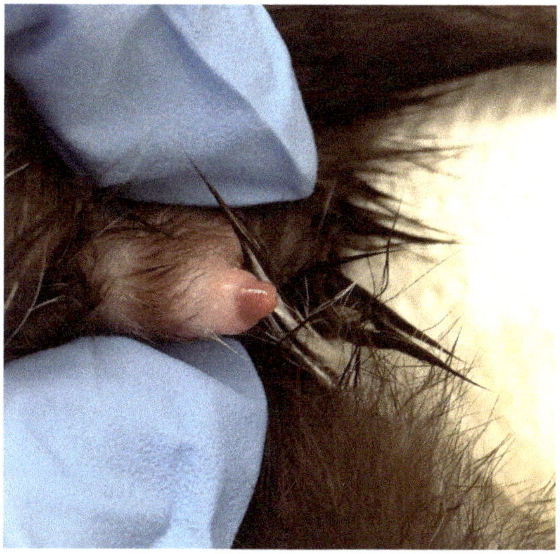

Fig. 22.3. The adhesion between the penis and prepuce is present in the prepubertal cat. This adhesion breaks down under the influence of androgens. When the breakdown is incomplete, a penile frenulum remains. (Image courtesy of Dr Aime Johnson.)

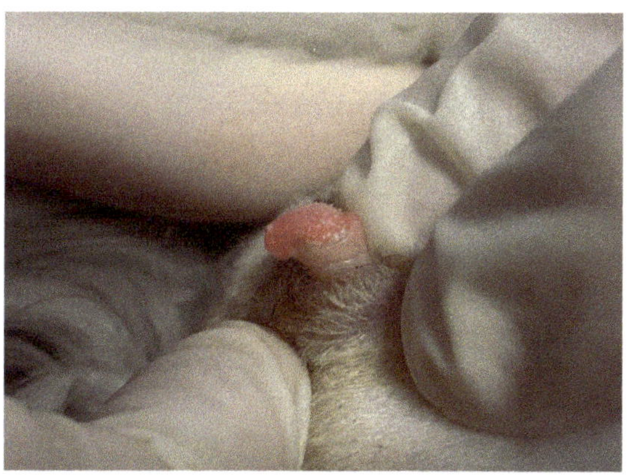

Fig. 22.4. A persistent frenulum in a tom. Note the remnant of the balanopostetic fold that failed to break down causing the penis to deviate to the left of the photo. (Image courtesy of G. Robiteau.)

opening) (Kutzler, 2011). Diagnosis is made by visual inspection. Histologic examination of gonadal tissue with karyotype evaluation is necessary to diagnose intersex condition. If indicated, penile hypoplasia can be treated by surgical shortening of the prepuce, enlargement of the preputial orifice, or penile amputation with urethrostomy.

Hypospadias

Hypospadias occurs from an incomplete fusion of the median raphe of the penis, prepuce, or scrotum, such that the urethral opening is in an abnormal location (Fig. 22.5). This is attributable to incomplete masculinization of the urogenital sinus during the process of male urethral development. Hypospadias has been reported in tomcats (Bloom, 1954). Hypospadias can be induced in female kittens by administering progestogens to the queen during pregnancy (fetal masculinization). Hypospadias can also be induced by feeding the pregnant queen a diet deficient in vitamin A (Ader and Hobson, 1978). The defect is named based upon where the urethral opening is, and are as follows: ventral to the tip of the penis (glandular hypospadias); ventral to the body of the penis (penile hypospadias); in the scrotal area (scrotal hypospadias); or in the perineal area (perineal hypospadias). The severity of the defect increases the further from the normal location the urethral opening is. For example, glandular hypospadias is often asymptomatic and typically requires no treatment. Penile, scrotal, and perineal hypospadias are often characterized by urinary incontinence, with urine scalding and inguinal dermatitis. In addition, these forms of hypospadias often occur with other congenital defects including penile/preputial hypoplasia and cryptorchidism.

Integrity of the urethra must be maintained when surgically repairing hypospadias. After placing a urinary catheter, the urethral mucosa is dissected and separated from the skin at the mucocutaneous junction. The incised edges of urethral mucosa are sutured, taking care not to place knots inside the urethral lumen (because this may serve as a nidus calculus formation). In the case of penile hypospadias, amputation of the penis and prepuce to the level of the urethral opening is performed. With scrotal or perineal hypospadias, complete penile amputation and either scrotal or perineal urethrostomy is required. Regardless of which form of hypospadias exists, castration should be performed.

Cloacal duplication

During embryologic development, duplication of the cloacal membrane may lead to duplication of the urogenital tubercle, resulting in duplication of the penis. This defect has been described in line bred Siamese cats (Axnér *et al.*, 1996).

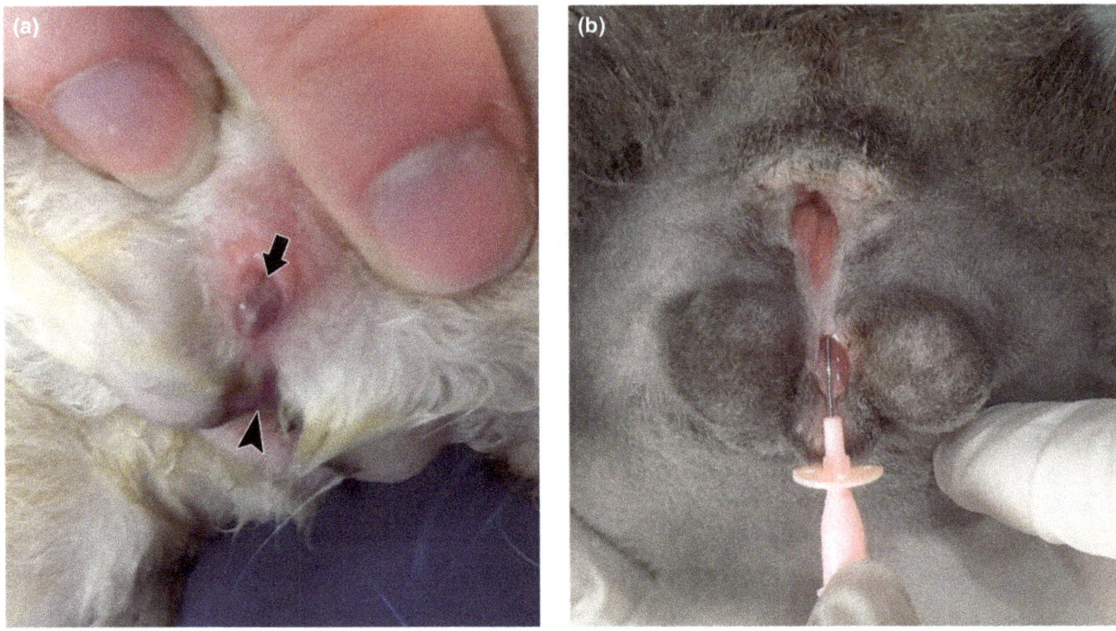

Fig. 22.5. **(a)** Hypospadias affecting the penis. The opening of the urethra extends the entire shaft of the penis rather than just the tip (arrow). Also note that the scrotum is split separating the left and right testicles (arrowhead), a common finding with hypospadias. (Image courtesy of Zuzanna Niewiadomska.) **(b)** A more severe form of hypospadias. The penile opening is under the handle of the probe distal to the testicles. The probe is placed into the defect that is located on midline between the testicles. Note here that the scrotum is split as was seen in fig. 22.5a. (Image courtesy of G. Robiteau.)

22.3 Acquired Disorders

22.3.1 Trauma

Injury to the prepuce and penis may occur from blunt force trauma (e.g. vehicular accidents); bite wounds; self-mutilation (e.g. secondary to separation anxiety); or during breeding. The need for surgical intervention depends on the existence of or potential for urethral obstruction or uncontrolled hemorrhage (Fig. 22.6).

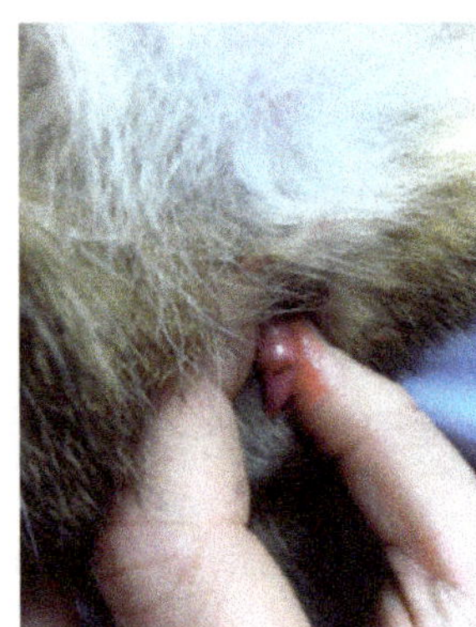

Fig. 22.6. The base of the penis has a laceration caused by self-mutilation. This wound was allowed to heal by second intention with careful follow-up to make sure an adhesion did not form. (Photo courtesy of Dr Aime Johnson and Ms Jessica Cannon.)

Punctures or lacerations of the prepuce and penis

Although punctures and lacerations of the prepuce may be readily apparent, injuries to the penis may be less obvious. Small volumes of blood may drip slowly and continuously from the preputial orifice. Minor injuries to the penis (e.g. punctures, minor lacerations) should be managed as open wounds, treated with topical and systemic antimicrobials, and allowed to heal by second intention. In cases in which urethral integrity may be compromised, placement of an indwelling urinary catheter until healed may deter stricture formation. For penile lacerations with significant hemorrhage, penile amputation with perineal urethrostomy may be necessary.

Fracture of the os penis

The feline os penis has a lower mineral density than other bones but can be visualized on radiographs (Piola et al, 2011) (Fig. 22.7). It should not be mistaken for a pathologic finding (e.g. urolithiasis or dystrophic mineralization). Fracture of the os penis may occur with a preputial or penile laceration. Clinical signs include hemorrhagic preputial discharge and/or hematuria and dysuria. Crepitus on palpation of the penis may be evident. Diagnosis may be confirmed via radiographs or computed tomography (Fig. 22.8). Urinary catheter placement before radiography or retrograde contrast urethrography can be used to determine if the urethral canal is impinged. Fractures of the os penis are most often simple fractures and can be managed conservatively with placement of an indwelling urinary catheter for at least 7 days to provide stability during healing. Systemic antimicrobial and anti-inflammatory medications should also be administered. Urethral obstruction associated with callus formation can occur as the os penis fracture heals, necessitating penile amputation with perineal urethrostomy.

22.3.2 Balanoposthitis

Balanoposthitis is inflammation of the penis (balanitis) and the prepuce (posthitis). This condition is uncommon in cats, but when it occurs, it is commonly associated with an underlying cause (e.g. urolithiasis, trauma) (Foster, 2012). A case of balanoposthitis was reported in a cat that was secondary to chronic prostatitis, cystitis, and pyelonephritis (Pointer and Murray, 2011). Balanoposthitis can also occur in the cat secondary to phimosis, especially if urine is accumulating within the prepuce. Clinical signs of balanoposthitis include excessive preputial licking/grooming, painful preputial swelling, and a mucopurulent preputial discharge (Davidson, 2016). If left untreated, balanoposthitis can cause preputial and penile mucosa ulceration and adhesion formation. Treatment of balanoposthitis includes systemic antimicrobial and anti-inflammatory medications in addition to treating the underlying cause to prevent recurrence.

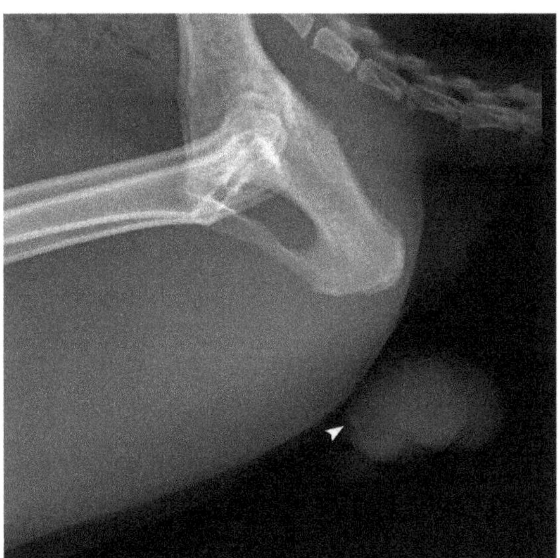

Fig. 22.7. Lateral radiograph of the pelvis in a male cat. The os penis can be identified ventral to the testicles and within the prepuce (arrow). (Image courtesy of Dr Aime Johnson.)

22.3.3 Hair ring

Hair rings can form around the base of the glans penis and are more common in long-haired cats (Zambelli and Levy, 2010). Hair rings are also more common in intact toms because the testosterone-dependent spines can trap hair and other fibers (Foster, 2012). The clinical signs associated with hair rings include intromission failure with intense and prolonged pelvic thrusting and persistent mounting (Hart and Peterson, 1971). Hair rings can also predispose tomcats to phimosis and paraphimosis,

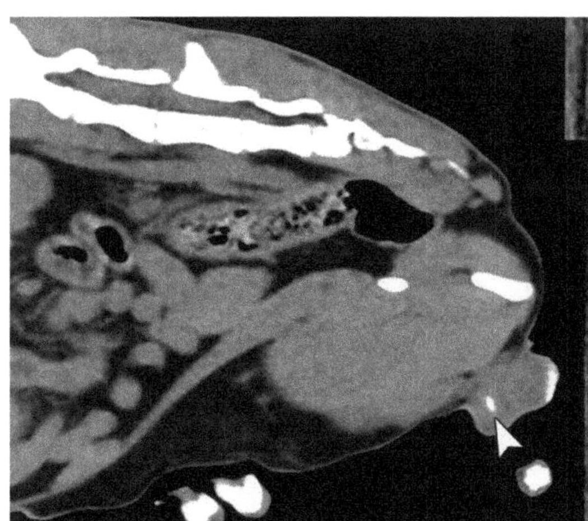

Fig. 22.8. Computed tomography image of a sagittal section showing a normal os penis (arrow) within the prepuce of an intact male tom. (Image courtesy of Dr Rachel Moon.)

which are associated with additional clinical signs (see Sections 22.3.4 and 22.3.5). For uncomplicated cases, removal of the hair ring will restore normal behavior and mating ability.

22.3.4 Phimosis

Phimosis is the inability to extrude the penis from the prepuce. Phimosis is an uncommon finding in cats. Phimosis can result from a congenital defect (e.g. abnormally small preputial opening) or an acquired condition secondary to penile or preputial inflammation or trauma, with the latter being the most common cause (Kirk, 1931; May and Hauptman, 2009). In long-haired cats, phimosis can occur secondary to an accumulation of circumferential penile hair rings (Romagnoli and Schlafer, 2006). Clinical signs of phimosis are variable. Often the problem is unnoticed until the cat attempts to mate and is unable to copulate. Excessive preputial licking/grooming or dribbling urine from the preputial opening after urination are common owner complaints. Hematuria and dysuria have also been a presenting sign of phimosis in an intact tomcat (Kirk, 1931). The diagnosis is made while attempting to examine the penis. There may be concurrent inflammation of the prepuce and ulceration at the preputial opening. Treatment depends on the existence of an underlying cause (e.g. hair ring, inflammation). If there is no underlying cause and the phimosis is symptomatic, preputial surgical enlargement is indicated. This can be accomplished by removing a V-shaped wedge of tissue at the level of the preputial orifice, which will prevent urine pooling and recurrent inflammation. The prognosis for most phimosis cases that have been subjected to corrective surgery is good to excellent with appropriate postsurgical care to prevent self-trauma.

22.3.5 Paraphimosis

Paraphimosis is the inability to completely withdraw the penis into the prepuce and is an emergency condition. Although paraphimosis is rare in cats, it can occur following breeding, penile entrapment from a hair ring, priapism, or following castration (Kirk, 1931; Swalec and Smeak, 1989). Priapism is a form of paraphimosis in which the penis is persistently erect. Feline priapism is most commonly reported in Siamese (Gunn-Moore *et al.*, 1995). Diagnosis is made by visual inspection of the penis protruding from the prepuce. Chronic protrusion of the penis causes the penile mucosa to become dry, congested, erythematous, inflamed, edematous, ischemic, excoriated, and painful, which may lead to self-mutilation. Radiographs should be performed to rule-out concurrent fracture of the os penis.

The goal of treatment is to replace the penis into the prepuce as soon as possible and prevent recurrence of the problem (Davidson, 2016). Urine production should be monitored closely. Before attempting manual replacement of the penis under general anesthesia, the clinician should clip or pluck the hair around the preputial opening and apply copious amounts of lubricant to the penile mucosa. If the tomcat is intact, castration is often performed to prevent erection that could result in recurrence of the paraphimosis. If the penis cannot be replaced manually, a preputiotomy with or without phallopexy should be performed. If the penis is severely damaged, penile amputation with perineal urethrostomy should be performed. The prognosis is good to guarded for resolution of paraphimosis, depending on the severity and duration of clinical signs.

22.3.6 Neoplasia

Preputial neoplasia is extremely rare in cats but has been reported. Cutaneous mast cell tumors on the prepuce appear as a solitary, raised, firm, well-circumscribed, hairless, dermal nodule (Govier, 2003). Siamese and Siamese-crosses are predisposed to developing mast cell tumors, with the average age of occurrence at 8 to 9 years (Miller *et al.*, 1991). Surgical excision with wide margins if possible is the treatment of choice. Although local recurrence is rare, one-third of cats will develop cutaneous mast cell tumors in other locations (Buerger and Scott, 1987). There have been no cases of penile neoplasia reported in cats.

22.4 References

Ader, P. L. and Hobson, H. P. (1978) Hypospadias: a review of the veterinary literature and a report of three cases. *Journal of the American Animal Hospital Association* 14, 721–727.

Axnér, E., Ström, B., Linde-Forsberg, C., Gustavsson, I., Lindblad, K., *et al.* (1996) Reproductive disorders in 10 domestic male cats. *Journal of Small Animal Practice* 37(8), 394–401. doi: 10.1111/j.1748-5827.1996.tb02427.x

Balogh, O., Berger, A., Pieńkowska-Schelling, A., Willmitzer, F., Grest, P., *et al.* (2015) 37,X/38,XY mosaicism in a cryptorchid Bengal cat with Müllerian duct remnants. *Sexual Development* 9, 327–332. doi: 10.1159/000443233

Bloom, F. (1954) Pathology of the dog and cat. In: *American Veterinary Publications*, Evanston, Illinois, pp.194–212.

Bredal, W. P., Thoresen, S. I., Kvellestad, A., and Lindblad, K. (1997) Male pseudohermaphroditism in a cat. *Journal of Small Animal Practice* 38(1), 21–24. doi: 10.1111/j.1748-5827.1997.tb02981.x

Buerger, R. G. and Scott, D. W. (1987) Cutaneous mast cell neoplasia in cats: 14 cases (1975–1985). *Journal of the American Veterinary Medical Association* 190, 1440–1444.

Centerwall, W. R. and Bernischke, K. (1975) An animal model for the XXY Klinefelter's syndrome in man: tortoiseshell and calico male cats. *American Journal of Veterinary Research* 32, 1275–1280.

Davidson, A. P. (2016) Reproductive diseases of the male small animal. In: Aiello, S. E. (ed.) *The Merck Veterinary Manual*, 11th edn. Merck & Co., Inc., Kenilworth, New Jersey, pp. 1400–1402.

Diegman, F. G., Loo, B. J., and Grom, P. A. (1978) Female pseudohermaphroditism in a cat. *Feline Practice* 8(5), 45.

Foster, R. A. (2011) Male reproductive system. In: Zachary, J. and McGavin, D. M. (eds) *Pathologic Basis of Veterinary Disease*, 5th edn. Elsevier Mosby, St. Louis, Missouri, pp. 1127–1152.

Foster, R. A. (2012) Common lesions in the male reproductive tract of cats and dogs. *Veterinary Clinics of Small Animal* 42, 527–545. doi: 10.1016/j.cvsm.2012.01.007

Govier, S. M. (2003) Principles of treatment for mast cell tumors. *Clinical Techniques in Small Animal Practice* 18(2), 103–106. doi: 10.1053/svms.2003.36624

Gunn-Moore, D. A., Brown, P. J., Holt, P. E., and Gruffydd-Jones, T. J. (1995) Priapism in seven cats. *Journal of Small Animal Practice* 36(6), 262–266. doi: 10.1111/j.1748-5827.1995.tb02912.x

Hart, B. L. and Peterson, D. M. (1971) Penile hair rings in male cats may prevent mating. *Laboratory Animal Science* 21,422.

Herron, M. A. and Boehringer, B. T. (1975) Male pseudohermaphroditism in a cat. *Feline Practice* 4, 30–32.

Hutchinson, J. A. (1973) Persistence of the penile frenulum in dogs. *Canadian Veterinary Journal* 14, 71.

Kirk, H. (1931) Phimosis and paraphimosis in the cat. *Veterinary Records* 11, 832.

Knighton, E. (2004) Congenital adrenal hyperplasia secondary to 11 beta-hydroxylase deficiency in a domestic cat. *Journal of the American Veterinary Medical Association* 225, 238–241. doi: 10.2460/javma.2004.225.238

Kutzler, M. A. (2011) The reproductive tract, In: Peterson, M. E. and Kutzler, M. A. (eds) *Small Animal Pediatrics: The First 12 Months of Life*. Elsevier, St. Louis, Missouri, pp. 405–417.

Malouf, N., Bernischke, K., and Hoefnagel, D. (1967) XX/XY chimerism in a tricolored male cat. *Cytogenetics* 6, 228–241.

May, L. R. and Hauptman, J. G. (2009) Phimosis in cats: 10 cases (2000-2008). *Journal of the American Animal Hospital Association* 45, 277–283. doi: 10.5326/0450277

Meyers-Wallen, V. N. (1993) Genetics of sexual differentiation and anomalies in dogs and cats. *Journal of Reproduction and Fertility Supplement* 47, 441–452.

Meyers-Wallen, V. N. and Patterson, D. F. (1989a) Sexual differentiation and inherited disorders of sexual development in the dog. *Journal of Reproduction and Fertility Supplement* 39, 57–64.

Meyers-Wallen, V. N. and Patterson, D. F. (1989b) Disorders of sexual development in dogs and cats. In: Kirk, R. W. (ed.) *Current Veterinary Therapy, Small Animal Practice XIII*. W. B. Saunders, Philadelphia, Pennsylvania, pp. 1261–1269.

Meyers-Wallen, V. N., Wilson, J. D., Griffin, J. E., Fisher, S., Moorhead, P. H., *et al.* (1989c) Testicular feminization in a cat. *Journal of the American Veterinary Medical Association* 195(5), 631–634.

Miller, M. A., Nelson, S. L., Turk, J. R., Pace, L. W., Brown, T. P., *et al.* (1991) Cutaneous neoplasia in 340 cats. *Veterinary Pathology* 28:389–395. doi: 10.1177/030098589102800506

Osborne, C. A., Johnston, G. R., Polzin, D. J., Kruger, J. M., Poffenbarger, E. M., *et al.* (1984) Redefinition of the feline urologic syndrome: feline lower urinary tract disease with heterogeneous causes. *Veterinary Clinics of North America Small Animal Practice* 14, 409–439. doi: 10.1016/s0195-5616(84)50051-5

Piola, V., Posch, B., Aghte, P., Caine, A., and Herrtage, M. E. (2011) Radiographic characterization of the os penis in the cat. *Veterinary Radiology and Ultrasound* 52, 270–272.

Pointer, E. and Murray, L. (2011) Chronic prostatitis, cystitis, pyelonephritis, and balanoposthitis in a cat. *Journal of the American Animal Hospital Association* 47, 258–261. doi: 10.5326/JAAHA-MS-5627

Priester, W. A., Glass, A. G., and Waggoner, N. S. (1970) Congenital defects in domesticated animals: general considerations. *American Journal of Veterinary Research* 31, 1871–1879.

Pyle, R. L., Patterson, D. F., Hare, W. C. D., Kelly, D. F., and Digiulia, T. (1971) XXY sex chromosome constitution in a Himalayan cat with tortoise-shell points. *Journal of Heredity* 62, 220–222. doi: 10.1093/oxfordjournals.jhered.a108154

Romagnoli, S. and Schlafer, D. H. (2006) Disorders of sexual differentiation in puppies and kittens: a diagnostic and clinical approach. *Veterinary Clinics of North American Small Animal Practice* 36, 573–606. doi: 10.1016/j.cvsm.2005.12.007

Schulman, J. and Levine, S. H. (1989) Pyometra involving uterus masculinus in a cat. *Journal of the American Veterinary Medical Association* 205, 690–691.

Swalec, K. M. and Smeak, D. D. (1989) Priapism after castration in a cat. *Journal of the American Veterinary Medical Association* 195(7), 963–964.

Szczerbal, I., Stachowiak, M., Dzimira, S., Sliwa, K., and Switonski, M. (2015) The first case of 38,XX (SRY-positive) disorder of sex development in a cat. *Molecular Cytogenetics* 8, 22. doi: 10.1186/s13039-015-0128-5

Szczerbal, I., Stachowiak, M., Nowacka-Woszuk, J., Dzimira, S., Szczepanska, K., *et al.* (2017) Disorder of sex development in a cat with chromosome mosaicism 37,X/38,X,r(Y). *Reproduction in Domestic Animals* 52, 914–917. doi: 10.1111/rda.12968

Szczerbal, I., Krzeminska, P., Dzimira, S., Tamminen, T. M., Saari, S., *et al.* (2018) Disorders of sex development in cats with different complements of sex chromosomes. *Reproduction in Domestic Animals* 53, 1317–1322. doi: 10.1111/rda.13263

Zambelli, D. and Levy, X. (2010) Clinical approaches to the infertile male. In: England, G. and von Heimendahl, A. (eds) *BSAVA Manual of Canine and Feline Reproduction and Neonatology*. BSAVA, Gloucester, Scotland, pp. 70–79.

23 Semen Cryopreservation

Daniele Zambelli and Marco Cunto

Animal Reproduction Unit, Department of Veterinary Medical Sciences, Alma Mater Studiorum, University of Bologna, Bologna, Italy

23.1 Introduction

Unlike the canine species where breeders frequently require the conservation of seminal material, among cat breeders this procedure is rarely requested and unfortunately it is also poorly known. Cryopreservation of dog sperm has been practiced for many years and has allowed the creation of sperm banks in several countries. In the domestic cat, the use of artificial insemination (AI) in practice is generally reduced and limited to the use of fresh sperm. This is likely due to the inability to obtain a sufficient quantity of good quality post-thawed sperm, combined with the difficulties of insemination. These factors reduce the request by the breeders and the proposal by the veterinarians to proceed with the cryopreservation of sperm. With an increase in the number of cats as companion animals, the interest in the collection, assessment, and cryopreservation of cat semen is increasing (Siemieniuch and Dubiel, 2007). The development of valid protocols for sperm cryopreservation in domestic cats is not only useful for use in breeding of domestic cats, but also for application of cryopreservation techniques to wild felids (Rijsselaere and van Soom, 2010). The Convention of International Trade of Endangered Species reported that 36 of the 37 existing feline species are threatened with extinction (CITES, 1973) and the most important cause of this situation is poor breeding performance induced mainly by a decrease in genetic diversity, caused by inbreeding due to geographical isolation and population contraction (Wildt, 1990).

Artificial insemination can be performed with fresh, cooled, or cryopreserved semen, the latter providing long-term storage for postponed use. The first pregnancies in domestic cats with frozen–thawed semen were obtained in 1978 (Platz *et al.*, 1978) and, after these, numerous freezing protocols and AI procedures have been reported.

Both ejaculated (Glover and Watson, 1985, 1987; Pope *et al.*, 1989, 1991; Pukazhenthi *et al.*, 1999) and epididymal spermatozoa (Goodrowe and Hay, 1993; Harris *et al.*, 2001) can be prepared for the cryopreservation process. It is also possible to cool the testicles and then flush the epididymides and vas deferens in order to collect spermatozoa and freeze at another location (Goodrowe and Hay, 1993; Hay and Goodrowe, 1993).

Cat semen has been frozen using vials (Lengwinat and Blottner, 1994), straws (Pope *et al.*, 1991; Hay and Goodrowe, 1993), and pellets (Platz *et al.*, 1976, 1978). In general, the cryopreservation protocols are associated with reduced motility, viability, acrosome loss (Pope *et al.*, 1991), and a reduction of fertilizing capacity (Pukazhenthi *et al.*, 2000). A decrease of motility of 76% has been observed when freezing in pellets leading to the conclusion that freezing in straws is more valuable than the pellet method (Pope *et al.*, 1991).

Numerous factors affect sperm quality during freezing–thawing process, such as extender composition (Axnér *et al.*, 2004; Thuwanut *et al.*, 2008; Zambelli *et al.*, 2010), cooling rates, and freezing protocols. The freeze–thaw procedure in particular is responsible for inducing severe spermatozoal damage, which diminishes fertilizing ability. Therefore, cold-induced damage represents a limiting factor for the conservation of spermatozoa, particularly spermatozoa from felids, which are often affected by teratospermia (Luvoni *et al.*, 2003b). In one study, 73.4 ± 3.5% of sperm was found to be morphologically normal. Multiple mating activities compensate for insufficient sperm morphology. In the same paper, the percentage of morphological defects in freezing–thawing semen increased and the average of morphologically normal sperm declined to 58.7 ± 3.8%. In other studies it has been reported that the percentage of normal

 Feline Reproduction (eds. A.K. Johnson and M.A. Kutzler)
DOI: 10.1079/9781789247107.0023

sperm declined from 76 ± 2.0% in fresh to 64 ± 2.6% in post-thaw epididymal sperm (Hay and Goodrowe, 1993).

23.2 Extenders

Extenders are added to semen to buffer changes in pH, to provide an energy source for spermatozoa, and to prevent bacterial growth and injury to spermatozoa during cooling, freezing, and thawing. The presence of seminal plasma negatively affects spermatozoal fertilizing ability in the cat (McLaughlin and Hamner, 1974). Sperm centrifugation at low speed (300 × *g*) and subsequent removal of seminal plasma significantly prolongs spermatozoal survival time (Luvoni *et al.*, 2003a). Better results can be achieved applying the swim-up process, which selects spermatozoa on the basis of motility and structural integrity (Howard *et al.*, 1990; Chatdarong *et al.*, 2010b).

According to the literature, in the absence of feline-specific commercial extenders, the TRIS-based extender is the hitherto most widely used for freezing feline sperm. Glycerol (Nelson *et al.*, 1999; Baran *et al.*, 2004), sodium dodecyl sulfate (Axnér *et al.*, 2004; Zambelli *et al.*, 2010), egg yolk (Glover and Watson, 1987; Hermansson and Axnér, 2007), and different types of sugar (Glover and Watson, 1987) have been added to feline extenders in different proportions to improve sperm cryopreservation results. Antibiotics as streptomycin sulfate and/or penicillin G potassium have been also included in the extender composition (Johnston *et al.*, 2001).

Good results in terms of maintaining motility and percentage of normal acrosomes after thawing have been reported using TRIS containing 20% egg yolk and 8% glycerol (Zambelli *et al.*, 2002). Soy lecithin has been reported to protect against cold shock similar to the low-density lipoprotein in egg yolk. Plant protein-based extenders have been used with sperm from primates (Li *et al.*, 2005), cows (Aires *et al.*, 2003), sheep (Forouzanfar *et al.*, 2010), and dogs (Beccaglia *et al.*, 2009), producing post-thaw sperm quality equal to or greater than traditional egg yolk extenders. In particular, soy-based medium used for domestic cat sperm cryopreservation resulted in good long-term motility and capacitation status of frozen–thawed sperm, maintaining fertilizing ability (Vick *et al.*, 2012).

Glycerol is often incorporated as cryoprotectant in freezing extenders, usually in a TRIS-based extender containing 20% (v/v) egg yolk. It protects spermatozoa from the consequences of ice formation by increasing the unfrozen water fraction. However, even its osmotic effect could affect membrane integrity. This compound is used at low concentration as cat spermatozoa appears to be particularly sensitive to high concentrations (Nelson *et al.*, 1999). A decline in motility has been also observed, likely due to changes in osmolality (Pukazhenthi *et al.*, 2000) and active transport and permeability of the plasma membrane in the tail region, combined with an alteration of energy availability or damage to the axonema elements (Watson, 1995). Glycerol is used at final concentrations of 3–8% (Hay and Goodrowe, 1993; Nelson *et al.*, 1999), with 4–5% most commonly used (Thuwanut *et al.*, 2010; Villaverde *et al.*, 2013). To achieve 5% glycerol in final concentration, glycerol is added in two steps of dilution (i.e. 3% and 7% glycerol, respectively) (Axnér *et al.*, 2004; Chatdarong *et al.*, 2010b), or it is added to freezing extenders used for the second step of dilution only (i.e. extenders for the first and second steps containing 0% and 10% glycerol, respectively) (Villaverde *et al.*, 2013). Temperature of glycerol addition has also been considered to influence post-thaw sperm quality (Thiangtum *et al.*, 2006). Glycerol is either added at room temperature or, to reduce its cytotoxicity, completely or partially at 4–5°C (after cooling).

Another aspect to consider is the necessity of mammalian spermatozoa to optimize energy consumption to enhance flagellar contractility and ensure adequate motility. Sugars have been included in sperm diluents as exogenous energy substrates, as osmotic components, and as cryoprotective agents (Watson, 1979). However, in order to prevent high sugar concentrations from saturating the energy-obtaining machinery of the spermatozoa, it is important to maintain moderate concentrations of these substances in the extender (Rigau *et al.*, 2001). Although most monosaccharides can be used, there may be differences between different species metabolism (Rikmenspoel and Caputo, 1966). Fructose and glucose are known to be the major energy source for ejaculated spermatozoa and are found naturally in the seminal plasma of many species. However, in all mammalian species, including the domestic cat (Johnston *et al.*, 1988; Ponglowhapan *et al.*, 2004), the seminal plasma does not contain monosaccharides. In these species, it has been proposed that exposure to these sugars occurs in the female genital tract, inducing sperm motility patterns after entering the female (Rigau *et al.*, 2001). When using artificial extenders, fructose (Cocchia *et al.*, 2010; Toyonaga *et al.*, 2010; Baran *et al.*, 2011) and glucose (Siemieniuch and Dubiel, 2007; Thuwanut *et al.*, 2008; Chatdarong *et al.*, 2010b; Zambelli *et al.*, 2010) are the sugars that are routinely added to feline sperm freezing extenders. The type of sugar added seems to have no effect on the morphology and motility of frozen–thawed cat sperm (Hay and Goodrowe, 1993).

Sodium dodecyl (lauryl) sulfate or SD(L)S, the active compound of the commercial products 'Orvus Es Paste (OEP)' and 'Equex-STM,' a water-soluble anionic surfactant that is frequently added to extenders used for semen cryopreservation in domestic cats and several other species (Jiménez, 1987; Peña *et al.*, 1998; Cheng *et al.*, 2004; Buranaamnuay *et al.*, 2009; Anakkul *et al.*, 2011). It modifies egg yolk lipoproteins contained in the extenders and protects sperm against toxic effects during the freezing–thawing process, improving sperm cryotolerance and quality after thawing (Martin *et al.*, 1979; Arriola and Foote, 1987). In cat sperm cryopreservation, both OEP (Tsutsui *et al.*, 2003; Martins *et al.*, 2009; Toyonaga and Tsutsui, 2012) and Equex-STM (Axnér *et al.*, 2004; Thuwanut and Chatdarong, 2009) have generally been included in freezing extenders at 0.5% to 1% final concentrations and are shown to provide improved frozen–thawed sperm motility (Mizutani *et al.*, 2010). A protective effect of Equex-STM paste on feline epididymal spermatozoal acrosomes has also been shown, although there were not significant differences in sperm viability variables (Tsutsui *et al.*, 2003). A negative effect on sperm membranes and motility has been reported during *in vitro* incubation (Axnér *et al.*, 2004), indicating a brief pre-freeze exposure has a more pronounced protective effect (Peña and Linde-Forsberg, 2000; Jiménez *et al.*, 2013). Both in epididymal cat sperm (Axnér *et al.*, 2004) and cat semen collected by electroejaculation (Zambelli *et al.*, 2010), more desirable results have been obtained with a 0.5% Equex-STM supplementation. In addition, Zambelli *et al.* (2010) reported that in vitro fertilizing capacity of frozen–thawed sperm was not affected by Equex-STM addition in the freezing extender used for the second dilution, before cooling at 5°C (Buranaamnuay, 2017).

The use of antioxidants (AOs) in feline semen freezing extenders and their effect on sperm quality has been tested with varying results. While addiction of 10 U/mL glutathione peroxidase to TRIS-egg yolk (TEY) provided positive effects on post-thaw epididymal cat sperm, the use of 200 U/mL catalase or 600 U/mL superoxide dismutase did not improve sperm motility or acrosome integrity immediately after thawing compared with the extender without supplementation (Thuwanut *et al.*, 2010). Likewise, extender supplemented with 400 U/mL of either catalase or superoxide dismutase did not improve the motility, viability, or acrosome integrity of frozen–thawed sperm (Thiangtum *et al.*, 2009).

Protective effects of antioxidants DL-cysteine (improved post-thaw motility and DNA integrity) and a water-soluble vitamin E analog (Trolox) (improved post-thaw motility, progressive motility and membrane integrity) on frozen–thawed epididymal cat sperm was reported when either of these compounds (at 5 mM) was added to a TEY-lactose extender (Thuwanut *et al.*, 2008). Furthermore, with epididymal cat sperm, sperm motility improvement, immediately and 2 hours after thawing, was obtained by supplementation of a TEY-glucose freezing extender with 25 mM L-carnitine (Manee-In *et al.*, 2014).

Other additives have been occasionally added to extenders used for cat sperm cryopreservation. Luvoni *et al.* (2002) supplemented TEY-glucose extender with 25–50 mM taurine, a sulfur-containing p-amino acid having a role in osmoregulation of sperm cells that stimulates sperm motility. A higher motility was reported with no difference between the two concentrations of taurine being reported. Similarly, addition of 75 mM taurine to skimmed milk-glucose extender containing 10% egg yolk was as effective as TEY-fructose extender in preserving motility and normal morphology of frozen–thawed sperm collected by electroejaculation.

The ability of several substances of plant origin to protect spermatozoa during cryopreservation has also been assessed. Aloe vera, for example, contains substances similar to conventional cryoprotectants (Souza *et al.*, 2014). The cryoprotective action of aloe vera has been identified in refrigeration of semen of goats (Aguiar *et al.*, 2012), cattle (Vargas, 2012), dogs (Melo *et al.*, 2014), and peccaries (Souza *et al.*, 2016). Other properties of aloe vera as an antioxidant and antimicrobial and in cellular regeneration have been considered to improve spermatozoa survival during cryopreservation (Estakhr and Javdan, 2011; Nejatzadeh-Barandozi, 2013;

Rozkot *et al.*, 2013; Freitas *et al.*, 2014). However, the use of crude aloe vera extract was not satisfactory on the cryopreservation of epididymal spermatozoa of domestic cats after thawing (Barbosa *et al.*, 2020).

Caffeine, pentoxifylline and 2′-deoxyadenosine have been used in cryopreservation processes for their dose-dependent effect as motility stimulants. These substances produce a hyperactivated motion of frozen–thawed cat epididymal spermatozoa reducing the decrease in motility by approximately 10% compared to the pre-freeze value (Stachecki *et al.*, 1994).

Different non-feline commercial extenders based on TEY, egg yolk or milk-free extenders (Jiménez *et al.*, 2013, Brusentsev *et al.*, 2018), skimmed milk–egg yolk (Jiménez *et al.*, 2013) or TRIS-based extenders requiring egg yolk addiction (Brusentsev *et al.*, 2018) have been assessed for cat sperm cryopreservation. TEY-based specifically-produced extenders generally result in better sperm cryoprotection, but sometimes commercial extenders remain a good option for ease of use and availability.

23.3 Cooling Rates and Techniques

The rate of cooling from body temperature to freezing temperatures is crucial to preserve integrity and fertilizing potential of spermatozoa (Luvoni *et al.*, 2003a). Prior to freezing, feline semen require an equilibration period at +5°C for about 20 minutes. The mechanism by which cold shock acts on the sperm cell is not entirely clear, but it is probably related to the phase transitions of membrane lipids, resulting in phase separations and loss of the selective permeability characteristics of living biological membranes (Watson, 1995). Ice crystals cause rupture of cellular membranes when the cells are exposed to a rapid rate of cooling (4°C/min) from body temperature to +5°C, while decreasing the cooling rate to 0.5°C/min minimizes the structural damage (Pukazhenthi *et al.*, 1999).

Once 5°C is reached, sperm is packaged in straws or ampules. Further temperature change may be programmed with a controlled freezer or by exposing to liquid nitrogen (LN2) vapor before immersion into liquid nitrogen and final storage (Pope *et al.*, 1991). The last method is more economical than using a programmable freezer and more convenient than using dry ice. Sperm-loaded straws are placed horizontally or vertically over the surface of LN2 for a period of time to allow the sample temperature to decrease from 4–5 °C to approximately −40°C (Zambelli *et al.*, 2002), −100°C (Wood *et al.*, 1993), −110°C (Baran *et al.*, 2004), −120°C (Siemieniuch and Dubiel, 2007) or −130°C (Schäfer *et al.*, 2000) before the samples are plunged in the LN2. Generally, horizontal placement is performed for samples loaded in 1.5 mL cryotubes (Stachecki *et al.*, 1994) and both 0.5 mL (Schäfer and Holzmann, 2000) and 0.25 mL (Luvoni *et al.*, 2002; Kashiwazaki *et al.*, 2005; Tebet *et al.*, 2006; Cocchia *et al.*, 2010) straws. Horizontal cryotubes/straws are placed at different distances from the surface of the LN2 on the basis of protocols reported in literature: 4 cm (Karja *et al.*, 2002; Baran *et al.*, 2011), 6 cm (Villaverde *et al.*, 2009; Cocchia *et al.*, 2010) or 7 cm (Toyonaga *et al.*, 2010) above the LN2 surface. When samples are placed vertically, the distance between straws (usually 0.25 mL) in a canister and LN2 surface in a tank is modified in three steps prior to plunging the straws in LN2 (Axnér *et al.*, 2004; Chatdarong *et al.*, 2009; Thuwanut and Chatdarong, 2009). This technique was first described for dog sperm cryopreservation where the top of the canister was held at 7, 13 and 20 cm below the opening of the tank for 2, 2 and 1 minutes, respectively (Rota *et al.*, 1997). Vertical cryopreservation of cat sperm is also described using a specialized type of vacuum flask (Dewar; SIO, Milan, Italy). Straws (0.25 mL) in a pre-cooled (5°C) stainless-steel cylinder (14 × 4 cm) are placed in the Dewar flask (25 cm in diameter and 47 cm in height) above the surface of LN2 at distances useful to obtain specific cooling rates (i.e. 3 cm above LN2 to achieve 3.85°C/min freezing rate). The cylinder is finally plunged in LN2 (Zambelli *et al.*, 2002, 2006, 2008, 2010). This cryopreservation technique, associated with a slow cooling rate (3.85°C/min), showed a higher motility and normal acrosome percentages after thawing than more rapid cooling rates (9, 22.8, 36 and 43°C/min; Zambelli *et al.*, 2002). Multi-step LN2 vapor cryopreservation was also performed by placing 0.25 mL straws on a multi-step rack above the surface of the LN2 at 7 cm for 1 minute and 3.5 cm for 1 minute before immersing the straws into LN2 (Vick *et al.*, 2012).

As mentioned above, production of cryopreserved cat epididymal and ejaculated sperm by using a programmable freezing machine has also been reported (Lengwinat and Blottner, 1994; Tsutsui *et al.*, 2000, 2003; Mizutani *et al.*, 2010).

The cooling rate was relatively slow during the initial stage of cryopreservation (i.e. –1 °C/min from 4°C to –1°C or –25°C), to minimize ice crystal formation in the cells, and thereafter was rapidly accelerated (i.e. –30°C/min or greater) until the final temperature of –100°C (Lengwinat and Blattner, 1994) or –196°C (Tsutsui *et al.*, 2000, 2003; Mizutani *et al.*, 2010) was reached. The cryopreserved samples were subsequently transferred to a LN2 container.

Successful cryopreservation of cat epididymal sperm was also reported after slow equilibration to 15 or 10°C. In particular, these temperatures were reached after 40 and 100 minutes, respectively, and then sperm was placed 2 cm above liquid nitrogen for 15 minutes. At a mean temperature of 167°C, samples were plunged into liquid nitrogen and transferred to the storage container (Klaus *et al.*, 2016).

23.4 Thawing

Like the cryopreservation process, the thawing procedure may also result in sperm damage (Holt *et al.*, 1992; Curry and Watson, 1994; Rota *et al.*, 1998). During thawing, recrystallization occurs, with the formation of large ice crystals which subsequently causes cell damage (Mazur *et al.*, 1981). Moreover, osmotic gradients are generated across the sperm membranes during thawing, causing cell membrane damage and cell death (Holt and North, 1994; Gilmore *et al.*, 1996). Different freezing processes often require different thawing rates to achieve optimum sperm survival. Generally, cells that undergo fast freezing require fast thawing. It has been reported that after rapid cooling, rapid rewarming limits the time for recrystallization to occur (Holt and North 1994). This may be the reason the thawing of some dog spermatozoa at 70°C resulted in higher sperm quality and less capacitation-like changes than thawing at 37°C (Rota *et al.*, 1998; Peña and Linde-Forsberg, 2000). Fast thawing may, however, also have negative effects as the spermatozoa are subjected to abrupt changes in osmolarity (Holt *et al.*, 1992; Gao *et al.*, 1997). Although there is a scarcity of reports on different thawing rates for cryopreserved cat spermatozoa, Rijsselaere *et al.* (2007) found that thawing epididymal cat spermatozoa for 5 seconds at 60°C resulted in fewer acrosome-reacted spermatozoa and fewer abnormal sperm heads than thawing at 37°C for 1 minute, whereas other sperm characteristics did not differ. Thawing at 37°C is likely to be more practical in practice as most clinic water baths are set at this temperature. Chatdarong *et al.* (2010a) reported that frozen cat semen can be thawed either at 37°C or 70°C with similar results, but a post-thaw dilution with TRIS buffer is recommended to reduce the toxic effect of some ingredients in the extender during post-thaw incubation.

23.5 Suggested Protocol

The authors use a previously reported protocol described by Zambelli *et al.* (2002) and successively modified in 2006 (Zambelli *et al.*, 2006). The semen is centrifuged at 300 × *g* for 5 minutes to remove excess plasma and to concentrate the semen. The sperm pellets are then extended with TRIS containing 20% egg yolk (Zambelli *et al.* 2000, 2006). A successive dilution in a 1:1 ratio using the same medium containing 8% glycerol and 1% Equex-STM paste (Zambelli *et al.*, 2006), allow to obtain doses of 200 µl containing 40 × 10^6 spermatozoa. The first and the second dilution are made by dropwise addition of the extender at room temperature (about 20°C). After loading into 0.25 mL straws, the spermatozoa are cooled to 5°C at a rate 0.2°C/s and maintained at that temperature for 25 minutes. The straws are frozen in vapor produced by liquid nitrogen contained in a Dewar flask. A stainless-steel cylinder, pre-cooled to 5°C, is loaded with 0.25 mL straws. The cylinder is placed in the Dewar flask at a distance from the liquid nitrogen to achieve cooling rates of 3.85°C/min. The cylinder is plunged into liquid nitrogen when it reaches –40°C. The straws are thawed in a 37°C water bath for 30 seconds.

23.6 References

Aguiar. G. V., Santos, B. M. B., Cavalcante, J. M. M., Rodrigues, F. R. N., Salgueiro, C. C. M., *et al.* (2012) Addition of Aloe vera to powder coconut water solution (ACP-101®) like cryoprotector of the goat semen cooled at 4°C. *Ciência Animal* 22, 292–295.

Aires, V. A., Hinsch, K. D., Mueller-Schloesser, F., Bogner, K., Mueller-Schloesser, S., *et al.* (2003) In vitro and in vivo comparison of egg yolk-based and soybean lecithin-based extenders for cryopreservation of bovine semen. *Theriogenology* 60, 269–279. doi: 10.1016/s0093-691x(02)01369-9

Anakkul, N., Suwimonteerabutr, J., Singlor, J., Phutikanit, N., Tharasanit, T., *et al.* (2011) Effect of Equex STM Paste on the quality and motility characteristics of post thawed cryopreserved goat semen. *The Thai Journal of Veterinary Medicine* 41, 345–351.

Arriola, J. and Foote, R. H. (1987) Glycerolation and thawing effects on bull spermatozoa frozen in detergent-treated egg yolk and whole egg extenders. *Journal of Dairy Science* 70, 1664–1670. doi: 10.3168/jds.s0022-0302(87)80194-7

Axnér, E., Hermansson, U., and Linde-Forsberg, C. (2004) The effect of Equex STM paste and sperm morphology on post-thaw survival of cat epididymal spermatozoa. *Animal Reproduction Science* 84, 179–191. doi: 10.1016/j.anireprosci.2003.11.003

Baran, A., Bacinoglu, S., Evecen, M., Sahin, B. E., Alkan, S., *et al.* (2004) Freezing of cat semen in straws with different glycerol levels containing Tris extender. *Turkish Journal of Veterinary and Animal Science* 28, 545–552.

Baran, A., Tek, C., Demir, K., Sabuncu, A., and Ozdas, O. B. (2011) Intrauterine insemination with cat semen frozen with various extenders. *Turkish Journal of Veterinary and Animal Science* 35, 311–318.

Barbosa, B. S., Santos, F. A., Macêdo, L. B., Izzo, R. G., Fernandes, D. P., *et al.* (2020) Effect of supplementation of Aloe vera extracts in cold storage media and cryopreservation of domestic cat epididymal spermatozoa. *Animal Reproduction* 17(1). doi: 10.21451/1984-3143-AR2019-0067

Beccaglia, M., Anastasi, P., and Luvoni, G. C. (2009) Freezing of canine semen in an animal-free protein extender. *Veterinary Research Communications* 33, 77–80. doi: 10.1007/s11259-009-9249-9

Brusentsev, E., Kizilova, E., Mokrousova, V., Kozhevnikova, V., Rozhkova, I., *et al.* (2018) Characteristics and fertility of domestic cat epididymal spermatozoa cryopreserved with two different freezing media. *Theriogenology* 110, 148–152. doi: 10.1016/j.theriogenology.2017.12.038

Buranaamnuay, K. (2017) Protocols for sperm cryopreservation in the domestic cat: A review. *Animal Reproduction Science* 183, 56–65. doi: 10.1016/j.anireprosci.2017.06.002

Buranaamnuay, K., Tummaruk, P., Singlor, J., Rodriguez-Martinez, H., and Techakumphu, M. (2009) Effects of straw volume and equex-STM® on boar sperm quality after cryopreservation. *Reproduction in Domestic Animals* 44, 69–73. doi: 10.1111/j.1439-0531.2007.00996.x

Chatdarong, K., Thuwanut, P., Suksamai, P., Patanatiradaj, S., and Sangwornrachasup, A. (2009) Survival of frozen-thawed cat spermatozoa pre-cooled in the epididymides. *Reproduction in Domestic Animals* 44 (2), 377–380. doi: 10.1111/j.1439-0531.2009.01412.x

Chatdarong, K., Thuwanut, P., Manee-in, S., Lohachit, C., and Axnér, E. (2010a) Effects of thawing temperature and post-thaw dilution on the quality of cat spermatozoa. *Reproduction in Domestic Animals* 45, 221–227. doi: 10.1111/j.1439-0531.2008.01218.x

Chatdarong, K., Thuwanut, P., and Morrell, J. M. (2010b) Single-layer centrifugation through colloid selects improved quality of epididymal cat sperm. *Theriogenology* 73, 1284–1292. doi: 10.1016/j.theriogenology.2009.12.009

Cheng, F. P., Wu, J. T., Chan, J. P. W., Wang, J. S., Fung, H. P., *et al.* (2004) The effect of different extenders on post-thaw sperm survival, acrosomal integrity and longevity on cryopreserved semen of Formosan Sika deer and Formosan Sambar deer. *Theriogenology* 61, 1605–1616. doi: 10.1016/j.theriogenology.2003.07.015

CITES (1973) Convention on International Trade in Endangered Species of Wild Flora and Fauna, part of the Endangered Species Act (PL 93-205, 93rd Congress) and in 50 appendices. *Code Fed. Reg.*, part 23.

Cocchia, N., Ciani, F., El-Rass, R., Russo, M., Borzacchiello, G., *et al.* (2010) Cryopreservation of feline epididymal spermatozoa from dead and alive animals and its use in assisted reproduction. *Zygote* 18, 1–8. doi: 10.1017/S0967199409990256

Curry, M. R. and Watson, P. F. (1994) Osmotic effects on ram and human sperm membranes in relation to thawing injury. *Cryobiology* 31, 39–46. doi: 10.1006/cryo.1994.1005

Estakhr, J. and Javdan, N. (2011) Spermatogenic activity of Aloe vera in adult male rats. *Pharmacology online* 2, 886–889.

Forouzanfar, M., Sharafi, M., Hosseini, S. M., Ostadhosseini, S., Hajian, M., *et al.* (2010) In vitro comparison of egg yolk-based and soybean lecithin-based extenders for cryopreservation of ram semen. *Theriogenology* 73, 480–487. doi: 10.1016/j.theriogenology.2009.10.005

Freitas, V. S., Rodrigues, R. A. F., and Gaspi, F. O. G. (2014) Propriedades farmacológicas da *Aloe vera* (L.). Burm. F. *Revista Brasileira Plantas Medicinais* 16(2), 299–307.

Gao, D. Y., Mazur, P., and Critser, J. K. (1997) Fundamental cryobiology of mammalian spermatozoa. In: Karow, A. M. and Critser, J. K. (eds) *Reproductive Tissue Banking*. Academic Press, San Diego, California, pp. 263–328.

Gilmore, J. A., Du, J., Tao, J., Peter, A. T., and Critser, J.K. (1996) Osmotic properties of boar spermatozoa and their relevance to cryopreservation. *Journal of Reproduction and Fertility* 107, 87–95. doi: 10.1530/jrf.0.1070087

Glover, T. E. and Watson, P. F. (1985) The effect of buffer osmolality on the survival of cat (*Felis catus*) spermatozoa at 5°C. *Theriogenology* 24, 449–456. doi: 10.1016/0093-691x(85)90051-2

Glover, T. E. and Watson, P. F. (1987) The effects of egg yolk, the low-density lipoprotein fraction of egg yolk, and three monosaccharides on the survival of cat (*Felis catus*) spermatozoa stored at 5°C. *Animal Reproduction Science* 13, 229–237. doi: 10.1016/0378-4320(87)90112-6

Goodrowe, K. L. and Hay, M. A. (1993) Characteristics and zona binding ability of fresh and cooled domestic cat spermatozoa. *Theriogenology* 40, 967–975. doi: 10.1016/0093-691x(93)90365-c

Harris, R. F., Pope, C. E., Gomez, M. C., Leibo, S. P., and Dresser, B. L. (2001) Storage of domestic cat spermatozoa for extended periods at 4°C. *Theriogenology* 55, 308.

Hay, M. A. and Goodrowe, K. L. (1993) Comparative cryopreservation and capacitation of spermatozoa from epididymides and vasa deferentia of the domestic cat. *Journal of Reproduction and Fertility Supplement* 47, 297–305.

Hermansson, U. and Axnér, E. (2007) Epididymal and ejaculated cat spermatozoa are resistant to cold shock but egg yolk promotes sperm longevity during cold storage at 4 degrees C. *Theriogenology* 67, 1239-1248. doi: 10.1016/j.theriogenology.2007.01.008

Holt, W. V. and North, R. D. (1994) Effects of temperature and restoration of osmotic equilibrium during thawing on the induction of plasma membrane damage in cryopreserved ram spermatozoa. *Biology of Reproduction* 51, 414–424. doi: 10.1095/biolreprod51.3.414

Holt, W. V., Head, M. F., and North, R. D. (1992) Freeze-induced membrane damage in ram spermatozoa is manifested after thawing: observations with experimental cryomicroscopy. *Biology of Reproduction* 46, 1086–1094. doi: 10.1095/biolreprod46.6.1086

Howard, J. G., Brown, J. L., Bush, M., and Wildt, D. E. (1990) Teratospermic and normospermic domestic cats: ejaculate traits, pituitary-gonadal hormones, and improvement of spermatozoa motility and morphology after swim up processing. *Journal of Andrology* 11, 204–215.

Jiménez, C. F. (1987) Effects of Equex STM and equilibration time on the pre-freeze and post thaw motility of equine epididymal spermatozoa. *Theriogenology* 28, 773–782. doi: 10.1016/0093-691X(87)90029-X

Jiménez, E., Pérez-Marín, C. C., Vizuete, G., Millán, Y., and Agüera, E. I. (2013) Effect of different extenders on in vitro characteristics of feline epididymal sperm during cryopreservation. *Reproduction in Domestic Animals* 48, 665–672. doi: 10.1111/rda.12142

Johnston, S. D., Osborne, C. A., and Lipowitz, A. J. (1988) Characterizations of seminal plasma, prostatic fluid, and bulbourethral gland secretions in the domestic cat. In: *Proceedings of the 11th International Congress Animal Reproduction AI.* Dublin, UK, pp.560.

Johnston, S. D., Root Kustriz, M. V., and Olson, P. N. S. (2001) Semen Collection and evaluation in the cat. In: Johnston, S. D., Root Kustriz, M. V., and Olson, P. N. S. (eds) *Canine and Feline Theriogenology.* W. B. Saunders Company, Philadelphia, Pennsylvania, pp. 508–520.

Karja, N. W., Otoi, T., Murakami, M., Fahrudin, M., and Suzuki, T. (2002) In vitro maturation, fertilization and development of domestic cat oocytes recovered from ovaries collected at three stages of the reproductive cycle. *Theriogenology* 57, 2289–2298. doi: 10.1016/s0093-691x(02)00905-6

Kashiwazaki, N., Yamaguchi, R., Uesugi, R., Hishiyama, N., Kim, M., *et al.* (2005) Sperm motility, plasma membrane integrity, and binding capacity to homologous zona pellucida of cryopreserved epididymal spermatozoa in the domestic cat. *Journal of Reproduction and Development* 51, 735–739. doi: 10.1262/jrd.17052

Klaus, C., Eder, S., Franz, C., and Müller, K. (2016) Successful cryopreservation of domestic cat (*Felis catus*) epididymal sperm after slow equilibration to 15 or 10°C. *Reproduction in Domestic Animals* 51, 195–203. doi: 10.1111/rda.12666

Lengwinat, T. and Blottner, S. (1994) In vitro fertilization of follicular oocytes of domestic cat using fresh and cryopreserved epididymal spermatozoa. *Animal Reproduction Science* 35, 291–301. doi: 10.1016/0378-4320(94)90044-2

Li, Y. H., Cai, K. J., Su, L., Guan, M., He, X. C., *et al.* (2005) Cryopreservation of cynomolgus monkey (*Macaca fascicularis*) spermatozoa in a chemically defined extender. *Asian Journal of Andrology* 7, 139–44. doi: 10.1111/j.1745-7262.2005.00039.x

Luvoni, G. C., Ruggiero, C., Marinoni, G., and Kalchschmidt, E. (2002) Effect of taurine-containing diluent for cryopreservation of domestic cat epididymal spermatozoa. *Theriogenology* 57, 466.

Luvoni, G. C., Kalschmidt, E., Leoni, S., and Ruggiero, C. (2003a) Conservation of feline semen. Part I: cooling and freezing protocols. *Journal of Feline Medicine and Surgery* 5, 203–208. doi: 10.1016/S1098-612X(03)00029-9

Luvoni, G. C., Kalchschmidt, E., and Marinoni, E. (2003b) Conservation of feline semen. Part II: Cold-induced damages on spermatozoal fertilizing ability. *Journal of Feline Medicine and Surgery* 5, 257–263. doi: 10.1016/S1098-612X(03)00030-5

Manee-In, S., Parmornsupornvichit, S., Kraiprayoon, S., Tharasanit, T., Chanapiwat, P., *et al.* (2014) L-Carnitine supplemented extender improves cryopreserved-thawed cat epididymal sperm motility. *Asian-Australasian Journal of Animal Science* 27(6), 791–796. doi: 10.5713/ajas.2013.13565

Martin, J. C., Klug, E., and Gunzel, A. R. (1979) Centrifugation of stallion semen and its storage in large volume straws. *Journal of Reproduction and Fertility Supplement* 27, 47–51.

Martins, J. L., Villaverde, A. I., Lima, A. F., Steagall, P. V., Ferreira, J. C., *et al.* (2009) Impact of 24-h cooling prior to freezing on the survival of domestic cat (*Felis catus*) epididymal sperm. *Reproduction in Domestic Animals* 44(2), 366–368. doi: 10.1111/j.1439-0531.2009.01432.x

Mazur, P., Rall, W. F., and Rigopoulos, N. (1981) Relative contribution of the fraction of unfrozen water and of salt concentration to the survival of slowly frozen human erythrocytes. *Biophysical Journal* 36, 653–675. doi: 10.1016/S0006-3495(81)84757-1

McLaughlin, K. C. and Hamner, C. E. (1974) A demonstration of cat seminal plasma antifertility activity. *Proceedings of the Society for Experimental Biology and Medicine* 145, 103–106. doi: 10.3181/00379727-145-37757

Melo, C. C. S., Oliveira, É. C. S., Ramos, R. P., Lima, C. F., Rodrigues, A. E. S., *et al.* (2014) Renovação do diluidor Tris com gema de ovo ou *Aloe vera* sp. Na viabilidade do sêmen canino refrigerado a 5°C–resultados preliminares. *Acta Veterinaria Brasilica* 8, 142–143.

Mizutani, T., Sumigama, S., Nagakubo, K., Shimizu, N., Oba, H., *et al.* (2010) Usefulness of addition of Orvus ES paste and sodium lauryl sulfate to frozen feline semen. *Journal of Veterinary Medical Science* 72, 23–27. doi: 10.1292/jvms.08-0332

Nejatzadeh-Barandozi, F. (2013) Antibacterial activities and antioxidant capacity of aloe vera. *Organic and Medical Chemistry Letters* 3(1), 1–8. doi: 10.1186/2191-2858-3-5

Nelson, K. L., Crichton, E. G., Doty, L., Volenec, D. E., Morato, R. G., *et al.* (1999) Heterologous and homologous fertilizing capacity of cryopreserved felid sperm: a model for endangered species. *Theriogenology* 51, 290.

Peña, A. I., Barrio, F., Quintela, L. A., and Herradon, P. G. (1998) Effects of sodium dodecyl sulphate on post-thaw dog semen quality during in vitro incubation at 39 °C and 22 °C. *Reproduction in Domestic Animals* 33, 393–398. doi: 10.1111/j.1439-0531.1998.tb01377.x

Peña, A. and Linde-Forsberg, C. (2000) Effects of Equex, one- or two-step dilution, and two freezing and thawing rates on post-thaw survival of dog spermatozoa. *Theriogenology* 54(6), 859–875. doi: 10.1016/S0093-691X(00)00397-6

Platz, C. C., Follis, T., Demorest, N., and Seager, S. W. J. (1976) Semen collection, freezing and insemination in the domestic cat. In: *Proceedings of VIII International Congress on Animal Reproduction and Artificial Insemination*, Cracow, Poland, pp. 1053–1056.

Platz, C. C., Wildt, D. E., and Seager, S. W. J. (1978) Pregnancy in the domestic cat after artificial insemination with previously frozen spermatozoa. *Journal of Reproduction and Fertility* 52, 279–282. doi: 10.1530/jrf.0.0520279

Ponglowhapan, S., Essen-Gustavsson, B., and Linde-Forsberg, C. (2004) Influence of glucose and fructose in the extender during longterm storage of chilled canine semen. *Theriogenology* 62, 1498–1517. doi: 10.1016/j.theriogenology.2004.02.014

Pope, C. E., Gelwicks, E. J., Wachs, K.B., Keller, G. L., and Dresser, B. L. (1989) In vitro fertilization in the domestic cat (Felis catus): a comparison between freshly collected and cooled semen. *Theriogenology* 31, 241.

Pope, C. E., Turner, J. L., Quatman, S. P., and Dresser, B. L. (1991) Semen storage in the domestic felid: a comparison of cryopreservation methods and storage temperature. *Biology of Reproduction* 44, 117.

Pukazhenthi, B., Pelican, K., Wildt, D. E., and Howard, J. G. (1999) Sensitivity of domestic cat (*Felis catus*) sperm from normospermic versus teratospermic donors to cold-induced acrosomal damage. *Biology of Reproduction* 61, 135–141. doi: 10.1095/biolreprod61.1.135

Pukazhenthi, B., Noiles, E., Pelican, K., Donoghue, A., Wildt, D., *et al.* (2000) Osmotic effects on feline spermatozoa from normospermic versus teratospermic donors. *Cryobiology* 40, 139–150. doi: 10.1006/cryo.2000.2233

Rigau, T., Farre, M., Ballester, J., Mogas, T., Pena, A., *et al.* (2001) Effects of glucose and fructose on motility patterns of dog spermatozoa from fresh ejaculates. *Theriogenology* 56, 801–815. doi: 10.1016/S0093-691X(01)00609-4

Rijsselaere, T., Pope, E., Wirtu, G., Filliers, M., Maes, D., *et al.* (2007) Effect of thawing temperature on survival of cooled, cryopreserved epididymal spermatozoa. In: *Proceedings of the Fifth Annual Symposium EVSSAR*, Estoril, European Veterinary Society of Small Animal Reproduction, Estoril, Portugal, pp. 106.

Rijsselaere, T. and van Soom, A. (2010) Semen collection, assessment and artificial insemination in the cat. *Vlaams Diergeneeskundig Tijdschrift* 79, 467-470.

Rikmenspoel, R. and Caputo, R. (1966) The Michaelis-Menten constant for fructose and for glucose of hexokinases in bull spermatozoa. *Journal of Reproduction and Fertility* 1, 437–444. doi: 10.1530/jrf.0.0120437

Rota, A., Ström, B., Linde-Forsberg, C., and Rodriguez-Martinez, H. (1997) Effects of Equex STM paste on viability of frozen-thawed dog spermatozoa during in vitro incubation at 38 degrees C. *Theriogenology* 47, 1093–1101. doi: 10.1016/s0093-691x(97)00066-6

Rota, A., Linde-Forsberg, C., Vannozzi, J., Romagnoli, S., and Rodriguez-Martinez, H. (1998) Cryosurvival of dog spermatozoa at different glycerol concentrations and freezing/thawing rates. *Reproduction in Domestic Animals* 33, 355–361. doi: 10.1111/j.1439-0531.1998.tb01370.x

Rozkot, M., Frydrychová, S., Benešová, N., and Opletal, L. (2013) Small molecules of natural origin as a source of antimicrobial agents in pig breeding – review. *Research in Pig Breeding* 7, 26–33.

Schäfer, S. and Holzmann, A. (2000) The use of transmigration and spermac stain to evaluate epididymal cat spermatozoa. *Animal Reproduction Science* 59, 201–211. doi: 10.1016/s0378-4320(00)00073-7

Siemieniuch, M. and Dubiel, A. (2007) Preservation of tomcat (*Felis catus*) semen in variable temperatures. *Animal Reproduction Science* 91, 135–144. doi: 10.1016/j.anireprosci.2006.04.049

Stachecki, J. J., Ginsburg, K. A., and Armant, D. R. (1994) Stimulation of cryopreserved epididymal spermatozoa of the domestic cat using the motility stimulants caffeine, pentoxifylline and 2#-deoxy-adenosine. *Journal of Andrology* 15, 157–164.

Souza, A. L. P., Lima, G. L., and Silva, A. R. (2014) Alternativas para o aperfeiçoamento dos protocolos de criopreservação de sêmen de animais selvagens. *Revista Brasileira Reproduo Animal* 38, 98–102.

Souza, A. L. P., Lima, G. L., Peixoto, G. C. X., Silva, A. M., Oliveira, M. F., *et al.* (2016) Use of Aloe vera-based extender for chilling and freezing collared peccary (*Pecari tajacu*) semen. *Theriogenology* 85(8), 1432–1438. doi: 10.1016/j.theriogenology.2016.01.007

Tebet, J. M., Martins, M. I. M., Chirinea, V. H., Souza, F. F., Campagnol, D., *et al.* (2006) Cryopreservation effects on domestic cat epididymal versus electroejaculated spermatozoa. *Theriogenology* 66, 1629–1632. doi: 10.1016/j.theriogenology.2006.02.013

Thiangtum, K., Swanson, W. F., Howard, J., Tunwattana, W., Tongthainan, D., *et al.* (2006) Assessment of basic seminal characteristics, sperm cryopreservation and heterologous in vitro fertilisation in the fishing cat (*Prionailurus viverrinus*). *Reproduction, Fertility, and Development* 18, 373–382. doi: 10.1071/rd05098

Thiangtum, K., Pinyopummin, A., Hori, T., Kawakami, E., and Tsutsui, T. (2009) Effect of catalase and superoxide dismutase on motility, viability and acrosomal integrity of frozen-thawed cat spermatozoa. *Reproduction in Domestic Animals* 44, 369–372. doi: 10.1111/j.1439-0531.2009.01420.x

Thuwanut, P. and Chatdarong, K. (2009) Incubation of post-thaw epididymal cat spermatozoa with seminal plasma. *Reproduction in Domestic Animals* 44(2), 381–384. doi: 10.1111/j.1439-0531.2009.01436.x

Thuwanut, P., Chatdarong, K., Techakumphu, M., and Axnér, E. (2008) The effect of antioxidants on motility, viability, acrosome integrity and DNA integrity of frozen-thawed epididymal cat spermatozoa. *Theriogenology* 70(2), 233–240. doi: 10.1016/j.theriogenology.2008.04.005

Thuwanut, P., Chatdarong, K., Johannisson, A., Bergqvist, A. S., Soderquist, L., *et al.* (2010) Cryopreservation of epididymal cat spermatozoa: effects of in vitro antioxidative enzyme supplementation and lipid peroxidation induction. *Theriogenology* 73, 1076–1087. doi: 10.1016/j.theriogenology.2010.01.007

Toyonaga, M. and Tsutsui, T. (2012) The quality of cryopreserved sperm collected from feline caudal epididymides using seminal plasma. *Journal of Veterinary Medical Science* 7, 1349–1353. doi: 10.1292/jvms.11-0175

Toyonaga, M., Sato, Y., Morita, M., Watanabe, M., Oba, H., *et al.* (2010) The qualities of cryopreserved epididymal sperm collected from feline epididymides stored at low temperature. *Journal of Veterinary Medical Science* 72, 777–780. doi: 10.1292/jvms.09-0260

Tsutsui, T., Tanaka, A., Takagi, Y., Nakagawa, K., Fujimoto, Y., *et al.* (2000) Unilateral intrauterine horn insemination of frozen semen in cats. *Journal of Veterinary Medical Science* 62, 1247–1251. doi: 10.1292/jvms.62.1247

Tsutsui, T., Wada, M., Anzai, M., and Hori, T. (2003) Artificial insemination with frozen epididymal sperm in cats. *Journal of Veterinary Medcal Science* 65, 397–399. doi: 10.1292/jvms.65.397

Vargas, W. D. E. (2012) Efecto de la adición de un surfactante natural (Aloe vera) al diluyente Triladyl® para crioconservación de semen bovino en toros reproductores de agso-genes, Quito-Pichincha (tesis). Universidad Técnica de Cotopaxi, Latacunga, pp. 155.

Vick, M. M., Bateman, H. L., Lambo, C. A., and Swanson, W. F. (2012) Improved cryopreservation of domestic cat sperm in a chemically defined medium. *Theriogenology* 78, 2120–2128. doi: 10.1016/j.theriogenology.2012.08.009

Villaverde, A. I., Melo, C. M., Martin, I., Ferreira, T. H., Papa, F. O., *et al.* (2009) Comparison of efficiency between two artificial insemination methods using frozen–thawed semen in domestic cat (*Felis catus*) Artificial insemination in domestic cats. *Animal Reproduction Science* 114, 434–442. doi: 10.1016/j.anireprosci.2008.10.008

Villaverde, A. I., Fioratti, E. G., Penitenti, M., Ikoma, M. R. V., Tsunemi, M. H., *et al.* (2013) Cryoprotective effect of different glycerol concentrations on domestic cat spermatozoa. *Theriogenology* 80, 730–737. doi: 10.1016/j.theriogenology.2013.06.010

Watson, P. F. (1979) The preservation of semen in mammals. In: Finn, C.A. (ed.) *Oxford Reviews of Reproductive Biology*, Vol. 1. Oxford University Press, Oxford, pp. 283–351.

Watson, P. F. (1995) Recent developments and concepts in the cryopreservation of spermatozoa and the assessment of their post-thawing function. *Reproduction, Fertility and Development* 7, 871–891. doi: 10.1071/rd9950871

Wildt, D. E. (1990) Potential applications of IVF technology for species conservation. In: Bavister, B. D., Cummins, J., and Roldan, E. R. S. (eds) *Fertilization in Mammals*. Serono Symposium, Norwell, Massachusetts, pp. 349–364.

Wood, T. C., Swanson, W. F., Davis, R. M., Anderson, J. E., and Wildt, D. E. (1993) Functionality of sperm from normo-versus teratospermic domestic cat cryopreserved in pellets or straw containers. *Theriogenology* 39, 342. doi: 10.1016/0093-691X(93)90197-D

Zambelli, D., Caneppele, B., Castagnetti, C., and Belluzzi, S. (2002) Cryopreservation of cat semen in straws: comparison of five different freezing rates. *Reproduction in Domestic Animals* 37, 310–313. doi: 10.1046/j.1439-0531.2002.00365.x

Zambelli, D., Merlo, B., Iacono, E., Prati, F., and Belluzzi, S. (2006) Fertilizing ability of electro-ejaculated cryopreserved semen in the domestic cat. *Reproduction in Domestic Animals* 41, 137–141. doi: 10.1111/j.1439-0531.2006.00654.x

Zambelli, D., Prati, F., Cunto, M., Iacono, E., and Merlo, B. (2008) Quality and in vitro fertilizing ability of cryopreserved cat spermatozoa obtained by urethral catheterization after medetomidine administration. *Theriogenology* 69:485–490. doi: 10.1016/j.theriogenology.2007.10.019

Zambelli, D., Iacono, D., Raccagni, R., and Merlo, B. (2010) Quality and fertilizing ability of electroejaculated cat spermatozoa frozen with or without Equex STM paste. *Theriogenology* 73, 886–892. 10.1016/j.theriogenology.2009.11.012

24 Use of Epididymal Sperm for Preservation of Genetics and Artificial Insemination

Riley E. Thompson[1], Fiona K. Hollinshead[1], and Budhan S. Pukazhenthi[2]

[1]Department of Clinical Sciences, Colorado State University, Fort Collins, Colorado, USA; [2]Center for Species Survival, Smithsonian Conservation Biology Institute, Front Royal, Virginia, USA

24.1 Introduction

There are many assisted reproductive technologies (ARTs) available for the cat to facilitate genetic banking, enhance population numbers of many wild felid species and, conversely, to reduce population numbers of many domestic/feral felids. Most of these ARTs focus on the use of live animals or reproductive tissues derived from spay or neuter procedures. In clinical practice, many domestic cats may die from underlying disease(s) or other health complications. Under these circumstances, owners may choose to collect and bank germplasm from their animal.

Collection and/or cryopreservation of viable sperm from the epididymis of male cats for use with other ARTs to propagate offspring is well described (Lengwinat and Blottner, 1994; Kunkitti *et al.*, 2016). Recovery of epididymal sperm following castration or loss of an animal is now routine in the reproductive management of rare and endangered wild felids (Silva *et al.*, 2004; Kunkitti *et al.*, 2016). Major considerations for successful collection of viable sperm from the epididymides include: (i) sexual maturity; (ii) time elapsed from castration/death; and (iii) storage conditions. In this chapter, we will discuss the current status of recovery methods, storage requirements, preservation, and use of epididymal sperm in domestic cats.

24.2 Fundamental Biology of the Epididymis

The epididymis further matures spermatozoa during its passage from the rete testis through to storage in the cauda epididymis. The average transit time (10–12 days) through the length of the epididymis is similar to other species (Axnér, 2006). The epididymis is composed of a single tortuous duct, and spermatozoa are transported by peristalsis (Courot, 1981). While the functional regions of the epididymis are far more complex (Axnér, 2006), gross anatomical characterization is the most clinically useful method to determine the maturation stage of the epididymal sperm recovered for preservation or use in an ART system. The epididymis is anatomically divided into the caput (head), corpus (body), and cauda (tail) (Fig. 24.1), which also is the route spermatozoa travel from the rete testis to the ductus deferens. During transit, a number of structural and functional changes occur to the spermatozoa including: (i) acrosome maturation with most sperm having abnormal acrosomes in the caput and normal acrosomes in the cauda epididymis (Axnér *et al.*, 1999); (ii) sperm motility is achieved (Axnér, 2006); and (iii) migration of the cytoplasmic droplet from a proximal location to a distal location on the sperm midpiece takes place in the transition region between the caput and corpus in the feline epididymis (Axnér *et al.*, 1999).

 Feline Reproduction (eds. A.K. Johnson and M.A. Kutzler)
DOI: 10.1079/9781789247107.0024

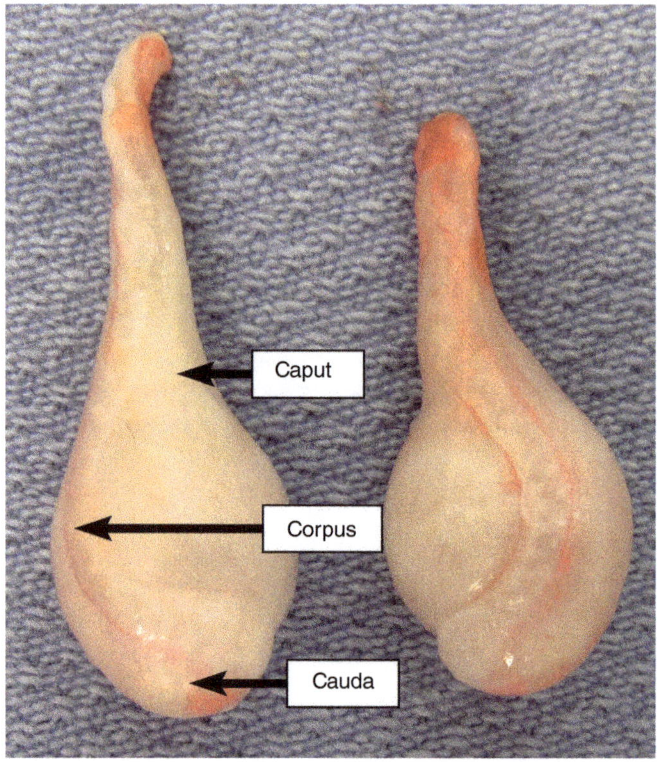

Fig. 24.1. Image depicting feline testes after castration with the caput, corpus and cauda epididymis indicated. (Image: author's own.)

Ejaculation causes loss of most distal droplets (Axnér *et al.*, 1998); therefore, sperm in the cauda epididymis tend to retain the distal cytoplasmic droplet. Importantly, although sperm derived from the testis is capable of fertilizing oocytes via intracytoplasmic sperm injection (Comizzoli *et al.*, 2006), sperm collected from the caput cannot fertilize oocytes following standard *in vitro* fertilization (IVF) or artificial insemination due to no or low progressive motility. In contrast, sperm collected from the cauda epididymis exhibit similar fertilizing rates compared to ejaculated sperm following artificial insemination (Axnér, 2006).

24.3 Collection, Storage, and Shipment of Testes

Most tomcats >6 months of age are suitable for epididymal sperm collection. To maximize recovery of good quality motile sperm, gonads must be recovered from deceased animals within 24 hours of death and the tissue stored at 4°C. It is also important that the excised gonads are kept moist with sterile saline or other defined tissue culture medium and maintained at 4°C for no longer than 24 hours (refrigeration) (Klaus *et al.*, 2016; Kunkitti *et al.*, 2016). Since there is no influence of season on tomcat sperm output or quality, viable sperm can be obtained from adult tomcats throughout the year (Spindler and Wildt, 1999). However, when animals die or are euthanized due to infectious diseases, caution must be used when determining if spermatozoa should be collected and banked for future use.

24.3.1 Removal of testes from tom cats

1. Perform routine closed surgical castration in a live male or remove testes with scrotum in a deceased animal if shipment over a long distance to the lab is required. Ligate the ductus deferens on the side closest to the testicle prior to removal. Remove a long section of ductus deferens.
2. If testicles are not being processed at the collection location, wrap each testis (with ductus deferens

ligated to prevent loss of spermatozoa) in sterile saline-soaked gauze, place in a sample bag and transport or ship in a Styrofoam cooler containing a frozen ice pack. Place paper towels between testes and ice pack to prevent direct contact. Alternatively, the testes can be shipped in containers designed for cooled transport of equine or canine sperm.

24.3.2 Procedure for epididymal sperm collection in laboratory (Table 24.1)

Dissection of testes and epididymides

1. Dissect the parietal vaginal tunic (Prochowska *et al.*, 2015) and carefully expose the testis and epididymis (Fig. 24.2a).

  a. Isolate the cauda epididymis from the testis by dissecting the proper ligament of the testis (Fig. 24.2b)

2. Bisect the epididymis between the cauda and corpus while keeping the ductus deferens attached to the cauda epididymis (Fig. 24.2c).

3. Using microdissection instruments, remove as many blood vessels as possible from the cauda epididymis without cutting into epididymal tissue. Use towels or sterile gauze to gently blot blood from tissue.

4. Place the cauda epididymis and the ductus deferens into a small petri dish containing the sperm collection medium (see below).

Sperm recovery

1. Recover sperm from the ductus deferens by one of two methods:

  a. Retrograde flushing – by injecting sperm collection media into the cut end of the ductus deferens using a blunt-tipped 25 G or tuberculin needle and syringe to flush sperm from

Table 24.1. Equipment and manufacturer required for epididymal sperm harvesting and cryopreservation.

Equipment and supplies	Manufacturer
Large (100 mm diameter) and small (35 mm diameter) petri dishes	e.g. Corning, Nunc
Scalpel blade and handle	e.g. #10 or #20 blade
Small sharp dissection scissors	
Mosquito forceps	
Clean disposable wipes	e.g. Kimwipes
Sperm collection media	Homemade: See below. Commercially available: TYB refrigeration medium (Irvine Scientific)
Sperm freezing media	Homemade: see the text Commercially available: TYB-freezing medium (Irvine Scientific)
0.25 mL semen freezing straws	e.g. Minitube, IMV Technologies
Straw labeler/straw labels	e.g. Brady BMP21 Label Printer and labels OR Hand label with a Sharpie
Pipettes and pipette tips (1000, 200, 20 µL) or plastic pipettors	
2 mL microcentrifuge tubes	
Sealer for semen straws	e.g. ULINE heat sealer OR polyvinyl alcohol (PVA) powder to seal
Refrigerator or ideally a cold room	
Water-filled container	e.g. large 250 mL beaker with 200 mL water
Styrofoam cooler	
Test tube rack (metal) or floating semen straw freezing rack	
Liquid nitrogen and tank	
Liquid nitrogen-safe forceps, goggles, gloves	
Centrifuge or microcentrifuge	

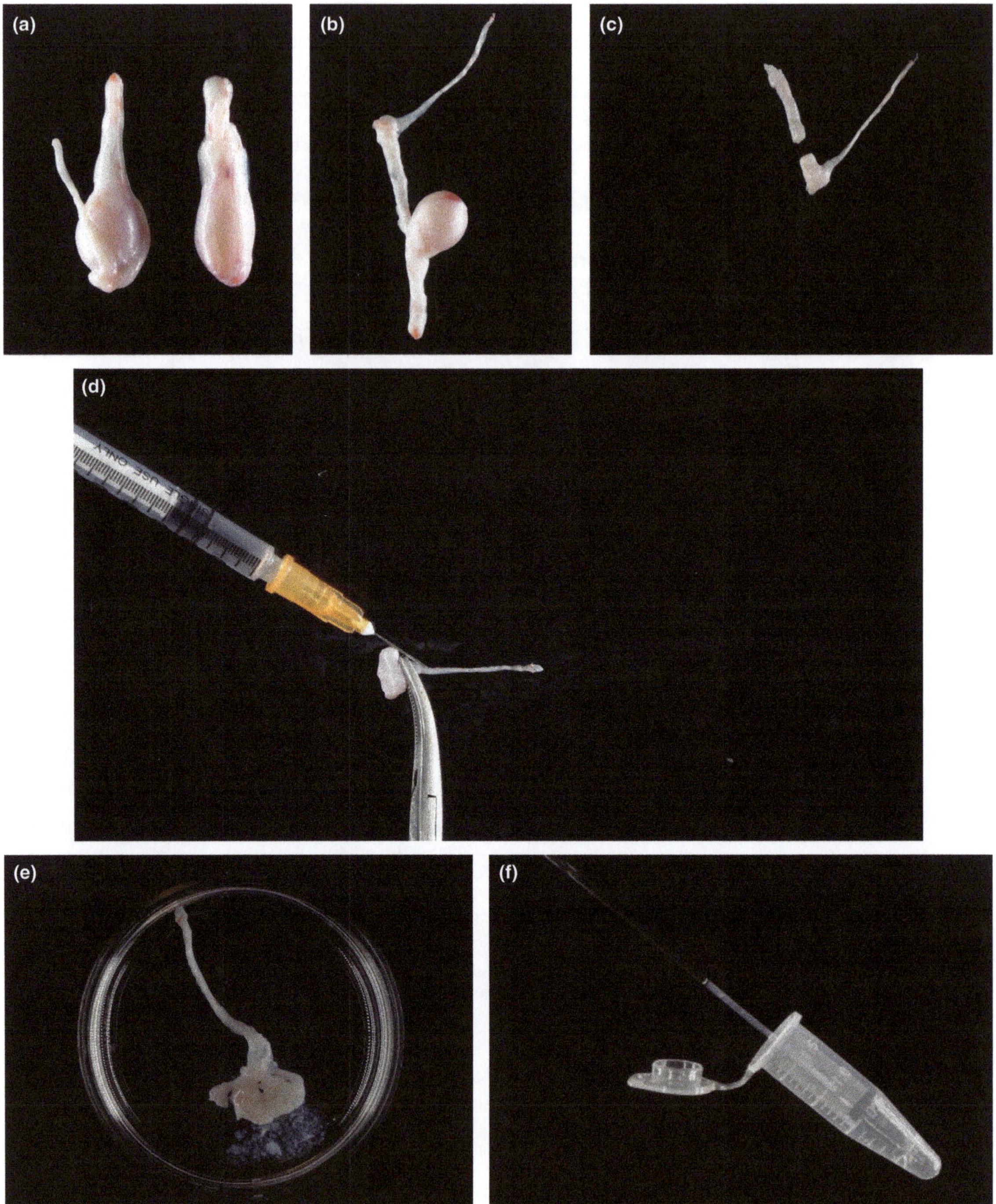

Fig. 24.2. Images depicting epididymal sperm collection procedure. **(a)** Left testis after removal of the vaginal tunic with the intact vaginal tunic on the right testis. **(b)** After transecting the proper ligament of the testis to separate the cauda and corpus of the epididymis from the testis. **(c)** Transection of the epididymis between the cauda and corpus with the ductus deferens attached to the cauda. **(d)** Anterograde flushing of the ductus deferens. **(e)** Sperm releasing into collection medium after cutting the cauda epididymis. **(f)** Transfer of sperm solution to microcentrifuge tube. (Images: author's own.)

the cauda epididymis. If flow through the epididymis cannot be established with gentle pressure, serial cuts into the cauda can be made until the sperm medium flows through and into the collection dish.
   b. Anterograde flushing – by first clamping the ductus deferens adjacent to the cauda epididymis with hemostats and inserting a 25 G or tuberculin needle into the lumen of the ductus deferens and flushing sperm collection medium into the ductus deferens toward the open end (Fig. 24.2d).
   c. Sperm recovered from the ductus deferens using the anterograde method can be cryopreserved separately or combined with cauda epididymal sperm.
2. Place the cauda epididymides in pre-warmed sperm collection medium and use a scalpel blade to create multiple cuts into cauda epididymis to release sperm into the collection medium. (Fig. 24.2e).
   a. Avoid cutting into any remaining blood vessels to minimize contamination with blood cells.
   b. Take care to not cut the tissue so vigorously that tissue chunks will be mixed in with the sperm.
3. Incubate dissected/macerated cauda epididymides for 5 minutes ideally on a warm stage to allow sperm to diffuse into the pre-warmed (37°C) collection medium. Periodically, agitate the tissue gently.
4. Remove the tissue from the petri dish and transfer the sperm collection medium and sperm mixture into sterile microcentrifuge tubes. (Fig. 24.2f). Rinse tissue with collection medium prior to removing it from the dish.

Sperm collection medium options

1. M199 (HEPES modification) culture medium (Klaus *et al.*, 2016).
2. Hams F-10 culture medium (Spindler and Wildt, 1999).
3. Tris buffer without glycerol (Zambelli, 1994; Zambelli *et al.*, 2000; Hermansson and Axnér, 2007).
4. Dulbecco's phosphate-buffered saline (Vizuete *et al.*, 2014).
5. Test yolk buffer – refrigeration medium (TYB; Irvine Scientific) or make up freezing medium in house - **part A** of 2-step freezing medium without glycerol (Spindler *et al.*, 2004; Pukazhenthi *et al.*, 2006; Thiangtum *et al.*, 2006).

24.4 Cryopreservation of Epididymal Sperm

The most common protocol for cryopreservation in felids is the 'two-step method.' The first step involves cooling sperm diluted in media without a cryoprotectant, and the second step involves adding a cryoprotectant, such as glycerol, prior to freezing with liquid nitrogen. For domestic cat sperm cryopreservation, test yolk buffer (TYB) is often used. This medium can be either purchased from commercial sources or a modification of a similar product can be prepared in the clinic or laboratory. Alternatively, small volumes of cat epididymal spermatozoa can be frozen using an ultra-fast freezing method for long-term storage using a soy lecithin medium (Swanson *et al.*, 2017).

Formulas for sperm freezing media

1. Commercial TYB; Irvine Scientific)
   a. Combine 2:1 TYB-freezing medium (contains 12% glycerol) and TYB refrigeration medium (contains 0% glycerol) to achieve 8% glycerol concentration. For cryopreservation, add pre-cooled TYB with 8% glycerol 1:1 to the sperm suspension to achieve 4% glycerol final concentration.
2. Homemade TEST buffer with 7.5% (v/v) glycerol and 15% (v/v) water-soluble fraction of hen's egg yolk (Lengwinat and Blottner, 1994).
   a. Prepare Tes-Tris buffer by adding 48.3 g TES:N tris (hydroxymethyl)(methyl-2-aminoethane) sulfonic acid, 11.6 g tris (hydroxymethyl aminomethane), and 2 g fructose per 1000 mL water. Osmolality of the buffer should be 325 mOsm/kg, pH=7.1–7.2 (Schmehl *et al.*, 1986).
   b. Add 15% (v/v) water-soluble fraction of hen's egg yolk to the Tes-Tris buffer.
   c. Add glycerol (7.5% v/v) to the Tes-Tris egg yolk solution.
3. Ultra-fast freezing solution (Swanson *et al.*, 2017; Vansandt *et al.*, 2021)
   a. Ultra-fast freezing medium: soy lecithin-based medium containing 0.2 M sucrose.
   b. Soy lecithin medium (Vick *et al.*, 2012): Tes-Tris stock buffers (TES 74 g/L and Tris HCl 39.68 g/L) are titrated to pH 7.3 (TEST). Then, add 480 mL TEST to 300 mL sodium citrate solution (33.84 g/L) with 220 mL double-distilled water, then fructose (14 g),

soybean lecithin (10 g), streptomycin sulfate (0.05 g), and penicillin-G (100 kIU) are added. Adjust to pH 7.0 and centrifuge at 2,900 × *g* for 15 minutes and filter the supernatant through 0.8 and 0.4 ∝m filters.

24.4.1 Procedure for sperm freezing

Two-step slow freeze (cryopreservation) method

1. Centrifuge recovered/flushed diluted epididymal sperm at 300 × *g* for 8 minutes. Remove the supernatant.
2. Slowly resuspend sperm pellet in TYB refrigeration medium (this does not contain glycerol) to achieve a final sperm concentration of 40 to 60 million sperm/mL (Cocchia *et al.*, 2010).
3. Place the resuspended spermatozoa in a 10- or 15-mL sterile test tube in a container with 500 mL of water at room temperature (~22°C) and cool the sperm solution in the container in a refrigerator until the water reaches 4°C for approximately 3 hours (until the water bath reaches 4°C) (Thiangtum *et al.*, 2006).
4. Slowly dilute the sperm solution 1:1 with pre-cooled (4°C) TYB-freezing medium containing 8% glycerol (following dilution the final concentration of cryoprotectant will be 4% v/v glycerol) at 4°C.
5. Allow the diluted sperm to equilibrate at 4°C for 15 minutes before loading and sealing the extended sperm in pre-cooled (4°C) 0.25 mL plastic straws.
6. Label all straws with the following information – animal ID, breed, and date of collection at the minimum. It is important to use liquid nitrogen-safe straw labels or hand label with a sharpie.
7. Load (0.25 mL) straws using a pipettor and seal the open end using a heat sealer or PVA powder.
8. Place straws on rack in cooler 7.5 cm above the surface of liquid nitrogen for 1 minute then 2.5 cm above liquid nitrogen for 1 minute (Spindler *et al.*, 2004; Thiangtum *et al.*, 2006).
9. Plunge the straws into liquid nitrogen (Cocchia *et al.*, 2010) and store the straws in a long-term liquid nitrogen tank.

Ultra-fast freezing (vitrification) method (Swanson et al., 2017)

1. Harvest sperm as described above.
2. Transfer sperm suspension to a sterile microcentrifuge tube and centrifuge (300 × *g*; 8 minutes) to pellet sperm.
3. Resuspend sperm pellet (1:3 v/v) with freezing solution.
4. Equilibrate at room temperature for 5 minutes.
5. Directly pipet 30 μl aliquots of sperm suspension into a bucket containing liquid nitrogen.
6. Using long forceps, transfer sperm pellets into pre-labeled cryo-vials, and store cryo-vials in liquid nitrogen.

24.4.2 Procedure for thawing/rewarming

Thawing (for slow freeze cryopreserved samples)

1. Remove the straw from liquid nitrogen with pre-chilled (ends in liquid nitrogen) forceps and transfer the straw immediately into a 37°C water bath and vigorously agitate for 30 seconds.
2. Slowly dilute thawed semen with 1 mL pre-warmed (37°C) Tris egg yolk extender without cryoprotectant (Cocchia *et al.*, 2010).

OR

Thawed sperm suspension can be diluted slowly (drop wise) with defined culture medium (see medium for sperm collection).

Rewarming vitrified sperm pellets (Swanson et al., 2017)

1. Remove the cryovial from liquid nitrogen storage and maintain in liquid nitrogen.
2. Open cryovial and transfer sperm pellet into liquid nitrogen.
3. Using pre-chilled metal forceps, transfer a single pellet into a glass test tube containing 0.1 mL of feline-optimized culture medium (FOCM; Herrick *et al.*, 2007) while holding the tube in a 37°C water bath.
4. After 30 seconds, transfer the sperm suspension into a sterile microcentrifuge tube and slowly add 0.2 mL of pre-warmed FOCM medium.
5. Centrifuge the tube at 300 × *g* for 5 minutes.
6. Remove the supernatant and resuspend the sperm pellet in pre-warmed fresh medium based on the artificial reproductive technique to be used.

24.5 Use of Epididymal Sperm for Breeding

Epididymal sperm has been used successfully for IVF and artificial insemination (Lengwinat and

Blottner, 1994; Tsutsui *et al.*, 2003) in felids. For further information, see chapters on artificial reproductive techniques.

24.6 Perspectives

Rather than isolating sperm from freshly collected epididymides, future research on cryopreservation/vitrification of intact epididymal tissue similar to ovarian tissue pieces (Brito *et al.*, 2018; Gorricho *et al.*, 2018) could determine if viable sperm may be isolated after tissue thawing for use with intracytoplasmic sperm injection or IVF system, which would save time if sperm processing cannot be performed immediately.

24.6.1 Practical perspectives

'DON'T':

- Ship or transport testes directly on top of ice or an ice block.
- Store testes in freezer (–20°C).

'DO':

- If shipping testes to a lab for processing, send with a label describing all animal details (name, breed, age, medical condition, etc.).
- Call ahead to make sure they are prepared to process the testes as soon as they arrive.

24.7 References

Axnér, E. (2006) Sperm maturation in the domestic cat. *Theriogenology* 66, 14–24. doi: 10.1016/j.theriogenology.2006.03.022

Axnér, E., Holst, B. S., and Linde-Forsberg, C. (1998) Morphology of spermatozoa in the cauda epididymidis before and after electroejaculation and a comparison with ejaculated spermatozoa in the domestic cat. *Theriogenology* 50, 973–979. doi: 10.1016/s0093-691x(98)00200-3

Axnér, E., Linde-Forsberg, C., and Einarsson, S. (1999) Morphology and motility of spermatozoa from different regions of the epididymal duct in the domestic cat. *Theriogenology* 52, 767–778. doi: 10.1016/S0093-691X(99)00170-3

Brito, D. C. C., Domingues, S. F. S., Rodrigues, A. P. R., Maside, C., Lunardi, F. O., *et al.* (2018) Cryopreservation of domestic cat (*Felis catus*) ovarian tissue: Comparison of two vitrification methods. *Theriogenology* 111, 69–77. doi: 10.1016/j.theriogenology.2018.01.015

Cocchia, N., Ciani, F., El-Rass, R., Russo, M., Borzacchiello, G., *et al.* (2010) Cryopreservation of feline epididymal spermatozoa from dead and alive animals and its use in assisted reproduction. *Zygote* 18, 1–8. doi: 10.1017/S0967199409990256

Comizzoli, P., Wildt, D. E., and Pukazhenthi, B. S. (2006) In vitro development of domestic cat embryos following intra-cytoplasmic sperm injection with testicular spermatozoa. *Theriogenology* 66, 1659–1663. doi: 10.1016/j.theriogenology.2006.01.038

Courot, M. (1981) Transport and maturation of spermatozoa in the epididymis of mammals. In: Bollack, C. and Clavert, A. (eds) *Progress in Reproductive Biology, Vol. 8, Epididymis and Fertility: Biology and Pathology*. S. Karger, Basle, Switzerland, pp. 67–79.

Gorricho, C. M., Tavares, M. R., Apparício, M., Fonseca-Alves, C. E., Macente, B. I., *et al.* (2018) Vitrification of cat ovarian tissue: Does fragment size matters? *Reproduction in Domestic Animals* 53, 125–132. doi: 10.1111/rda.13357

Hermansson, U. and Axnér, E. (2007) Epididymal and ejaculated cat spermatozoa are resistant to cold shock but egg yolk promotes sperm longevity during cold storage at 4 degrees C. *Theriogenology* 67, 1239–1248. doi: 10.1016/j.theriogenology.2007.01.008

Herrick, J. R., Bond, J. B., Magarey, G. M., Bateman, H. L., Krisher, R. L., *et al.* (2007) Toward a feline-optimized culture medium: Impact of ions, carbohydrates, essential amino acids, vitamins, and serum on development and metabolism of in vitro fertilization-derived feline embryos relative to embryos grown in vivo. *Biology of Reproduction* 76, 858–870. doi: 10.1095/biolreprod.106.058065

Klaus, C., Eder, S., Franz, C., and Müller, K. (2016) Successful cryopreservation of domestic cat (*Felis catus*) Epididymal sperm after slow equilibration to 15 or 10° C. *Reproduction in Domestic Animals* 51, 195–203. doi: 10.1111/rda.12666

Kunkitti, P., Axnér, E., Bergqvist, A. S., and Sjunnesson, Y. (2016) In vitro fertilization using frozen-thawed feline epididymal spermatozoa from corpus and cauda regions. *Theriogenology* 86, 1403–1408. doi: 10.1016/j.theriogenology.2016.04.085

Lengwinat, T. and Blottner, S. (1994) In vitro fertilization of follicular oocytes of domestic cat using fresh and cryopreserved epididymal spermatozoa. *Animal Reproduction Science* 35, 291–301. doi: 10.1016/0378-4320(94)90044-2

Prochowska, S., Niżański, W., Ochota, M., and Partyka, A. (2015) Characteristics of urethral and epididymal semen collected from domestic cats—A retrospective study of 214 cases. *Theriogenology* 84, 1565–1571. doi: 10.1016/j.theriogenology.2015.08.005

Pukazhenthi, B., Laroe, D., Crosier, A., Bush, L.M., Spindler, R., *et al.* (2006) Challenges in cryopreservation of clouded leopard (*Neofelis nebulosa*) spermatozoa. *Theriogenology* 66, 1790–1796. doi: 10.1016/j.theriogenology.2006.02.020

Schmehl, M. K., Anderson, S. P., Vazquez, I. A., and Graham, E. F. (1986) The effect of dialysis of extended ram semen prior to freezing on post-thaw survival and fertility. *Cryobiology* 23, 406–414. doi: 10.1016/0011-2240(86)90025-8

Silva, A. R., Morato, R. G., and Silva, L. D. (2004) The potential for gamete recovery from non-domestic canids and felids. *Animal Reproduction Science* 81, 159–175. doi: 10.1016/j.anireprosci.2003.10.001

Spindler, R. E. and Wildt, D.E. (1999) Circannual variations in intraovarian oocyte but not epididymal sperm quality in the domestic cat. *Biology of Reproduction* 61, 188–194. doi: 10.1095/biolreprod61.1.188

Spindler, R. E., Huang, Y., Howard, J. G., Wang, P., Zhang, H., *et al.* (2004) Acrosomal integrity and capacitation are not influenced by sperm cryopreservation in the giant panda. *Reproduction* 127, 547–556. doi: 10.1530/rep.1.00034

Swanson, W. F., Bateman, H. L., and Vansandt, L. M. (2017) Urethral catheterization and sperm vitrification for simplified semen banking in felids. *Reproduction in Domestic Animals* 52, 255–260. doi: 10.1111/rda.12863

Thiangtum, K., Swanson, W. F., Howard, J., Tunwattana, W., Tongthainan, D., *et al.* (2006) Assessment of basic seminal characteristics, sperm cryopreservation and heterologous in vitro fertilisation in the fishing cat (*Prionailurus viverrinus*). *Reproduction, Fertility and Development* 18, 373–382. doi: 10.1071/rd05098

Tsutsui, T., Wada, M., Anzai, M., and Hori, T. (2003) Artificial insemination with frozen epididymal sperm in cats. *Journal of Veterinary Medical Science* 65, 397–399. doi: 10.1292/jvms.65.397

Vansandt, L. M., Bateman, H. L., Miller, A. G., Herrick, J. R., Moresco, A., *et al.* (2021) Cross-species efficacy of a chemically-defined, soy lecithin-based cryomedium for semen banking in imperiled wild felids. *Theriogenology* 159, 108–115. doi: 10.1016/j.theriogenology.2020.10.021

Vick, M. M., Bateman, H. L., Lambo, C. A., and Swanson, W. F. (2012) Improved cryopreservation of domestic cat sperm in a chemically defined medium. *Theriogenology* 78, 2120–2128. doi: 10.1016/j.theriogenology.2012.08.009

Vizuete, G., Jiménez, E., Agüera, E. I., and Pérez-Marín, C. C. (2014) Impact of ultra-rapid freezing on the motility, morphology, viability and acrosome integrity of epididymal cat sperm diluted in sucrose-based extenders. *Reproduction in Domestic Animals* 49, e5–e8. doi: 10.1111/rda.12253

Zambelli, D. (1994) Study of sperm morphology and preservation in the cat and of reproductive physiologic parameters in the female for the use in the AI. PhD Thesis, University of Perugia, pp.69–70.

Zambelli, D., Bergonzoni, M. L., and Caneppele, B. (2000) Long and short term sperm preservation in the cat using chilling or freezing. In: *SISVet Proceedings*, Riva del Garda (TN), Italy, pp.121–122.

25 Clinical Approach to Infertility

Sandra Goericke-Pesch

Reproductive Unit – Clinic for Small Animals, University of Veterinary Medicine Hannover, Foundation, Hannover, Germany

25.1 Introduction

Causes of infertility and abortion are numerous and have been presented in detail for the queen in Chapters 5 and 7 and for the tom in Chapter 19. This chapter is a discussion of how to approach a case of infertility in practice.

For the clinician, different approaches are possible to identify infertility reasons in queens and tomcats. A limitation is that breeders are usually urgently needing an answer (namely the reason of 'infertility'), but often not willing to pay excessive amounts of money for the diagnostics. Consequently, structured analysis of the case is required to limit expenses and to (hopefully) provide an answer. Infertility can be broken into several main categories which allow the practitioner to better choose diagnostics and treatment options. For the queen, failure to cycle, failure to allow mating, failure to ovulate, and failure to become pregnant are the main categories. For the tom, erection/breeding failure, ejaculation failure, and failure to achieve pregnancies should be investigated. Following the signalment of the animal, a detailed history should be obtained, followed by a physical and gynecological examination. Very often an ultrasound examination is required. Sampling of swabs for bacteriological examination, complete semen evaluation, or other further examinations such as serum hormone testing or viral infections might be useful. The history, physical, and gynecological examinations are always required as a baseline. Asking the 'right' questions during a detailed history will provide a starting place to help figure out where the exact problem is located.

25.2 The Queen

See Table 25.1 for a summary of procedures when investigating an 'infertile queen'.

25.2.1 History

A detailed history is vital to allow the practitioner information and guide diagnostics. Consequently, the following questions need to be addressed:

Whether the queen:

1. Has been in estrus before (what age she initially cycled, how often she did cycle – the age and breed of the queen as well as the current season and the season of her birth should be considered)?
2. Has/had been cycling on a regular basis (including asking about the interval between the estrus cycles – in general and after (suspected) matings)?
3. Had been pregnant before (including obtaining information about mating – if observed, the course of the previous pregnancy/pregnancies, parturition(s) and the postpartum period(s); number of kittens and survival rates)?
4. Was exposed to a proven fertile male (has that male produced kittens recently or are there confirmed pregnancies from that male)?
5. Was mated at all, if so when and how often mating occurred in estrus (with the intention to figure out if the mating(s) had been observed and if she was mated frequently enough to induce ovulation)?
6. Conceived and how this was proven (e.g. by clinical signs, such as swelling and reddening of the nipples, by abdominal palpation or by ultrasound examination) or if it was just assumed by the breeder?
7. Showed signs of abortion/stillbirth, etc., including presence of vaginal discharge earlier or after the last mating before presentation?

All these questions should be asked to obtain the necessary information about the reproductive background of the individual cat, but also several 'general' questions should be addressed concerning the cattery and management (see Chapter 4). Information to gather should include how many

DOI: 10.1079/9781789247107.0025

total cats live in the cattery (intact queens, kittens, and tomcats) and whether only one queen is affected by infertility or several (and in the latter case, how many). In cases where several females are affected, were they mated to a single tom, and is the tom from the cattery or was the queen brought to an 'external' tom? Are the cats solely housed indoors, do they have outdoor access in a fenced area, do they have contact to other animals or cats from other households? Diet is important as certain problems are more likely with raw feed (thyroidal gland addition can lead to the downregulation of luteinizing hormone (LH); inadequate composition of vitamins/minerals/trace elements; bacteria, e.g. salmonellosis can lead to dysbiosis causing diarrhea, *Salmonella typhimurium* from raw chicken causing stillbirth). Some commercially available dry or canned feed can also be problematic if it is the wrong composition, too old, or incorrectly stored because it can lead to reactive oxygen species formation or heavy metal contamination. Information about the general health status of the cat should be obtained at the time of presentation but also at the time of and prior to mating. As viral infections such as feline parvovirus and feline leukemia virus can negatively affect fertility and cause abortion and stillbirth, the vaccination protocol of the cattery is highly relevant. Furthermore, previous and current medications should be identified, such as antifungal treatment against ringworm (might interfere with estrus), deworming (time point and medication), contraceptives (progestins, melatonin, gonadotropin-releasing hormone (GnRH) agonist implants), or any other medications are also of interest as specific drugs might have detrimental effects on the estrous cycle and early pregnancy.

Table 25.1. Overview about the procedure with an 'infertile female feline patient'. (Author's own table.)

History	
Signalment	Breeding name, breed, ID (microchip/tattoo), date of birth
Physical examination	Entire body (nose to tail)
Gynecological examination	Inspection of the external genitalia (discharge?) Vaginal cytology
Ultrasound examination	Vagina (if visible) Uterus Ovaries
Further examinations (if required)	Bacteriological examination of a vaginal swab Hormone testing Proof of virus infections (Serology/PCR) Karyotyping
Diagnosis, evaluation and treatment approaches	

The detailed history is very important, if not the most important tool to make the decision of which diagnostics should be performed to identify the cause of infertility of the queen.

25.2.2 Gynecological examination

A gynecological examination is crucial in all feline gynecological patients presented for failure to cycle, to conceive, or to maintain pregnancy. The gynecological examination of the cat must include inspection of the vulva to identify any sign of vaginal discharge. In long-haired cats, veterinarians should also check for signs of vaginal discharge at the 'trousers' (hind legs) and under the tail (Fig. 25.1). In case the queen is particularly fastidious, a second quick look for vaginal discharge at the end of the

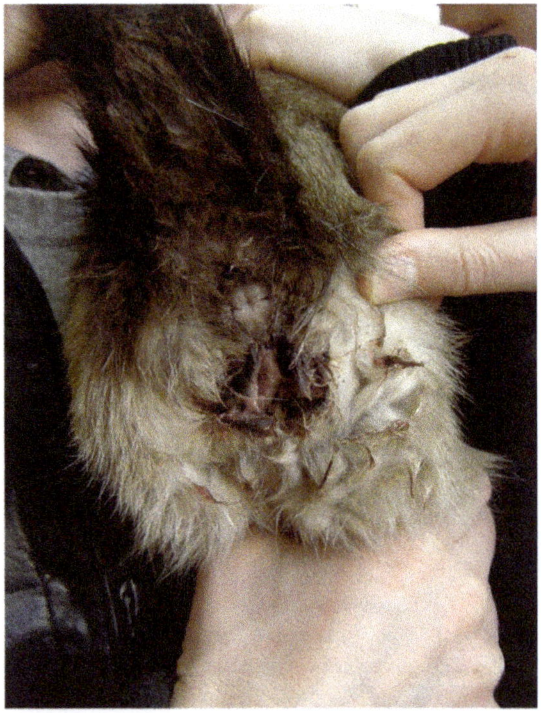

Fig. 25.1. During gynecological examination the anogenital region must be inspected for the presence of vaginal discharge. In the present case, vaginal discharge was the only clinical sign of fetal death. (Image: author's own.)

examination may show discharge that was emitted during her examination. Assessing vaginal swabs for bacteriology and cytological examination is suitable for evaluation of the stage of the estrus cycle as well as for suspicion of bacterial infection and/or pyometra. Before sampling, the vulva should be briefly cleaned with some dry paper or a paper moistened with some 'mucosal-friendly' disinfectant (not alcohol!). Tiny cotton swabs (Fig. 25.2),

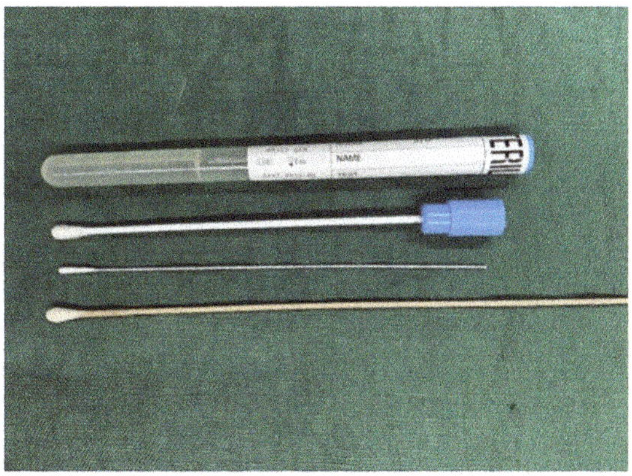

Fig. 25.2. Different cotton swabs are available for sampling of vaginal cytologies. In cats, only the thin cotton swab is suitable for sample collection. In case of bacteriological examination, the swab can be placed in appropriate tubes with Amies medium. (Image: author's own.)

e.g. human urethral swabs, are introduced as far as possible into the vagina of the queen, gently rubbed against the mucosa of the dorsal vagina and removed. The first swab can be taken for bacteriological examination and the second for vaginal cytology. The second swab is then rolled in subsequent lanes on a glass slide. After air drying, the smear can be stained with a standard blood cell stain, such as Hemacolour® (Figs 25.3 and 25.4) or DiffQuick®. These stains are readily available and easy to use and evaluate. Papanicolaou stain allows for easy visualization of estrogenic influence by orange staining of the cells compared to dark green staining in cells not exposed to estradiol-17ß, but the time and effort required for this staining does not make it a commonly used stain in daily clinical routine.

The stage of the cycle should be identified for each queen presenting for infertility. Normal vaginal cytology is discussed in Chapter 2. Davidson and Baker (2009a) provide guidance on ultrasound findings in the queen. Bacteria found on a vaginal cytology do not necessarily indicate infection, but in cases of infertility, a swab should be submitted for bacteriological examination for adequate evaluation of bacteria present. Presence of numerous leucocytes (Fig. 25.5) is often indicative of inflammation. Absence of leucocytes with presence of vaginal discharge might indicate a non-infectious

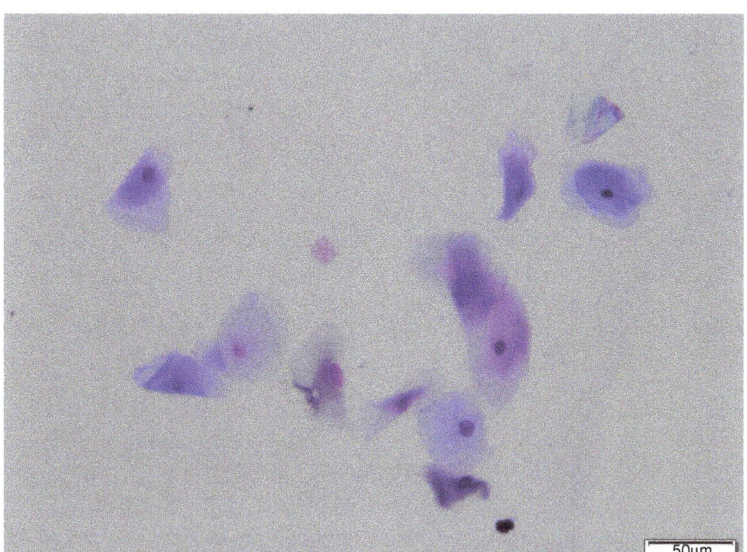

Fig. 25.3. Vaginal cytology smear stained with Hemacolour® mainly revealing superficial cells – with normal and pycnotic nucleus as well as some a nucleated cells. (The smear was obtained from a queen in estrus.) (Image: author's own.)

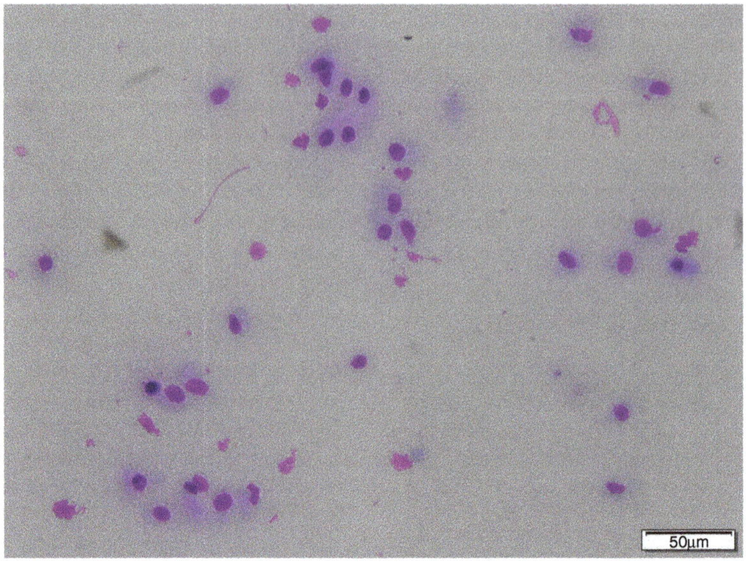

Fig. 25.4. Vaginal cytology smear stained with Hemacolour® mainly revealing parabasal and small intermediate cells. Some cell detritus and mucus are visible. (The smear was obtained from a pregnant cat.) (Image: author's own.)

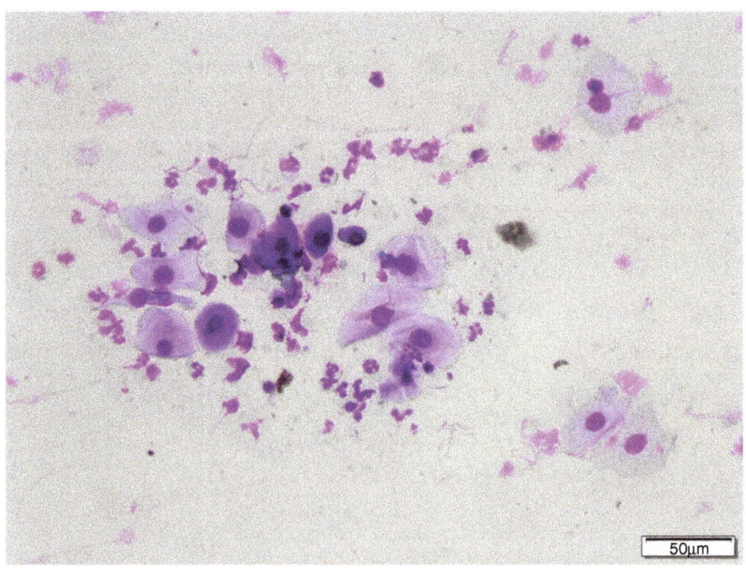

Fig. 25.5. Vaginal cytology smear stained with Hemacolour® mainly revealing leucocytes, small and large intermediate cells, some mucus is also visible. (The smear was obtained from a pregnant cat with vaginal discharge. Fetal death caused by high growth of *E. coli* var. *hem.* was proven.) (Image: author's own.)

cause of vaginal discharge or partial abortion (with the remaining pregnancy to be continuing to term). Even though direct correlations between altered fertility and bacterial infections are difficult to identify, a bacteriological examination of a vaginal swab is recommended. In cases of heavy growth and/or pure culture of ß-hemolytic streptococci or *Escherichia coli* var. *hem.* treatment according to the antibiogram is recommended as these bacteria have been shown to be associated with endometritis and pyometra, but also placentitis (ß-hemolytic streptococci), abortion (*E. coli* var. *hem.*), neonatal death (*S. typhimurium*; Reilly *et al.*, 1994), and neonatal septicemia (ß-hemolytic streptococci, *E. coli* var. *hem.*) (Pretzer, 2008; own clinical experiences). Further bacteria that have been associated with reproductive tract disorders and discussed in relation to sub- and infertility are *Mycoplasma* spp. (McKinney, 1973), *Ureaplasma* spp., *Chlamydia* spp., and *Coxiella burnetti*. These bacteria require specific culture conditions and therefore PCR is usually performed instead. *Chlamydophila felis*, caused persistent salpingitis after experimental infection, but was also found in the genital tract after conjunctivitis and natural infection without any reproductive clinical signs. Final evaluation of the clinical relevance of those bacteria is difficult.

Figure 25.6 provides an overview about underlying reasons, possible history and diagnostic procedures in queens presented for infertility.

25.2.3 Failure to cycle

Failure to cycle may be due to primary or secondary anestrus. In the case of primary anestrus, the queen has never been in estrus before, whereas secondary anestrus indicates that the queen had been cycling, but the interval since the last estrus is prolonged. Silent heat, physiological hormonal changes according to estrus without any clinical estrus signs, and behavior is a possible differential to anestrus that needs to be ruled out. Ultrasound examination of the ovaries helps confirm the presence of ovarian follicles (Fig. 25.7). Queens with silent heat are fertile and can be co-housed over longer periods with a known fertile tomcat. Changing the environment and reducing stress might contribute to more obvious estrus behavior in affected cats.

Primary anestrus is due to failure of puberty (or a queen that is still too young) mainly because of chromosomal and/or developmental abnormalities, malnutrition or even disease. Puberty can occur as early as 4 months of age. However, large, often long-haired breeds, such as Norwegian Forrest cats or Maine Coon go into puberty later compared to small, short-haired breeds, such as Siamese and can be up to 21–24 months at the first estrus. Certain color patterns, such as calico and tortoiseshell, have been associated with genetic abnormalities (X0 and XXY genome) causing infertility. Karyotyping should be considered in case of primary anestrous, especially when anatomical deviations are also identified during physical examination.

Secondary anestrus can be related to unknown history of neutering, pregnancy, contraceptive medication (progestins, slow-release GnRH agonist implants, melatonin), but also prolonged luteal phase due to progesterone producing ovarian cysts/cystic corpora lutea, disease, and malnutrition. Rarely, other medication can prevent cyclicity, such as high concentrations of glucocorticoids. Taking a good history is necessary to verify recent (or long-term) medication use. Even though blood concentrations of some progestins can be analyzed in the lab, this is not a routine procedure in the daily clinic making it almost impossible to verify progestin medication in case of unknown history (such as change of owner). To rule out earlier surgical sterilization, the ventral midline and both flank areas of the abdominal wall should be carefully checked for any sign of a scar. Abdominal ultrasound can rule out pregnancy as a cause of failure to cycle (Fig. 25.8). Abdominal ultrasound also helps with identifying cystic corpora lutea on the ovary preventing the return to estrus. Cystic corpora lutea can be identified by their increased size, anechogenic filling and thickened wall combined with the lack of estrus.

Hormone analysis is especially helpful in diagnosing failure of cyclicity or ovulation. Progesterone can be used to detect recent ovulation in cases where anestrus or silent estrus is suspected. Repeated progesterone analysis helps confirm the suspicion of prolonged progesterone production. Analysis of anti-Müllerian hormone (AMH) and LH is suitable to confirm presence/absence of ovarian tissue. Progesterone can be analyzed from serum or plasma. Prior to collection, the veterinarian should identify the preferred sample type of the laboratory where the sample will be submitted. Even though progesterone is relatively stable once the serum or plasma is removed from the red blood cells (4 days at room temperature, about 1 week after cooling to +4°C), shipping cooled is best. As diurnal variation of progesterone concentrations as demonstrated in the bitch (Thuróczy *et al.*, 2003) seems possible in queens too, sampling in the morning or, in case of repeated samples, around the same time of the day is preferable. The glycoprotein AMH is secreted by Sertoli cells and granulosa cells and can consequently be used as proof of presence

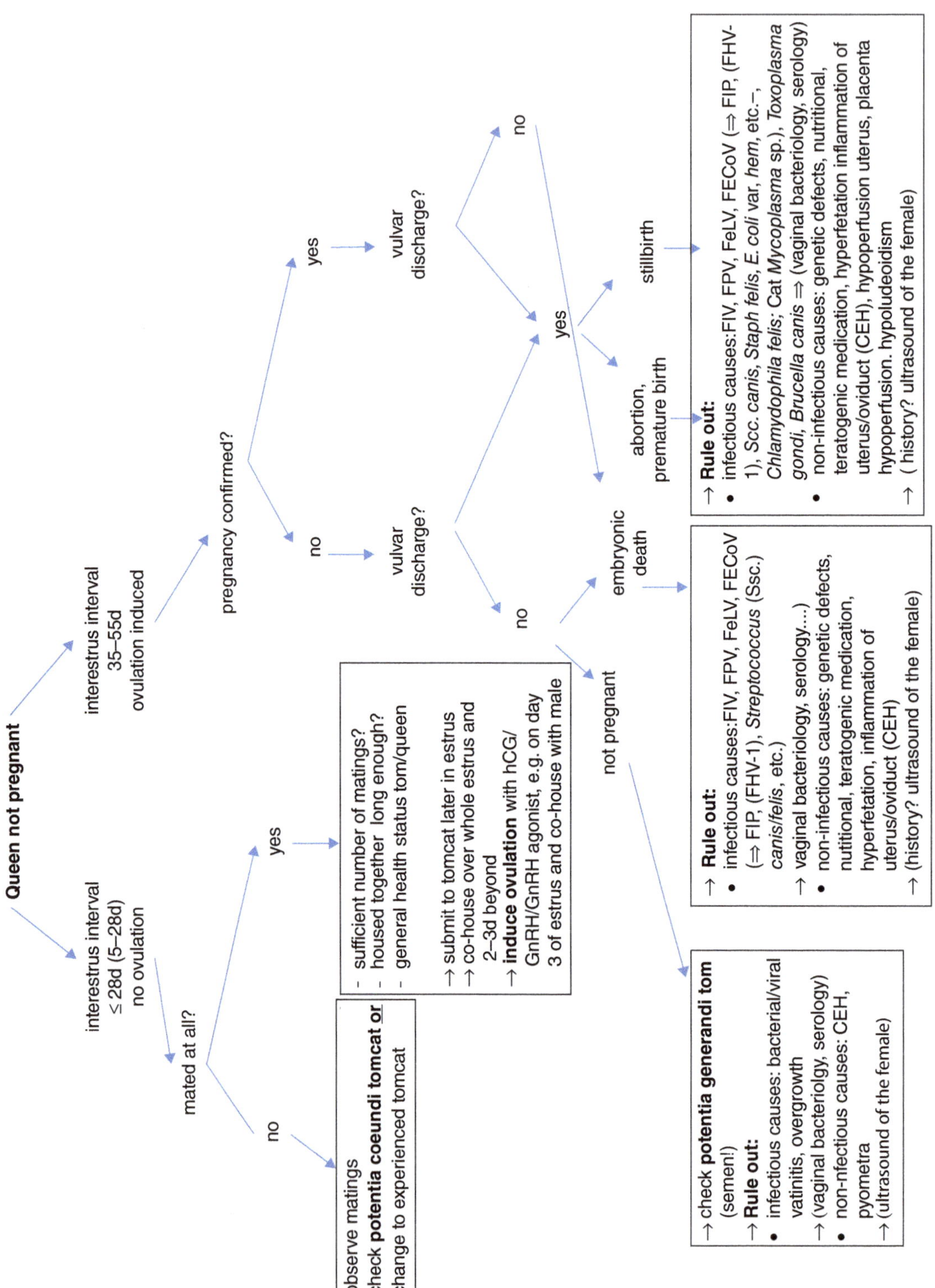

Fig. 25.6. 'Not pregnant queen': what to ask and do if the queen is not pregnant.

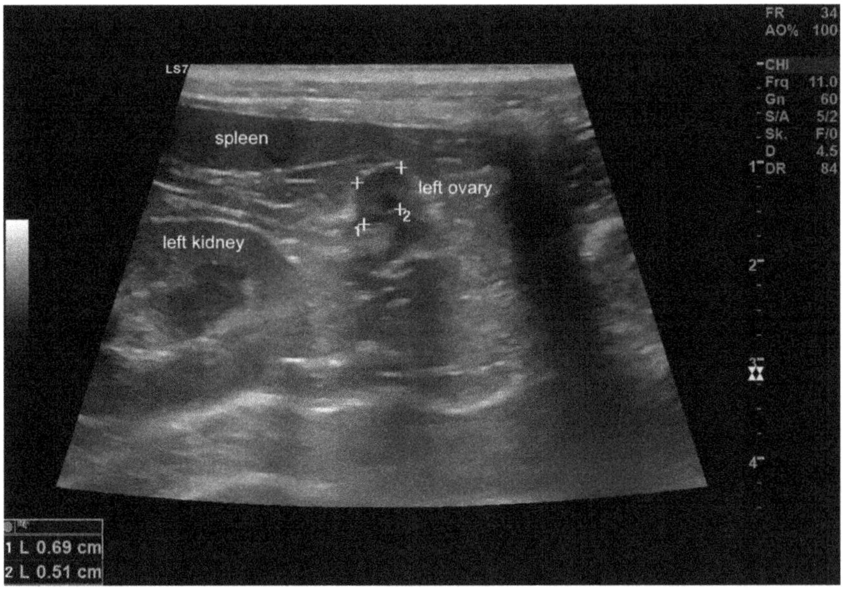

Fig. 25.7. Ultrasound image from an ovary obtained from an estrous queen. Two anechogenic structures are clearly visible. (Image: author's own.)

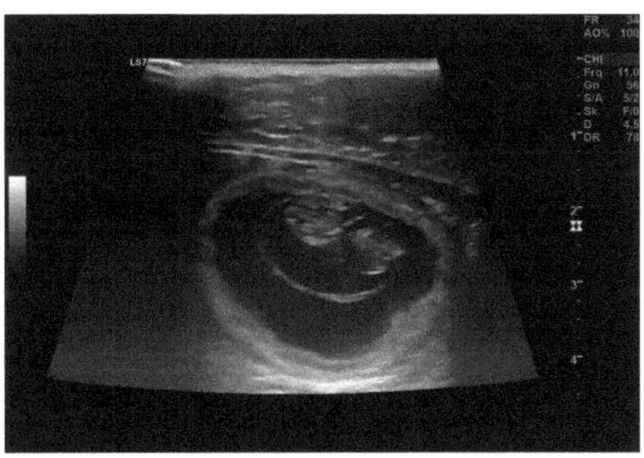

Fig. 25.8. Ultrasound finding in early pregnancy, the uterine wall, the embryo and the fetal membranes are clearly visible. (Image: author's own.)

of germinative tissue in male and female prepubertal and post-pubertal animals (Walter, 2020). As the hormone is stable for about 3 days at room temperature and for about 5 days at 2–8°C, samples should be shipped cooled to the laboratory. Early (unknown) ovariohysterectomy is the most common cause for ovarian absence. Spayed females have low concentrations of AMH (human-based test: <0.1 ng/mL (Place *et al.*, 2011) or <0.14 ng/mL (Axnér and Ström Holst, 2015)). Intact animals have significantly higher AMH concentrations (human-based test: 0.7–10 ng/mL (Place *et al.*, 2011) or 1.3–19 ng/mL (Axnér and Ström Holst, 2015)). With these threshold levels, no false-positive and false-negative results have been reported (Walter, 2020). Interestingly, AMH concentrations seem to be age dependent in intact queens with highest values in kittens up to 3 months of age (Snoeck *et al.*, 2017).

Repeated LH analysis can be performed using a semiquantitative test (e.g. Witness® LH) instead of AMH to detect the presence of mature ovaries. Low LH concentrations indicate presence of ovarian tissue. The use of an in-house analysis makes this test easier to perform clinically. Shipment for an LH test is difficult due to its instability (one day at 2–8°C). High LH might be present in intact animals at the time of LH peak or in neutered animals due to the lack of negative feedback. If an elevated LH is obtained, this can be repeated in 2-3 days and in the intact animal, the LH will again be low.

Treatment options

In cases of primary and secondary anestrous, estrus induction can be attempted after prepubertal age, underlying health conditions, anatomic or genetic abnormalities, and diestrus have been ruled out. Light-regime management (> 14 hours of light) and exposure to other estrus queens and intact toms are non-invasive means to induce estrus. More frequently, hormonal options are applied, either GnRH, GnRH analogs, follicle-stimulating hormone (FSH) or FSH-analogs (see Chapter 3). Most frequently, estrus is medically induced by a single dose of 100–150 IU equine chorion gonadotropin (eCG) IM (Kutzler, 2007). The queen should be allowed to mate while in estrus for induction of ovulation. Alternatively, ovulation can be induced by a single dose of 75–100 IU human chorion gonadotropin (hCG) IM 80–88 hours after eCG (Donoghue *et al.*, 1992; Swanson *et al.*, 1997) or by a single dose of 25 µg/cat IM cystorelin (Kutzler, 2007), or 50 µg/cat gonadorelin (Ferré-Dolcet *et al.*, 2021). Estrus can also be induced by SQ application of a slow-release GnRH agonist as a 4.7 mg Suprelorin® implant (Zambelli *et al.*, 2015). In this case, the implant should be removed after successful estrus induction.

25.2.4 Failure to allow mating

Failure to allow mating is most often associated with behavioral causes, such as overly aggressive or shy queens. Congenital (or acquired) vaginal abnormalities are rare but should be ruled out. Behavioral causes can be treated by changing the breeding management. Moving the tom to the queen's housing may give her more confidence or trying another male to see if there is an incompatibility factor. Some queens might be more receptive when they are at the peak of estrus around day 3 to 4. Bringing the queen to the male early in estrus to get accustomed to the new environment might be beneficial in other queens. Causes of pain during mating (back or hind limb pain, vaginal scaring, etc.) should also be assessed and treated appropriately. Only healthy animals should be submitted to breeding. If changes in breeding management are not successful, pharmacological induction of ovulation and artificial insemination can be considered.

25.2.5 Failure to ovulate

Failure to ovulate can be suspected when queens allow mating or are in estrus every 8–10 days. Management of the cattery should be assessed to determine if matings of the queen have been observed. The mating behavior should include the appropriate posture, yowling when intromission occurs, and the 'after reaction' of rolling, licking, etc. immediately after mating. If these behaviors are not occurring, it is likely that the tom is failing to actually achieve intromission and he should be examined as the potential problem. Additionally, the number of matings should be assessed as multiple matings (more than four) are required to induce ovulation. Failure to ovulate can be diagnosed by observing matings between the tom and the queen, and assaying progesterone 4–7 days later. If ovulation has occurred, the progesterone will rise (above 2 ng/mL). If progesterone is still baseline (less than 0.2 ng/mL), ovulation did not occur. If the queen is allowing mating before a preovulatory follicle is present, the male can be allowed access to the queen for a longer period of time so breeding during her optimal follicular period. Primary ovulation failure can be treated by inducing ovulation pharmacologically, e.g. by 75–100 IU hCG, and allowing the queen and tom to mate afterwards, or artificial insemination can be performed. After ovulation is induced, progesterone can be assayed approximately 1 week later to ensure ovulation did occur (progesterone will rise).

Persistent estrus

Persistent estrus is also related to the failure to ovulate and clinical signs are related to persistent estrogen production. Specific breeds, such as Siamese, or individual cats can present with short interestrus intervals and the owner may perceive this as persistent heat. A thorough history and repeated gynecological examinations with assessment of vaginal cytology provides clarification between short interestrus or prolonged estrus.

Ovarian/follicular cysts are a common cause of persistent estrus and ovulation failure. Though rare, granulosa cell tumors can present as persistent estrus, too. Vaginal cytology is consistent with the presence of estrogen (cornified epithelium, Fig. 25.3). Abdominal ultrasound is suitable to identify follicular cysts and granulosa cell tumor. Follicular cysts are characterized as large fluid-filled, anechogenic structures present on the ovary. They can be distinguished from follicles by their size (usually significantly bigger, often >10 mm) and/or persistence (repeated ultrasound examination within a respective time frame, e.g. 5–7 days, reveals the same structure(s)). Granulosa cell tumors appear as inhomogeneous ovarian texture with hyperechogenic and hypoechogenic areas and possible calcification. AMH analysis has been postulated to be beneficial for identification of granulosa cell tumors in queens (Heaps *et al.*, 2017; Walter, 2020), similar to the situation in dogs where significantly higher AMH concentrations are associated with the presence of granulosa cell tumors (Walter *et al.*, 2018).

As a note, paraovarian cysts are fluid-filled structures in the surrounding area of the ovaries that do not cause clinical signs or require treatment/action. Typically, they are incidental findings, but can be mistaken for follicular cysts.

Whereas ovariohysterectomy, either partial or total, is the treatment of choice in cases of a granulosa cell tumor, induction of ovulation either by repeated vaginal stimulation with a cotton swab or medically by 75–100 IU hCG/cat IM or 25–50 μg GnRH/cat IM can be attempted in cases of follicular cysts. If vaginal stimulation or medical treatment is not successful, surgical removal of the cyst(s) or unilateral ovariectomy (in case of unilateral presence of follicular cysts) can be performed. If all options fail, surgical neutering is required. Progestin treatment to induce regression of cysts is not recommended due to the increased risk of pyometra.

25.2.6 Failure to become pregnant

Failure to become pregnant may be a queen or tom issue. History is typically that the queen allowed mating, was not observed in estrus for 40–45 days, but then returned to estrus before the expected gestational period. Alternative history is that the queen was mated successfully but was then determined not to be pregnant at about 30 days. Confirmation of an elevated progesterone following mating helps to differentiate failure to become pregnant from ovulation failure. In general, noninfectious and infectious causes of pregnancy failure have to be considered. However, failure to become pregnant is most frequently noninfectious. Uterine pathology, such as cystic endometrial hyperplasia (CEH)-pyometra complex, is most common (Fig. 25.9). Mating with an infertile tomcat, nutritional deficits, and rare developmental disorders, such as aplasia of selected parts of the genital tract and/or malformation of the genital tract have to be considered as noninfectious causes. Systemic illness, reduced general condition, malnutrition, or obesity can have an impact on reproductive performance.

If uterine pathology is present, the prognosis for future fertility is low. If the queen is young, medical management of pyometra may be attempted. Diagnosis and treatment of pyometra is discussed in Chapter 14. Mating of the breeding queen with a proven fertile tomcat in the next estrus after successful and completed treatment is considered beneficial to maximize chances for a subsequent pregnancy and to reduce the risk for a pyometra relapse.

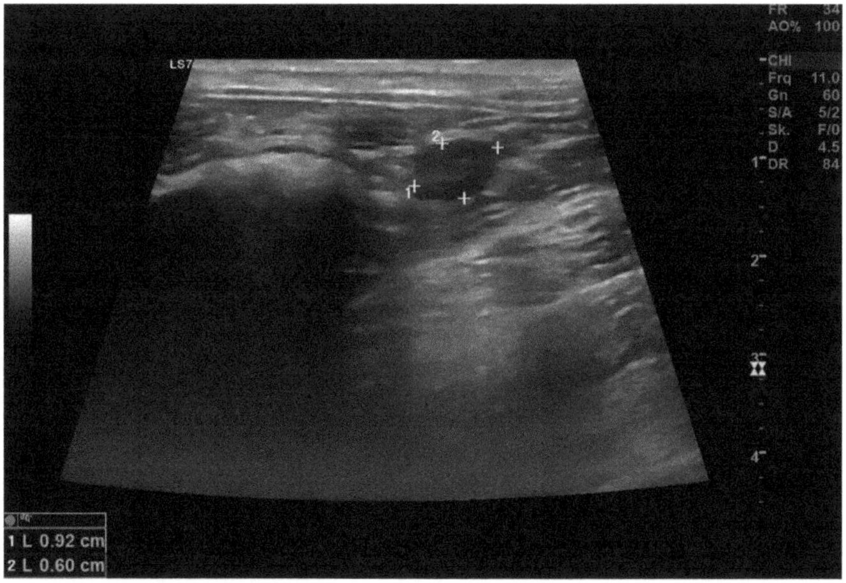

Fig. 25.9. Ultrasound examination from the uterus of a queen not conceiving. The uterine wall is slightly thickened and shows slight signs of cystic endometrial hyperplasia. (Image: author's own.)

Now, in times of increased 'biologically appropriate raw food' and home-made diet feeding, nutritional deficits are again more frequently observed. Reproductive performance is affected by inadequate essential fatty acids and low energy contents underlining the need for optimum nutrition of breeding queens. Nutritional imbalances, insufficient taurine, arachidonate and copper, but also inadequate essential fatty acids and energy content can negatively affect reproductive performance. Taurine deficiency can result in increased fetal resorption. Clinical history and diet analysis can help identifying the cause of infertility.

25.2.7 Failure to carry pregnancy to term – early embryonic loss, fetal death and stillbirth

As discussed earlier, failure to maintain pregnancy can be noninfectious or infectious (Table 25.2) with infectious causes more common and disastrous to a breeding program. Early pregnancy loss is often unnoticed and without clinical signs except for a prolonged interestrus interval, making differentiation between early embryonic loss and pregnancy failure difficult. Later pregnancy loss is associated with bloody or brownish vulvar discharge, expulsion of fetuses/fetal parts/fetal membranes, and possibly signs of general illness. Table 25.2 provides insights into the time points when pregnancy is disrupted, either at the time of embryogenesis, during fetal development, or at the time of parturition as stillbirth.

Viral infections require proper diagnosis and includes serology testing or antigen proof by PCR. Viral infections could be causative alone, but also with concomitant other causes. Regarding bacteriological examination, a vaginal swab is suggestive of the cause in case of bacterial overgrowth (high numbers) of a single organism. When infectious and degenerative changes of the uterus are suspected, histopathological and bacteriological examinations of uterine biopsies are required. Antibiotic choice should fit with the causative agent based on culture and susceptibility. In cases of *Chlamydophila felis* and *Coxiella burnetti*, systemic infection must be considered requiring treatment with doxycycline or fluroquinolons before establishing pregnancy. In cases of severe recurrent systemic problems (conjunctivitis, etc.), vaccination with a *Chlamydophila felis* killed vaccine should be considered if available.

Luteal failure or hypoluteoidism is the inability to produce sufficient progesterone to maintain pregnancy. This diagnosis is regularly postulated in breeding queens, especially Maine Coon cats, but

Table 25.2. Noninfectious and infectious causes for failure to maintain pregnancy and time point(s) when pregnancy is disturbed: (i) embryonic death; (ii) abortion/fetal death; (iii) stillbirth; and (iv) fetal defects. (Author's own table.)

Infectious causes	Noninfectious causes
Early embryonic loss	Early embryonic loss
Viral infections	Genetic defects i, ii, iii, iv
Feline immunodeficiency virus (FIV) i, ii, iii, iv	Nutritional deficits: i, ii, iv
Feline infectious peritonitis virus (FIPV) = feline enteric corona virus i, ii, iii	Lack of taurin
	Lack of vitamin A
Feline leukemia virus (FeLV) i, ii	Lack of vitamin E
Feline panleucopenia virus (FPLV) i, ii, iv[a]	Teratogenic drugs i, ii, iii, iv
Feline herpes virus (FHV-1) i	Hyperfetation i, ii, iii
Bacterial infections:	Inflammation of the oviduct/uterus i
Streptococci lancefield group G (*Streptococcus canis*) ii, iii	Endometrial hypotrophy/placental insuffi ciency ii, iii
	Hypoluteoidism/luteal failure ii
E. coli var. *hem.* ii, iii	
Campylobacter jejuni ii	
Salmonella typhimurium ii, iii	
Brucella canis ii?, iii?	
Mycoplasma /Ureaplasma sp. ii	
Chlamydophila felis ii, iii	
Parasites:	
Toxoplasma gondii ii, iii	

[a]Cerebellar hypoplasia.

published proof of the existence of true hypoluteoidism in queens is lacking. One possible reason might be that progesterone is produced not only by the corpora lutea, but also by the placenta in late pregnancy. Repeated weekly blood samplings for progesterone analysis during the course of pregnancy in case of suspicion can provide a diagnosis. Supplementation with progesterone or synthetic progestins has been suggested in cases of luteal failure/hypoluteoidism. Progesterone is given as described in dogs: either 2 mg/kg SQ (progesterone in oil) every other day or 5 mg/kg PO (micronized progesterone) three times daily. Alternatively, synthetic progestins, such as medroxyprogesterone acetate (0.1 mg/kg orally once daily) or altrenogest (0.088 mg/kg orally once daily), can be administered. Supplementation should not be instituted until after finalized organ development (approximately day 45 of gestation), since earlier use is associated with the risk of masculinization in female offspring and possibly cryptorchidism in male offspring (Wilkins, 1960; Curtis and Grant, 1964). Progesterone therapy can be considered if the serum progesterone drops – depending on the method of analysis – below 2 ng/mL or is dropping rapidly within a short period of time (several days). The consideration that luteal failure/hypoluteoidism might be a hereditary condition makes further use of affected breeding queens questionable.

25.3 The Tomcat

Literature about infertility in tomcats is even more limited than in queens. Some information is gained from endangered wild felids or domestic felids as a model for their wild relatives. Infertility may be acquired or hereditary but it is difficult to determine between the two unless the tom was once fertile. The basic clinical approach to handle the 'infertile' tom is very similar regardless of what the problem is and includes a complete reproductive work-up including semen collection and evaluation. Once this is complete, the practitioner will have more information to determine additional diagnostics needed. The minimum data base for an infertile tomcat is described in Table 25.3.

25.3.1 History

A detailed history is required to identify if infertility is related to impotentia coeundi (if the tomcat is unable to mate) or impotentia generandi (if the tomcat mates normally, but mated queens do not conceive). Impotentia coeundi might be due to early age (sexual immaturity, late puberty as described in Persians and related breeds) or caused by fear/bad experiences such as dominant queens, wrong conditioning (too close relation to the owner, hand-raising without contact to sexual partners), not optimum

Table 25.3. Diagnostic plan for an infertile male feline patient. (Author's own table.)

History		
Signalement	Breeding name, breed, ID (microchip/tattoo), date of birth	
Physical examination		
Andrological examination	Scrotum	Position, size, symmetry, injuries, inflammation, adhesions, thickness of skin, adhesions, spermatic cords
	Testes	Size, consistency, inflammation signs, tumor
	Epididymes	Size, consistency, inflammation signs, tumor
	Spermatic cords	(If they can be reached)
	Prepuce	Discharge, inflammation signs, tumor
	Penis	
Ultrasound examination	Testes	
	Epididymes	
	Spermatic cords (if possible)	
	Accessory sex glands (if possible)	
Semen collection and evaluation		
Further examinations (if required)	Bacteriological examination of the semen	
	Virological examination of the semen, PCR, serology, if required	
	Seminal plasma analysis (alkaline phosphatase)	
	Hormone testing	
	Karyotyping	
Diagnosis, evaluation, and treatment approaches		

housing, social stress, pain and/or neurological lesions in the lumbar, pelvic, or hind leg region, or anatomical/skeletal malformations.

Questions related to the reproductive history and general health of the individual tomcat and conditions in the cattery need to be asked. Special consideration should be given to determine the health status of the tom within the past 2 months, as events during this time period would affect spermatogenesis. An important question relates to the number of queens mated and the origin of the queens, namely if they come from the same cattery or from external catteries.

In detail, the following questions about the reproductive history should be asked:

1. Number and origin of mated queens (own/external cattery)?
2. Number of queens conceiving/not pregnant? Litter size over time? (Pregnancy or lack of pregnancy confirmed by inspection of the mammary nipples, by abdominal palpation or ultrasound?)
3. Has the tom been bred to previously fertile queens that gave birth to healthy litters?
4. Is libido present?
5. Have mating(s) been observed? Did the queen(s) show 'normal' behavior during and after mating (yowling at intromission of the penis, 'after reaction' such as licking, rolling, etc.)?
6. How often has the individual queen(s) been mated and when had she/they been mated in relation to the time that queens had been in estrus at presentation? How long had the queens been in estrus after the suspected 'mating(s)'?
7. When did last (successful) mating occur (in regard to time to presentation)?
8. Has the tom presented before for andrological examination and semen evaluations? Results from previous examinations?
9. Any illness, injury, or fever, especially within the past 2 months?
10. Is the tom currently receiving any medications or did he within the past 2 months?

General cattery questions are similar to what has been addressed in the queen.

25.3.2 Physical and andrological examination

The aim of the physical examination is to identify any current diseases and health issues, but also to obtain relevant information about the general and nutritional condition of the cat. Gingivitis, stomatitis, and other painful conditions of the mouth can prevent the tomcat from neck biting, a necessary reflex during coitus. The veterinarian should specifically look for signs of lumbar, pelvic, or hind leg pain, or neurologic problems that may interfere with normal mating. Neuropathies related to diabetes mellitus might also be a cause for ejaculation failure.

During andrological examination, the scrotum, testes, epididymides, spermatic cords, prepuce, and penis should be evaluated by visual inspection and palpation. Examination should include careful examination of the position of the testes, size, symmetry, if the scrotal skin can be moved freely above the testes, and if any signs of inflammation or injury are present. Fighting of cats might result in bite injuries and consequently abscessation in the scrotum. Severe old scrotal insults can be associated with periorchitis and scar tissue formation, resulting in a decreased mobility of the scrotal skin. Increase of scrotal temperature due to inflammation or inability for thermoregulation due to restricted movement within the scrotum is detrimental for semen quality. The size can be evaluated by a measuring caliper (manual/digital; Fig. 25.10) or ultrasound, and the length, width and height should be taken for each testis individually. In general, repeated measurements should be taken under sedation to increase the accuracy. Care should be taken not to compress the tissue during the measuring process with the caliper or ultrasound. Even though current reference values are limited to domestic shorthair cats, comparison with those in relation to the body weight of the respective tomcat might provide useful information. Testicular volume of adult, sexually mature tomcats with normal semen quality (body weight 3.9–6.4 kg) taken with a digital caliper is in mean 3.1 mm^3 (range 2.1–4.3 mm^3; own unpublished observations). Testicular hypoplasia and hypotrophy are known to be associated with reduced spermatogenic output. Similarly, testicular consistency provides relevant information about the spermatogenic capacity. Overly firm testes might indicate a testicular tumor (very rare in cats, however) or acute orchitis, and soft/soft-elastic testes might indicate reduced spermatogenic activity. Figure 25.11 shows normal-sized testes of a tomcat with a high total sperm count and of a patient with azoospermic ejaculates. Both tomcats have a similar body weight. Note the reduced size of the testicles. The epididymis is

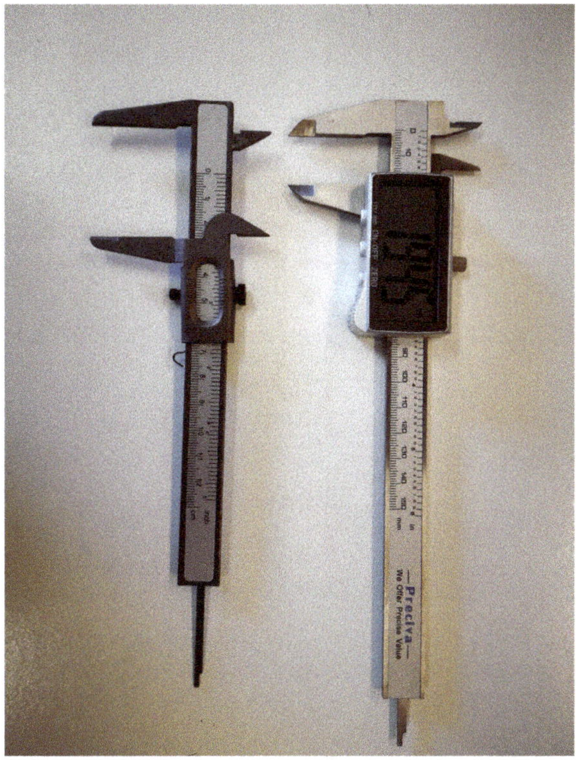

Fig. 25.10. Digital and manual caliper as well as measuring tape to measure testicular dimensions. (Image: author's own.)

firmly attached to the testicle and cannot be easily differentiated unless there is significant disease (enlargement caused by inflammation or neoplasia). Evaluation of the spermatic cords is challenging but published literature about abnormalities of the spermatic cords is rare. Inflammation of the spermatic cord, or funiculitis, has been reported after castration (Araújo *et al.*, 2012) or associated with tuberculosis.

Examination of the penis is not always possible in the non-sedated tom but can be definitively performed after/during sedation/anesthesia for semen collection. The external genitalia should be thoroughly examined for gross lesions such as ulceration, discoloration, or discharge. The size of penile spines may be decreased in cases of hypotestosteronemia due to pituitary hypogonadism or iatrogenic contraceptive treatment with GnRH agonist implants (Fig. 25.12). Congenital or acquired phimosis or strictures of the penis by hair rings in long-haired cats could prevent successful breeding. Anatomical deviations of the penis resulting in altered direction of the penis during erection are rarely observed, but should be evaluated, especially in cases of erection or intromission failure. Accessory sex glands of the cat (prostate and bulbourethral gland) can be examined by ultrasound, but examination may require some training due to their usually small size and the location within the pelvis. Reports about diseases in the feline accessory sex glands are rare.

On ultrasound, the testicular parenchyma should be of homogeneous texture with the mediastinum testes located centrally (Fig. 25.13). Davidson and Baker (2009b) provide guidance on ultrasound findings in the tomcat. Mixed echogenicity may indicate orchitis, often associated with periorchitis and thickening of the skin. Anechogenic areas can be present in case of testicular cysts, dilatation of the seminiferous tubules, or the mediastinum testis. Varicoceles, or dilatation of testicular veins, have been reported to cause pain and infertility in humans (Paick and Choi, 2019), but have not been reported in tomcats to the best of the author's knowledge. The use of Doppler ultrasound is advisable in cases of

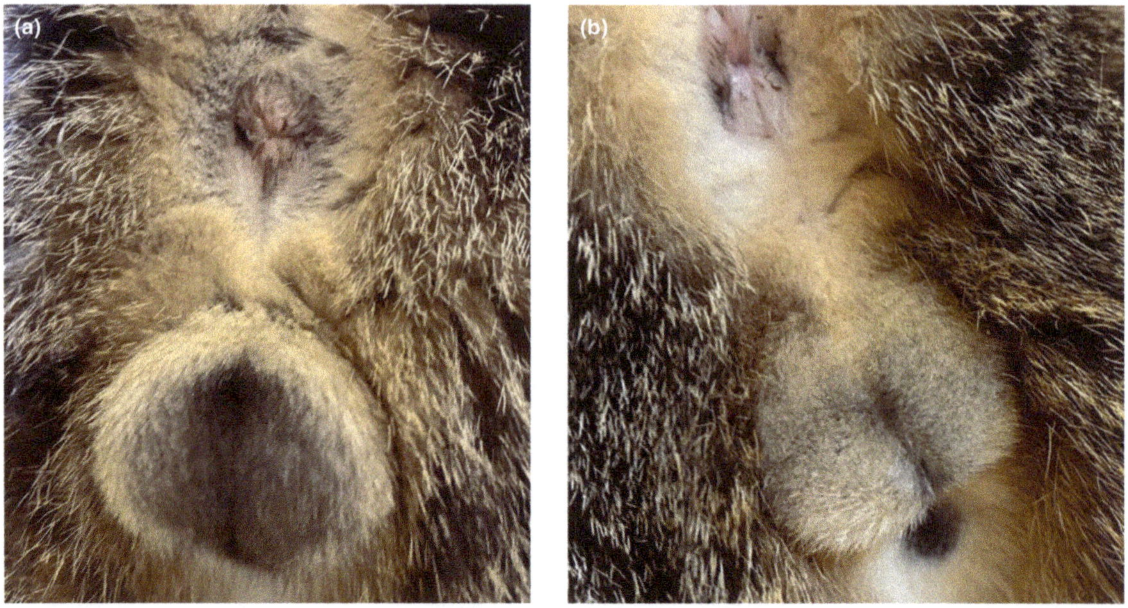

Fig. 25.11. **(a)** Normal testis size (from a fertile tomcat), compared to **(b)** small testis size (from an azoospermic tomcat), both tomcats are Domestic Shorthair breed. (Images: author's own.)

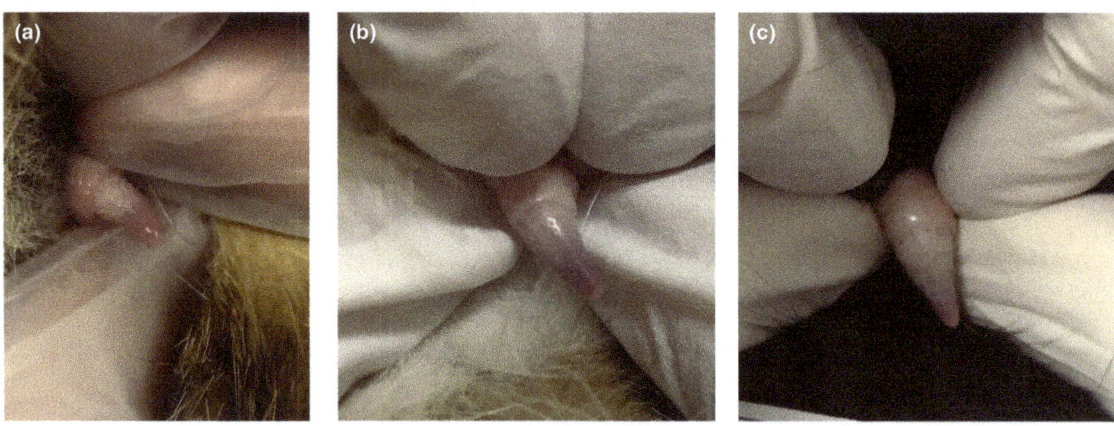

Fig. 25.12. The presence of penile spines will be evaluated during andrological examination. **(a)** Normal-sized, prominent penile spines are present in intact male cats. **(b)** They are absent following surgical neutering or during successful hormonal castration using a GnRH agonist implant, but also due to, e.g., pituitary hypogonadism. **(c)** Presence of small penile spines might indicate low testosterone concentrations. (Images: author's own.)

anechogenic areas to assess blood flow and identify dilated veins or arteries. Hyperechogenic areas indicate fibrosis and/or possibly calcification. Significant changes within the parenchyma might indicate permanent alterations and consequently severe effects on spermatogenesis.

25.3.3 Semen collection and evaluation

Semen collection and evaluation are crucial for diagnosis of infertility and possible causes. Macroscopic evaluation of the semen sample for color and consistency can provide initial insights: a transparent color of the ejaculate collected

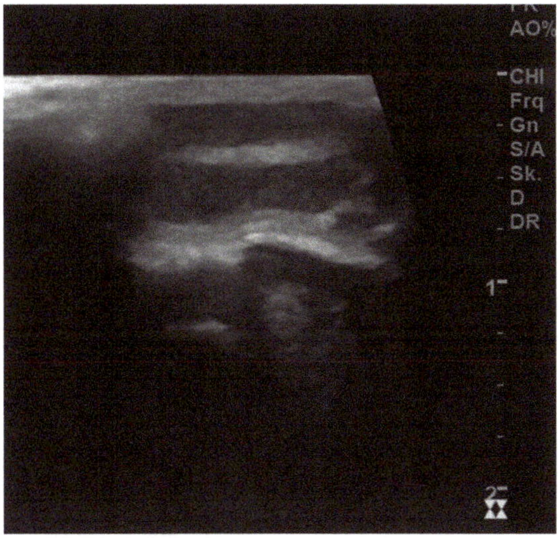

Fig. 25.13. Ultrasound image of a feline testis. Note the thickened, hyperechogenic mediastinum testis. (Image: author's own.)

might indicate azoospermia or severe oligozoospermia. Based on the extremely variable results of feline ejaculates described in the literature, with certain dependency on the collection method (artificial vagina/transurethral catheterization/electroejaculation) (Figs 25.14 and 25.15), conclusions about the fertility of the examined tomcat are difficult. Teratozoospermia is common in cats and can also be associated with normal fertility (Pukazhenthi *et al.*, 2001; Neubauer *et al.*, 2004). Azoospermia, the lack of spermatozoa, can be differentiated from incomplete ejaculation testing for alkaline phosphatase (ALP) in the seminal plasma. As in other species, ALP derives from the epididymis and high concentrations (>5,000 IU/L) in the seminal plasma indicate emptying of the epididymal tail (= complete ejaculation). Similarly to other species, seminal plasma ALP concentrations are often >20,000 IU/L. In cases of azoospermic ejaculates and high ALP seminal plasma, the diagnosis is non-obstructive azoospermia and the tomcat can be considered as infertile at that time point. Often (non-obstructive) azoospermia is associated with other clinical findings such as soft testes and/or irregular testicular parenchyma on ultrasound examination. A follow-up examination with semen collection and evaluation should be performed 2–3 months later. This interval is related to the duration of spermatogenesis (46.8 days) and the duration of epididymal maturation (10–14 days). In cases of low ALP seminal plasma, either incomplete ejaculation (usually due to semen collection method) or obstructive azoospermia (bilateral) should be considered. Obstructive azoospermia is related to an obstruction or pathology of the epididymal, vasal, or ejaculatory duct. It can be related to genitourinary infection or congenital abnormality or surgical vasectomy. Clinically, obstructive azoospermia is an extremely rare diagnosis with only one case report (Umbach *et al.*, 2020).

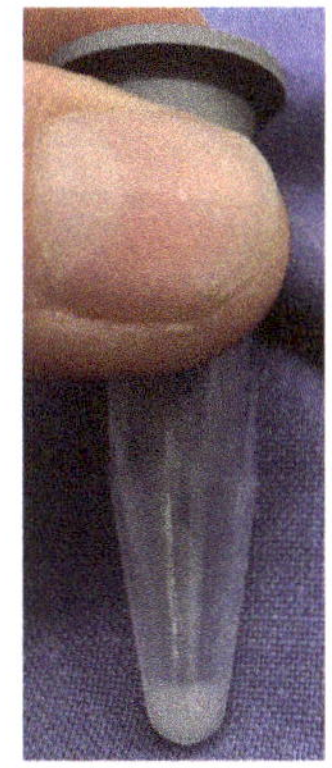

Fig. 25.14. Artificial vagina for semen collection: a rubber is attached to an Eppendorf tube. The ejaculate collected manually is in the tube. (Image: author's own.)

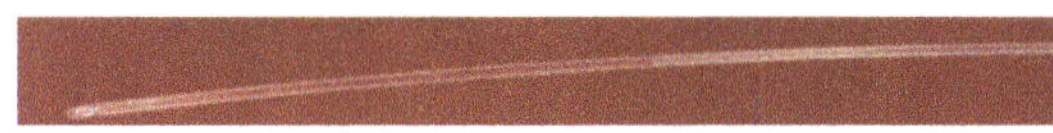

Fig. 25.15. Azoospermic ejaculate collected following sedation with dexmedetomidine/methadone using transurethral catheterization. Note: The tip of the catheter is not cut to avoid traumatization of the penile urethra. In this case it is important not to insert the last 2 cm into the urethra. Alternatively, the tip of the catheter can be cut. (Image: author's own.)

25.3.4 Additional examinations

Bacteriological/virological examination of the semen

Bacteriological examination of the semen sample should be considered in cases where semen evaluation does not provide an indication for infertility in the tomcat, and in cases with a history of repeated resorption/abortion/stillbirth in queens mated by the respective tomcat. Physiologically, aerobic and anaerobic bacteria are considered the normal flora of a feline ejaculate, but also of the prepuce. Our own unpublished data shows that semen samples collected by transurethral catheterization represent a physiological mixed flora, often including low to moderate growth of different, apathogenic and facultative pathogenic species (*E. coli* var. *hem.*, staphylococci, streptococci, *Pasteurella* spp., *Proteus* spp., *Enterococcus* spp.). Pure culture and heavy growth of specifically *E. coli* var. *hem.* or ß-hemolytic. streptococci, and *Streptococcus canis*, has been associated with a few cases of otherwise unexplained infertility and therefore treatment would be advisable. Vaginal swabs from mated queens not conceiving and/or aborting queens can be collected and sent for bacteriological examination to compare with the semen culture. To the best of the author's knowledge, no information about the presence and pathogenicity of *Chlamydophilaceae*, *Mycoplasma*, and *Ureaplasma* spp. in feline semen is available. But as these have been identified as part of the physiological flora and facultative pathogens in queens, and in semen of other male species, it seems likely that they are present in tomcat semen, too. Feline orchitis has been reported with tuberculosis and *Brucella canis*. Both diseases have zoonotic potential.

Even though herpesvirus (FHV-1) transmission via semen is possible, there are no reports about feline herpes virus transmission via semen and/or seminal fluids. Furthermore, researchers did not identify FHV-1 DNA in ejaculates from FHV-1 affected Pallas cats over a 3-year period, indicating that transmission via semen is unlikely (Swanson *et al.*, 2006). However, as infection is oronasal, transmission might only be avoided when semen collection and artificial insemination of the queen is performed therefore avoiding any contact between breeding partners. Feline infectious peritonitis (FIP) is an immune-mediated disease initiated by feline coronavirus (FCoV) infection. Even though orchitis had been described with FIP (Foster *et al.*, 1996; Sigurdardóttir *et al.*, 2001), a recent study was unable to show transmission of FCoV by semen (Stranieri *et al.*, 2020). Different to this, several studies showed that feline immunodeficiency virus (FIV) is spread by natural mating and artificial insemination as FIV is present in the seminal plasma of semen samples (Jordan *et al.*, 1998, 1999). Virus infection can be diagnosed by paired serum samples for serology or PCR.

Hormone analysis

Determination of serum testosterone is useful to identify cryptorchidism, hypogonadism and testicular atrophy. Due to the pulsatile secretion pattern, a single analysis is not sufficient in the tomcat. Whereas a single testosterone analysis might provide correct conclusions in the dog, it poses a relatively high risk for false-negative results in tomcats as intact tomcats can have basal testosterone concentrations ($T < 0.1$ ng/mL). Consequently, a GnRH stimulation test with one serum sample before GnRH stimulation, administration of a GnRH analog, such as buserelin acetate (25 µg/cat (Goericke-Pesch *et al.*, 2013) or 0.4 µg/kg (Stempel and Goericke-Pesch, 2020)) IV and one to three samples after stimulation (30, 60, and 90 minutes) are recommended. Alternatively, a hCG stimulation test can be performed by an initial blood sample (basal), then administering 500 IU hCG IV (Memon *et al.*, 1992) or IM followed by another sample 30, 60 and 120 minutes later. In clinical practice, reduced sampling frequency is often sufficient with one sample 'before' and one 'after' stimulation sample (GnRH 60 minutes, hCG 60 or 90 minutes). Presence of functional testicular tissue is indicated by a significant increase of testosterone concentrations of at least 1.5 times. The lack of a testosterone increase following GnRH administration can be related to pituitary hypogonadism. This can be congenital (primary), but also secondary, e.g. by application of a GnRH agonist implant. Spontaneous secondary pituitary hypogonadism is known in humans but has not been described in cats.

Luteinizing hormone can be evaluated using a semiquantitative in-house rapid test for determination of the neutering state and for confirmation of incomplete castration. Low LH is indicative for an intact hypothalamus-pituitary-gonadal axis, whereas repeatedly high LH concentrations confirm earlier castration. The presence of penile spines, high AMH, and an increase of testosterone concentrations following GnRH stimulation test will also confirm an intact male. The glycoprotein AMH, produced by Sertoli cells, is the key hormone for sex differentiation in the male. Presence of AMH confirms presence of gonadal tissue and neutered male and female animals have extremely low concentrations (below the detection limit, <0.02 ng/mL, depending on the laboratory). Interestingly, highest AMH concentrations were found in dogs with Sertoli cell tumors, cryptorchid cases, and intersex conditions. To the best of the author's knowledge, there is no current publication about the use of AMH to diagnose feline testicular tumors.

Karyotyping

Disorders of the sexual development (DSD) can be the cause of infertility making karyotyping a useful additional diagnostic tool. Physiologically domestic cats (*Felis catus*) have a diploid set of chromosomes 2n, 38,XX or 38,XY. With coat colors, the color orange is located on the X chromosome and is dominant over all colors except for white loci. Consequently, male cats can be orange or orange-white. Other color patterns in the male such as calico or tortoiseshell can be associated with abnormal sexual development. Typically, they have a XXY chromosome set (formerly Klinefelter) or mosaic cells with 38,XX and 38,XY, but are infertile due to the lack of spermatogenesis. Several reports exist in the literature with a male phenotype: XX/XY chimeras with ovary and testis or ovotestes and are rarely fertile. Other rare reports include XY-DSD with persistent Müllerian duct, hypospadias, or isolated cryptorchidism. XX-DSD (formerly sex reversal) affected cats have a male phenotype, but no visible testes.

Figure 25.16 provides an overview about underlying reasons, possible history and diagnostic procedures in tomcats presented for infertility.

25.3.5 Common problems and possible treatment approaches

Failure to mate and failure to achieve an erection

Failure to mate is named impotentia coeundi. Tomcats can fail to mate due to sexual immaturity, disturbances of the general conditions, orthopedic problems, or other health issues, such as stomatitis, gingivitis, etc. Pain due to any cause, also due to bite injuries and abscessation, can result in loss of libido and consequently failure to mate. Dominant queens exposed to inexperienced males can also be the reason why mating is not successful. History and physical as well as andrological examination might provide a cause for the mating failure. Late puberty has been described in Persians, Maine Coon and Norwegian Forrest cats. If no abnormality or disease can be detected, behavioral issues and/or lack of experience should be considered. In these cases, the tomcat should be exposed to a receptive, experienced queen in mid estrus. It is rather difficult to verify failure to achieve an erection in the tomcat due to the size of the penis and the mating behavior itself. Congenital phimosis, hair rings, or orchitis can also cause mating failure.

In the case of primary diseases, treatment of the primary problem is crucial. In the case of orthopedic problems or any other cause of pain, pain medication can provide some success. In case of sexual immaturity patience is necessary until animals are sexually mature. Treatment of impotentia coeundi is challenging if no underlying disease is present. In cases of reduced libido, improving environmental conditions, co-housing with experienced queens in estrus, or placing with the female already in estrus should be tried. In other species, GnRH agonists (buserelin acetate 25 µg/cat) or LH-analogs (hCG, 250 IU/cat) can be administered to increase testosterone and therefore libido. However, there are no reports about the use of these for this purpose in the tom.

Failure to induce ovulation

Failure to induce ovulation is either associated with the inability to mate correctly (impotentia coeundi) or with insufficient numbers of matings during estrus. For further diagnostic and treatment approaches in the queen see Chapter 5.

Failure to achieve pregnancy

Failure to achieve pregnancy can be due to impotentia coeundi and/or impotentia generandi, the lack of fertilizing the queen after successful matings and induction of ovulation. Impotentia coeundi is described in the section on 'Failure to mate and failure to achieve an erection'.

Subfertility can be associated with slight deviations from the reference range of semen parameters, so called dysspermia. Pathospermia, one or more significantly altered semen parameter(s), is usually associated with subfertility or infertility. Oligozoospermia, a reduced total sperm count, can be due to sexual immaturity, spontaneous, or iatrogenic hormonal suppression, e.g. by contraceptive agents, infectious diseases, or orchitis, but also inherited testicular hypoplasia. Clinically, small, soft testes or firm testes are often present. Asthenozoospermia

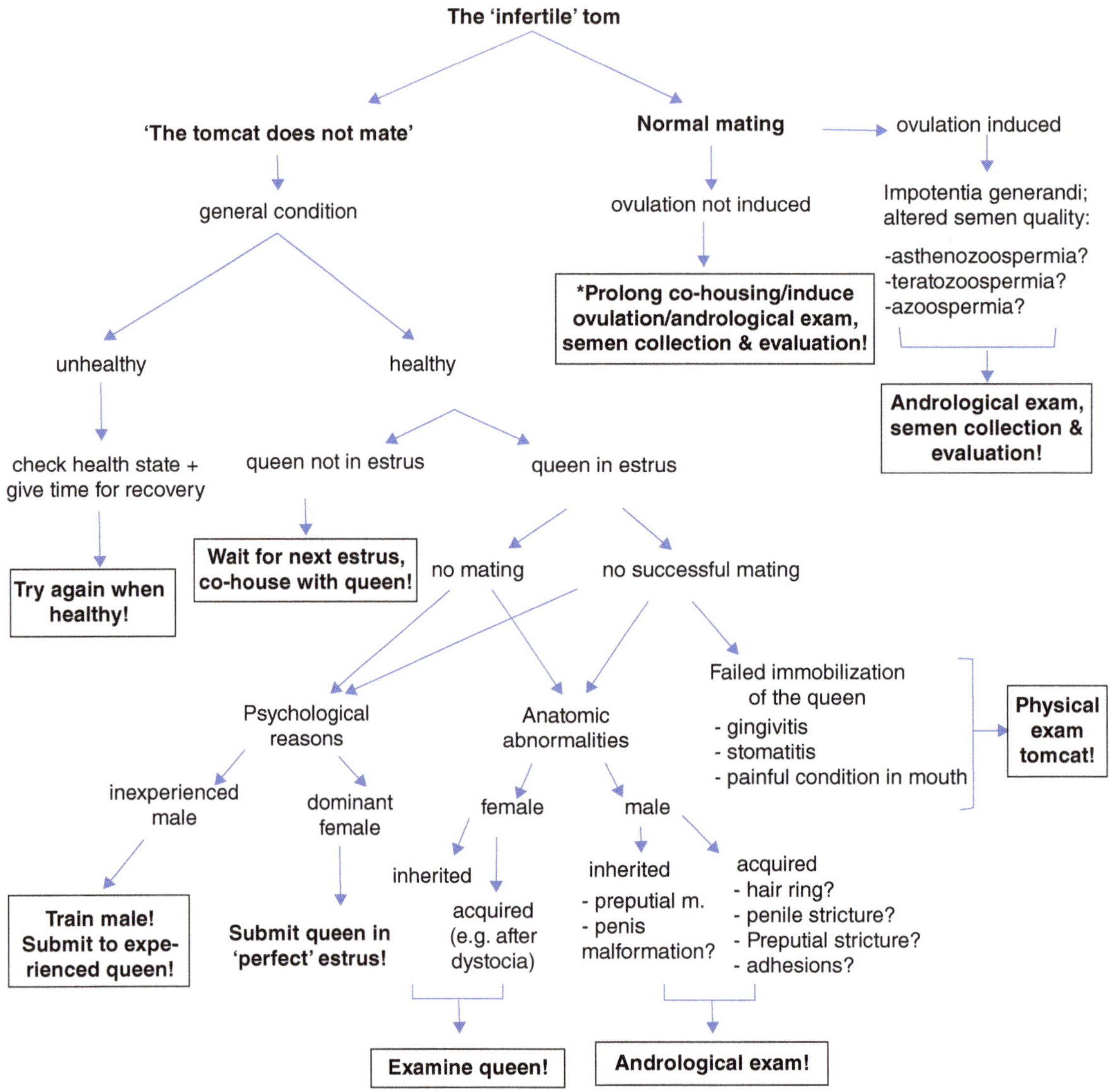

Fig. 25.16. 'The infertile tom': how to proceed with an infertile tom in the reproduction clinic.

(<70% progressive motility), often associated with teratozoospermia (>60% morphologically abnormal sperm), can be related to infections of the genital tract or to general infectious diseases with fever, urine contamination – as often observed with excessive stimulation with electroejaculation (urospermia). As described above, teratozoospermia is common in cats (Pukazhenthi *et al.*, 2001; Neubauer *et al.*, 2004) but often does not affect fertility in a natural mating situation making it difficult to estimate the impact on fertility of the respective tomcat.

Azoospermia, the lack of spermatozoa in an ejaculate, can be related to incomplete ejaculation, insufficient release of sperm due to insufficient use of α2-agonists with transurethral catheterization or inadequate electric stimulation, or 'real' azoospermia. 'Real' azoospermia can be pretesticular due to, for example, lack of adequate stimulation (hypogonadism), testicular non-obstructive, or post-testicular obstructive. Non-obstructive (testicular) azoospermia is most common and can be genetic (possibly associated with calico or tortoiseshell color pattern), congenital (bilateral abdominal cryptorchidism or Sertoli cell only syndrome), or acquired (testicular trauma, injury or tumor). Obstructive azoospermia, caused by an obstruction in the efferent ways, is rare and only one case report exists (Umbach *et al.*, 2020). As in other species, it can be diagnosed by low ALP activity in seminal plasma. Andrological examination including ultrasound, hormone analysis, karyotyping, and determination of the ALP in seminal plasma are helpful tools to identify the possible cause.

To test for the reversibility of observed changes and for further evaluation of the long-term impact on fertility, another semen collection should be performed 2–3 months after the initial examination. In case of orchitis, prognosis is poor. If only one testicle is affected, and orchitis is not related to a viral infection (e.g. FIP), *Brucella canis*, or tuberculosis, unilateral castration at the time of diagnosis can be considered to preserve fertility. If chronic, the associated inflammation in the affected testicle may lead to testicular degeneration in the remaining testicle, further lowering fertility. In cases of leukospermia, antimicrobial treatment according to the antibiogram is recommended with cases of heavy or pure cultures. If no bacterial infection or hypogonadism is identified, prognosis is often poor as only nonspecific treatment is possible. Nonspecific treatment includes a well-balanced diet as unbalanced diets were shown to result in oligozoospermia (or even azoospermia) in felids (Howard and Allen, 2007). Compared to dogs, few studies are published about the benefits of dietary supplements on semen quality in the tom, but, as with other species (Salas-Huetos *et al.*, 2018), there may be some benefit.

25.4 References

Araújo, N. L. de S., Carneiro, R. S., da Nóbrega Neto, P. I., and Araújo A. L. (2012). Funiculitis is a cat – a case report. *Ciência Animal* 22, 550–552.

Axnér, E. and Ström Holst, B. (2015) Concentrations of anti-Müllerian hormone in the domestic cat. Relation with spay or neuter status and serum estradiol. *Theriogenology* 83(5), 817–821. doi: 10.1016/j.theriogenology.2014.11.016

Curtis, E. M. and Grant, R. P. (1964) Masculinization of female pups by progestogens. *Journal of the American Veterinary Medical Association* 144, 395–398.

Davidson, A. P. and Baker, T. W. (2009a) Reproductive ultrasound of the bitch and the queen. *Topics in Companion Animal Medicine* 24(2), 55–63. doi: 10.1053/j.tcam.2008.11.002

Davidson, A. P. and Baker, T. W. (2009b) Reproductive ultrasound of the dog and tom. *Topics in Companion Animal Medicine* 24(2), 64–70. doi: 10.1053/j.tcam.2008.11.003

Donoghue, M., Johnston, L. A., Munson, L., Brown, J. L., and Wildt, D.E. (1992) Influence of gonadotropin treatment interval on follicular maturation, in vitro fertilization, circulating steroid concentrations, and subsequent luteal function in the domestic cat, *Biology of Reproduction* 46(5), 972–980. doi: 10.1095/biolreprod46.5.972

Ferré-Dolcet, L., Frumento, P., Abramo, F., and Romagnoli, S. (2021) Disappearance of signs of heat and induction of ovulation in oestrous queens with gonadorelin: a clinical study. *Journal of Feline Medicine and Surgery* 23(4):344–350. doi: 10.1177/1098612X20951284

Foster, R. A., Caswell, J. L., and Rinkardt, N. (1996) Chronic fibrinous and necrotic orchitis in a cat. *Canadian Veterinary Journal* 37, 681–682.

Goericke-Pesch, S., Georgiev, P., Fasulkov, I., Vodenicharov, A., and Wehrend, A. (2013) Basal testosterone concentrations following the application of a slow release GnRH agonist implant are associated with a loss of response to buserelin, a short-term GnRH agonist, in the tom cat. *Theriogenology* 80, 65–69. doi: S0093-691X(13)00110-6

Heaps, L. A., Scudder, C. J., Lipscomb, V. J., Steinbach, S. M., Priestnall, S. L., *et al.* (2017). Serum anti-Müllerian hormone concentrations before and after treatment of an ovarian granulosa cell tumour in a cat. *Journal of Feline Medicine and Surgery Open Reports* 3, 2055116917722701. doi: 10.1177/2055116917722701

Howard, J. and Allen M. E. (2007) Nutritional factors affecting semen quality in felids. *Zoo and Wild Animal Medicine: Current Therapy* VI, 272–283.

Jordan, H. L., Howard, J., Barr, M. C., Kennedy-Stoskopf, S., Levy, J. K., *et al.* (1998) Feline immunodeficiency virus is shed in semen from experimentally and naturally infected cats. *AIDS Research in Human Retroviruses* 14, 1087–1092. doi: 10.1089/aid.1998.14.1087

Jordan, H. L., Liang, Y., Hudson, L. C., and Tompkins, W. A. (1999) Shedding of feline immunodeficiency virus in semen of domestic cats during acute infection. *American Journal of Veterinary Research* 60(2), 211–215.

Kutzler, M. A. (2007) Estrus induction and synchronization in canids and felids. *Theriogenology.* 68(3), 354–374. doi: 10.1016/j.theriogenology.2007.04.014

McKinney, H. R. (1973) A study of toxoplasma infections in cats. *Veterinary Medicine Small Animal Clinician* 68, 493–495.

Memon, M. A., Ganjam, V. K., Pavletic, M. M. and Schelling, S. H. (1992) Use of human chorionic gonadotropin stimulation test to detect a retained testis in a cat. *Journal American Veterinary Medicine Association* 201, 1602.

Neubauer, K., Jewgenow, K., Blottner, S., Wildt, D. E., and Pukazhenthi, B. S. (2004) Quantity rather than quality in teratospermic males: a histomorphometric and flow cytometric evaluation of spermatogenesis in the domestic cat (*Felis catus*). *Biology of Reproduction* 71, 1517–1524. doi: 10.1095/biolreprod.104.031062

Paick, S. and Choi, W. S. (2019). Varicocele and testicular pain: a review. *World Journal of Mens Health* 37, 4–11. doi: 10.5534/wjmh.170010

Place, N. J., Hansen, B. S., Cheraskin, J. L., Cudney, S. E., Flanders, J. A., Newmark, A.D., Barry, B., Scarlett, J. M. (2011) Measurement of serum anti-Müllerian hormone concentration in female dogs and cats before and after ovariohysterectomy. *Journal of Veterinary Diagnostic Investigation.* 23(3), 524–527. doi: 10.1177/1040638711403428.

Pretzer, S. D. (2008) Bacterial and protozoal causes of pregnancy loss in the bitch and queen. *Theriogenology* 70, 320–326. doi: 10.1016/j.theriogenology.2008.04.03

Pukazhenti, B., Wildt, D. E., and Howard, J. G. (2001) The phenomenon and significance of teratozoospermia in felids. *Journal of Reproduction and Fertility* 57, 423–433.

Reilly, G. A., Bailie, N. C., Morrow, W. T., McDowell, S. W., and Ellis, W. A. (1994) Feline stillbirths associated with mixed salmonella typhimurium and leptospira infection. *Veterinary Records* 135, 608.

Salas-Huetos, A., Rosique-Esteban, N., Becerra-Tomás, N., Vizmanos, B., Bulló, M., *et al.* (2018) The effect of nutrients and dietary supplements on sperm quality parameters: a systematic review and meta-analysis of randomized clinical trials. *Advances in Nutrition* 9, 833–848. doi: 10.1093/advances/nmy057

Sigurdardóttir, O. G., Kolbjørnsen, O., and Lutz, H. J. (2001) Orchitis in a cat associated with coronavirus infection. *Comparative Pathology* 124, 219–222. doi: 10.1053/jcpa.2000.0443

Snoeck, F., Sarrazin, S., Wydoogh, E., and Soom, V. (2017). Age and anti-Müllerian hormone levels predict the success of in vitro maturation of cat oocytes. *Reproduction in Domestic Animals* 52, 98–102. doi: 10.1111/rda.12827

Stempel, S. and Goericke-Pesch, S. (2020) Castration and GnRH-agonists in small animal practice - what do we know 13 years after EU registration? *Tierärztliche Praxis Kleintiere/Heimtiere* 48: 420–432. DOI 10.1055/a-1274-9268 (German)

Stranieri, A., Probo, M., Pisu, M. C., Fioletti, A., Meazzi, S., *et al.* (2020) Preliminary investigation on feline coronavirus presence in the reproductive tract of the tom cat as a potential route of viral transmission. *Journal of Feline Medicine and Surgery* 22, 178–185. doi: 10.1177/1098612X19837114

Swanson, W. F., Wolfe, B. A., Brown, J. L., Martin-Jimenez, T., Riviere, J. E., *et al.* (1997) Pharmokinetics and ovarian-stimulatory effects of equine and human chorionic gonadotropins administered singly and in combination in the domestic cat. *Biology of Reproduction* 57, 295–302. doi: 10.1095/biolreprod57.2.295

Swanson W. F., Maggs, D. J., Clarke H. E., Newell A. E., Bond J. B., *et al.* (2006) Assessment of viral presence in semen and reproductive function of frozen-thawed spermatozoa from Pallas' cats (*Otocolobus manul*) infected with feline herpesvirus. *Journal of Zoo and Wildlife Medicine* 37, 336–346. doi: 10.1638/05-073.1

Thuróczy, J., Wölfling, A., Tibold, A., Balogh, L., Jánoki, G. A., *et al.* (2003). Effect of anticoagulants and sampling time on results of progesterone determination in canine blood samples. *Reproduction in Domestic Animals* 8, 386–389. doi: 10.1046/j.1439-0531.2003.00450.x

Umbach, A.K., Spennes, J., Goericke-Pesch, S. (2020) Azoospermia and suspicion of obstruction of the efferent ducts in a ragdoll breeding male tomcat, *Congress Proceedings DVG-DGK* Berlin, 15.-17.10.2020, pp. 229–230.

Walter, B. (2020) Anti-Müllerian hormone in dogs and cats reproduction. *Reproduction in Domestic Animals* 55, 26–31. doi: 10.1111/rda.13603

Walter, B., Coelfen, A., Jaeger, K., Reese, S., Meyer-Lindenberg, A., and Aupperle-Lellbach, H. (2018). Anti-Muellerian hormone concentration in bitches with histopathologically diagnosed ovarian tumours and cysts. *Reproduction in Domestic Animals* 53, 784–792. doi:10.1111/rda.13171

Wilkins, L. (1960). Masculinization of female fetus due to use of orally given progestins. *Journal of the American Medical Association* 172, 1028–1032. doi: 10.1001/jama.1960.03020100036007

Zambelli, D., Bini, C., Küster, D.G., Molari, V., and Cunto, M. (2015) First deliveries after estrus induction using deslorelin and endoscopic transcervical insemination in the queen. *Theriogenology* 84, 773–778. doi: 10.1016/j.theriogenology.2015.05.010

26 Options for Contraception in Female and Male Felids

Cristina Gobello

Director Center of Reproductive Physiology, Veterinary Sciences, National University of La Plata and National Research Council, La Plata, Argentina

26.1 Introduction

Domestic cats are prolific breeders that can produce litters from puberty (as early as 4 months of age) until late in life. Although cats are long-day breeders, many domestic felids can reproduce throughout the year (Faya *et al.*, 2011a). Furthermore, intact female cats are more difficult to confine than most other domestic animals and even those with responsible owners produce unwanted litters.

In domestic felids, temporary reversible control of reproduction, i.e. contraception, is often requested by cat owners and breeders. Contraception can also reduce unwanted sexually dimorphic behavior such as roaming, fighting, and calling (Goericke-Pesch, 2017). In addition, it has been shown that suppressing endogenous ovarian activity before artificial insemination or *in vitro* fertilization/embryo transfer improves pregnancy rates (Stewart *et al.*, 2015). However, continuous contraceptive treatment with current treatment options may induce cyclicity and uterine issues long term and therefore it is not indicated in breeding animals.

26.2 Females

26.2.1 Progestins

Progestins are synthetic derivatives of progestogens that, although more potent than endogenous progesterone, act in the same manner by decreasing gonadotropin-releasing hormone (GnRH) pulsatility, which in turn decreases gonadotrophin secretion. The most widely used progestins in domestic felids are medroxyprogesterone acetate (17α-hydroxy-6α-methylprogesterone acetate), megestrol acetate (6-methyl-6-dehydro-17α-acetoxyprogesterone), and proligestone (14α,17α-propylidene-dioxyprogesterone). Other progestins tested with some degree of success for reproductive control in cats include levonorgestrel, chlormadinone acetate, delmadinone acetate, and altrenogest. Progestins are marketed as both long-acting suspensions for parenteral injection and oral formulations (tablet or liquid) (Romagnoli and Concannon, 2003).

Progestin administration requires precise dosing and fixed treatment schedules to minimize the potential for side effects that can be observed with high doses, prolonged use, and females with previous subclinical problems. Thus, the lowest dose and frequency needed to suppress estrus should always be recommended. However, a higher dose might be needed to interrupt an already commenced estrous cycle (Jöchle and Jöchle, 1975). Contact with male cats should be avoided until all estrus signs have ceased.

The ideal progestin is one that has high anti-gonadotrophic activity with low progestogenic effects. Medroxyprogesterone acetate has both high anti-gonadotrophic and progestogenic activity, making it an efficient but less safe option. Proligestone is a third-generation progestin with weaker stimulus on the endometrium and on the mammary epithelium as compared to other progestins (Evans and Sutton, 1989; Findik *et al.*, 1999). Although long-acting injectable progestins are convenient, low doses of oral megestrol acetate offer the possibility to discontinue the medication immediately if side effects develop.

The appearance of side effects can also vary depending on the stage of the estrous cycle in which the progestin treatment is administered. Progestins are safer to administer during anestrus or seasonal interestrus than in estrus when the progestogenic activity could be exaggerated by high

 Feline Reproduction (eds. A.K. Johnson and M.A. Kutzler)
DOI: 10.1079/9781789247107.0026

concentrations of endogenous estradiol (Chen *et al.*, 2001). Queens with an unknown reproductive history should have the stage of cycle confirmed by vaginal cytology and progesterone serum concentrations before treatment. Although prepubertal queens have been traditionally excluded from progestin treatments because of the potential consequences on the immature gonadal axis, there is no evidence of this adverse effect (Lopez Merlo *et al.*, 2016). It is generally believed that healthy young, post-pubertal, anestrous queens undergoing low-dose treatments for short durations rarely experience any side effects.

Undesirable reproductive side effects of progestins include cystic endometrial hyperplasia, pyometra, benign mammary gland hyperplasia, and mammary neoplasia. However, the side effects of progestins are not limited to the genital tract and can include adrenocortical suppression, hyperglycemia and diabetes mellitus, polyphagy, obesity, lethargy, apathy, immunosuppression, and even skin problems at the injection site (e.g. hair discoloration, alopecia, skin atrophy, calcinosis circumscripta) (Tomlinson *et al.*, 1984; Romagnoli and Concannon, 2003).

Megestrol acetate

Megestrol acetate (MA) is the shortest-acting progestin and is available in an oral formulation in most countries (Oen, 1977). The dose when administered during anestrus is 5 mg/cat orally every 2 weeks or 2.5 mg/cat orally every week (Oen, 1977; Romagnoli and Concannon, 2003). When administered during the breeding season, the dose of MA is 2 mg/cat orally every day for 2 weeks when initiated during interestrus or at a dose of 5 mg/cat orally once day for 4 days when initiated during proestrus or estrus (Romagnoli and Concannon, 2003). After the initial treatment protocol, estrus suppression can be prolonged during the breeding season using the anestrus dose.

Medroxyprogesterone acetate

Medroxyprogesterone acetate (MPA) is available in both parenteral and oral formulations in most countries. The half-life of MPA is 12–17 hours following an oral dose or 40–50 days following an intramuscular injection (Romagnoli, 2015). MPA can be administered during anestrus or during the breeding season. The dose for MPA is a single 25 –100 mg injection every 4–6 months or an oral treatment of 0.05 mg/kg/day for 12 months (Harris and Wolchuk, 1963; Romagnoli, 2015). If the female is in heat (estrus), a 5-day oral course of 5.0 mg/day should precede the previous protocols (Romagnoli, 2015).

Proligestone

The subcutaneous dose of proligestone is 100–250 mg/cat (approximately 25–30 mg/kg) when administered at the onset of proestrus, during interestrus, or anestrus at a frequency of every 3, 4, or 5 months, respectively (Findik *et al.*, 1999; Romagnoli and Concannon, 2003). According to the manufacturer, when administered during proestrus, estrus signs disappear in 1–7 days after treatment. The manufacturer also recommends that breeding females go through a normal cycle between injections.

26.2.2 GnRH agonists

GnRH agonists are produced by making amino acid substitutions of the native GnRH molecule resulting in greater potency and longer duration of efficacy. Long-term administration of GnRH agonists desensitizes and down-regulates pituitary GnRH receptors which inhibits gonadotropin synthesis and secretion. However, GnRH agonist treatment does have an initial short stimulatory effect (referred to as 'flare up'), which is the main disadvantage of its use in female animals (discussed further in the last paragraph of this section) (Gobello, 2012).

The GnRH agonist, deslorelin, has been used for estrus suppression in cats (Munson *et al.*, 2001; Ackermann *et al.*, 2012; Toydemir *et al.*, 2012). The estrus suppression effects of a 4.7 mg deslorelin acetate implant were shown to be reversible in queens (Ackermann *et al.*, 2012) with normal fertility restored (Gobello, 2012). The duration of estrus suppression in queens after deslorelin implant insertion varies widely between 16 and 37 months (Goericke-Pesch *et al.*, 2013). Estrus suppression was reported to last for 18.5 months following administration of a 9.5 mg deslorelin implant (Toydemir *et al.*, 2012). However, the efficacy and safety of repeated treatments with GnRH agonist implants in queens still needs to be investigated.

The safety and efficacy of deslorelin implants has been evaluated in prepubertal and postnatal kittens.

Administration of a 4.7 mg deslorelin acetate implant at 50% of adult body weight (approximately 4 months of age) postponed puberty in queens until an average of 10 months of age (range: 6–15 months of age) (Risso *et al.*, 2012). Administration of a deslorelin implant to 3- to 9-month-old kittens resulted in estrus suppression until 21–36 months of age (Cecchetto *et al.*, 2017). Prepubertal GnRH agonist treatment did not alter growth rate but may result in early estrus induction (Risso *et al.*, 2012; Cecchetto *et al.*, 2017). Pyometra was reported following administration to one prepubertal kitten (Risso *et al.*, 2012). Postnatal administration of deslorelin (1.6 mg) delayed puberty in both female and male kittens until 281.2 ± 21.6 days old (range 180–428 days; Carranza *et al.*, 2014). Further investigation is required to determine the effect of administering different deslorelin dosages on puberty postponement as well as the possibility of adverse long-term effects.

As previously mentioned, an initial undesirable increase in estradiol concentrations occurred in queens after inserting the deslorelin implant. However, administration of MA (5 mg) at 14 days and 12 hours before and 14 days after administration of a 9.5 mg deslorelin implant prevented estrus behavior associated with the flare up but did not prevent an increase in estradiol in most queens (Toydemir *et al.*, 2012). It is important to mention that it was not established whether progestin treatment was necessary both before and after deslorelin implant insertion to suppress estrus during the flare up or if the progestin treatment should vary depending on estrous cycle stage when the deslorelin implant is inserted.

Note: deslorelin implants are not currently available in the US for use in the cat.

26.2.3 Melatonin

Melatonin (N-acetyl-5-methoxytryptamine), a pineal gland hormone secreted during periods of darkness, regulates the hypothalamic-pituitary-ovarian axis in cats. Melatonin reaches peak concentrations during anestrus and interestrus (Leyva *et al.*, 1984, 1989). The reproductive effects of administration of exogenous melatonin (generic oral tablets for humans, subcutaneous implants labeled for sheep) have been investigated in cats.

Administration of long-term release melatonin implants (18 mg) or oral melatonin tablets (4 mg/cat/day) to queens exposed to 14 hours of light resulted in estrus suppression for 63.8 ± 5 days (Faya *et al.*, 2011b). In a separate study administering the same implants during estrus or interestrus, estrus was suppressed 61.1 ± 6.8 and 113.3 ± 6.1 days, respectively (Gimenez *et al.*, 2009). In another study where the same melatonin implants were administered to queens during interestrus, estrus was only suppressed in 68% (13/19) and one of the queens that displayed estrus was mated, became pregnant, and delivered kittens (Schäfer-Somi, 2017). Research in purebred queens had similar results with 81% (22/27) experiencing estrus suppression for an average of 103.9 days (Schäfer-Somi, 2017). However, when administered to prepubertal queens (weighing 1.5–1.9 kg), estrus suppression was not significantly different from that of the controls (Faya *et al.*, 2011b). It is important to mention that there have been no clinically detectable side effects, including growth rate in prepubertal cats, associated with melatonin administration.

26.2.4 Other

Other contraceptive options such as gene silencing, targeted delivery of cytotoxins, and immunocontraception are still being investigated. Immunocontraception, via vaccination against GnRH, the luteinizing hormone receptor, or zona pellucida proteins, has been described in this species. Initial zona pellucida vaccines did not prevent gestation (Levy *et al.*, 2005). Granulomatous reactions to the adjuvant were also a problem for this vaccine (Munson *et al.*, 2005).

GonaCon™ is a GnRH-hemocyanin conjugate immunocontraceptive vaccine against GnRH registered in wild mammalian species. When the early formulation of this product was used in contraceptive trials in female domestic cats, it showed an effect that exceeded a mean of 3 years. Since these initial studies, there have been formulation composition changes in the vaccine. Thus, a new formula consisting of a different antigen-carrier protein and increased antigen concentration produced a strong humoral immune response as well as self-limiting masses at the site of the injection in some cats (Vansandt *et al.*, 2017). More recently, a single dose of GonaCon (USDA APHIS National Wildlife Research Center, Fort Collins CO) provided contraception lasting for a minimum of 1 year in 30% of 20 treated female cats (Fischer *et al.*, 2018). This level of contraception induced is not sufficiently effective to be recommended for use in queens.

26.3 Males

26.3.1 GnRH agonists

Deslorelin (4.7 mg) implants have been administered to tom cats and will decrease serum dihydrotestosterone (DHT) concentration within 23–30 days (Gültiken *et al.*, 2017) and serum testosterone to basal concentrations within 11 weeks (Goericke-Pesch *et al.*, 2011). Serum dihydrotestosterone concentrations will remain low for 26.5 ± 7.42 months (Gültiken *et al.*, 2017). In response to the reduction in testosterone, penile spines disappear within 9.4 ± 1.0 weeks after implant insertion (Goericke-Pesch *et al.*, 2011). After an initial stimulation in sexually dimorphic behaviors in response to implant insertion (Goericke-Pesch *et al.*, 2011), libido, mating behavior, and urine marking are suppressed for 88.7 ± 12.4 weeks (Goericke-Pesch *et al.*, 2014b) or 115.1 ± 32.2 weeks (Gültiken *et al.*, 2017).

Within 36 weeks of a deslorelin implant (4.7 mg) insertion, testicular volume was reduced by about 73% (Goericke-Pesch *et al.*, 2011), which was accompanied by azoospermia and a variable degree of spermatogenic suppression (Novotny *et al.*, 2015). The duration of implant efficacy varies between reports from 78.8 ± 12.9 weeks (range: 61.7–100.7 weeks) (Goericke-Pesch *et al.*, 2014a) to 95.6–108.6 weeks (Favre *et al.*, 2018). When administered to prepubertal tom cats (3 months old), reproductive function was suppressed for over 48 weeks (Mehl *et al.*, 2016). The induced infertility was reversible with fertile matings and normal testicular histology returning 7–42 weeks and 13.6–47.6 weeks after the last basal testosterone concentration, respectively (Goericke-Pesch *et al.*, 2014b).

Implants containing different concentrations of deslorelin have also been investigated. Using a deslorelin implant containing 9.4 mg, semen quality increased slightly during the first month after treatment, and then decreased to complete sterility within 40–72 days after implant insertion (Romagnoli *et al.*, 2017). At this dose, induced infertility persisted for 750–850 days (Romagnoli *et al.*, 2017). Postnatal administration of a deslorelin implant containing 1.6 mg delayed puberty until 281.2 ± 21.6 days of age (Carranza *et al.*, 2014). Regardless of deslorelin concentration, the site of administration (intrascapular vs periumbilical) does not affect treatment efficacy (Romagnoli *et al.*, 2019). With the exception of the initial stimulation in sexually dimorphic behavior, no side effects were observed in any deslorelin-treated toms.

26.3.2. Melatonin

Subcutaneous melatonin implants (18 mg) labeled for sheep and used off-label in queens for estrus suppression have been shown to decrease sperm quality for 120 ± 15 days after implant insertion without altering testosterone concentrations or causing undesirable effects (Favre *et al.*, 2014).

26.3.3 Other non-steroid options

RTI-4587-073(l) is an indenopyridine derivative that when administered orally to male cats, severely disrupted spermatogenesis during the first 24 hours after treatment and returning to normal in approximately one spermatic cycle and without any other clinical side effects (D'Francisco *et al.*, 2019). Further refinement, including repeated doses and eventual long-term adverse effects, follow-up of this indenopyridine should be carried out before their field implementation could be widely recommended.

Sclerosing agents, such as calcium chloride dehydrate, zinc gluconate, chlorhexidine digluconate have been injected intratesticular and intraepididymal to induce orchitis and sclerosis with sterilizing purposes. Due to their permanent effects, they will not be discussed further in this chapter.

26.4 References

Ackermann, C. L., Volpato, R., Destro, F. C., Trevisol, E., Sousa, N. R., *et al.* (2012) Ovarian activity reversibility after the use of deslorelin acetate as a short-term contraceptive in domestic queens. *Theriogenology* 78, 817–822. doi: 10.1016/j.theriogenology.2012.03.030

Carranza, A., Faya, M., Merlo, M. L., Batista, P., and Gobello, C. (2014) Effect of GnRH analogs in postnatal domestic cats. *Theriogenology* 82, 138–143. doi: 10.1016/j.theriogenology.2014.03.012

Cecchetto, M., Salata, P., Baldan, A., Milani, C., Mollo, A., *et al.* (2017) Postponement of puberty in queens treated with deslorelin. *Journal of Feline Medicine and Surgery* 19, 1224–1230. doi: 10.1177/1098612X16688406

Chen, Y. M., Wright, P. J., and Lee, C. S. (2001) A model for the study of cystic endometrial hyperplasia in bitches. *Journal of Reproduction and Fertility Supplement*, 57, 407–414.

D'Francisco, F., Merlo, M. L., Vercellini, R., Blanco, P., Barbeito, C., *et al.* (2019) Effect of the indenopyridine RTI-4587-073 (l) on feline testicle. *Animal Reproduction Science* 205, 10–17. doi: 10.1016/j.anireprosci.2019.03.014

Evans, J. M., and Sutton, D. J. (1989) The use of hormones, especially progestagens, to control oestrus in bitches. *Journal of Reproduction and Fertility Supplement* 39, 163–173.

Favre, R. N., Bonaura, M. C., Praderio, R., Stornelli, M. C., de la Sota, R. L., *et al.* (2014) Effect of melatonin implants on spermatogenesis in the domestic cat (*Felis silvestris catus*). *Theriogenology*, 82, 851–856. doi: 10.1016/j.theriogenology.2014.06.013

Favre, R. N., García, M. F., García Mitacek, M. C., Rearte, R., Fontaine, C., *et al.* (2018) Reestablishment of sperm quality after long-term deslorelin suppression in tomcats. *Animal Reproduction Science* 195, 302–308. doi: 10.1016/j.anireprosci.2018.06.008

Faya, M., Carranza, A., Priotto, M., Abeya, M., Diaz, J.D., *et al.* (2011a) Domestic queens under natural temperate photoperiod do not manifest seasonal anestrus. *Animal Reproduction Science* 129, 78–81. doi: 10.1016/j.anireprosci.2011.10.007

Faya, M., Carranza, A., Priotto, M., Graiff, D., Zurbriggen, G., *et al.* (2011b) Long-term melatonin treatment prolongs interestrus, but does not delay puberty, in domestic cats. *Theriogenology*, 75, 1750–1754. doi: 10.1016/j.theriogenology.2011.01.015

Findik, M., Erunal Maral, N. and Asian, S. (1999) The use of proligestone, megestrol acetate and GnRH on queens with the aim of hormonal contraception. *Turkish Journal of Veterinary Animal Science* 23:455–460.

Fischer, A., Benka, V. A., Briggs, J. R., Driancourt, M. A., Maki, J., *et al.* (2018). Effectiveness of GonaCon as an immunocontraceptive in colony-housed cats. *Journal of Feline Medicine and Surgery* 20(8), 786–792. doi: 10.1177/1098612X18758549

Gimenez, F., Stornelli, M. C., Tittarelli, C. M., Savignone, C. A., and Dorna, I. V. (2009) Suppression of estrus in cats with melatonin implants. *Theriogenology* 72(4), 493–499. doi: 10.1016/j.theriogenology.2009.04.004

Gobello, C. (2012) Effects of GnRH antagonists vs agonists in domestic carnivores, a review. *Reproduction in Domestic Animals* 47, 373–376. doi: 10.1111/rda.12025

Goericke-Pesch, S. (2017) Long-term effects of GnRH agonists on fertility and behaviour. *Reproduction in Domestic Animals* 52, 336–347. doi: 10.1111/rda.12898

Goericke-Pesch, S., Georgiev, P., Antonov, A., Albouy, M., and Wehrend, A. (2011) Clinical efficacy of a GnRH-agonist implant containing 4.7 mg deslorelin, Suprelorin, regarding suppression of reproductive function in tomcats. *Theriogenology* 75, 803–810. doi: 10.1016/j.theriogenology.2010.10.020

Goericke-Pesch, S., Georgiev, P., Atanasov, A., Albouy, M., Navarro, C., *et al.* (2013) Treatment of queens in estrus and after estrus with a GnRH-agonist implant containing 4.7 mg deslorelin; hormonal response, duration of efficacy, and reversibility. *Theriogenology* 79, 640–646. doi: 10.1016/j.theriogenology.2012.11.018

Goericke-Pesch, S., Georgiev, P., Antonov, A., Vodenicharov, A., Navarro, C., *et al.* (2014a) Reversibility of germinative and endocrine testicular function after long-term contraception with a GnRH-agonist implant in the tom – a follow-up study. *Theriogenology* 81, 941–946. doi: 10.1016/j.theriogenology.2014.01.015

Goericke-Pesch, S., Wehrend, A., and Georgiev, P. (2014b) Suppression of fertility in adult cats. *Reproduction in Domestic Animals*, 49, 33–40. doi: 10.1111/rda.12301

Gültiken, N., Aslan, S., Ay, S. S., Gülbahar, M. Y., Thuróczy, J., *et al.* (2017) Effect of deslorelin on testicular function, serum dihydrotestosterone and oestradiol concentrations during and after suppression of sexual activity in tom cats. *Journal of Feline Medicine and Surgery* 19, 123–131. doi: 10.1177/1098612X15615381

Harris, T. W. and Wolchuk, N. (1963) The suppression of estrus in the dog and cat with long term administration of synthetic progestational steroids. *American Journal of Veterinary Research* 24, 1003–1006.

Jöchle, W. and Jöchle, M. (1975) Reproductive and behavioral control in the male and female cat with progestins: long-term field observations in individual animals. *Theriogenology* 3, 179–185. doi: 10.1016/0093-691x(75)90002-3

Levy, J. K., Mansour, M., Crawford, P. C., Pohajdak, B., and Brown, R. G. (2005) Survey of zona pellucida antigens for immunocontraception of cats. *Theriogenology* 15(63), 1334–1341. doi: 10.1016/j.theriogenology.2004.07.015

Leyva, H., Addiego, L., and Stabenfeldt, G. (1984) The effect of different photoperiods on plasma concentrations of melatonin, prolactin, and cortisol in the domestic cat. *Endocrinology* 115, 1729–1736. doi: 10.1210/endo-115-5-1729

Leyva, H., Madley, T., and Stabenfeldt, G. H. (1989) Effect of light manipulation on ovarian activity and melatonin and prolactin secretion in the domestic cat. *Journal of Reproduction and Fertility Supplement* 39, 125–133.

Lopez Merlo, M., Faya, M., Blanco, P. G., Carranza, A., Barbeito, C., *et al.* (2016) Failure of a single dose of medroxyprogesterone acetate to induce uterine infertility in postnatally treated domestic cats. *Theriogenology* 85(4), 718–723. doi: 10.1016/j.theriogenology.2015.10.013

Mehl, N. S., Khalid, M., Srisuwatanasagul, S., Swangchan-Uthai, T., and Sirivaidyapong, S. (2016) GnRH-agonist implantation of prepubertal male cats affects their reproductive performance and testicular LH receptor and FSH receptor expression. *Theriogenology* 85, 841–848. doi: 10.1016/j.theriogenology.2015.10.031

Munson, L., Bauman, J. E., Asa, C. S., Jöchle, W., and Trigg, T. E. (2001) Efficacy of the GnRH analogue deslorelin for suppression of oestrous cycles in cats. *Journal of Reproduction and Fertility Supplement* 57, 269–273.

Munson, L., Harrenstien, L. A., Acton, A. E., Graham, P. A., Chassy, L. M., *et al.* (2005) Immunologic responses and adverse reactions to Freund's-adjuvanted porcine zona pellucida immuno-contraceptives in domestic cats. *Vaccine* 23(48-49), 5646–5654. doi: 10.1016/j.vaccine.2005.05.044

Novotny, R., Vitasek, R., Bartoskova, A., Cizek, P., Prinosilova, P., *et al.* (2015) Azoospermia with variable testicular histology after 7 months of treatment with a deslorelin implant in toms. *Theriogenology* 83, 1188–1193. doi: 10.1016/j.theriogenology.2014.12.026

Oen E. O. (1977) The oral administration of megestrol acetate to postpone oestrus in cats. *Nordisk Veterinaermedicin* 29, 287–291.

Risso, A., Corrada, Y., Barbeito, C., Diaz, J. D., and Gobello, C. (2012) Long-term-release GnRH agonists postpone puberty in domestic cats. *Reproduction in Domestic Animals* 47, 936–938. doi: 10.1111/j.1439-0531.2012.01994.x

Romagnoli, S. (2015) Progestins to control feline reproduction: Historical abuse of high doses and potentially safe use of low doses. *Journal of Feline Medicine and Surgery* 17, 743–752. doi: 10.1177/1098612X15594987

Romagnoli, S. and Concannon. P. (2003) Clinical use of progestins in bitches and queens: A review. In: Concannon, P., England, G., Verstegen, J., and Linde-Forsberg, C., (eds) *Recent Advances in Small Animal Reproduction*. International Veterinary Information Service, USA.

Romagnoli, S., Baldan, A., Righetti, C., Milani, C., Mollo, A., *et al.* (2017) Semen quality and interval to sterility in tom cats treated with a 9.4 mg deslorelin implant. *Journal of Feline Medicine and Surgery* 19, 194–199. doi: 10.1177/1098612X15623985

Romagnoli, S., Baldan, A., Ferro, S., Righetti, C., Scenna, L., *et al.* (2019) Length of efficacy and effect of implant location in adult tom cats treated with a 9.4 mg deslorelin subcutaneous implant. *Journal of Feline Medicine and Surgery* 21, 507–519. doi: 10.1177/1098612X18788157

Schäfer-Somi, S. (2017) Effect of melatonin on the reproductive cycle in female cats: a review of clinical experiences and previous studies. *Journal of Feline Medicine and Surgery* 19, 5–12. doi: 10.1177/1098612X15610369

Stewart, R. A., Crosier, A. E., Pelican, K. M., Pukazhenthi, B. S., Sitzmann, B. D., *et al.* (2015) Progestin priming before gonadotrophin stimulation and AI improves embryo development and normalises luteal function in the cat. *Reproduction, Fertility and Development*, 27, 360–371. doi: 10.1071/RD13274

Tomlinson, M. J., Barteaux, L., Ferns, L. E., and Angelopoulos, E. (1984). Feline mammary carcinoma: a retrospective evaluation of 17 cases. *The Canadian Veterinary Journal* 25, 435–439.

Toydemir, T. S., Kılıçarslan, M. R., and Olgaç, V. (2012) Effects of the GnRH analogue deslorelin implants on reproduction in female domestic cats. *Theriogenology* 77, 662–674. doi: 10.1016/j.theriogenology.2011.07.046

Vansandt, L. M., Kutzler, M. A., Fischer, A. E., Morris, K. N., and Swanson, W. F. (2017) Safety and effectiveness of a single and repeat intramuscular injection of a GnRH vaccine (GonaCon™) in adult female domestic cats. *Reproduction in Domestic Animals* 52(2), 348–353. doi: 10.1111/rda.12853

27 Assisted Reproduction Techniques in the Domestic Cat

Jennifer B. Nagashima and Budhan S. Pukazhenthi

Smithsonian Conservation Biology Institute, National Zoological Park, Front Royal, Virginia, USA

27.1 Introduction

Assisted reproductive technology (ART) is a term which encompasses all procedures aimed at improving or managing fertility. ARTs include, but are not limited to, induction of estrus with exogenous hormone treatments (Chapter 3), sperm collection (Chapter 18) and cryopreservation (Chapter 23), oocyte collection and cryopreservation, *in vitro* fertilization (IVF) or intracytoplasmic sperm injection (ICSI), artificial insemination (AI), and embryo transfer (ET). There have been significant efforts in recent decades to develop and optimize many of these techniques in the domestic cat. Beyond the interests of cat breeders, these technologies are of critical importance to research. The domestic cat is not only the ideal model for the development of fertility-preserving methods for its wild and endangered relatives, but the cat has also historically been a biomedical research model for human physiology and diseases. Per the Online Mendelian Inheritance in Animals, which catalogs inherited disorders and genes, the domestic cat shares over 200 genetic traits/disorders which are potential models for human disease (Nicholas, n.d.). The ability to precisely manage domestic cat reproduction has the potential to both reduce the numbers of animals needed for research and hasten the speed of work in understanding the causes and developing appropriate treatments for diseases shared by cats and humans alike. In this chapter, we will discuss the current status of key ARTs for domestic cats, including genome rescue methods (oocyte, embryo, and ovarian/testicular tissue collection, preservation, and culture) and embryo production technologies (IVF, ICSI, and cloning).

27.2 Genome Rescue Methods

In situations where a genetically valuable animal dies before successful breeding, or where physical or behavioral obstacles prevent the production of offspring, there may be interest in rescuing and preserving the genetic potential of the individual for later re-introduction into the population. For example, pregnancies have been achieved with frozen–thawed domestic cat epididymal sperm. Specifically, Toyonaga *et al.* (2011) reported 80% pregnancy rates after unilateral intrauterine insemination with spermatozoa recovered and cryopreserved from epididymides that were stored at refrigeration temperature. Although there are no reports of successful pregnancies with cryopreserved sperm recovered posthumously in wild felids, Howard *et al.* (2015) achieved pregnancies with cryopreserved spermatozoa collected over 20 years earlier from the endangered Black-footed ferrets (*Mustela nigripes*). This demonstrates the utility of collection and preservation of spermatozoa for achieving genetic rescue. The preservation of the male gamete is covered in Chapter 23 (Semen Cryopreservation) and estrus induction in felids is covered in Chapter 3. Here, we will focus on oocyte, ovarian tissue, and testicular tissue preservation, including outlining the general equipment and supplies necessary to consider implementing genome rescue technologies in a new clinical or laboratory setting (Table 27.1).

27.2.1 Oocytes

Antral stage follicles are observable in ovaries of kittens estimated to be <20 days of age, and culture and IVF of oocytes collected from 100- to 120-day-old kittens have successfully produced blastocyst-stage

 Feline Reproduction (eds. A.K. Johnson and M.A. Kutzler)
DOI: 10.1079/9781789247107.0027

Table 27.1. General equipment, supplies necessary for genome rescue and preservation work

Method	Equipment	General supplies
Oocyte collection – isolated ovaries	Dissecting or stereomicroscope (oocytes/embryos) Scalpel Forceps Pipette/tips or mouth pipette or Wiretrol (oocytes/embryos)	Petri dishes Cell medium (MEM, M199)
Oocyte collection - *in situ* aspiration	Surgical facilities with tilting table Laparoscope Verres needle Insufflator machine Trocars Aspiration needle (20G) Silicone or polyethylene tubing Vacuum pump for aspiration	Exogenous gonadotropins (ovarian stimulation) Anesthesia drugs Medium (Kreb's Ringer Bicarbonate[1], TL Hepes[2], Ham's F10[3,a])
Cryopreservation or vitrification	Forceps Pipette/tips or mouth pipette or Wiretrol Refrigerator (4°C) Freezer (–80°C) LN2 storage LN2 gloves, eye protection	Medium (TCM 199[4], MEM[5], Ham's F10[6]) Cryoprotectant Liquid nitrogen

[1]Goodrowe *et al.* (1988); [2]Pope (2004); [3]Crosier *et al.* (2020); [4]Thuwanut and Chatdarong (2012); [5]Lima *et al.* (2017); [6]Lima *et al.* (2018).
[a]Cheetah

embryos, albeit at a lower rate than oocytes from mature cats (13.3 versus 31.8%) (Uchikura *et al.*, 2010). The advantage of this, however, is that developmentally competent oocytes appear to be salvageable from most age cats throughout the year. Collection of these ova from ovaries (i.e. in the event of spay and/or after the death of an animal) is a straightforward process of shallowly slicing the surface of the ovary with a scalpel in a Petri dish filled with collection medium (Table 27.1), and observing the oocytes thus released from ovarian follicles under a dissecting/stereomicroscope. High-quality oocytes are typically (100–115 µm diameter) homogenously dark, round, and with several layers of surrounding cumulus cells (Reynaud *et al.*, 2009).

Oocytes can also be collected via laparoscopic aspiration from antral follicles. Detailed methodology for this technique has previously been published (Pope, 2004). Briefly, 20 G aspiration needles connected to silicone tubing are inserted via trocars placed above each ovary to puncture and provide suction (75 mmHg, via specialized vacuum pump) to 2–4 mm diameter follicles. Donor cats are typically stimulated via exogenous follicle-stimulating hormone/luteinizing hormone administration for optimal procedure timing and number of oocytes collected (see Chapter 3 on estrus induction). Though in the hands of skilled laparoscopy users, the risks associated with this procedure are fairly low but may include injury to nearby organs or the formation of adhesions, along with the potential for complications with anesthesia and ovarian stimulation protocols. However, if well-timed and executed, high-quality, mature oocytes can be fairly non-invasively obtained via laparoscopic aspiration in domestic cats.

Successful cryopreservation of cat oocytes is challenged by the high surface area/volume ratio of oocytes in general – unlike in the previously discussed sperm work, the large size of ova make reduction of water volume to prevent ice formation during preservation particularly difficult. Further, domestic cat ova have high intracellular lipid content compared with some other species (e.g. human, mouse), resulting in increased sensitivity to chilling and freezing (Galiguis *et al.*, 2014). In striving to reach the optimal balance of cryoprotectant concentrations, exposure time, and, specifically, cooling/warming rates, recent work in this field has focused on minimal volume vitrification (Zhang *et al.*, 2011). Vitrification, as opposed to slow or controlled-rate freezing, requires the ultra-rapid cooling of the sample such that it instantly transitions to a 'glass-like' state rather than freezing, thereby reducing the potential for ice-associated damage to the cell(s). Minimal volume vitrification typically takes the form of loading oocytes or embryos into a device (Fig. 27.1a), such as open or closed, very thin (i.e. 'pulled') straws (e.g. CryoTip, Irvine Scientific, USA), nanometer-diameter loop (e.g. Mounted CryoLoop™, Hampton Research, USA), or narrow strip of film (e.g. CryoTop™, Kitazato, Japan) in very small volumes of vitrification solution and plunging the loaded device into liquid nitrogen (LN2) to achieve sample vitrification. A visual example of cat oocyte collection and minimal volume vitrification has previously been published (Colombo and Luvoni, 2020), as well as a detailed review of cat gamete preservation work prior to 2006 (Luvoni, 2006).

Live offspring have been produced from *in vitro* matured (IVM), vitrified cat oocytes, following warming and ICSI (Pope *et al.*, 2012). In that study by Pope *et al.* (2012), four kittens were born (to two surrogates) out of 30 presumptive zygotes and four 2-cell embryos transferred (or 11.7% live-birth rate per IVM-vitrified-ICSI embryo transferred). No offspring were obtained from simultaneously transferring nine ICSI embryos produced from *in vivo* matured, vitrified oocytes. Despite this apparent difference, Sowińska *et al.* (2020) recently compared the developmental competence of cat oocytes vitrified both before and after IVM and found no difference in embryo development between the groups following ICSI. Kittens have also been born following warming and IVF of partially-polarized (lipid contents centrifuged to one pole of the gamete) IVM oocytes (Galiguis *et al.*, 2014) (Table 27.2). In that study, one kitten was born of 35 2- to 6-cell embryos transferred to two surrogates (2.8%), and another four kittens were born from 39 zygotes produced from non-polarized, ICSI-fertilized oocytes (10.2%).

Toward improving these rates, significant research in the last decade has focused on improving vitrification methods and evaluating the developmental competence of the oocytes in *in vitro* culture. Blastocyst-stage embryos have been reported following the warming and fertilization of oocytes cryopreserved with a variety of vitrification methods (Table 27.2), with blastocyst development rates ranging from 0–30.2%.

27.2.2 Embryos

Live offspring from frozen–thawed domestic cat embryos were first described in 1988 with *in vivo*-produced, blastocyst-stage embryos (Dresser *et al.*, 1988). In that study, 139 freshly-flushed embryos (obtained via laparotomy) were slow frozen (closed straws) in DPBS with glycerol. Following thawing and short-term incubation for embryo recovery, a total of 116 blastocysts were transferred into recipient uteri with 17 kittens born – or a live-birth success rate of 14.7%. Gómez *et al.* (2003) also successfully produced live births from embryos cryopreserved 4–5 days following *in vitro* fertilization. In this study, a total of 122 day 4 and 5 embryos (morula stage, produced via IVM/IVF) were transferred and two live kittens were born – yielding a live-birth rate of 1.7%. Two kittens have also been born from 209 frozen–thawed embryos which were produced via ICSI using sperm collected

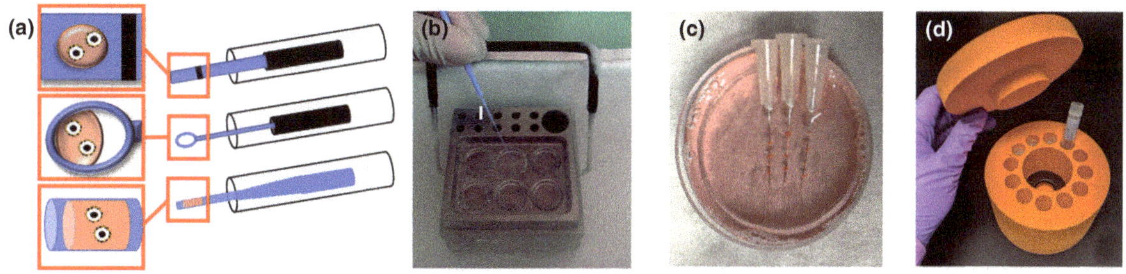

Figure 27.1. Methods for preservation of domestic cat oocytes, embryos and tissues, with schematic of various minimal volume vitrification strategies in: **(a)** including CryoTop, loop, and straw (top to bottom) (image: author's own), and preservation approaches for larger samples in **(b)** solid surface vitrification from (Wang *et al.*, 2009); **(c)** needle immersion vitrification (image: author's own); and **(d)** controlled-rate slow freezing (image: used with permission from the Society for Reproduction and Fertility/Bioscientifica).

Table 27.2. Reference table for oocyte cryopreservation/vitrification methods, success rates, with cryoprotectants dimethylsulfoxide (DMSO), ethylene glycol (EG), 1,2-propanediol (PrOH), and propylene glycol (PG) and success percentages reflecting proportion of each developmental benchmark relative to total oocytes in the treatment with highest rates per study.

Approach	Base medium	Cryoprotectant details	Warming	Success
Immature oocytes				
Slow freezing – closed straw	n/a	Equilibration in 9.3% EG and 0.2 M sucrose → programmable freezer	1 M sucrose solution → sucrose gradient dilution, washing	Meiosis resumption: 60.9%[1]
Vitrification – open cryoloop	DPBS	Equilibration in 5–10% EG, DMSO Vitrification in 20% EG, DMSO with 1.5 M trehalose and ± 10% Ficoll	1.5 M trehalose ± 10% Ficoll → gradient dilution, washing	Oocyte survival: 25–41%[2]
Vitrification – open straw	MEM, SOF, TCM199	Equilibration in 7.5–10% EG and DMSO Vitrification in 16.5–20% EG and DMSO with 1M sucrose (± Gap26 peptide[3] and resveratrol[4])	1 M sucrose solution →sucrose gradient dilution, washing	Maturation success: 19.0[3] to 69.0%[4] Embryo (IVF) production: 18.6[5] to 61.7%[4] Embryo (Parthenote) production: 3–9%[3] Blastocyst development: 0[4] to 4.3%[5] Blastocyst (Parthenote) development: 0–2.2%[3]
Vitrification – closed straw: VitKit, Syngro[a]	TCM199 or proprietary	Equilibration in 7.5% EG and DMSO Vitrification in 15 EG and DMSO, and 0.5 M sucrose (± 20% dextran[6])	1 M sucrose solution (± 20% dextran[6]) →Sucrose gradient dilution, washing	Meiosis resumption: 37.5%[1,a] Maturation success: 10.1%[6] Embryo production: 22.2%[6] Morula development: 0%[6]
Vitrification – open strip: Kitazato CryoTop[a], IZW Freeze	MEM, TCM199	Equilibration in 7.5–10% EG and DMSO Vitrification in 15–20% EG and DMSO with 0.5 M sucrose (± 10% Ficoll and 1.5 M trehalose[6])	1 M sucrose or 1.5 M trehalose and 10% Ficoll solutions → gradient dilution, washing	Maturation success: 17.9[7] to 38.7%[6] Embryo production: 18.4%[8] to 25.0[9,b] to 28.6[6] Blastocyst development: to 0[9,a] to 1.0[8] to 2.1[6]
Mature oocytes				
Vitrification – open cryoloop	DPBS, HSOF	Equilibration in 5–10% EG and DMSO or in increasing (5–10%) EG[9] Vitrification in 20% EG, DMSO with 1.5 M trehalose and ± 10% Ficoll or in 40% EG with 0.3 M sucrose and 1% Ficoll[9]	0.5 M sucrose or 1.5 M trehalose ± 10% Ficoll solution → Gradient dilution, washing	Oocyte survival: 41–52%[2] Embryo production: 16.2%[10] Blastocyst development: 5.9%[10]
Vitrification – open straw	TCM199	Equilibration in 10% EG and DMSO or 20% EG or DMSO Vitrification in 20% EG and DMSO or 40% EG or DMSO with 0.5 M sucrose	Sucrose solution → sucrose gradient, washing	Maturation rate: 19.2–37.6%[11] Embryo production: 24.8%[11] Blastocyst production: 7.5%[11] Implantation rate: (4- to 8-cell embryos) two fetal hearts (resorbed) from six embryos transferred (total 242 embryos)[11]

Continued

Table 27.2. Continued.

Approach	Base medium	Cryoprotectant details	Warming	Success
Vitrification – open strip: CryoTop, CryoTech[a]	DPBS, TCM199	Equilibration in 5–10% EG and DMSO Vitrification in high 15–20% EG and DMSO with either 0.5 M sucrose or 1.5 M trehalose and 10% Ficoll	1 M sucrose or 1.5 M trehalose, 30% Ficoll → gradient dilution, washing	Oocyte survival: 51[2] to 62%[12,a] Embryo (Parthenote) production: 46%[12] Embryo (IVF/ICSI) production: 21[9,a] to 68%[13] Blastocyst (IVF/ICSI) rate: 0%[9,b] to 3.9%[14] to 5.2%[13] Live-birth rates: 10.2%[13] (4 from 34 embryos transferred) to 11.8[14]

[1]Apparicio *et al.* (2013); [2]Mikołajewska *et al.* (2012); [3]Snoeck *et al.* (2018); [4]Comizzoli *et al.* (2009); [5]Cocchia *et al.* (2010); [6]Fernandez-Gonzalez and Jewgenow (2017); [7]de Almeida Monteiro Melo Ferraz *et al.* (2020); [8]Colombo *et al.* (2019); [9]Sowińska *et al.* (2020); [10]Merlo *et al.* (2008); [11]Tharasanit *et al.* (2011); [12]Nowak *et al.* (2020); [13]Pope *et al.* (2012); [14]Galiguis *et al.* (2014).
[a]Compositions of commercial vitrification solutions proprietary.
[b]Not all vitrified-warmed oocytes selected for ICSI.

from slow frozen then thawed testicular tissues (~1% live-birth rate). As these examples indicate, the chances of producing litters become increasingly challenging the more *in vitro* technologies/steps must be applied. In more recent years, research has focused on optimizing embryo survival post-thaw/warming (Table 27.3) and evaluating either their subsequent ability to develop to the blastocyst stage *in vitro* (if a 2- to 8-cell embryo), or the blastocoel cavity's ability to re-expand *in vitro* following warming (if a blastocyst). In general, embryo viability post-warming hovers around 70-80%, depending on the study and embryo developmental stage (Table 27.3); however, preserved 2- to 8-cell embryos display reduced capacity to develop to the blastocyst stage *in vitro*, regardless of slow freezing versus vitrification strategy (range from 13–53%).

27.2.3 Ovarian and testicular tissue

As previously mentioned, live kittens have been produced from mature sperm rescued from cryopreserved testicular tissue (Tharasanit *et al.*, 2012). However, the focus of this section will be the preservation of prepubertal testicular tissue where no mature spermatids are immediately available in fresh tissues. As of yet, live offspring have not been produced from cryopreserved or vitrified immature ovarian or testicular tissue from the domestic cat. Limited research has been done in this area, although vitrification, needle immersion vitrification, slow freezing, and two-step freezing protocols have been evaluated.

During vitrification, tissue pieces are incubated in equilibration solution and vitrification solution and then directly plunged into liquid nitrogen and transferred to cryo-vials for storage. Cat ovarian tissues have been vitrified in both open, solid-surface (Fig. 27.1b) and closed, stainless steel cylindrical structure conditions using EG, DMSO, and trehalose as cryoprotectants (Brito *et al.*, 2018). In that study, 19% of follicles maintained normal morphology following solid surface vitrification (SSV) in the presence of all cryoprotectants following warming and 7-day *in vitro* culture (Brito *et al.*, 2018).

In the needle immersion vitrification approach (Fig. 27.1c), ovarian or testicular tissue pieces are threaded on to a 30 G needle and serially immersed in equilibration and vitrification solution (Mouttham and Comizzoli, 2017; Lima *et al.*, 2018). After removing the excess vitrification solution using a sterile absorbent tissue, the needle with the tissues is plunged directly into liquid nitrogen. Samples are then transferred into pre-chilled cryo-vials for storage. When vitrified testicular tissues were warmed at 50°C for 5 seconds, seminiferous tubule structure, somatic cell and germ cell viability, and cell function (mitochondrial membrane potential and germ cell progression) were better compared with 37°C thawing (Lima *et al.*, 2018). For cat ovarian tissues, approximately 20% of follicles maintained normal morphology following needle immersion vitrification, warming, and 7-day

Table 27.3. Reference table for embryo cryopreservation/vitrification methods, success rates, with cryoprotectants dimethylsulfoxide (DMSO), ethylene glycol (EG), 1,2-propanediol (PrOH), and propylene glycol (PG). Success percentages reflect proportion of each developmental benchmark relative to total embryos in the treatment with highest rates per study.

Approach	Cryoprotectant details	Warming	Success
2- to 8-cell embryos			
Slow freezing – closed straws	Stepwise equilibration in increasing PG, sucrose and dextran 70 or PG and sucrose Vitrification in 1.4 M PG, 0.125 M sucrose, and 10% dextran 70 or 10% PG and 0.125 M sucrose OR Equilibration in 0.125 M trehalose, then increasing EG (2.5 to 5%) Vitrification in 10% EG with 0.125 M trehalose	Warming at 22°C → Dilution, washing	Embryo survival: 78.2%[1] Blastocyst development: ~2–4 cell = 20.0[1] to 21.3[2,a] to 40.7[3] to 46.4%[4] and ~8-cell to morula = 54.4%[4] Live-birth rate: ~2- to 4-cell = 0%[4] to 1.0[2], and ~8-cell to morula = 1.7%[4]
Vitrification – open strip	Equilibration in 7.5% DMSO and PrOH with 0.5 M sucrose and 10% Ficoll Vitrification in 15% DMSO and PrOH with- 1 M sucrose and 10% Ficoll) OR Equilibration in 10% PG and DMSO Vitrification in 20% PG and DMSO with 1 M sucrose	Warming in sucrose solution (0.3–1 M, ± Ficoll), then gradient dilution, washing	Embryo survival: ~2- to 4-cell = 73.3 - 76.9%[5], and ~8-cell to morula = 72.7 - 93.3%[5] Blastocyst development: 13.3% (4- to 8- cell)[5] to 26.7% (>8-cell)[5] to 28.6% (2- to 4-cell)[1]
Blastocysts			
Vitrification – open strip	Equlibration in 7.5% DMSO and PrOH with 0.5 M sucrose and 10% Ficoll, Vitrification in 15% DMSO and PrOH with 1 M sucrose and 10% Ficoll Or Equilibration in 7.5% EG and DMSO Vitrification in 15% EG, DMSO, with 0.5 M sucrose	Warming in sucrose solution (0.5–1 M, 10% Ficoll), then sucrose gradient dilution, washing	Blastocyst survival (expansion): 38.5[5] or 64.3% (punctured blastocyst)[4] to 73.8%[6]

[1]Mokrousova *et al.* (2020); [2]Tharasanit *et al.* (2012); [3]Pedersen *et al.* (2008); [4]Gómez *et al.* (2003); [5]Ochota *et al.* (2017); [6]Tsujioka *et al.* (2008).
[a]Not all cryopreserved embryos cultured.

in vitro culture (Mouttham and Comizzoli, 2017). As with oocytes and embryos, there have been some comparisons of slow freezing versus vitrification methods for gonadal tissue in the cat. Tanpradit *et al.* (2015) found that a slow freezing method, wherein tissues were cooled at a rate of −1°C/min to −80°C in a specialized controlled-rate freezing container (as in Fig. 27.1d) overnight prior to being immersed in liquid nitrogen (Fig. 27.1c) was superior to an open vitrification system in maintaining normal ovarian follicles.

Two-step freezing involved placing tissue pieces on the wall side of a pre-cooled cryo-vial and then placing the vials over liquid nitrogen vapor (4 cm above the liquid) for 10 minutes and plunging into liquid nitrogen. Tissues are warmed by placing the cryo-vials at ambient temperature for 30 seconds and then transferring the tissues into ambient temperature medium. Although most approaches yield greater than 50% cell survival, conditions to support *in vitro* spermatogenesis are poorly developed except for the laboratory mice (Yokonishi *et al.*, 2014).

27.2.4 Future perspectives on genome rescue from tissues

Use of preserved testicular and ovarian tissues remains limited. Immature/prepubertal cat testicular tissue may be grafted into immunodeficient mice (Fig. 27.2a), which has previously supported the progression of spermatogenesis and production of mature, elongating spermatids (Yeunhee *et al.*, 2007). Similarly, xenografts of cryopreserved cat ovarian cortical tissue into immunodeficient mice display evidence of antral follicle development (Bosch *et al.*, 2004). Though results are promising for both types of gonadal tissue, these *in vivo* systems require fairly specialized infrastructure to use, as immunodeficient rodent models need particular care.

An alternative to the *in vivo* incubation systems is *in vitro* culture. In smaller mammals (i.e. the laboratory mouse) testicular and ovarian tissues, or isolated ovarian follicles from immature animals have been grown *in vitro* to produce mature gametes for use in IVF. Unfortunately, these technologies have not yet been translated to the domestic cat. For example, murine neonatal testicular tissue has been cultured on an agarose gel block (Fig. 27.2b) to produce mature sperm *in vitro* (Sato *et al.*, 2011). Application of a similar culture system to domestic cat testicular tissue found some germ cells survived 6-week culture, but they displayed no evidence of differentiation (Silva *et al.*, 2018). Much more research is needed to understand the requirements to support spermatogenesis *in vitro* in the cat. Similarly, prepubertal ovarian tissue has not yet advanced to a stage where mature, fertilizable oocytes can be grown from large mammalian species. This is likely due to the prolonged incubation necessary to grow large mammalian follicles from the earliest (primordial) stage through to preovulatory – estimated to take about 100 days in species like the cat, cow, and human compared with ~20 days in smaller mammals like the laboratory mouse (Picton *et al.*, 2008). Further, during this time the ~40 µm diameter primordial follicles grow to a preovulatory size of >3 mm (Reynaud *et al.*, 2009) (compared with ~0.5 mm in the mouse; Picton *et al.*, 2008). The cat follicle's nearly 100 times expansion in size comes with significant changes in physical, hormonal, and nutrient requirements which are challenging to recapitulate *in vitro*.

Owing to these challenges, recent research has focused on the development of more 'biomimetic' culture systems. One primary example is the implementation of bioreactor and microfluidic chip culture methods, wherein culture medium is designed to 'flow' through the tissue culture chamber to better mimic nutrient availability and waste exchange rates that the tissue would be exposed to via circulation *in vivo*. On the male side, this organ-on-a-chip technology has been used to support murine spermatogenesis *in vitro* for 6 months, including producing live offspring from sperm developed in the system (Komeya *et al.*, 2016). As yet, there have been no published reports of similar technology being applied to domestic cat testicular tissue culture. On the female side, our laboratory has developed prototype microfluidic ovary-on-a-chip (Fig. 27.2c) for the *in vitro* culture of domestic cat ovarian tissue and isolated follicles (Nagashima *et al.*, 2018). This dynamic culture method was equivalent to the gold-standard agarose gel system for short-term culture, and research is ongoing in the cat and other large mammalian models to fine-tune this and other novel culture methods to support *in vitro* folliculogenesis.

27.3 Embryo Production Technologies

This section is organized such that we begin by discussing the least invasive/technically challenging methods and expand from there. Nevertheless, some specialized laboratory equipment and/or consumable supplies are required for these ARTs, which we have outlined in Table 27.4.

27.3.1 IVM, IVF, ICSI and beyond

Oocytes collected from immature follicle stages via ovarian cortical tissue slicing require maturation *in vitro* prior to fertilization. IVM has been accomplished via incubation of groups of oocytes (with attached cumulus cells; Sowińska *et al.*, 2017) in maturation media (typically TCM199) containing a protein source (e.g. bovine serum albumin),

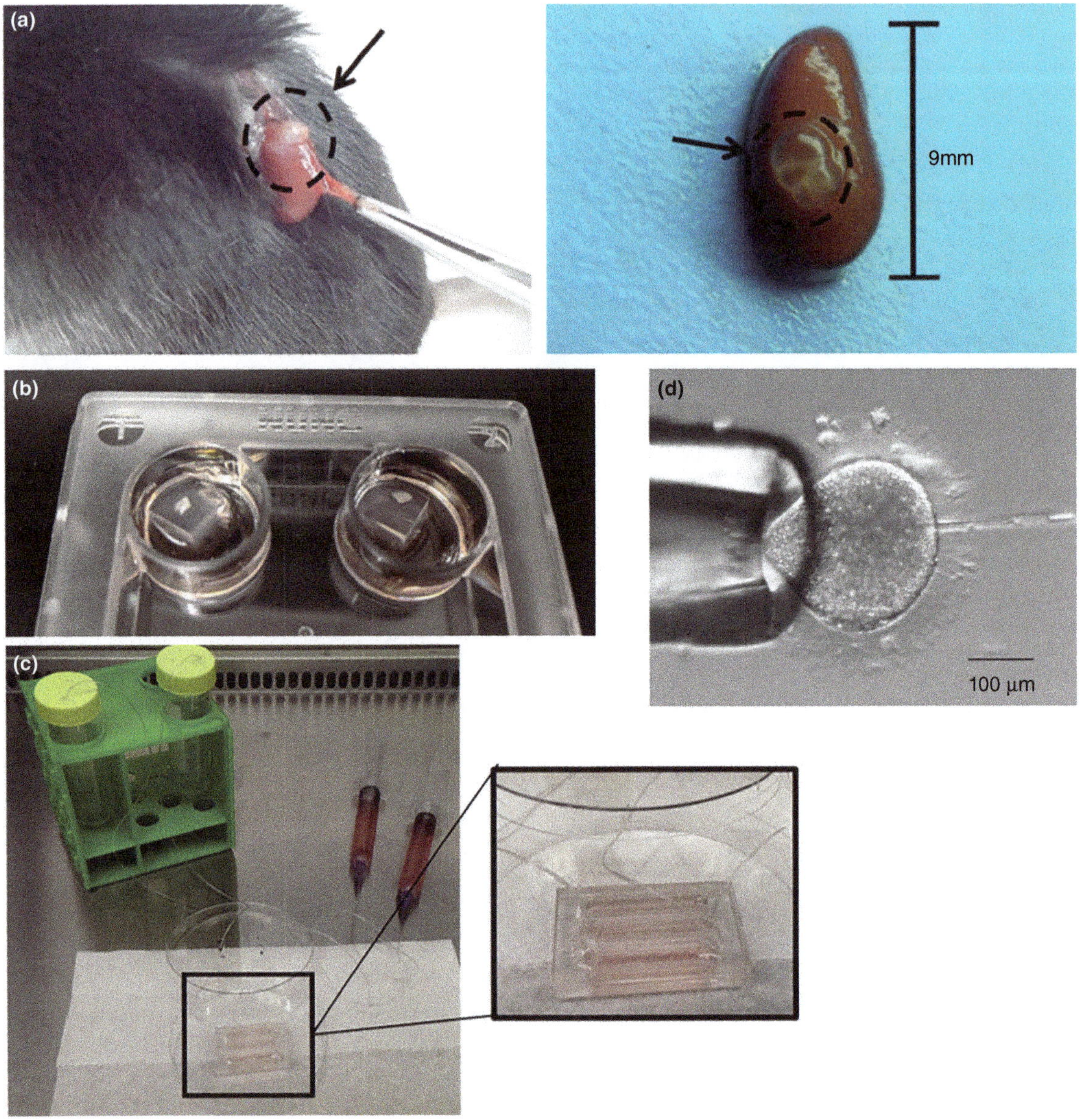

Figure 27.2. Gamete and embryo production technologies, with: **(a)** xenografted ovarian tissue under the kidney capsule of an immunodeficient mouse (left), with evidence of antral follicle development (right) (adapted with permission from dos Santos *et al.* 2016). **(b)** Example of agarose gel block tissue culture (image: author's own); **(c)** dynamic flow chip culture (image: author's own); and **(d)** cat ICSI (used with permission from Gómez *et al.*, 2000/CSIRO Publishing).

follicle-stimulating hormone and luteinizing hormone or eCG/hCG, with incubation at 37–38°C and 5% CO_2 for 24–36 hours and resulting in oocytes resuming meiosis and reaching a fertilizable Metaphase II. Utilizing both *in vivo* and *in vitro* matured, IVF and ICSI have been used to produce live offspring in the domestic cat. In IVF, matured oocytes are co-incubated with domestic cat sperm at 37–38°C and 5% CO_2 for up to 24 hours (for detailed technical methods on cat IVM and IVF see

Herrick, 2019). *In vitro* production rates of 2-cell embryos vary based on use of cryopreserved gametes and the season and/or reproductive stage during which the oocytes were collected (Freistedt *et al.*, 2001; Karja *et al.*, 2002). Nevertheless, IVM/IVF and embryo culture can be performed fairly readily in the cat given access to gametes and an incubator (Table 27.4). In ICSI, sperm are directly injected into an oocyte via micromanipulation (Figure 27.2d). Production of 2-cell embryos via ICSI ranges from 30-80% (Gómez *et al.*, 2000; Pope *et al.*, 2012; Tharasanit *et al.*, 2012). Transfer of ICSI-derived embryos has resulted in live-birth rates of ~1 to 11% of embryos transferred (Gómez *et al.*, 2000; Pope *et al.*, 2012; Tharasanit *et al.*, 2012). It should be noted that the variability in these rates is likely due to other factors, including sperm and oocyte handling (cryopreserved versus fresh) and developmental stage of embryos transferred (zygote versus morula stage). Beyond this, a skilled technician and specialized micromanipulation equipment is necessary to perform this procedure (Table 27.4).

Cloning, otherwise referred to as somatic cell nuclear transfer (SCNT) involves the transfer of somatic cell nuclei into enucleated oocytes and then activation to resume development. Interestingly, several commercial entities now offer this service for a fee. Unlike AI and IVF/ET, efficiency of producing cloned embryos and live offspring via cloning is less than 1%. This approach also requires more complex infrastructure and a large number of recipients to ensure success. Although an increasing number of pet owners are interested in cloning their cats, there are several ethical considerations that must be evaluated. First, the production of a cloned animal does not occur in a vacuum – one or more surrogate queens must undergo ovarian stimulation for specifically-timed estrus and then subjected to ET procedures. The source, well-being, and ultimate fate of the surrogate must be considered as well. Second, pet owners should be strongly advised that a cloned offspring will not likely exhibit the whole range of behaviors or even physical attributes (coat colors, patterning) that the donor animal might have exhibited. Finally, with the low rates of success in conjunction with these above factors, clients also may need to be encouraged to adopt animals to rescue cats in place of pursuing cloning. However, in the event a client requests the cloning of their cat, referring them to commercial vendors may yield the best outcome.

That said, cloning does hold the potential to offer a wide range of benefits for the research community. Cloned cats are often used to investigate new therapies wherein the donor effects (genotype) may be minimized, similar to the advantage of the homogenous laboratory mouse. Further, cloning (as well as transgenesis, which is beyond the scope of this chapter but we refer the reader to Asfaw and

Table 27.4. General equipment and supplies necessary for *in vitro* culture and embryo production technologies. Equipment and supplies listed in earlier rows assumed necessary for subsequent rows as well. (Author's own table.)

Method	Equipment	General supplies
Oocyte/embryo/tissue culture	Dissecting or stereomicroscope with warming plate (oocytes/embryos) Forceps Pipette/tips or mouth pipette or Wiretrol (Oocytes/embryos) CO_2 incubator Sterile work zone Refrigerator (4°C) Freezer (–20°C)	Petri dishes Cell medium CO_2 source
ICSI	Dissecting or stereomicroscopes with warming plates Inverted microscope with micromanipulation equipment CO_2 incubator Sterile work zone	Petri dishes Cell medium CO_2 source Holding and injection ICSI pipettes
Cloning	Dissecting or stereomicroscopes with warming plates Inverted microscope with micromanipulation equipment CO_2 incubator Sterile work zone	Petri dishes Cell medium CO_2 source Holding and injection ICSI pipettes Recipient cats

Assefa, 2019) might be utilized to increase populations of specific biomedical research model cats. As previously mentioned, the domestic cat shares over 200 genetic traits/disorders which are potential models for human disease (Nicholas, n.d.); however, obtaining enough individuals to develop robust studies on potential therapies can be challenging for rare diseases. Producing litters composed entirely of cats with the specific genetic traits of interest, rather than hoping for one or two individuals per litter would be useful to increase research efficiency and reduce the number of animals produced in breeding colonies for research.

27.4 Conclusion

Significant advances have been achieved in the development and application of assisted reproductive technologies for domestic cats. These advances have been made possible by research conducted in both academic and clinical settings. Despite this, the overall success of producing live offspring in domestic cats via ARTs remains low. It is evident that more research is warranted to improve these technologies. A major challenge to achieving improved pregnancy rates is attributed to individual variation in responses to hormonal stimulation. With respect to AI, both nonsurgical and laparoscopic approaches are well developed. However, the latter approach requires advanced instrumentation and extensive training. *In vitro* embryo production is also well advanced in felids. But achieving pregnancies via ET remain highly variable and could benefit from additional research. More cutting-edge technologies (*in vitro* culture systems for oocytes, and gonadal tissues) are in various stages of development for domestic cats. In the context of veterinary practitioners, technologies described here could enable veterinarians to offer various ARTs to pet owners, but one should also consider the pros and cons of these technologies especially in the context of producing surplus domestic cats when several thousand kittens and adult cats are available annually for adoption.

27.5 References

Apparicio, M., Ruggeri, E. and Luvoni, G. (2013) Vitrification of immature feline oocytes with a commercial kit for bovine embryo vitrification. *Reproduction in Domestic Animals* 48, 240–244. doi: 10.1111/j.1439-0531.2012.02138.x

Asfaw, A. B. and Assefa, A. (2019) Animal transgenesis technology: A review. *Cogent Food & Agriculture* 5, 1686802. doi: 10.1080/23311932.2019.1686802

Bosch, P., Hernandez-Fonseca, H. J., Miller, D. M., Wininger, J. D., Masser, J. B. *et al.* (2004) Development of antral follicles in cryopreserved cat ovarian tissue transplanted to immunodeficient mice. *Theriogenology* 61, 581–594. doi: 10.1016/S0093-691X(03)00244-9

Brito, D. C. C., Domingues, S. F. S., Rodrigues, A. P. R., Maside, C., Lunardi, F. O., *et al.* (2018) Cryopreservation of domestic cat (*Felis catus*) ovarian tissue: Comparison of two vitrification methods. *Theriogenology* 111, 69–77. doi: 10.1016/j.theriogenology.2018.01.015

Cocchia, N., Ciani, F., Russo, M., El Rass, R., Rosapane, I., *et al.* (2010) Immature cat oocyte vitrification in open pulled straws (OPSs) using a cryoprotectant mixture. *Cryobiology* 60, 229–234. doi: 10.1016/j.cryobiol.2010.01.003

Colombo, M., Luvoni, G. C. (2020) Minimum Volume Vitrification of Immature Feline Oocytes. *Journal of Visualized Experiments* 160. doi: 10.3791/61523

Colombo, M., Morselli, M. G., Tavares, M. R., Apparicio, M., and Luvoni, G. C. (2019) Developmental competence of domestic cat vitrified oocytes in 3D enriched culture conditions. *Animals* 9, 329–342. doi: 10.3390/ani9060329

Comizzoli, P., Wildt, D. E., and Pukazhenthi, B. S. (2009) *In vitro* compaction of germinal vesicle chromatin is beneficial to survival of vitrified cat oocytes. *Reproduction in Domestic Animals* 44, 269–274. doi: 10.1111/j.1439-0531.2009.01372.x

Crosier, A.E., Lamy, J., Bapodra, P., Rapp, S., Maly, M., *et al.* (2020) First birth of cheetah cubs from *in vitro* fertilization and embryo transfer. *Animals* 10, 1811. doi: 10.3390/ani10101811

de Almeida Monteiro Melo Ferraz, M., Fujihara, M., Nagachima, J. B., Noonan, M. J., Inoue-Murayama, M., *et al.* (2020) Follicular extracellular vesicles enhance meiotic resumption of domestic cat vitrified oocytes. *Scientific Reports* 10, 8619. doi:10.1038/s41598-020-65497-w

dos Santos, F. A., Pimental, M. M. L., Teixeira, A. C. G., Cosmo, C. Í., Lima, M. A., *et al.* (2016) Follicular right shift: Xenografting queens' ovarian tissue into severe combined immunodeficiency mice and its responses to exogenous gonadotropin. *Theriogenology* 86, 1811–1817. doi: 10.1016/j.theriogenology.2016.05.034

Dresser, B., Gelwicks, E., Wachs, K., and Keller, G. (1988) First successful transfer of cryopreserved feline (*Felis catus*) embryos resulting in live offspring. *Journal of Experimental Zoology* 246, 180–186. doi: 10.1002/jez.1402460210

Fernandez-Gonzalez, L. and Jewgenow, K. (2017) Cryopreservation of feline oocytes by vitrification using commercial kits and slush nitrogen technique. *Reproduction in Domestic Animals* 52, 230–234. doi: 10.1111/rda.12837

Freistedt, P., Stojkovic, M., and Wolf, E. (2001) Efficient *in vitro* production of cat embryos in modified synthetic oviduct fluid medium: Effects of season and ovarian status. *Biology of Reproduction* 65, 9–13. doi: 10.1095/biolreprod65.1.9

Galiguis, J., Gómez, M. C., Leibo, S., and Pope, C. E. (2014) Birth of a domestic cat kitten produced by vitrification of lipid polarized *in vitro* matured oocytes. *Cryobiology* 68, 459–466. doi: 10.1016/j.cryobiol.2014.02.012

Gómez, M. C., Pope, C. E., Harris, R. Davis, A., Mikota, S., *et al.* (2000) Births of kittens produced by intracytoplasmic sperm injection of domestic cat oocytes matured *in vitro*. *Reproduction Fertility and Development* 12, 423–433. doi: 10.1071/rd00126

Gómez, M. C., Pope, E., Harris, R., Mikota, S., and Dresser, B. L. (2003) Development of *in vitro* matured, *in vitro* fertilized domestic cat embryos following cryopreservation, culture and transfer. *Theriogenology* 60, 239–251. doi: 10.1016/s0093-691x(03)00004-9

Goodrowe K. L., Howard, J., and Wildt, D. E. (1988) Comparison of embryo recovery, embryo quality, oestradiol-17β and progesterone profiles in domestic cats (*Felis catus*) at natural or induced oestrus. *Reproduction* 82(2), 553–561. doi: 10.1530/jrf.0.0820553

Herrick, J. R. (2019) *In vitro* culture of embryos from domestic cats. In: Herrick, J. (ed.) *Comparative Embryo Culture. Methods in Molecular Biology*. Humana, New York, pp 229–246. doi: 10.1007/978-1-4939-9566-0_17

Howard, J. G., Lynch, C., Santymire, R. M., Marinari, P. E., and Wildt, D. E. (2016) Recovery of gene diversity using long-term cryopreserved spermatozoa and artificial insemination in the endangered black-footed ferret. *Animal Conservation* 19, 102–111.

Karja, N. W. K., Otoi, T., Murakami, M., Fahrudin, M., and Suzuki, T. (2002) *In vitro* maturation, fertilization and development of domestic cat oocytes recovered from ovaries collected at three stages of the reproductive cycle. *Theriogenology* 57, 2289–2298. doi: 10.1016/S0093-691X(02)00905-6

Komeya, M., Kimura, H., Nakamura, H., Yokonishi, T., Sato, T. *et al.* (2016) Long-term ex vivo maintenance of testis tissues producing fertile sperm in a microfluidic device. *Scientific Reports* 6, 1–10. doi: 10.1038/srep21472

Lima, D. B. C., Silva, T. F. P., Morais, G. B. Aquino-Cortez, A., Evangelista, J. S. A. M., *et al.* (2017) Different associations of cryoprotectants for testicular tissue of prepubertal cats submitted to vitrification. *Reproduction in Domestic Animals* 52, 235–241. doi: 10.1111/rda.12833

Lima, D. B. C., da Silva, L. D. M., and Comizzoli, P. (2018) Influence of warming and reanimation conditions on seminiferous tubule morphology, mitochondrial activity, and cell composition of vitrified testicular tissues in the domestic cat model. *PloS One* 13, e0207317. doi: 10.1371/journal.pone.0207317

Luvoni, G. C. (2006) Gamete cryopreservation in the domestic cat. *Theriogenology* 66, 101–111. doi: 10.1016/j.theriogenology.2006.03.012

Merlo, B., Iacono, E., Regazzini, M., and Zambelli, D. (2008) Cat blastocysts produced in vitro from oocytes vitrified using the cryoloop technique and cryopreserved electroejaculated semen. *Theriogenology* 70, 126–130. doi: 10.1016/j.theriogenology.2008.03.009

Mikołajewska, N., Müller, K., Niżański, W., and Jewgenow, K. (2012) Vitrification of domestic cat oocytes – effect on viability and integrity of subcellular structures. *Reproduction in Domestic Animals* 47, 295–299. doi: 10.1111/rda.12044

Mokrousova, V. I., Okotrub, K. A., Brusentsev, E. Y., Kizilova, E. A, Surovtsev, N. V., *et al.* (2020) Effects of slow freezing and vitrification on embryo development in domestic cat. *Reproduction in Domestic Animals* 55, 1328–1336. doi: 10.1111/rda.13776

Mouttham, L. and Comizzoli, P. (2017) Presence of sucrose in the vitrification solution and exposure for longer periods of time improve post-warming follicle integrity in cat ovarian tissues. *Reproduction in Domestic Animals* 52, 224–229. doi 10.1111/rda.12847

Nagashima, J., El Assal, R., Songsasen, N. and Demirci, U. (2018) Evaluation of an ovary-on-a-chip in large mammalian models: Species specificity and influence of follicle isolation status. *Journal of Tissue Engineering and Regenerative Medicine* e1926–e1935.

Nicholas, F. W. (n.d.) OMIA – Online Mendelian Inheritance in Animals. Available at: https://www.omia.org/home/ (accessed 30 December 2021).

Nowak, A., Kochan, J., Świętek, E., Barbara, K., Prochowska, S., *et al.* (2020) Survivability and developmental competences of domestic cat (*Felis catus*) oocytes after Cryotech method vitrification. *Reproduction in Domestic Animals* 55, 992–997. doi: 10.1111/rda.13741

Ochota, M., Wojtasik, B. and Niżański, W. (2017) Survival rate after vitrification of various stages of cat embryos and blastocyst with and without artificially collapsed blastocoel cavity. *Reproduction in Domestic Animals* 52, 281–287. doi: 10.1111/rda.12826

Pedersen, M. J., Watson, C. A., Blevins, B. A., and Loskutoff, N. M. (2008) 163 Domestic cat (*Felis catus*) embryo cryopreservation: slow freezing versus vitrification. *Reproduction, Fertility and Development* 21, 180–181. doi: 10.1071/RDv21n1Ab163

Picton, H. M., Harris, S. E., Muruvi, W. and Chambers, E. L. (2008) The *in vitro* growth and maturation of follicles. *Reproduction* 136, 703–715. doi: 10.1530/rep-08-0290

Pope, C.E. (2004) *In vitro* fertilization and embryo transfer in felids. In: Schatten, H. (ed.) *Germ Cell Protocols: Molecular Embryo Analysis, Live Imaging, Transgenesis, and Cloning, Vol. 2, Methods in Molecular Biology*, v. 254. Humana Press, Totowa, New Jersey, pp. 227–244.

Pope, C., Gómez, M. C., Kagawa, N., Kuwayama, M., Leibo, S. P., *et al.* (2012) *In vivo* survival of domestic cat oocytes after vitrification, intracytoplasmic sperm injection and embryo transfer. *Theriogenology* 77, 531–538. doi:10.1016/j.theriogenology.2011.08.028

Reynaud, K., Gicquel, C., Thoumire, S., Chebrout, M., Ficheux, C., *et al.* (2009) Folliculogenesis and morphometry of oocyte and follicle growth in the feline ovary. *Reproduction in Domestic Animals* 44, 174–179. doi: 10.1111/j.1439-0531.2007.01012.x

Sato, T., Katagiri, K., Gohbaram A., Inoue, K., Ogonuki, N., *et al.* (2011) *In vitro* production of functional sperm in cultured neonatal mouse testes. *Nature* 471, 504–507. doi: 10.1038/nature09850

Silva, A. F., Escada-Rebelo, S., Amaral, S., Tavares, R. S., Schlatt, S., *et al.* (2018) Can we induce spermatogenesis in the domestic cat using an *in vitro* tissue culture approach? *PLOS ONE* 13, e0191912. doi: 10.1371/journal.pone.0191912

Snoeck, F., Szymanska, K. J., Sarrazin, S., Ortiz-Escribano, N., Leybaert, L., *et al.* (2018) Blocking connexin channels during vitrification of immature cat oocytes improves maturation capacity after warming. *Theriogenology* 122, 144–149. doi: 10.1016/j.theriogenology.2018.09.011

Sowińska, N. Frankowska, K., Filipczyk, A., Adamaszek, A., Fic, K., *et al.* (2017) The effect of cumulus cells on domestic cat (*Felis catus*) oocytes during *in vitro* maturation and fertilization. *Reproduction in Domestic Animals* 52, 108–113. doi: 10.1111/rda.12895

Sowińska, N., Zahmel, J., Wojciech, N., Hribal, R., Fernandez-Gonzalez, L., *et al.* (2020) Meiotic status does not affect the vitrification effectiveness of domestic cat oocytes. *Animals* 10, 1371. doi: 10.3390/ani10081371

Tanpradit, N., Comizzoli, P., Srisuwatanasagul, S., and Chatdarong, K. (2015) Positive impact of sucrose supplementation during slow freezing of cat ovarian tissues on cellular viability, follicle morphology, and DNA integrity. *Theriogenology* 83, 1553–1561, doi: 10.1016/j.theriogenology.2015.01.035

Tharasanit, T. Manee-In, S., Buarpung, S., Chatdarong, K., Lohachit, C., *et al.* (2011) Successful pregnancy following transfer of feline embryos derived from vitrified immature cat oocytes using 'stepwise' cryoprotectant exposure technique. *Theriogenology* 76(8) 1442–1449. doi: 10.1016/j.theriogenology.2011.06.014

Tharasanit, T., Buarpung, S., Manee-In, S., Thongkittidilok, C., Tiptanavattana, N., *et al.* (2012) Birth of kittens after the transfer of frozen–thawed embryos produced by intracytoplasmic sperm injection with spermatozoa collected from cryopreserved testicular tissue. *Reproduction in Domestic Animals* 47, 305–308. doi: 10.1111/rda.12072

Thuwanut, P. and Chatdarong, K. (2012) Cryopreservation of cat testicular tissues: Effects of storage temperature, freezing protocols and cryoprotective agents. *Reproduction in Domestic Animals* 47, 777–781. doi: 10.1111/j.1439-0531.2011.01967.x

Toyonaga, M., Sato, Y., Sasaki, A., Kaihara, A., and Tsutsui, T. (2011) Artificial insemination with cryopreserved sperm from feline epididymides stored at 4°C. *Theriogenology* 76, 532–537. doi: 10.1016/j.theriogenology.2011.03.005

Tsujioka, T., Otzdorff, C., Braun, J., and Hochi, S. (2008) Effect of post-IVF developmental kinetics on *in vitro* survival of vitrified-warmed domestic cat blastocysts. *Reproduction in Domestic Animals* 43, 323–327. doi: 10.1111/j.1439-0531.2007.00902.x

Uchikura, K., Nagano, M., and Hishinuma, M. (2010) Evaluation of follicular development and oocyte quality in pre-pubertal cats. *Reproduction in Domestic Animals* 45, e405–e411. doi: 10.1111/j.1439-0531.2010.01590.x

Wang, X., Catt, S., Pangestu, M., and Temple-Smith, P. D. (2009) Live offspring from vitrified blastocysts derived from fresh and cryopreserved ovarian tissue grafts of adult mice. *Reproduction* 138, 527–535. doi: 10.1530/REP-09-0148

Yeunhee, K., Vimal, S., Budhan, P., and Alexander, J. T. (2007) Effect of donor age on success of spermatogenesis in feline testis xenografts. *Reproduction, Fertility and Development* 19, 869–876. doi: 10.1071/rd07056

Yokonishi, T., Sato, T., Komeya, M., Katagiri, K., Kubota, Y., *et al.* (2014) Offspring production with sperm grown *in vitro* from cryopreserved testis tissues. *Nature Communications* 5, 4320.

Zhang, X., Catalano, P. N., Gurkan, U. A., Khimji, I., and Demirci, U. (2011) Emerging technologies in medical applications of minimum volume vitrification. *Nanomedicine* 6, 1115–1129. doi: 10.2217/nnm.11.71

28 Application of Assisted Reproductive Technology (ART) in Non-Domestic Felids

William F. Swanson

Center for Conservation and Research of Endangered Wildlife (CREW), Cincinnati Zoo and Botanical Garden, Cincinnati, OH, USA

28.1 Introduction

Over the past 10 million years of Earth's history, wild felids have evolved to become one of its most successful taxa, consisting today of 38 recognized species inhabiting five continents and still filling their respective ecological niches as apex predators (IUCN, 2020). Although no species-level extinctions have occurred among felids during the past 10,000 years, most extant wild cat species are now facing growing threats to their continued survival in nature, primarily due to the direct ramifications of human population growth, excess resource consumption and related habitat destruction and climate change. Almost all non-domestic felid populations are declining in the wild, with 25 entire species classified under some degree of imperilment (i.e. critically endangered to near threatened) on the International Union for the Conservation of Nature's Red List (IUCN, 2020) and numerous IUCN-assessed (and many more non-assessed) subspecies edging closer to extinction (Table 28.1).

To counter this loss of biodiversity, nearly 600 zoological parks, accredited either by the United States-based Association of Zoos and Aquariums (AZA) or the European Association of Zoos and Aquaria (EAZA), have established cooperative breeding programs to maintain assurance populations for many of these threatened cat species. The AZA's Species Survival Plans (SSPs) and EAZA's European Endangered species Programs (EEPs) use demographic and genetic analyses of pedigree data from studbooks to create breeding plans that strive to maximize demographic and genetic viability (Swanson, 2006). Currently, the AZA oversees SSPs for 14 cat species whereas the EAZA has EEPs for 13 species, with 11 species managed by both zoo organizations (Table 28.1). Unfortunately, the vast majority (>75%) of zoo-based cat populations are not sustainable for even the next 100 years if dependent on natural breeding alone within traditional management programs (Swanson, 2006). The loss of managed populations in zoos would eliminate a vital safety net for some species and deprive scientists of a valuable research resource that may be necessary for conserving others.

Securing the long-term sustainability of non-domestic felid populations under human care will be extremely challenging, but this prospect can be significantly enhanced through the broader application of reproductive sciences, including assisted reproductive technologies (ART). For wild felids, the priority reproductive techniques for conservation within zoos are still the most basic, comprising semen collection and analyses, in vitro fertilization (IVF), embryo transfer (ET), artificial insemination (AI), and sperm and embryo cryopreservation. More advanced reproductive techniques, such as somatic cell nuclear transfer or creation of sperm and oocytes from induced pluripotent stem cells, often are promoted for their conservation potential, but any applied benefit exists many years into the future for wildlife. Unfortunately, wild cat species lack the luxury of waiting for these emerging scientific technologies to effectively address their pressing conservation needs. The survival of felid species within zoos ultimately hinges on producing enough viable offspring to offset deaths from aging, injury and disease, constrained by the limited physical space, low genetic diversity and restricted financial

DOI: 10.1079/9781789247107.0028

Table 28.1. Conservation status and population management programs for wild felids.

Common name	Genus/species	Conservation status (IUCN)[a]	Management program	
			AZA[b]	EAZA[c]
Tiger	*Panthera tigris*	EN	SSP	EEP
Lion	*Panthera leo*	VU	SSP	EEP
Jaguar	*Panthera onca*	NT	SSP	EEP
Leopard	*Panthera pardus*	VU	SSP	EEP
Snow leopard	*Uncia*	VU	SSP	EEP
Clouded leopard	*Neofelis nebulosa*	VU	SSP	EEP
Cheetah	*Acinonyx jubatus*	VU	SSP	EEP
Fishing cat	*Prionailurus viverrinus*	VU	SSP	EEP
Pallas' cat	*Otocolobus manul*	NT	SSP	EEP
Sand cat	*Felis margarita*	LC	SSP	EEP
Black-footed cat	*Felis nigripes*	VU	SSP	EEP
Canada lynx	*Lynx canadensis*	LC	SSP	–
Serval	*Leptailurus serval*	LC	SSP	–
Ocelot	*Leopardus pardalis*	LC	SSP	–
Margay	*Leopardus wiedii*	NT	–	EEP
Geoffroy's cat	*Leopardus geoffroyi*	LC	–	EEP

[a]IUCN Red List species-level classification: EN, endangered; VU, vulnerable; NT, near threatened; LC, least concern.
[b]Association of Zoos and Aquariums, Species Survival Plan.
[c]European Association of Zoos and Aquaria, European Endangered species Program.

resources inherent to managing most zoo-based populations. If ART is to have a meaningful impact on maintaining these cat species, its efficacy and applicability to population management must be substantially improved within the next 10 to 20 years. Time really has become the most critical factor in applying ART to conservation of felid species within zoos and the wild.

Our ability to apply any of these techniques successfully to wild felids is dependent on initial research conducted in their most appropriate reproductive model, the domestic cat. Domestic cats (*Felis silvestris catus*) were tamed by humans from wild cats only ~10,000 years ago and retain many physiological and genetic similarities with their wild counterparts. Most of our basal knowledge of felid reproduction is derived from laboratory studies in domestic cats, and all ART now used successfully in wild felids was first developed, refined and applied with this domesticated population (Sojka *et al.*, 1970; Platz and Seager, 1978; Kraemer *et al.*, 1979). Wild felid populations in zoos, in turn, have provided scientists with a vital resource to investigate the cross-species extrapolation of these techniques. One prerequisite for applying ART to wild cats is characterization of species-specific reproductive traits, discerning similarities and differences on a species-by-species basis through semen collection and analysis and, most importantly, non-invasive endocrine monitoring via fecal hormone analysis (Brown *et al.*, 1994). Although wild felids and domestic cats obviously differ substantially via evolutionary divergence, enough reproductive commonalities exist that the applied use of ART is now gaining some traction as a population management strategy for wild cats (unlike the current situation with ART in most other wildlife taxa).

28.2 Semen Collection, Analysis and Cryopreservation

Semen collection of felids is essential for assessment of male basal reproductive traits as well as procurement of semen for application to cryopreservation, in vitro fertilization, and artificial insemination. Fortunately, for felids, there are several methods available for semen collection that have proven safe and effective across species. For wild felids, electroejaculation of anesthetized males represents the most widely used approach, having been successfully applied for semen recovery in almost every wild felid species maintained in zoos over the past 40 years (Platz and Seager, 1978). For this technique, a lubricated rectal probe, with either longitudinal or circumferential electrodes and a probe diameter adjusted for the cat's body size (i.e. approximately the diameter of the species typical stool sample), is inserted into the rectum (Fig. 28.1). An electrostimulator, connected to the rectal probe, elicits ejaculation by delivering a controlled series of low voltage (2–6 V) stimuli, typically fractionated in two or three sets of 20–30 stimuli each. A warmed, sterile plastic cup, placed over the glans penis, permits recovery of the ejaculated sample (Fig. 28.2a). Most recently, an alternative approach for semen collection has been described for cats, using an open-ended urinary catheter inserted into the urethra (to the depth of the prostate) to recover highly concentrated semen (Fig. 28.2b) (Zambelli *et al.*, 2008). For this method, males require anesthesia with an alpha 2 agonist drug (e.g. medetomidine, dexmedetomidine) to induce sperm release from the vas deferens into the distal urethra. Catheter diameter (3.5 or 5 French) and depth of insertion (range, 6–30 cm) varies based on differences in body sizes typical for each species. Depending on species and individual, total sperm recovery with urethral catheterization may equal that obtained with electroejaculation and good quality samples have been recovered from lions (Lueders *et al.*, 2012) and at least ten other wild cat species using this approach. In rare cases, semen also can be collected voluntarily using an artificial vagina in non-anesthetized wild felids (e.g. cheetah, tiger) but only if males have received intensive operant conditioning by their human handlers. Last, semen may be recovered from most felids after death by flushing the vas deferens and caudal epididymides with culture medium. For many individuals, viable samples may be obtained up to 24 hours after death if tissues are kept chilled during storage and transport.

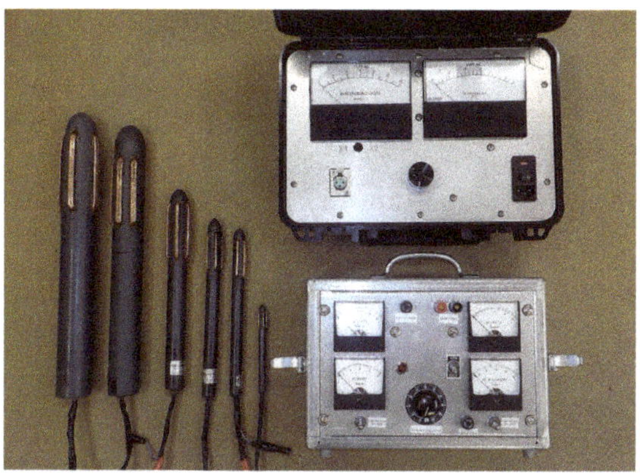

Fig. 28.1. Semen collection equipment: electrostimulators and rectal probes (1.0 cm to 4.2 cm, diameter) used for electroejaculation of domestic cats and wild felids (ranging in size from black-footed cats to Amur tigers). (Image: author's own.)

Comprehensive semen analyses provide insight into the fertility status of individual cats as well as determination of normative seminal parameters typical for each cat species (Herrick *et al.*, 2010). Following semen recovery, cat samples typically are evaluated for several basal characteristics, specifically volume, seminal pH, sperm concentration, progressive motility, rate of progressive movement, and sperm morphology, using standard microscopic methods commonly applied to other mammalian species. Seminal traits can vary substantially among individual cats, but consistent differences are often observed in sperm numbers and morphology

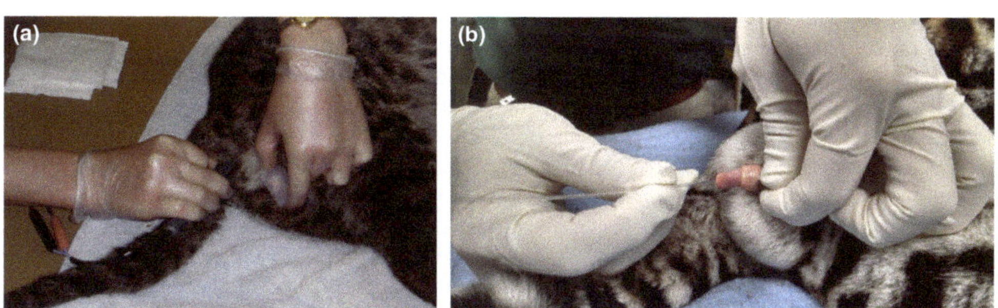

Fig. 28.2. Semen collection methods in felids. **(a)** Electroejaculation of a fishing cat using a 1.6 cm diameter rectal probe and polypropylene collection cup (image: author's own). **(b)** Urethral catheterization of an ocelot using a 5 Fr open-ended polypropylene catheter following medetomidine/ketamine-induced anesthesia. (Image: author's own.)

traits between species. In general, smaller cats provide fewer sperm per ejaculate (often <50 million) compared to larger cats (>100 million), limiting sperm availability in small felids for freezing or AI. Certain species, such as cheetahs and clouded leopards, exhibit very poor sperm morphology (<30% normal) and are classified as teratospermic whereas other species, such as ocelots and tigers, routinely have >60% normal sperm, with most other species falling in between those two extremes. Of importance, teratospermia can severely affect both sperm function and cryosensitivity, confounding the use of ART with these affected species.

With wild felids, reproductive studies are often conducted in collaboration with multiple zoos dispersed geographically, requiring long-distance travel and limiting transport of complex laboratory equipment. For this reason, a 'mobile lab' approach is frequently required, with a preference for lab equipment that is compact, lightweight, and durable that potentially may affect study design. For example, sperm motility traits in wild cat studies are often evaluated subjectively to bypass use of more cumbersome computer-assisted sperm analysis systems, although easily portable systems are now becoming available. Other sperm traits such as acrosome status, viability, capacitation status, and mitochondrial function may be assessed from fixed samples using specialized colorimetric (e.g. rose Bengal/fast green) or fluorescent (e.g. Hoescht, FITC-PNA) stains. More advanced parameters assessed in wild cats may include sperm metabolism, chromatin fragmentation, and sperm functionality, particularly through use of heterologous *in vitro* fertilization. Among felids, cross-species reproductive barriers are absent at the gamete level, allowing sperm from any wild felid to penetrate and fertilize domestic cat oocytes in vitro. Domestic cat oocytes are readily available and easily matured using ovaries acquired from spay clinics, eliminating the challenge of obtaining homologous oocytes from wild cats for these sperm function studies. While heterologous IVF has value for assessing fertility of individual males, it has proven most beneficial for comparative evaluation of sperm function in conjunction with semen cryopreservation studies (Herrick *et al.*, 2010).

Semen cryopreservation is a cornerstone for applying ART to endangered species conservation and management. The ability to cryopreserve and store felid sperm for decades or centuries creates an invaluable resource to maintain most genetic diversity of managed populations within liquid nitrogen tanks rather than as living animals, potentially doubling or tripling the number of cat species that can be effectively conserved within zoos. Further, frozen semen allows gene flow to be established between zoos and countries, as well as between *in situ* and *ex situ* populations, as an alternative to stressful transport of living cats (Swanson *et al.*, 2007). However, for this potential to become reality, cat semen samples must be processed and frozen in a manner to recover adequate viability and function to produce offspring, either through IVF or AI. Unfortunately, despite decades of research, cat semen remains relatively difficult to cryopreserve effectively.

Historically, cryopreservation of domestic cat sperm involved diluting samples in an egg-yolk-based extender containing glycerol and, following short-term cooling in a refrigerator, rapid freezing by pelleting onto dry ice blocks. Application of this approach to wild felids allowed recovery of a moderate percentage of viable, motile sperm after thawing but longevity was often abbreviated, and only a handful of offspring were ever produced following AI with semen frozen using this method. Refinement of semen freezing over the years has involved numerous studies investigating alterations of extenders, cryoprotectants, cooling rates, packaging methods and thawing rates. Many semen samples from wild felids are still frozen using a commercially available egg-yolk-based extender with glycerol, but methodology has evolved to include slow cooling of samples prior to freezing followed by stepwise cryopreservation in straws over liquid nitrogen vapor or within a dry shipper container.

Recent research has shown the superiority of freezing domestic cat and wild felid semen in a soy-lecithin-based extender (with glycerol) to reduce batch-to-batch variability, infectious disease concerns, and regulatory barriers associated with using egg-yolk-based products (Vick *et al.*, 2012). Comparative studies in jaguars, ocelots, Pallas' cats, fishing cats, black-footed cats, and sand cats have found that the soy lecithin-based medium provides similar post-thaw motility and function (with heterologous IVF) as observed with egg-yolk-based medium. As one variation on this approach, the feasibility of ultra-rapid freezing of cat semen directly into liquid nitrogen (in a soy-lecithin-based extender containing sucrose instead of glycerol) has been demonstrated, including the birth of viable kittens following AI. This method, when combined with urethral catheterization for semen collection, provides a rapid field-friendly semen banking approach that requires minimal equipment and can be used by zoo veterinarians or wildlife biologists working with felid populations *ex situ* or *in situ* (Swanson *et al.*, 2016). However, despite some improvements in cat semen cryopreservation methods in recent years, post-thaw parameters in many wild felids are still less than ideal for ART and represent a major hindrance to incorporating routine semen banking and standard insemination techniques into population management programs.

28.3 Artificial Insemination

Artificial insemination is the most direct method available to produce living offspring in wild felids and has been promoted as the most relevant ART for wildlife management (Pukazhenthi and Wildt, 2004). Artificial insemination is the most valuable tool for propagating wild cats that are behaviorally or physically incompatible, creating genetic exchange between cats housed in different zoos and establishing gene flow between cats living within zoos and the wild (Swanson, 2006; Howard and Wildt, 2009). In domestic cats, AI was first used to produce kittens over 50 years ago (Sojka *et al.*, 1970) and, with recent refinements in AI strategies, now provides a consistently effective method for generating kittens with both freshly collected and frozen-thawed semen (Swanson, 2019). Vaginal and transcervical AI in wild felids has resulted in a handful of pregnancies over the past 40 years, but has not been consistently productive, primarily due to suspected anesthetic interference to sperm transport in sedated females (Table 28.2). More recent transcervical AI attempts have produced several pregnancies in three species (lion, golden cat, Persian leopard) inseminated following ovulation induction during natural estrous phases. However, this approach requires relatively high sperm numbers for conception and, with its dependence on scheduling during natural estrus, is poorly amenable to population management across institutions.

The incorporation of laparoscopy, a minimally invasive surgical technique, into reproductive studies of domestic cats substantially benefited AI development in felids (Fig. 28.3) (Wildt *et al.*, 1977). A laparoscopic uterine AI (LU-AI) method, developed in the late 1980s, improved pregnancy success in domestic cats treated with exogenous gonadotropins (eCG, hCG) and its extrapolation to wild felids resulted in pregnancies in eight species (Fig. 28.4a) (Howard and Wildt, 2009). With this approach, females typically are treated with a single injection of equine chorionic gonadotropin (eCG) to induce ovarian follicular growth followed 3 to 4 days later by human chorionic gonadotropin (hCG) to induce ovulation, with AI conducted 36 to 45 hours after hCG injection. Determination of proper gonadotropin dosages and timing of AI required species-by-species adjustments, with larger cats generally ovulating at a later time point post-hCG and ovarian sensitivity to eCG/hCG dosages varying substantially by species, but with little relation to body weight. For cheetahs and ocelots, multiple pregnancies have been produced by LU-AI, including with frozen-thawed sperm in both species. However, AI success in other species has been limited, in part because LU-AI, as with transcervical AI, requires relatively robust sperm numbers to achieve conception that also may be severely compromised by sperm freezing.

Recent improvements in AI strategies in domestic cats and wild felids have involved multiple alterations in the standard laparoscopic AI protocol, including changes in exogenous gonadotropin regimens, site of insemination and control of ovarian function (Conforti *et al.*, 2013; Swanson, 2019). Although eCG and hCG are highly effective for inducing ovarian activity and ovulation, the circulatory persistence of hCG stimulates post-ovulatory follicle growth and associated endocrine disruption, adversely affecting embryo migration and fetal development. Substitution of porcine luteinizing hormone (pLH) for hCG produces consistent ovulation induction without causing secondary ovarian stimulation. Further, the preferred site of insemination was shifted from the uterus to the oviduct, depositing sperm directly into the ampulla where fertilization occurs and greatly reducing total sperm numbers and/or quality needed for successful AI (Fig. 28.4b). Laparoscopic oviductal AIs (LO-AIs) now are routinely performed across species with just 2 to 4 million motile sperm. Last, exogenous gonadotropin treatments for AI procedures in the past often were conducted without consideration of underlying ovarian activity in selected females, producing inconsistent ovarian responses in many individuals (Howard and Wildt, 2009; Thongphakdee *et al.*, 2018). With the current LO-AI protocol, ovarian activity in female cats

Table 28.2. Successful artificial insemination and embryo transfer in wild felids.

		Artificial insemination		Embryo transfer		
Common name	Genus/species	Approach[a]	Semen status[b]	Embryo Source[c]	Transfer method[d]	Embryo status[e]
Tiger	*Panthera tigris*	V/LU/LO	F	IVF	SO	F
Lion	*Panthera leo*	TC	F			
Jaguar	*Panthera onca*	LO/LU	F			
Leopard	*Panthera pardus*	TC	F			
Snow leopard	*Uncia*	LU	F			
Clouded leopard	*Neofelis nebulosa*	LU/LO	F/FT			
Cheetah	*Acinonyx jubatus*	LU	F/FT	IVF	LO	F
Puma	*Puma concolor*	SU/LU	F			
Fishing cat	*Prionailurus viverrinus*	LO	F	IVF	SU	F
Pallas' cat	*Otocolobus manul*	LO	F/FT			
Sand cat	*Felis margarita*	LO	FT	IVF	LO	F
Ocelot	*Leopardus pardalis*	LU/LO	F/FT	IVF	LO	FT
Tigrina	*Leopardus tigrinus*	LU	F			
Golden cat	*Catopuma temminckii*	TC	F			
Leopard cat	*Prionailurus bengalensis*	LU	F/FT			
Black-footed cat	*Felis nigripes*			IVF	LO/LOi	FT
Caracal	*Caracal*			IVF	SU	F/FT
Serval	*Leptailurus serval*			IVF	SU	F
Wild cat	*Felis silvestris*			IVF	SU	F/FT

[a]Approach: V, vaginal; TC, transcervical; SU, surgical uterine; LU, laparoscopic uterine; LO, laparoscopic oviductal; [b]Semen status: F, fresh; FT, frozen-thawed; [c]Embryo source: IVF, in vitro fertilization; [d]Transfer method: SU, surgical uterine; SO, surgical oviductal; LO, laparoscopic oviductal; i, interspecies; [e]Embryo status: F, fresh; FT, frozen-thawed.

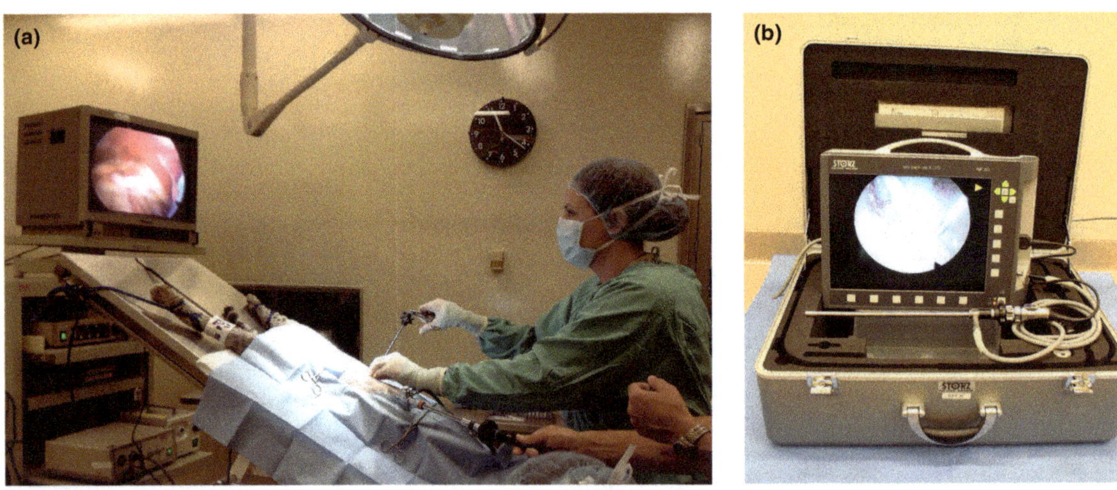

Fig. 28.3. Laparoscopy in felids. **(a)** Standard laparoscopic equipment tower used for LO-AI at home institutions. **(b)** Portable laparoscopic equipment used for 'mobile lab' reproductive procedures during travel to distant institutions. (Images: author's own.)

typically is suppressed prior to gonadotropin treatment by daily feeding of low-dose progesterone (altrenogest) for 30 to 55 consecutive days, depending on species (Swanson, 2019). Following 5 to 7 days of progesterone withdrawal, females are injected with eCG/pLH and inseminated using a fixed-time LO-AI procedure. With this approach, 70-80% of domestic cats conceive with both

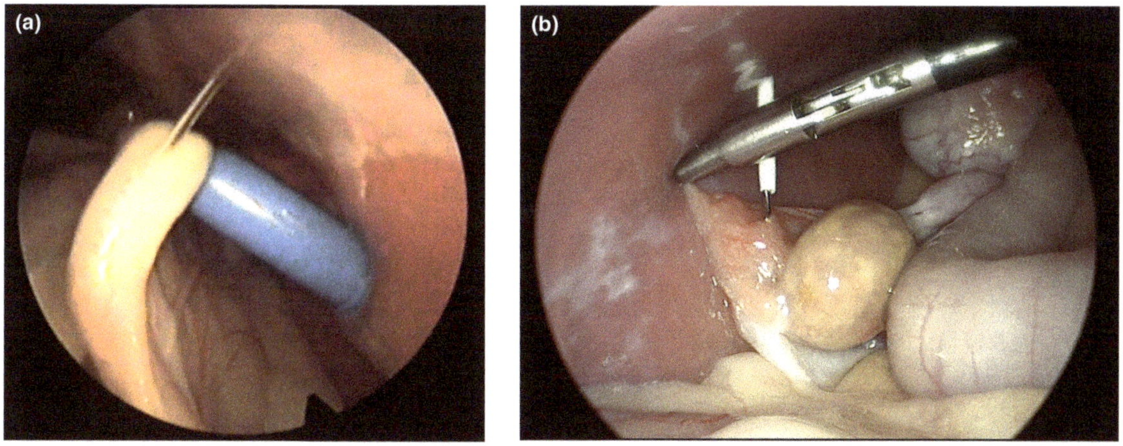

Fig. 28.4. Laparoscopic AI. **(a)** LU-AI of a domestic cat showing insertion of the AI catheter into the lumen of the distal uterine horn. **(b)** LO-AI of an ocelot showing placement of the blunted AI needle deep into the oviductal ampulla. (Images: author's own.)

freshly collected and frozen-thawed sperm and offspring have been produced in six wild felid species, including multiple pregnancies in ocelots with fresh and frozen semen (Table 28.2). In ocelots, LO-AI has provided a substantial boost to SSP population numbers and significantly enhanced genetic diversity by producing multiple ocelot litters using frozen semen from a non-represented founder male. Of the 14 SSPs managed by the AZA, the ocelot SSP has received the most benefit from applied ART and serves as a prospective model for incorporating LO-AI into management programs for other felids.

28.4 *In Vitro* Fertilization, Embryo Culture and Cryopreservation

In vitro fertilization studies in domestic cats have provided important insights into reproductive function in felids, facilitating studies of gonadotropin-induced folliculogenesis, oocyte maturation, sperm capacitation, gamete interaction, and embryo developmental kinetics and culture requirements. IVF research also has provided the opportunity to investigate the potential use of embryo transfer for population management by eliminating the challenge of recovering *in vivo*-generated embryos after natural breeding or AI, and amplifying the number of embryos that can be produced by each female (Goodrowe *et al.*, 1988; Pope, 2014). As with AI, exogenous gonadotropin treatment has been a central factor in advances made with IVF technologies. In domestic cats and wild felids, eCG or porcine follicle stimulating hormone (pFSH) have been routinely used to hyperstimulate ovarian follicular growth followed by pLH or hCG to induce follicular maturation prior to aspiration. Oocyte recovery typically is conducted at ~24–27 hours after pLH or hCG treatment via laparoscopy and most oocytes usually complete nuclear maturation (to meiosis II) within 1 to 2 hours post-collection. As with AI, ovarian stimulation protocols developed in domestic cats for IVF have shown some effectiveness among most wild felid species with species-specific adjustments of gonadotropin dosages. Across species, felid sperm readily undergoes capacitation in most protein-supplemented culture media and high to moderate fertilization percentages *in vitro* have been reported for nearly 20 wild cat species to date (Fig. 28.5a) (Swanson, 2006, Pope, 2019). IVF also requires much fewer sperm numbers (~20–50 × 10^6 motile sperm per IVF drop) than even LO-AI, and often can produce adequate fertilization percentages despite using compromised frozen-thawed semen (Fig. 28.5b).

IVF research also has facilitated initiation of embryo culture studies, allowing comparison of developmental kinetics for *in vitro* and *in vivo* generated embryos and cross-species assessment of IVF-produced embryo development. Multifactorial investigation of media formulations and stage-specific metabolic needs have permitted refinement of embryo culture systems in domestic cats to produce more consistent blastocyst formation within physiologically normal developmental time frames (Herrick *et al.*, 2007). Routine production of uterine-stage embryos simplifies embryo transfer by potentially allowing transcervical embryo deposition, but findings from transfer studies suggest that prolonged embryo culture still may adversely affect viability *in vivo* (Pope, 2014). Last, IVF techniques have enabled detailed studies of embryo cryopreservation at both early (two to eight cell) and late (morula/blastocyst) stages of development. Embryo cryopreservation methods used in other mammalian species, including slow straw freezing and vitrification, have proven effective in domestic cats as well as a few wild cat species (Pope, 2014, 2019). As with sperm freezing and AI, the existence of reliable embryo freezing protocols is a prerequisite for any future application of embryo transfer for conservation management of wild felids.

28.5 Embryo Transfer

From an applied perspective, the most valuable attribute of IVF is its capacity to routinely generate viable embryos for transfer to produce offspring in wild felid species. Compared to AI, ET is a more complex ART, requiring separate laparoscopic procedures for oocyte recovery and transfer, and frequently necessitating embryo cryopreservation to permit subsequent synchronization of ET recipients. However, ET does provide a more direct means for securing the genetic potential of female cats, either through scheduled oocyte retrieval/IVF procedures for prospective management or following unexpected mortality events and IVF of *in vitro* matured oocytes for genetic rescue. Early embryo transfer studies in domestic cats demonstrated the feasibility of producing kittens following surgical uterine transfer of *in vivo*-derived embryos (Kraemer *et al.*, 1979). Surgical embryo transfer of IVF embryos was the primary method of ET for wild felids for over a decade, with pregnancies produced in five species (tiger, wild cat, fishing cat, caracal, serval), including successful pregnancies from frozen embryos in the wild cat and caracal (Table 28.2). However, with the increased use of laparoscopic oocyte collection and AI approaches and the growing preference for oviductal transfers of early-stage IVF embryos, laparoscopic oviductal ET (LO-ET) techniques subsequently were developed in domestic cats to replace more invasive laparotomy procedures (Swanson, 2012; Pope, 2014). Comparative studies in wild felids have shown that LO-ET has cross-species utility, with pregnancies and full-term offspring subsequently produced with IVF embryos in four species (ocelots, sand cats, black-footed cats, cheetahs), including five pregnancies in ocelots following transfer of frozen-thawed embryos (Table 28.2). However, at present, IVF and ET does not play a meaningful role in the management of any wild felid population.

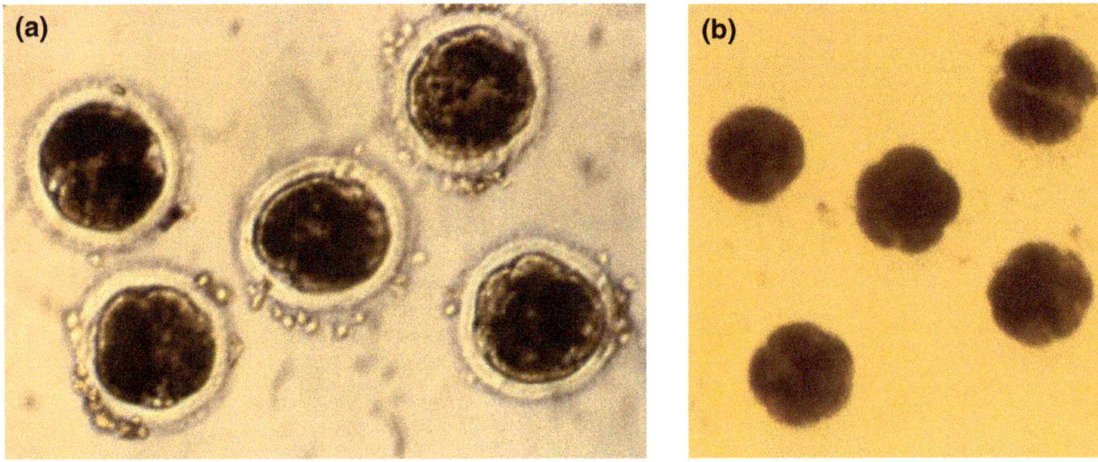

Fig. 28.5. In vitro fertilization and embryo culture in felids. **(a)** Ocelot embryos (2 to 8 cell) at 48 hours post-insemination of ocelot oocytes with homologous sperm. **(b)** Ocelot-domestic hybrid embryos (2 to 8 cell) at 48 hours post-insemination of domestic cat oocytes with frozen-thawed ocelot sperm. (Images: author's own.)

Although LO-ET of early-stage embryos has proven feasible in several wild cat species, embryo culture systems and recipient synchronization methods still require further investigation if efficacy is to be improved for applied use. One confounding factor involves the interaction of embryo viability with the maternal reproductive milieu, creating difficulties in separating the impact of embryo culture deficiencies, especially with prolonged culture, from abnormalities in the oviductal or uterine environment possibly resulting from exogenous gonadotropin treatment. Until these issues are addressed, it may prove difficult to transition from LO-ET to a less invasive transcervical ET approach that could allow IVF/ET to have broader utility for population management as one alternative to LO-AI.

28.6 References

Brown, J.L., Wasser, S.K., Wildt, D.E., and Graham, L.H. (1994) Comparative aspects of steroid hormone metabolism and ovarian activity in felids, measured noninvasively in feces. *Biology of Reproduction* 51, 776–786. doi: 10.1095/biolreprod51.4.776

Conforti, V.A., Bateman, H.L., Schook, M.M., Newsom, J., Lyons, L.A., *et al.* (2013) Laparoscopic oviductal artificial insemination improves pregnancy success in exogenous gonadotropin-treated domestic cats as a model for endangered felids. *Biology of Reproduction* 89, 1–9. doi: 10.1095/biolreprod.112.105353

Goodrowe, K.L., Wall, R.J., O'Brien, S.J., Schmidt, P.M., and Wildt, D.E. (1988) Developmental competence of domestic cat oocytes after fertilization in vitro. *Biology of Reproduction* 39, 355–372. doi: 10.1095/biolreprod39.2.355

Herrick, J.R., Bond, J.B., Magarey, G.M., Bateman, H.L., Krisher, R.L., *et al.* (2007) Toward a feline-optimized culture medium: Impact of ions, carbohydrates, essential amino acids, vitamins, and serum on development and metabolism of in vitro fertilization-derived feline embryos relative to embryos grown in vivo. *Biology of Reproduction* 76, 858–870. doi: 10.1095/biolreprod.106.058065

Herrick, J.R., Campbell, M., Levens, G., Moore, T., Benson, K., *et al.* (2010) In vitro fertilization and sperm cryopreservation in the black-footed cat (*Felis nigripes*) and sand cat (*Felis margarita*). *Biology of Reproduction* 82, 552–562. doi: 10.1095/biolreprod.109.081034

Howard, J.G. and Wildt, D.E. (2009) Approaches and efficacy of artificial insemination in felids and mustelids. *Theriogenology* 71, 130–148. doi: 10.1016/j.theriogenology.2008.09.046

IUCN (2020) International Union for Conservation of Nature's red list of threatened species. Version 2020-1. Available at: https://www.iucnredlist.org. (accessed 2 June 2020).

Kraemer, D.C., Flow, B.L., Schriver, M.D., Kinney, G.M., and Pennycook, J.W. (1979) Embryo transfer in the nonhuman primate, feline and canine. *Theriogenology* 11, 51–62. doi: 10.1016/S0093-691X(79)80018-7

Lueders, I., Luther, I., Scheepers, G., and Van der Horst, G. (2012) Improved semen collection for wild felids: urethral catheterization yields high sperm quality in African lions (*Panthera leo*). *Theriogenology* 78, 696–701. doi: 10.1016/j.theriogenology.2012.02.026

Platz, C.C. and Seager, S.W.J. (1978) Semen collection by electroejaculation in the domestic cat. *Journal of the American Veterinary Medical Association* 173, 1353–1155.

Pope, C.E. (2014) Aspects of in vivo oocyte production, blastocyst development and embryo transfer in the cat. *Theriogenology* 81,126–137. doi: 10.1016/j.theriogenology.2013.09.006

Pope, C.E. (2019) Forty years of assisted reproduction research in non-domestic, wild and endangered mammals. *Revista Brasileira de Reprodução Animal* 43, 160–167.

Pukazhenthi, B.S. and Wildt, D.E. (2004) Which reproductive technologies are most relevant to studying, managing and conserving wildlife? *Reproduction, Fertility and Development* 16, 33–46. doi: 10.10371/RD03076

Sojka, N.J., Jennings, L.L., and Hamner, C.E. (1970) Artificial insemination in the cat (*Felis catus L.*). *Laboratory Animal Care* 20, 198–204.

Swanson, W.F. (2006) Application of assisted reproduction for population management in felids: the potential and reality for conservation of small cats. *Theriogenology* 66, 49–58. doi: 10.1016/j.theriogenology.2006.03.024

Swanson, W.F. (2012) Laparoscopic oviductal embryo transfer and artificial insemination in felids: Challenges, strategies and successes. *Reproduction in Domestic Animals* 47(6), 136–140. doi: 10.1111/rda.12069

Swanson, W.F. (2019) Practical application of laparoscopic oviductal artificial insemination for propagation of domestic cats and wild felids. *Reproduction, Fertility and Development* 31, 27–39. doi: 10.1071/RD18350

Swanson, W.F., Stoops, M.A., Magarey, G.M., and Herrick, J. (2007) Sperm cryopreservation in endangered felids: developing linkage of in situ–ex situ populations. In: Roldan, E. and Gomenido, M. (eds) *Spermatology*. Nottingham University Press, Nottingham, UK, pp. 417–432.

Swanson, W.F., Bateman, H.L., and Vansandt, L.M. (2016) Urethral catheterization and sperm vitrification for simplified semen banking in felids. *Reproduction in Domestic Animals* 52(2), 255–260. doi: 10.1111/rda.12863

Thongphakdee, A., Tipkantha, W., Punkong, C., and Chatdarong, K. (2018) Monitoring and controlling

ovarian activity in wild felids. *Theriogenology* 109, 14–21. doi: 10.1016/j.theriogenology.2017.12.010
Vick, M. M., Bateman, H. L., Lambo, C. A., Swanson, W. F. Improved cryopreservation of domestic cat sperm in a chemically defined medium. *Theriogenology* 78(9), 2120–2128. doi: 10.1016/j.theriogenology.2012.08.009
Wildt, D.E., Kinney, G.M., and Seager, S.W.J. (1977) Laparoscopy for direct observation of internal organs in the domestic cat and dog. *American Journal of Veterinary Research* 38, 1429–1432.
Zambelli, D., Prati, F., Cunto, M., Iacono, E., and Merlo, B. (2008) Quality and in vitro fertilizing ability of cryopreserved cat spermatozoa obtained by urethral catheterization after medetomidine administration. *Theriogenology* 69, 485–490. doi: 10.1016/j.theriogenology.2007.10.019

Index

Note: The page numbers in italics and bold represents figures and tables respectively.

www.ingramcontent.com/pod-product-compliance
Lightning Source LLC
LaVergne TN
LVHW070849210926
848482LV00016B/901
* 9 7 8 1 7 8 9 2 4 7 0 8 4 *